Fabry disease

Perspectives from 5 years of FOS

Edited by
**Atul Mehta, Michael Beck and
Gere Sunder-Plassmann**

Fabry disease
Perspectives from 5 years of FOS

Edited by Atul Mehta, Michael Beck
and Gere Sunder-Plassmann

With a foreword by Hermann Fabry

Contributions by

*Sélim Aractingi, John D Aubert, Frank Bähner, Miguel Barba, Frédéric Barbey, Karin Baron,
Ditmar Basalla, Michael Beck, Soumeya Bekri, Roscoe O Brady, Guido Conti,
Timothy M Cox, Patrick B Deegan, Sian Evans, Manuela Födinger, Maria Fuller, Andreas Gal,
Dominique P Germain, Volkmar Gieselmann, Urs Giger, Lionel Ginsberg, Daniel Hajioff,
Mark E Haskins, Stefan Hegemann, Elizabeth Hernberg-Ståhl, Björn Hoffmann,
John J Hopwood, Derralynn A Hughes, Alex Ioannidis, Roland Jaussaud,
Christoph Kampmann, Annerose Keilmann, Satish Keshav, Christine Lavery, Olivier Lidove,
Aleš Linhart, Françoise Livio, Atul Mehta, Peter J Meikle, Alan Milligan, David F Moore,
Matthias J Müller, Elizabeth F Neufeld, Rosella Parini, Donald F Patterson,
Guillem Pintos-Morell, Susanne Pitz, Uma Ramaswami, Linda Richfield, Markus Ries,
Imke Rohard, Paul Saftig, Ellen Schäfer, Raphael Schiffmann, Andreas Schwarting,
Rashmi R Shah, Andrea Sodi, Gere Sunder-Plassmann, Ravi Thadhani, Catharina Whybra,
Urs Widmer, Bryan Winchester, Elisabeth Young*

Oxford PharmaGenesis™ Ltd

Editors:

Dr Atul Metha
Department of Academic Haematology, Royal Free and University College Medical School, London, UK

Professor Michael Beck
Universitäts-Kinderklinik, Mainz, Germany

Professor Gere Sunder-Plassmann
Division of Nephrology and Dialysis, Department of Medicine III, Medical University Vienna, Vienna, Austria

ISBN 1-903539-03-X

British Library Cataloguing-in-Publication Data

A catalogue record for this book is available from the British Library.

Published by Oxford PharmaGenesis™ Ltd, 1 Tubney Warren Barns, Tubney, Oxford OX13 5QJ, UK.

© 2006 Oxford PharmaGenesis™ Ltd

Printed and bound in the UK by Biddles Ltd, England.

The opinions expressed in this publication are those of the authors and do not necessarily reflect the opinions or recommendations of the publisher. The dosages, indications and methods of use for the products referred to by the authors are not necessarily the same as indicated in the package inserts for these products and may reflect the clinical experience of the authors or may be derived from the professional literature or other clinical sources.

The publisher can give no guarantee for information about drug dosage and application thereof contained in this publication. In every individual case, the respective user must check its accuracy by consulting other pharmaceutical literature.

Acknowledgements
We are grateful to the following people for permission to use the images on the front cover. Clockwise from top left:

The heart in a female patient with Fabry disease, showing storage, vacuolization, and hypertrophy and disarray of muscle fibres – Milan Elleder (University Hospital Prague, Prague, Czech Republic).

Magnetic resonance imaging showing a left cerebellar hemisphere stroke caused by vertebral artery occlusion in a patient with Fabry disease – Raphael Schiffmann (NIH, Bethesda, Maryland, USA) and David F Moore (University of Manitoba, Winnipeg, Canada).

Typical dermatological lesions around the umbilicus – Thomas Jansen (Ruhr University, Bochum, Germany).

Cornea verticillata – Andrea Sodi (University of Florence, Florence, Italy).

Foreword

Hermann Fabry

Bochum, Germany

Since the earliest descriptions of Fabry disease by William Anderson and my uncle, Johannes Fabry, in 1898, we have come a long way in understanding the clinical manifestations of the disease, as well as the pathophysiological and biochemical processes underlying this debilitating disorder. Anderson and Fabry described a disease that was characterized by angiokeratomas, proteinuria and lymphoedema; more than 100 years later, we know that Fabry disease is an X-linked inherited sphingolipidosis in which a mutation in the gene encoding the enzyme α-galactosidase A leads to the progressive accumulation of globotriaosylceramide within lysosomes. Symptoms are wide-ranging and multisystemic, including renal, cardiac and cerebrovascular complications; quality of life is severely impaired and affected individuals have a significantly reduced life-expectancy.

Until very recently, treatment of Fabry disease was symptomatic; however, the sequencing of the gene encoding α-galactosidase A in 1989 by Kornreich *et al.* paved the way to producing recombinant enzyme and, eventually, to the advent of enzyme replacement therapy (ERT). The licensing of ERT in 2001 heralded a revolution in therapy, leading to the possibility that disease progression could be halted, or even reversed, and quality of life improved.

FOS – the Fabry Outcome Survey – was developed in 2001 to gain further understanding of the nature of Fabry disease and to improve the clinical management of patients with the disorder. Its strengths lie in the fact that it is a multinational, multicentre database, allowing large quantities of data to be collected on the natural history of Fabry disease and the beneficial effects of ERT. The success of FOS is a testament to the great value of international collaboration in increasing awareness and understanding of rare diseases such as Fabry disease, and it is an excellent model for the development of databases for other orphan diseases. As experience within FOS grows, I hope that the future for those individuals and families affected by Fabry disease will be brighter.

It remains for me to thank the many clinicians and researchers who have contributed to FOS, the FOS Executive Committee and, most importantly, the patients themselves for allowing their data to be entered into FOS. I would also like to congratulate the editors and authors for their hard work in producing such an excellent publication.

Contents

Section 1: General aspects of lysosomal storage diseases

Section 2: Development of FOS – the Fabry Outcome Survey

Section 3: Fabry disease: clinical features and natural course

Section 4: Selected aspects of the clinical management of Fabry disease

Contributors

Sélim Aractingi
Department of Dermatology–Allergy, Hôpital Tenon, 75020 Paris, France

John D Aubert
Pneumology Division, University Hospital (CHUV), 1011-Lausanne, Switzerland

Frank Bähner
Universitäts-Kinderklinik, Langenbeckstrasse 1, D-55101 Mainz, Germany

Miguel Barba
Internal Medicine Department, Albacete University Hospital, 37 Hermanos Falcó Street, 02006 Albacete, Spain

Frédéric Barbey
Nephrology Division, University Hospital (CHUV), 1011-Lausanne, Switzerland

Karin Baron
Universitäts-Kinderklinik, Langenbeckstrasse 1, D-55101 Mainz, Germany

Ditmar Basalla
Morbus Fabry Selbsthilfegruppe e.V. (MFSH), Cologne, Germany

Michael Beck
Universitäts-Kinderklinik, Langenbeckstrasse 1, D-55101 Mainz, Germany

Soumeya Bekri
Medical Biochemistry Laboratory, Rouen CHU, Hôpital Charles Nicolle, Anneau Central, 76031 Rouen, Cedex, France

Roscoe O Brady
Developmental and Metabolic Neurology Branch, National Institute of Neurological Disorders and Stroke, Building 10, Room 3D03, National Institutes of Health, Bethesda, MD 20892-1260, USA

Guido Conti
ENT Clinic, Catholic University of the Sacred Heart, Rome, Italy

Timothy M Cox
Department of Medicine, University of Cambridge, Addenbrooke's Hospital, Hills Road, Cambridge CB2 2QQ, UK

Patrick B Deegan
Department of Medicine, University of Cambridge, Addenbrooke's Hospital, Hills Road, Cambridge CB2 2QQ, UK

Sian Evans
Lysosomal Storage Disorders Unit, Department of Academic Haematology, Royal Free and University College Medical School, Rowland Hill Street, London NW3 2PF, UK

Manuela Födinger
Clinical Institute of Medical and Chemical Laboratory Diagnostics, Medical University Vienna, Währinger Gürtel 18–20, A-1090 Vienna, Austria

Maria Fuller

Lysosomal Diseases Research Unit, Department of Genetic Medicine, Children, Youth and Women's Health Service, North Adelaide, South Australia 5006, Australia

Andreas Gal

Institut für Humangenetik, Universitätsklinikum Hamburg-Eppendorf, Butenfeld 42, 22529 Hamburg, Germany

Dominique P Germain

Assistance Publique – Hôpitaux de Paris, Paris, France

Volkmar Gieselmann

Institut für Physiologische Chemie, Rheinische Friedrich-Wilhelms-Universität, Bonn 53115, Germany

Urs Giger

Laboratory of Pathology and Section of Medical Genetics, School of Veterinary Medicine, University of Pennsylvania, 3800 Spruce Street, Philadelphia, PA 19104-6051, USA

Lionel Ginsberg

Department of Neurology, Royal Free Hospital, Pond Street, London NW3 2QG, UK

Daniel Hajioff

Royal National Throat, Nose & Ear Hospital, London, UK

Mark E Haskins

Laboratory of Pathology and Section of Medical Genetics, School of Veterinary Medicine, University of Pennsylvania, 3800 Spruce Street, Philadelphia, PA 19104-6051, USA

Stefan Hegemann

University Hospital Zurich, Department of ORL HNS, Zurich, Switzerland

Elizabeth Hernberg-Ståhl

Fabry Outcome Survey, TKT Europe AB, Rinkebyvägen 11B, SE-182 36, Danderyd, Sweden

Björn Hoffmann

Department of General Pediatrics, Heinrich-Heine-University, Moorenstrasse 5, D-40225 Düsseldorf, Germany

John J Hopwood

Lysosomal Diseases Research Unit, Department of Genetic Medicine, Children, Youth and Women's Health Service, North Adelaide, South Australia 5006, Australia

Derralynn A Hughes

Lysosomal Storage Disorders Unit, Department of Academic Haematology, Royal Free and University College Medical School, Rowland Hill Street, London NW3 2PF, UK

Alex Ioannidis

Department of Ophthalmology, Royal Free Hospital, Pond Street, London NW3 2QG, UK

Roland Jaussaud

Department of Internal Medicine and Infectious Diseases, Robert Debré Hospital, Reims, France

Christoph Kampmann

Universitäts-Kinderklinik, Langenbeckstrasse 1, D-55101 Mainz, Germany

Annerose Keilmann

Department of Communication Disorders, University of Mainz, Langenbeckstrasse 1, D-55101 Mainz, Germany

Satish Keshav — Department of Medicine, Royal Free and University College Medical School, Rowland Hill Street, London NW3 2PF, UK

Christine Lavery — Society for Mucopolysaccharide and Related Diseases, MPS House, White Lion Road, Amersham, Bucks HP7 9LP, UK

Olivier Lidove — Department of Internal Medicine, Bichat Hospital, 75877 Paris, France

Aleš Linhart — 2nd Department of Internal Medicine, 1st School of Medicine, Charles University, U Nemocnice 2, CZ-128 08 Prague 2, Czech Republic

Françoise Livio — Clinical Pharmacology Department, University Hospital (CHUV), 1011-Lausanne, Switzerland

Atul Mehta — Lysosomal Storage Disorders Unit, Department of Academic Haematology, Royal Free and University College Medical School, Rowland Hill Street, London NW3 2PF, UK

Peter J Meikle — Lysosomal Diseases Research Unit, Department of Genetic Medicine, Children, Youth and Women's Health Service, North Adelaide, South Australia 5006, Australia

Alan Milligan — Lysosomal Storage Disorders Unit, Department of Academic Haematology, Royal Free and University College Medical School, Rowland Hill Street, London NW3 2PF, UK

David F Moore — Section of Neurology, Department of Internal Medicine, University of Manitoba, Winnipeg, Canada

Matthias J Müller — Department of Psychiatry, University of Mainz, D-55101 Mainz, Germany, and Clinic for Psychiatry and Psychotherapy Marburg-Sued, D-35039 Marburg, Germany

Elizabeth F Neufeld — Department of Biological Chemistry, David Geffen School of Medicine at UCLA, Los Angeles, CA 90095-1737, USA

Rosella Parini — Department of Paediatrics, S. Gerardo Hospital, Monza, Italy

Donald F Patterson — Laboratory of Pathology and Section of Medical Genetics, School of Veterinary Medicine, University of Pennsylvania, 3800 Spruce Street, Philadelphia, PA 19104-6051, USA

Guillem Pintos-Morell — Department of Paediatrics, University Hospital 'Germans Trias i Pujol', Badalona, Spain

Susanne Pitz — Department of Ophthalmology, University of Mainz, Langenbeckstrasse 1, 55101 Mainz, Germany

Uma Ramaswami — Department of Paediatric Endocrinology, Diabetes and Metabolism, Box 181, Addenbrooke's Hospital, Cambridge CB2 2QQ, UK

Linda Richfield

Lysosomal Storage Disorders Unit, Department of Academic Haematology, Royal Free and University College Medical School, Rowland Hill Street, London NW3 2PF, UK

Markus Ries

Developmental and Metabolic Neurology Branch, National Institute of Neurological Disorders and Stroke, Building 10, Room 3D03, National Institutes of Health, Bethesda, MD 20892-1260, USA

Imke Rohard

Institut für Humangenetik, Universitätsklinikum Hamburg-Eppendorf, Butenfeld 42, 22529 Hamburg, Germany

Paul Saftig

Biochemical Institute, Christian-Albrechts-University Kiel, Olshausenstrasse 40, D-24098 Kiel, Germany

Ellen Schäfer

Institut für Humangenetik, Universitätsklinikum Hamburg-Eppendorf, Butenfeld 42, 22529 Hamburg, Germany

Raphael Schiffmann

Developmental and Metabolic Neurology Branch, National Institute of Neurological Disorders and Stroke, Building 10, Room 3D03, National Institutes of Health, Bethesda, MD 20892-1260, USA

Andreas Schwarting

Department of Nephrology, University of Mainz, Langenbeckstrasse 1, 55101 Mainz, Germany

Rashmi R Shah

Gerrards Cross, Buckinghamshire, SL9 7JA, UK

Andrea Sodi

Department of Ophthalmology, University of Florence, Florence, Italy

Gere Sunder-Plassmann

Division of Nephrology and Dialysis, Department of Medicine III, Medical University Vienna, Währinger Gürtel 18–20, A-1090 Vienna, Austria

Ravi Thadhani

Harvard Medical School, Boston, MA, USA

Catharina Whybra

Universitäts-Kinderklinik, Langenbeckstrasse 1, D-55101 Mainz, Germany

Urs Widmer

Department of Internal Medicine, University Hospital Zurich, CH-8091 Zurich, Switzerland

Bryan Winchester

Biochemistry, Endocrinology and Metabolism Unit, UCL Institute of Child Health, Great Ormond Street Hospital, University College London, London, WC1N 1EH, UK

Elisabeth Young

Biochemistry, Endocrinology and Metabolism Unit, UCL Institute of Child Health, Great Ormond Street Hospital, University College London, London, WC1N 1EH, UK

List of abbreviations

A	Adenine	**DTPA**	Diethylenetriaminepentacetic acid
ACE	Angiotensin-converting enzyme	**EC**	European Commission
ACKD	Acquired cystic kidney disease	**ECG**	Electrocardiography
		EDTA	Ethylenediamine tetraacetic acid
ACMG	American College of Medical Genetics	**EDTA**	European Dialysis and Transplant Association
AIDS	Acquired immunodeficiency syndrome	**eGFR**	Estimated glomerular filtration rate
AP	Adaptor proteins	**EMEA**	European Medicines Agency
AV	Atrioventricular	**eNOS**	Endothelial nitric oxide synthase
Aδ	Small myelinated nerve fibres	**EQ-5D**	European Quality of Life questionnaire
BMI	Body mass index	**ER**	Endoplasmic reticulum
BMJ	British Medical Journal	**ERA**	European Renal Association
BMT	Bone marrow transplantation	**ERT**	Enzyme replacement therapy
bp	Base pairs	**ESI-MS/MS**	Electrospray ionization tandem mass spectrometry
BPI	Brief Pain Inventory		
C	Cytosine	**ESRD**	End-stage renal disease
C1q	Complement component 1q	**ESRF**	End-stage renal failure
C3	Complement component 3	**EtDO-P4**	Ethylenedioxy-1-phenyl-2-palmitoylamino-3-pyrrolidino-1-propanol
cAMP	Cyclic AMP		
cDNA	Complementary DNA		
CHMP	Committee for Medicinal Products for Human Use	**EU**	European Union
		FDA	Food and Drug Administration
CHO	Chinese hamster ovary		
CI	Confidence interval	**FEV$_1$**	Forced expiratory volume in 1 second
CKD	Chronic kidney disease		
CLN	Neuronal ceroid lipofuscinosis	**FIRE**	Fabry International Research Exchange
CNS	Central nervous system		
COMP	Committee for Orphan Medicinal Products	**FLAIR**	Fluid-attenuated inversion recovery
		FOS	Fabry Outcome Survey
COPD	Chronic obstructive pulmonary disease	**FOS-MSSI**	Fabry Outcome Survey adaptation of the Mainz Severity Score Index
CT	Computed tomography		
Cys	Cysteine		
D313Y	Pseudodeficiency allele		
DGJ	Deoxygalactonojirimycin	**FVC**	Forced vital capacity
DHPLC	Denaturing high-performance liquid chromatography	**G**	Guanine
		GAG	Glycosaminoglycan
		GalNAc	*N*-acetylgalactosamine
DSM-IV	Diagnostic and Statistical Manual of Mental Disorders – Fourth Edition	**Gb$_3$**	Globotriaosylceramide
		gDNA	Genomic DNA

GFR	Glomerular filtration rate	**LSD**	Lysosomal storage disease
GH	Growth hormone	**LV**	Left ventricle
GL-3	Globotriaosylceramide (also abbreviated to Gb_3)	**LVH**	Left ventricular hypertrophy
		LVM	Left ventricular mass
GLA	α-galactosidase A gene	**M6P**	Mannose-6-phosphate
GlcNAc	*N*-acetylglucosamine	**MDRD**	Modification of Diet in Renal Disease
GOLD	Global Initiative on Obstructive Lung Disease	**MFSH**	Morbus Fabry Selbsthilfegruppe e.V.
HAMD	Hamilton Depression Rating Scale	**MHC**	Major histocompatibility complex
HAWIE	Hamburg-Wechsler Intelligence Test for Adults	**MHLW**	Japanese Ministry of Health, Labour and Welfare
HbA$_{1c}$	Glycosylated haemoglobin	**MHRA**	Medicines and Healthcare Products Regulatory Agency
HGV Society	Human Genome Variation Society		
HPTLC	High-performance thin-layer chromatography	**MPBT**	Manufacturer's price before taxes
HRQoL	Health-related quality of life	**MPS**	Mucopolysaccharidosis
HRT	Hormone replacement therapy	**MRI**	Magnetic resonance imaging
HUD	Humanitarian Device Exemptions	**MSSI**	Mainz Severity Score Index
i.v.	Intravenous	*NAGA*	Gene encoding α-galactosidase B
IBS	Irritable bowel syndrome		
I-cell disease	Inclusion-cell disease	*N*B-DNJ	*N*-butyldeoxynojirimycin
iGb$_3$	Isoglobotriaosylceramide	**Nd:YAG**	Neodymium:yttrium– aluminium–garnet
IND	Investigational New Drug		
IQ	Intelligence quotient	*N*GNA	*N*-glycolyneuraminic acid
ISO	International Organization for Standardization	**NHS**	National Health Service
		NICE	National Institute for Health and Clinical Excellence
JND	Just noticeable difference (units for measuring sensory detection thresholds)	**NIH**	National Institutes of Health
		NKT	Natural killer T lymphocytes
		NPC	Niemann–Pick disease type C
KIGS	Pfizer International Growth Database	**NO**	Nitric oxide
KIKO	Japanese Organization for Pharmaceutical Safety and Research	**NSVT**	Non-sustained ventricular tachycardia
		NYHA	New York Heart Association
KIMS	Pfizer International Metabolic Database	**OMIM**	Online Mendelian Inheritance in Man
K$_m$	Michaelis constant	**ONOO⁻**	Peroxynitrite
LAMP	Lysosome-associated membrane protein	**OOPD**	Office of Orphan Products Development
LGP-85	Lysosomal membrane glycoprotein-85	**PARC**	Pulmonary and activation-regulated chemokine
LIMP	Lysosomal integral membrane protein	**PCR**	Polymerase chain reaction

PET	Positron emission tomography	**SAWP**	Scientific Advice Working Party
PGP	Protein gene product	**SD**	Standard deviation
PMDA	Pharmaceutical and Medical Devices Agency	**SELDI**	Surface-enhanced laser desorption ionization
PPCA	Protective protein/ cathepsin A	**SEM**	Standard error of the mean
PPIT	Public price including taxes	**SF-36**	Short-Form-36 questionnaire
PPRS	Pharmaceutical Price Regulation Scheme	**SNP**	Single nucleotide pair
		SRT	Substrate reduction therapy
PPV	Positive predictive values	**SSL**	Secure Socket Layer
PRIND	Prolonged reversible ischaemic neurological deficit	**SUMF1**	Sulphatase-modifying factor 1
		T	Thymine
QoL	Quality of life	**TGN**	Trans-Golgi network
QSART	Quantitative sudomotor axon reflex test	**TIA**	Transient ischaemic attack
		TNFα	Tumour necrosis factor-α
RER	Rough endoplasmic reticulum	**TRAP**	Tartrate-resistant acid phosphatase
RF	Renal function	**US**	Ultrasound
ROS	Reactive oxygen species	**USRDS**	United States Renal Data System
s.c.	Subcutaneous	**VAT**	Value-added tax

Preface

If I have seen further it is by standing on the shoulders of giants
Isaac Newton (1642–1727)

As a therapeutic concept, enzyme replacement therapy (ERT) is deceptively simple: if the cause of a disease is identified as an enzyme deficiency, then replacing the enzyme should restore normal metabolism and health. However, it took some 70 years from the first description of Fabry disease in 1898 to demonstrate the enzymatic defect, and a further 30 years to develop a therapeutic enzyme preparation.

This book charts the remarkable scientific achievements of this period that led eventually, in 2001, to the introduction of ERT. But foremost, it is a celebration of the clinical progress made in the past 5 years as a result of FOS – the Fabry Outcome Survey. The small number of patients with this rare disease who were involved in the initial clinical trials on safety and efficacy meant that it was very important for patients to be carefully followed up, in a structured and consistent way, and for their clinical progress to be closely documented. To achieve this, close collaboration at an international level was paramount, with comprehensive data collection guided by a common framework for the evaluation of signs and symptoms of the disease. Thus, FOS was created, and over the previous 5 years has been responsible for collection and analysis of the wide range of clinical safety and efficacy data reported in this volume.

The value of the database is evidenced by the many peer-reviewed publications based on FOS data. This success is a testament to the enormous effort and enthusiasm of numerous individuals, not least the patients and their families, who have agreed to contribute their data, and participating physicians and other healthcare providers, who have devoted their time and expertise to patient care and accurate data reporting.

One of the major strengths of FOS is that the scientific direction is governed by the various National Boards, the International Board and the Executive Committee, all of which consist of elected physicians who are active participants in FOS. We would like to thank present and past members of these bodies who have helped to shape the database into what we see today. Roberta Ricci and Urs Widmer deserve special thanks for their previous unstinting contributions to the work of the Executive Committee.

We would also like to acknowledge the expert help of our colleagues in reviewing the manuscripts for this publication. The multisystemic nature of Fabry disease has not made our task as Editors of this publication an easy one, and we are indebted to Aleš Linhart, Urs Widmer and Rolf Gunnarsson for their editorial input.

Finally, it has been a privilege to be involved in this publication. We have learnt much from reviewing the excellent contributions of our colleagues, and we thank them for their endeavours. As practising physicians, we hope that the knowledge assembled here will provide the inspiration for continued research into Fabry disease and its treatment, to the ultimate benefit of current and future patients.

May 2006

Atul Mehta, London, UK
Michael Beck, Mainz, Germany
Gere Sunder-Plassmann, Vienna, Austria

Section 1:

General aspects of lysosomal storage diseases

1 History of lysosomal storage diseases: an overview

Atul Mehta[1], Michael Beck[2], Aleš Linhart[3], Gere Sunder-Plassmann[4] and Urs Widmer[5]

[1]Lysosomal Storage Disorders Unit, Department of Academic Haematology, Royal Free and University College Medical School, Rowland Hill Street, London NW3 2PF, UK; [2]Universitäts-Kinderklinik, Langenbeckstrasse 1, D-55101 Mainz, Germany; [3]2nd Department of Internal Medicine, 1st School of Medicine, Charles University, U Nemocnice 2, CZ-128 08 Prague 2, Czech Republic; [4]Division of Nephrology and Dialysis, Department of Medicine III, Medical University Vienna, Währinger Gürtel 18–20, A-1090 Vienna, Austria; [5]Department of Internal Medicine, University Hospital Zurich, CH-8091 Zurich, Switzerland

Lysosomal storage diseases (LSDs) comprise a group of related conditions characterized by inappropriate lipid storage in lysosomes, due to specific enzyme deficiencies. Gaucher disease was the first of these disorders to be described, in 1882, followed by Fabry disease in 1898. The latter is now known to be due to deficiency of the enzyme α-galactosidase A. This leads to lysosomal storage of the glycosphingolipid globotriaosylceramide in tissues throughout the body, and progressively results in end-organ failure and premature death. Increased understanding of the LSDs has resulted in recent years in the introduction of enzyme replacement therapy, which aims to halt the natural progression of these metabolic disorders.

Introduction

The lysosomal storage diseases (LSDs) are a group of distinct genetic disorders, each of which is the result of a specific defect in a lysosomal enzyme. The reduced or absent enzyme activity results in the lysosomal accumulation of superfluous glycolipids that would normally be degraded. The diseases are classified according to the type of material that is accumulated; for example, lipid storage disorders, mucopolysacchari-doses and glycoproteinoses (Table 1) [1]. The first disease to be described that was later recognized as an LSD was Gaucher disease in 1882 [2], followed by Fabry disease in 1898 [3, 4]. Many of the conditions show significant similarities. Indeed, disruption of a single metabolic pathway can lead to a number of related diseases, depending on where in the pathway the defect occurs. Common features of the LSDs include bone abnormalities, organomegaly and disorders of the central and peripheral nervous systems.

Most LSDs are characterized by their progressive course, often resulting in severe disease manifestations and early death. Individually, the LSDs are rare, with reported incidences ranging from 1 in 57 000 live births for Gaucher disease to 1 in 4.2 million for sialidosis [5]. Overall, their incidence has been estimated as 1 in 7000 to 1 in 8000 live births [5, 6].

This chapter will provide a brief overview of the history of research into the LSDs, with particular reference to Fabry disease.

Recognition of the lysosome as central to storage diseases

In the late 1950s and early 1960s, de Duve and colleagues, using cell fractionation

Table 1. Classification of the lysosomal storage diseases. From Vellodi [1].

Mucopolysaccharidoses (MPS)	Krabbe disease
MPS I*	Metachromatic leukodystrophy
MPS II†	Niemann–Pick disease,
MPS IIIA	types A and B
MPS IIIB	**Other lipidoses**
MPS IIIC	Niemann–Pick disease,
MPS IIID	type C
MPS IVA	Wolman disease
MPS IVB	Neuronal ceroid lipofuscinosis
MPS VI*	**Glycogen storage disease**
MPS VII	Glycogen storage disease,
Glycoproteinoses	type II (Pompe disease)*
Aspartylglucosaminuria	**Multiple enzyme deficiency**
Fucosidosis	Multiple sulphatase deficiency
α-Mannosidosis	Galactosialidosis
β-Mannosidosis	Mucolipidosis II/III
Mucolipidosis I (sialidosis)	Mucolipidosis IV
Schindler disease	**Lysosomal transport defects**
Sphingolipidoses	Cystinosis
Fabry disease*	Sialic acid storage disease
Farber disease	**Other disorders due to defects in**
Gaucher disease*	**lysosomal proteins**
GM1-gangliosidosis	Danon disease
Tay–Sachs disease	Hyaluronidase deficiency
Sandhoff disease	

*Enzyme replacement therapy available.
†Enzyme replacement therapy under development.

techniques, cytological studies and biochemical analyses, identified and characterized the lysosome as a cellular organelle responsible for intracellular digestion and recycling of macromolecules [7–10]. This was the scientific breakthrough that would lead to the understanding of the physiological basis of the LSDs. Pompe disease was the first disease to be identified as an LSD in 1963, with Hers and co-workers [11, 12] reporting the cause as a deficiency of α-glucosidase. They also suggested that other diseases, such as the mucopolysaccharide storage diseases, might be due to enzyme deficiencies [13].

In 1965, an electron microscopy study by Hashimoto et al. revealed the presence of bodies in endothelial cells, smooth muscle cells, fibrocytes and perivascular cells of patients with Fabry disease [14]. Referring to these structures as "extremely overcrowded lysosomes", he concluded that there was a disturbance of lysosomal enzymes as a result of a genetic abnormality. In the same year, investigation of a family with four affected and four possibly affected males over four generations led Dempsey and colleagues to conclude that a sex-linked deficient gene with occasional penetrance in heterozygous females and constant penetrance in homozygous males was the cause [15]. More recent studies, however, have shown that heterozygous females may be affected as severely as hemizygous males, due to the

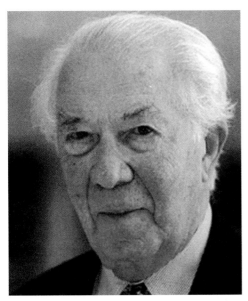

Christian de Duve

process of random inactivation of the normal X chromosome [16].

After establishing the lysosome and lysosomal enzymes as responsible for these rare metabolic disorders, Gaucher disease – the most common of the LSDs – became the focus of research. The underlying metabolic abnormality in Gaucher disease was established some four decades ago, with the demonstration that the enzymatic defect was insufficient activity of the enzyme glucocerebrosidase, which catalyses the hydrolytic cleavage of glucose from glucocerebroside [17, 18]. This information was rapidly utilized to develop widely used enzymatic assays for the diagnosis [19], carrier detection [20] and prenatal identification of this condition [21].

Treatment of LSDs

Enzyme replacement therapy (ERT) was first introduced for the treatment of Gaucher disease some 15 years ago, and is now being used successfully for the treatment of Fabry disease, mucopolysaccharidosis type I (MPS I), MPS VI and Pompe disease, and is under development for MPS II (Hunter syndrome). The develop-

ment of ERT will be described in Chapters 10 and 36, and possible future treatments in Chapter 43.

Before the introduction of ERT, treatment for LSDs was essentially palliative and aimed at alleviating specific symptoms, such as the neuropathic pain of Fabry disease, without targeting the underlying pathological condition. Previously, the only available treatment that could potentially alter the natural course of the disease was transplantation. For example, in Gaucher disease, bone marrow transplantation has proved successful, although this procedure is associated with a mortality of about 10% [22]. Likewise, renal transplantation in Fabry disease may be a successful alternative to dialysis but cannot correct the other multi-organ manifestations of the disease.

First description of Fabry disease

Fabry disease is now known to be an X-linked lysosomal storage disorder with estimated incidences ranging from as high as 1 in 40 000 live male births to 1 in 117 000 live male births [5, 23]. It is caused by the lysosomal accumulation of neutral glycosphingolipids, primarily globotriaosylceramide, due to deficiency of the enzyme α-galactosidase A. Progressive accumulation of substrate is associated with a wide range of disease signs and symptoms, including renal failure, cardiovascular dysfunction, neuropathy, stroke and dermatological manifestations in the form of angiokeratomas [24]. Life expectancy is reduced by an average of 15 years in female patients [25] and 20 years in males [26].

The first descriptions of Fabry disease were made in 1898 by two physicians. Working independently of each other, William Anderson and Johannes Fabry described patients with 'angiokeratoma corporis diffusum', the red–purple maculopapular skin lesions that are now recognized as a characteristic feature of the disorder [3, 4, 27, 28]. William Anderson,

Table 2. *Milestones in the discovery and treatment of lysosomal storage diseases (LSDs).*

Investigator(s)	Discovery	Year
Gaucher [2]	Description of a patient with Gaucher disease	1882
Anderson [3] and Fabry [4]	Description of a patient with Fabry disease (angiokeratoma corporis diffusum)	1898
Lieb [30]	Demonstration of accumulation of cerebroside in Gaucher disease	1924
Aghion [31]	Demonstration that glucocerebroside was the accumulating lipid in Gaucher disease	1934
de Duve [7]	First description of the lysosome	1959
Hers [11]	Identification of Pompe disease, the first LSD	1963
Sweeley and Klionsky [32]	Demonstration of globotriaosylceramide (ceramidetrihexoside) accumulation in Fabry disease	1963
de Duve [9]	Enzyme replacement therapy (ERT) proposed for the treatment of LSDs	1964
Brady *et al.* [17, 18]	Demonstration that insufficient activity of glucocerebrosidase was the metabolic defect in Gaucher disease	1965
Brady [33]	ERT proposed for the treatment of patients with Gaucher disease	1966
Brady *et al.* [34]	Demonstration of the enzymatic defect in Fabry disease	1967
Johnson and Brady [35]	Purification of α-galactosidase A from human placenta	1972
Brady *et al.* [36]	Biochemical effects of placental α-galactosidase A demonstrated in patients with Fabry disease	1973
Pentchev *et al.* [37]	Purification of glucocerebrosidase from human placenta	1973
Brady *et al.* [38]	Biochemical effects of placental glucocerebrosidase demonstrated in patients with Gaucher disease	1974
Pentchev *et al.* [39]	Demonstration of prolonged effect of glucocerebrosidase in patients with Gaucher disease	1975
Furbish *et al.* [40]	Large-scale preparation of placental glucocerebrosidase	1977
Furbish *et al.* [41]	Targeting glucocerebrosidase to macrophages	1981
Calhoun *et al.* [42]	Isolation of a cDNA clone encoding human α-galactosidase A	1985
Barton *et al.* [43]	First demonstration of a clinical response to ERT in a patient with Gaucher disease	1990
Barton *et al.* [44]	Demonstration of extensive clinical benefits of ERT in patients with Gaucher disease	1991
Grabowski *et al.* [45]	Demonstration of equivalence of placental and recombinant glucocerebrosidase	1995
Schiffmann *et al.* [46]	Demonstration that ERT reduces globotriaosylceramide storage in patients with Fabry disease	2000
Schiffmann *et al.* [47]	Clinical efficacy of ERT demonstrated in a randomized controlled trial in patients with Fabry disease	2001
Eng *et al.* [48]	Demonstration of safety and efficacy of recombinant α-galactosidase A replacement therapy in Fabry disease	2001
Amalfitano *et al.* [49]	ERT for Pompe disease	2001
Kakkis *et al.* [50]	ERT for Hurler syndrome	2001
Muenzer *et al.* [51]	ERT for Hunter syndrome	2002
Harmatz *et al.* [52]	ERT for Maroteaux–Lamy syndrome	2004

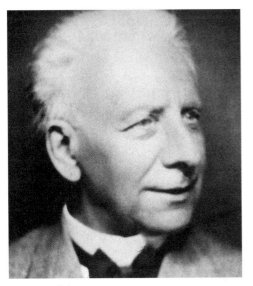

Johannes Fabry

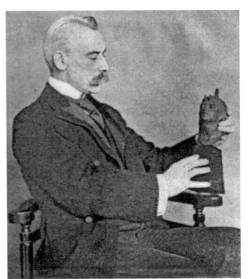

William Anderson

who trained at St Thomas' Hospital in London, first saw his patient in 1897, and described the dermatological symptoms without commenting on the possible cause. Johannes Fabry, who studied dermatology at the University of Bonn, also saw his first patient in 1897. The patient was 13 years of age at the time, and 4 years previously had developed cutaneous eruptions in the hollow of his left knee, which spread to the left thigh and trunk. It was suggested that the disease might represent a form of naevus or developmental defect.

Although the disorder is now commonly known simply as Fabry disease, it is also referred to as Anderson–Fabry disease in recognition of the original descriptions made in 1898 by Anderson and Fabry.

After these initial case reports of angio-keratoma corporis diffusum, other associated symptoms were described [29] before the lysosome was identified as the key organelle responsible for the pathology of Fabry disease and other LSDs.

Conclusions

We have come a long way since the first description of LSDs (Table 2). However,

although we now know the underlying biochemical basis for these diseases, much remains to be discovered about how excess lysosomal storage translates into organ dysfunction and premature death. Furthermore, we are only just starting to be able to address the underlying cause of some of these diseases using ERT. It is to be hoped that the insights gained over the previous 100 years will be continued for the benefit of patients with these devastating metabolic disorders.

References

1. Vellodi A. Lysosomal storage disorders. *Br J Haematol* 2005;128:413–31

2. Gaucher PCE. De l'épithélioma primitive de la rate. Thèse de Paris; 1882

3. Anderson W. A case of "angeio-keratoma". *Br J Dermatol* 1898;10:113–17

4. Fabry J. Ein Beitrag zur Kenntnis der Purpura haemorrhagica nodularis (Purpura papulosa haemorrhagica Hebrae). *Arch Dermatol Syph* 1898;43:187–200

5. Meikle PJ, Hopwood JJ, Clague AE, Carey WF. Prevalence of lysosomal storage disorders. *JAMA* 1999;281:249–54

6. Poorthuis BJ, Wevers RA, Kleijer WJ, Groener JE, de Jong JG, van Weely S *et al*. The frequency of lysosomal storage diseases in The Netherlands. *Hum Genet* 1999;105:151–6

7. de Duve C. Lysosomes, a new group of cytoplasmic particles. In: Hayashi T, editor. Subcellular particles. New York: Ronald Press; 1959. p. 128–59

8. de Duve C. Exploring cells with a centrifuge. *Science* 1975;189:186–94

9. de Duve C. From cytases to lysosomes. *Fed Proc* 1964;23:1045–9

10. de Duve C. Lysosomes revisited. *Eur J Biochem* 1983;137:391–7

11. Hers HG. α-Glucosidase deficiency in generalized glycogen storage disease (Pompe's disease). *Biochem J* 1963;86:11–6

12. Baudhuin P, Hers HG, Loeb H. An electron microscopic and biochemical study of type II glycogenosis. *Lab Invest* 1964;13:1139–52

13. Sly WS. Enzyme replacement therapy: from concept to clinical practice. *Acta Paediatr Suppl* 2002;439:71–8

14. Hashimoto K, Gross BG, Lever WF. Angiokeratoma corporis diffusum (Fabry). Histochemical and electron microscopic studies of the skin. *J Invest Dermatol* 1965;44:119–28

15. Dempsey H, Hartley MW, Carroll J, Balint J, Miller RE, Frommeyer WB, Jr. Fabry's disease (angiokeratoma corporis diffusum): case report on a rare disease. *Ann Intern Med* 1965;63:1059–68

16. Lyon MF. X-chromosome inactivation and human genetic disease. *Acta Paediatr Suppl* 2002;91:107–12

17. Brady RO, Kanfer JN, Shapiro D. Metabolism of glucocerebrosides. II Evidence of an enzymatic deficiency in Gaucher's disease. *Biochem Biophys Res Commun* 1965;18:221–5

18. Brady RO, Kanfer JN, Bradley RM, Shapiro D. Demonstration of a deficiency of glucocerebroside-cleaving enzyme in Gaucher's disease. *J Clin Invest* 1966;45:1112–15

19. Kampine JP, Brady RO, Kanfer JN, Feld M, Shapiro D. Diagnosis of Gaucher's disease and Niemann–Pick disease with small samples of venous blood. *Science* 1967;155:86–8

20. Brady RO, Johnson WG, Uhlendorf BW. Identification of heterozygous carriers of lipid storage diseases. Current status and clinical applications. *Am J Med* 1971;51:423–31

21. Schneider EL, Ellis WG, Brady RO, McCulloch JR, Epstein CJ. Infantile (type II) Gaucher's disease: in utero diagnosis and fetal pathology. *J Pediatr* 1972;81:1134–9

22. Beutler E, Grabowski G. Gaucher disease. In: Scriver CR, Beaudet AL, Sly WS, Valle D, editors. The metabolic and molecular bases of inherited disease. 8th edn. New York: McGraw-Hill; 2001. p. 3635–68

23. Desnick RJ, Ioannou YA, Eng CM. α-Galactosidase A deficiency: Fabry disease. In: Scriver CR, Beaudet AL, Sly WS, Valle D, editors. The metabolic and molecular basis of inherited disease. 8th edn. New York: McGraw-Hill; 2001. p. 3733–74

24. Mehta A, Ricci R, Widmer U, Dehout F, Garcia de Lorenzo A, Kampmann C et al. Fabry disease defined: baseline clinical manifestations of 366 patients in the Fabry Outcome Survey. *Eur J Clin Invest* 2004;34:236–42

25. MacDermot KD, Holmes A, Miners AH. Anderson–Fabry disease: clinical manifestations and impact of disease in a cohort of 60 obligate carrier females. *J Med Genet* 2001;38:769–75

26. MacDermot KD, Holmes A, Miners AH. Anderson–Fabry disease: clinical manifestations and impact of disease in a cohort of 98 hemizygous males. *J Med Genet* 2001;38:750–60

27. Fabry J. Zur Klinic und Aetiologie des Angio-keratoma. *Arch Dermatol Syph* 1916;123:294–307

28. Fabry J. Weiterer. Beitrag zur Klinik des Angio-keratoma naeviforme. *Dermatol Wochenschr* 1930; 90:339ff

29. Fabry H. Angiokeratoma corporis diffusum – Fabry disease: historical review from the original description to the introduction of enzyme replace-ment therapy. *Acta Paediatr Suppl* 2002;439:3–5

30. Lieb H. Cerebrosidespeicherung bei Splenomegalie Typus Gaucher. *Ztschr Physiol Chem* 1924;140:305–13

31. Aghion H. La maladie de Gaucher dans l'enfance. Thèse de Paris; 1934

32. Sweeley CC, Klionsky B. Fabry's disease: classifi-cation as a sphingolipidosis and partial characteri-zation of a novel glycolipid. *J Biol Chem* 1963; 238:3148–50

33. Brady RO. The sphingolipidoses. *N Engl J Med* 1966;275:312–8

34. Brady RO, Gal AE, Bradley RM, Martensson E, Warshaw AL, Laster L. Enzymatic defect in Fabry's disease. Ceramidetrihexosidase deficiency. *N Engl J Med* 1967;276:1163–7

35. Johnson WG, Brady RO. Ceramidetrihexosidase from human placenta. *Methods Enzymol* 1972;XXVIII: 849–56

36. Brady RO, Tallman JF, Johnson WG, Gal AE, Leahy WR, Quirk JM et al. Replacement therapy for inherited enzyme deficiency. Use of purified ceramidetrihexosidase in Fabry's disease. *N Engl J Med* 1973;289:9–14

37. Pentchev PG, Brady RO, Hibbert SR, Gal AE, Shapiro D. Isolation and characterization of glucocerebrosidase from human placental tissue. *J Biol Chem* 1973;248:5256–61

38. Brady RO, Pentchev PG, Gal AE, Hibbert SR, Dekaban AS. Replacement therapy for inherited enzyme deficiency. Use of purified gluco-cerebrosidase in Gaucher's disease. *N Engl J Med* 1974;291:989–93

39. Pentchev PG, Brady RO, Gal AE, Hibbert SR. Replacement therapy for inherited enzyme deficiency. Sustained clearance of accumulated glucocerebroside in Gaucher's disease following infusion of purified glucocerebrosidase. *J Mol Med* 1975;1:73–8

40. Furbish FS, Blair HE, Shiloach J, Pentchev PG, Brady RO. Enzyme replacement therapy in Gaucher's disease: large-scale purification of glucocere-brosidase suitable for human administration. *Proc Natl Acad Sci USA* 1977;74:3560–3

41. Furbish FS, Steer CJ, Krett NL, Barranger JA. Uptake and distribution of placental glucocerebrosidase in rat hepatic cells and effects of sequential deglycosylation. *Biochim Biophys Acta* 1981;673: 425–34

42. Calhoun DH, Bishop DF, Bernstein HS, Quinn M, Hantzopoulos P, Desnick RJ. Fabry disease: isolation of a cDNA clone encoding human α-galactosidase A. *Proc Natl Acad Sci USA* 1985;82:7364–8

43. Barton NW, Furbish FS, Murray GJ, Garfield M, Brady RO. Therapeutic response to intravenous infusions of glucocerebrosidase in a patient with Gaucher disease. *Proc Natl Acad Sci USA* 1990; 87:1913–16

44. Barton NW, Brady RO, Dambrosia JM, Di Bisceglie AM, Doppelt SH, Hill SC *et al*. Replacement therapy for inherited enzyme deficiency – macrophage-targeted glucocerebrosidase for Gaucher's disease. *N Engl J Med* 1991;324:1464–70

45. Grabowski GA, Barton NW, Pastores G, Dambrosia JM, Banerjee TK, McKee MA *et al*. Enzyme therapy in type 1 Gaucher disease: comparative efficacy of mannose-terminated glucocerebrosidase from natural and recombinant sources. *Ann Intern Med* 1995;122:33–9

46. Schiffmann R, Murray GJ, Treco D, Daniel P, Sellos-Moura M, Myers M *et al*. Infusion of α-galactosidase A reduces tissue globotriaosylceramide storage in patients with Fabry disease. *Proc Natl Acad Sci USA* 2000;97:365–70

47. Schiffmann R, Kopp JB, Austin HA, 3rd, Sabnis S, Moore DF, Weibel T *et al*. Enzyme replacement therapy in Fabry disease: a randomized controlled trial. *JAMA* 2001;285:2743–9

48. Eng CM, Guffon N, Wilcox WR, Germain DP, Lee P, Waldek S *et al*. Safety and efficacy of recombinant human α-galactosidase A replacement therapy in Fabry's disease. *N Engl J Med* 2001;345:9–16

49. Amalfitano A, Bengur AR, Morse RP, Majure JM, Case LE, Veerling DL *et al*. Recombinant human acid α-glucosidase enzyme therapy for infantile glycogen storage disease type II: results of a phase I/II clinical trial. *Genet Med* 2001;3:132–8

50. Kakkis ED, Muenzer J, Tiller GE, Waber L, Belmont J, Passage M *et al*. Enzyme-replacement therapy in mucopolysaccharidosis I. *N Engl J Med* 2001;344: 182–8

51. Muenzer J, Lamsa JC, Garcia A, Dacosta J, Garcia J, Treco DA. Enzyme replacement therapy in muco-polysaccharidosis type II (Hunter syndrome): a preliminary report. *Acta Paediatr Suppl* 2002;439:98–9

52. Harmatz P, Whitley CB, Waber L, Pais R, Steiner R, Plecko B *et al*. Enzyme replacement therapy in mucopolysaccharidosis VI (Maroteaux–Lamy syndrome). *J Pediatr* 2004;144:574–80

2 Epidemiology of lysosomal storage diseases: an overview

Maria Fuller, Peter J Meikle and John J Hopwood
Lysosomal Diseases Research Unit, Department of Genetic Medicine, Children, Youth and Women's Health Service, North Adelaide, South Australia 5006, Australia

Lysosomal storage diseases (LSDs) comprise a group of at least 50 distinct genetic diseases, each one resulting from a deficiency of a particular lysosomal protein/ activity or, in a few cases, from non-lysosomal activities that are involved in lysosomal biogenesis or protein maturation. Fabry disease is the second most common of the LSDs, after Gaucher disease. The reported epidemiological data are likely to be underestimates, due to missed diagnoses of these rare disorders. The positive and negative outcomes of newborn screening for Fabry disease and LSDs in general are considered. Early diagnosis and intervention before the onset of irreversible pathology will provide a substantial benefit to many of these newborns, as well as providing the opportunity for parents to receive genetic counselling. However, there can also be potential harm to the parent/newborn relationship as a consequence of knowing that the baby has an incurable disorder.

Introduction

A significant problem in gathering epidemiological data is the clinical heterogeneity present in all lysosomal storage diseases (LSDs). This leads to missed diagnoses and diagnostic confusion, which results in poor epidemiological data and an underestimation of the impact of LSDs in the community. Accurate epidemiological data are essential in order to appreciate both the specific and overall impact of LSDs on patients, families and the community, and to enable the introduction of policies that will effectively reduce this impact.

Genes and proteins

LSDs comprise a group of at least 50 distinct genetic diseases [1], each one resulting from a deficiency of a particular lysosomal protein/activity or, in a few cases, from non-lysosomal activities that are involved in lysosomal biogenesis or protein maturation.

The number of recognized LSDs is increasing as new disorders are characterized biochemically and genetically. Over the past decade, a deficiency of cathepsin K has been described, which results in an LSD called pycnodysostosis [2], and several of the genes and proteins involved in the neuronal ceroid lipofuscinoses (Batten disease family) have been characterized. Infantile neuronal ceroid lipofuscinosis, also known as Santavuori disease, has been shown to result from a deficiency of palmitoyl protein thioesterase [3], and classic late-infantile neuronal ceroid lipofuscinosis (Jansky–Bielschowsky disease) has been shown to result from a deficiency of tripeptidyl peptidase I [4], both of which are lysosomal enzymes. At least eight genes are thought to be involved in this group of LSDs, but only six have been identified to date [5]. In addition, the protein deficiency leading to Danon disease was recently identified as the lysosome-associated membrane protein LAMP-2 [6]. Undoubtedly, many more proteins and genes are involved in LSDs but are yet to be characterized.

Most LSDs are inherited in an autosomal recessive manner, with the exception of Hunter syndrome or mucopolysaccharidosis type II (MPS II), which shows X-linked recessive inheritance; Danon disease, which is X-linked dominant; and Fabry disease, which, with a high proportion of affected females, should not be described as X-linked recessive.

Although each LSD results from mutations in a different gene and a consequent deficiency of enzyme activity or protein function, all LSDs share one common biochemical characteristic: they result in an accumulation of substrates within lysosomes. The particular substrates that are stored and the site(s) of storage vary. The substrate type is used to group the LSDs into broad categories, including the mucopolysaccharidoses, the lipidoses, the glycogenoses and the oligosaccharidoses [7]. Despite this categorization, many clinical similarities are observed between groups as well as within each group. Common clinical features of many LSDs include bone abnormalities, organomegaly, central nervous system dysfunction and coarse hair and facies.

Some LSDs have been classified into clinical subtypes (such as the Hurler/Scheie definitions of MPS I or the infantile-/juvenile-/adult-onset forms of Pompe disease), but it is clear that most LSDs have a broad continuum of clinical severity and age at presentation.

Incidence and prevalence

Limited numbers of studies have investigated the incidence of LSDs, defined as the total number of cases diagnosed within a certain period of time, divided by the total number of live births in the same period (Table 1). One of the main problems associated with obtaining accurate epidemiological data for these individually rare disorders is that, in most countries, there are numerous diagnostic centres, which compounds the problem of collecting and correlating diagnoses. In Australia, two diagnostic centres serve the entire country, as well as covering New Zealand and a portion of South-East Asia. The National Referral Laboratory for Lysosomal, Peroxisomal and Related Genetic Disorders at the Children, Youth and Women's Health Service, North Adelaide diagnoses approximately 80% of LSD patients in Australia, while the Division of Chemical Pathology at the Royal Brisbane Hospitals, Brisbane covers the remainder.

In a retrospective case study, Meikle *et al.* reported on the incidence of LSDs in Australia [8]. Over the period January 1980 to December 1996, 470 diagnoses of LSDs were made, representing 27 different disorders. Based on these figures, the incidence of LSDs ranges from 1 in 57 000 for Gaucher disease to as low as 1 in 4.2 million for sialidosis. The incidence of LSDs as a group was calculated to be 1 in 7700; if prenatal diagnoses were not considered, the incidence of LSDs was 1 in 9000 births. However, the neuronal ceroid lipofuscinoses were not included in this study. Estimates of the global incidence of neuronal ceroid lipofuscinoses as high as 1 in 12 500 have been reported [9]. Based on Australian diagnoses made during the period 1998–2003, the combined incidence of the three most prevalent forms of neuronal ceroid lipofuscinoses (infantile, late-infantile and juvenile) has been estimated at approximately 1 in 60 000 (personal communication, MJ Fietz; Children, Youth and Women's Health Service, North Adelaide, Australia). Furthermore, there are likely to be other LSDs that are yet to be clinically and biochemically described, suggesting that the combined incidence of LSDs may be as high as 1 in 5000.

Table 1. *Incidence/prevalence of lysosomal storage diseases.*

Disease	Clinical phenotype	OMIM number	Enzyme deficiency	Incidence*/prevalence[†]		
				Australia [8]	The Netherlands [10]	Northern Portugal [12]
α-N-Acetylgalactosaminidase deficiency	Schindler disease; Kanzaki disease	104170	α-N-Acetylgalactosaminidase	–	1:500 000	–
Acid lipase deficiency	Cholesterol ester storage disease; Wolman disease	278000	Acid lipase	1:528 000	–	–
Aspartylglucosaminuria	Aspartylglucosaminuria	208400	Aspartylglucosaminidase	1:2 111 000	1:769 000	1:58 000
Cystinosis	Cystinosis	219800	Cystine transporter	1:192 000	–	–
Danon disease	Danon disease	300257	LAMP-2	–	–	–
Fabry disease	Fabry disease	301500	α-Galactosidase A	1:117 000[‡]	1:476 000	1:833 000[‡]
Farber lipogranulomatosis	Farber disease	228000	Acid ceramidase	–	–	–
Fucosidosis		230000	α-L-Fucosidase	> 1:2 000 000	1:2 000 000	–
Galactosialidosis types I/II		256540	Protective protein		1:2 500 000	1:130 000
	Gaucher disease type I	230800	β-Glucocerebrosidase	1:57 000	1:86 000	1:74 000
	Gaucher disease type II	230900				
	Gaucher disease type III	231000				
Atypical Gaucher disease	Atypical Gaucher disease	176801	Saposin C	–	–	–
Globoid cell leukodystrophy	Krabbe disease	245200	β-Galactocerebrosidase	1:201 000	1:74 000	1:82 000
Glycogen storage disease II	Pompe disease	232300	α-Glucosidase	1:146 000	1:50 000	1:588 000
GM1-gangliosidosis types I/II/III		230500	β-Galactosidase	1:384 000	1:243 000	1:161 000
GM2-gangliosidosis type AB		272750	GM2-activator deficiency	–	–	–
GM2-gangliosidosis type I (B variant)	Tay–Sachs disease	272800	β-Hexosaminidase A	1:201 000	1:243 000	1:32 000
GM2-gangliosidosis type II (O variant)	Sandhoff disease	268800	β-Hexosaminidase A and B	1:384 000	1:294 000	1:67 000

continued

Table 1. *Incidence/prevalence of lysosomal storage diseases (continued).*

Disease	Clinical phenotype	OMIM number	Enzyme deficiency	Incidence*/prevalence†		
				Australia [8]	The Netherlands [10]	Northern Portugal [12]
α-Mannosidosis types I/II		248500	α-D-Mannosidase	1:1 056 000	1:1 111 000	1:833 000
β-Mannosidosis		248510	β-D-Mannosidase	–	1:769 000	1:833 000
Metachromatic leukodystrophy		250100	Arylsulphatase A	1:92 000	1:70 000	1:54 000
Metachromatic leukodystrophy		249900	Saposin B	–	–	–
Mucolipidosis type I	Sialidosis types I/II	256550	Neuraminidase	1:4 222 000	1:2 000 000	–
Mucolipidosis types II/III	I-cell disease; pseudo-Hurler polydystrophy	252500 252600	N-Acetylglucosamine-1-phosphotransferase	1:325 000	1:416 000	1:37 000
Mucolipidosis type IIIC	Pseudo-Hurler polydystrophy	252605	N-Acetylglucosamine-1-phosphotransferase γ-subunit			
Mucolipidosis type IV		252650	Mucolipin 1	–	–	–
MPS type I	Hurler/Scheie syndrome	607014 607015 607016	α-L-Iduronidase	1:88 000	1:84 000	1:75 000
MPS type II	Hunter syndrome	309900	Iduronate-2-sulphatase	1:136 000‡	1:149 000‡	1:92 000‡
MPS type IIIA	Sanfilippo syndrome	252900	Heparan-N-sulphatase	1:114 000	1:86 000	–
MPS type IIIB	Sanfilippo syndrome	252920	α-N-Acetylglucosaminidase	1:211 000	1:238 000	1:139 000
MPS type IIIC	Sanfilippo syndrome	252930	AcetylCoA:glucosamine-N-acetyltransferase	1:1 407 000	1:476 000	1:833 000
MPS type IIID	Sanfilippo syndrome	252940	N-Acetylglucosamine-6-sulphatase	1:1 056 000	1:1 000 000	–
MPS type IVA	Morquio syndrome	253000	N-Acetylgalactosamine-6-sulphatase	1:169 000	1:455 000	1:167 000
MPS type IVB	Morquio syndrome	253010	β-Galactosidase	–	1:714 000	–

continued

Table 1. Incidence/prevalence of lysosomal storage diseases (continued).

Disease	Clinical phenotype	OMIM number	Enzyme deficiency	Incidence*/prevalence†		
				Australia [8]	The Netherlands [10]	Northern Portugal [12]
MPS type VI	Maroteaux–Lamy syndrome	253200	N-Acetylgalactosamine-4-sulphatase	1:235 000	1:666 000	1:238 000
MPS type VII	Sly syndrome	253220	β-Glucuronidase	1:2 111 000	1:416 000	–
MPS type IX		601492	Hyaluronidase 1	–	–	–
Multiple sulphatase deficiency		272200	Formylglycine-generating enzyme	1:1 407 000	1:2 000 000	1:208 000
Neuronal ceroid lipofuscinosis 1, infantile (CLN1)	Santavuori disease	256730	Palmitoyl protein thioesterase 1	1:60 000§	–	1:588 000
Neuronal ceroid lipofuscinosis 2, late-infantile (CLN2)	Jansky–Bielschowsky disease	204500	Tripeptidyl peptidase I	1:60 000§	–	1:1 429 000
Neuronal ceroid lipofuscinosis 3, juvenile (CLN3)	Batten disease	204200	CLN3p (function unknown)	1:60 000§	–	1:208 000
Neuronal ceroid lipofuscinosis 5 (CLN5)	Finnish variant late-infantile neuronal ceroid lipofuscinosis	256731	CLN5p (function unknown)	–	–	–
Neuronal ceroid lipofuscinosis 6 (CLN6)	Variant late-infantile neuronal ceroid lipofuscinosis	601780	CLN6p (function unknown)	–	–	1:70 000
Neuronal ceroid lipofuscinosis 8 (CLN8)	Northern epilepsy	600143	CLN8p (function unknown)	–	–	–

continued

Table 1. *Incidence/prevalence of lysosomal storage diseases (continued).*

Disease	Clinical phenotype	OMIM number	Enzyme deficiency	Incidence*/prevalence†		
				Australia [8]	The Netherlands [10]	Northern Portugal [12]
Niemann–Pick disease type A/B	Niemann–Pick disease	257200 607616	Acid sphingomyelinase	1:248 000	1:189 000	1:167 000
Niemann–Pick disease type C1	Niemann–Pick disease	257220	NPC1 protein (involved in cholesterol trafficking)			
Niemann–Pick disease type C2	Niemann–Pick disease	607625	NPC2 protein (involved in cholesterol trafficking)	1:211 000	1:286 000	1:45 000
Prosaposin deficiency		See 176801		–	–	–
Pycnodysostosis		265800	Cathepsin K	–	–	–
Sialic acid storage disease	Infantile free sialic acid storage disease; Salla disease	269920 604369	Sialin (sialic acid transporter)	1:528 000	1:1 428 000	–
Sialuria		269921	UDP-N-acetylglucosamine 2-epimerase	–	–	–

LAMP-2, lysosome-associated membrane protein 2; MPS, mucopolysaccharidosis; OMIM, Online Mendelian Inheritance in Man.
*Incidence in Australia defined as the total number of cases diagnosed within a certain period of time divided by the total number of births in the same period.
†Birth prevalence in The Netherlands and Portugal defined as the total number of diagnosed cases born within a certain period of time divided by the total number of births in the same period.
‡Values for hemizygotes only.
§Combined incidence of CLN1, CLN2 and CLN3 [1].

Meikle *et al.* reported the incidence of Fabry hemizygotes as 1 in 117 000 [8]. No data on heterozygotes were obtained, but the incidence determined in hemizygotes could be extrapolated to give a combined incidence of 1 in 58 000.

The incidence of LSDs in Australia is not dissimilar to other countries. Poorthuis *et al.* [10] reported on the frequency of LSDs in The Netherlands based on 963 diagnosed cases over the period 1970–96. The combined birth prevalence for all LSDs, defined as the total number of diagnosed cases born within a certain period of time divided by the total number of live births in the same period, was calculated to be 1 in 7100 live births, with glycogen storage disease type II being the most prevalent at 1 in 50 000. The prevalence of Fabry disease was estimated at 1 in 476 000 in this population, lower than in the Australian population, and Gaucher disease was calculated to be 1 in 86 000, also somewhat lower than the Australian figure and representing 8% of all reported LSDs.

A report from Italy on inborn errors of metabolism gave a combined LSD incidence of 1 in 8275, with Gaucher disease at 1 in 40 247 (21% of all reported LSDs) [11]. A recent report from Portugal estimated the combined birth prevalence of all LSDs to be 1 in 4000 births, with Gaucher disease at 1 in 74 000 births (5% of all reported LSDs) [12]. Ozkara and Topcu reported the combined birth prevalence of the sphingolipidoses in Turkey at 1 in 21 500, with Gaucher disease at 1 in 185 000 and Fabry disease 1 in 6 700 000 [13]. However, their study included only children under 5 years of age with neurological symptoms, thereby excluding most patients with Fabry disease. Bähner and colleagues recently reported that the incidence of MPS in Germany (1 in 28 000) is similar to that reported in other populations; however, different frequencies of individual MPS subtypes were observed [14].

There have also been several reports on the incidence of particular disorders in specific populations: values as high as 1 in 18 500 for aspartylglucosaminuria in the Finnish population [15] and 1 in 3900 for Tay–Sachs disease in the Ashkenazi Jewish population [16] have been reported.

In the UK, the prevalence of Fabry disease was reported to be 1 in 366 000 [17]. This figure was based on notifications of patients seen in UK clinics who had low α-galactosidase activities. Many patients with Fabry disease are likely to have been omitted and therefore the prevalence figure is probably an underestimate.

High-risk populations

Although LSDs have a low incidence in most populations, there are a number of exceptions. The Ashkenazi Jewish population is at high risk for a number of LSDs, including Gaucher disease, which is thought to have an incidence as high as 1 in 855 Ashkenazi Jewish births [18], Tay–Sachs disease and Niemann–Pick disease [19]. The Finnish population has been reported to have a high incidence of aspartylglucosaminuria (1 in 18 500 births) [15] and infantile (1 in 13 000 births) and juvenile (1 in 21 000 births) neuronal ceroid lipofuscinosis [20]. Both communities represent populations that have been, and to some extent still are, genetically isolated either culturally or geographically. This has contributed to the founder effects that have led to the relatively high incidence of specific LSDs in these populations.

Interpretation of data

For diseases that are very rare, even a single missed diagnosis can make a large difference to the calculated birth prevalence. In addition, the methods used to calculate incidence and birth prevalence figures must also be considered when comparing data from separate studies. In the Australian study, the period used to determine the total number of births was the period in which the diagnoses were made; the assumption was made that late-onset patients diagnosed during the study (and born before the study period) were representative of late-onset patients born within the study period who had not yet presented clinically [8]. In the Dutch and Portuguese studies, the period used to calculate the birth prevalence was based on the age of the patient; thus, the assumption was made that all patients born prior to the last patient in the subgroup were identified [10, 12]. There are limitations to both methods and it is likely that ascertainment of the late-onset LSD patients was incomplete, leading to underestimation of incidence and birth prevalence. In Australia, the incidence of Pompe disease was estimated to be approximately 1 in 146 000. However, studies based on carrier detection in normal populations have indicated that the incidence may be as high as 1 in 40 000 births in both the USA [21] and The Netherlands [22]. On the basis of their findings, Martiniuk and colleagues [21] predict that many mild adult cases remain undiagnosed.

Burden of illness

The burden of LSDs on the individual and family is undoubtedly enormous, although there is relatively little documentation in this area. The cost to the community in terms of medical treatment and support is also poorly defined. Therapy is likely to be available for several LSDs in the near future. In addition, a number of technologies for newborn screening have been proposed. If the current cost of these disorders to public health systems is to be assessed accurately, thereby allowing the cost-effectiveness of therapy and/or newborn screening to be investigated, accurate prevalence values will be required. The introduction of newborn screening for LSDs will provide such accurate prevalence data.

Fabry disease

Fabry disease has been reported to be the second most common LSD, after Gaucher disease, although reported incidence and birth prevalence figures vary considerably. These figures are likely to be underestimated due to missed diagnoses, because the disease presentation can be non-specific and signs and symptoms are often mistakenly attributed to other disorders.

Renal insufficiency is a key clinical feature of Fabry disease, and it is believed that the birth prevalence and incidence of Fabry disease in patients with end-stage renal failure is underestimated [23]. In a retrospective study of 105 male patients with Fabry disease, of whom 94 were Caucasian, 74% had renal disease [24]. Linthorst *et al.* [23] estimated the prevalence of Fabry disease in patients on dialysis at 0.22%. Consequently, screening for Fabry disease in large renal dialysis clinics has been suggested. In France, 106 patients on haemodialysis were screened for α-galactosidase activity. One patient was identified with Fabry disease and a further seven family members of this index case carried the same mutation [25]. A study in Japan reported that 1.2% of males receiving renal dialysis were affected with Fabry disease [26].

Progressive left ventricular hypertrophy is a common cardiac manifestation of Fabry disease, and the heart may be the only organ affected in the 'cardiac variant' of the disease. It has been estimated that 3% of males suffering from left ventricular hypertrophy and 6% of males with late-onset hypertrophic cardiomyopathy have Fabry disease [27, 28]. Up to 12% of females with late-onset hypertrophic cardiomyopathy may have Fabry disease [29]. Cardiac involvement is extensive and progressive in Fabry disease, and mitral valve prolapse is believed to occur in 50% of affected males [30]. Rolfs and colleagues have also reported a high prevalence of Fabry disease in acute stroke patients: from a cohort of 721 patients, biologically significant mutations were identified in 4.9% of males and 2.4% of females [31].

The majority of reports of Fabry disease are in Caucasians, but isolated cases have been reported in Asian populations. The results of a survey in Japan estimated the frequency of Fabry disease to be 1 in 200 000 [32]. In this study, renal failure was detected in 43% of Fabry patients over the age of 30 years, while cardiac disease was present in 60% of patients over the age of 40 years. Two point mutations have been described in Chinese patients with Fabry disease [33, 34].

It is generally believed that the majority of males with Fabry disease experience multiple clinical manifestations and suffer pain throughout their lives. However, although pain is considered the major clinical symptom of Fabry disease, it has been estimated that between 10% and 20% of patients lack this manifestation [35].

Newborn screening for Fabry disease and other LSDs

Newborn screening can be described as a population-based public health programme applied regionally to reduce the morbidity, severity or mortality of specific genetic disorders. Whether we should screen neonates for Fabry disease raises the question of the potential good versus the potential harm that may result from such a programme. The positive and negative outcomes from population-based screening have been debated extensively [36, 37] and many of the same considerations apply to screening for LSDs. For many LSDs, it is clear that early diagnosis and intervention before the onset of irreversible pathology will provide a substantial benefit to the newborn. There are also other potential benefits. Early diagnosis will enable parents to receive genetic counselling and provide them with reproductive choices. In families affected by an LSD, it is not uncommon to have two or more affected children before the first is diagnosed. Early diagnosis, as provided by a newborn screening programme, would also avoid the prolonged and stressful process of

diagnosis that is currently experienced by many patients and families. These benefits are primarily directed to the family rather than the newborn, but are nonetheless significant. On the other hand, the potential harm to the parent/newborn relationship that can result from the knowledge that the baby has an incurable disorder and the concept of depriving families of a 'normal' child for the period of time until the child presents clinically must be considered. These are difficult issues to define and quantify but must be addressed by the community before screening can commence.

Newborn screening involves diagnosis of a genetic disease to enable therapy to be given to prevent or slow the expression of the disease. Currently, there are no newborn screening programmes for Fabry disease or any other LSDs; however, a number of technologies are under development [38, 39]. Chamoles et al. [40] has described diagnostic assays using dried blood spots for the detection of α-galactosidase activity against a 4-methylumbelliferyl substrate in the presence of a high concentration of N-acetylgalactosamine (see also Chapter 17). Fuller et al. [41] reported the immunoquantification of α-galactosidase from dry blood spots, which was also diagnostic for Fabry hemizygotes. The capability of this assay to identify heterozygotes was improved when combined with the immunoquantification of saposin C. Heterozygotes and hemizygotes with Fabry disease, and unaffected controls, were able to be separated using urinary lipid profiling that included the glycolipid substrate ceramidetrihexoside (globotriaosylceramide) [42]. Importantly, measurement of ceramidetrihexoside in dry blood spots allowed clear separation of newborn Fabry hemizygotes from unaffected controls [39].

The cost of screening each LSD individually would in most cases be prohibitive, because of their low prevalence. However, several strategies have been proposed to enable the simultaneous screening of multiple LSDs. An estimate of the combined prevalence of LSDs in the Australian population is conservatively given as 1 in 5000, making simultaneous screening for multiple LSDs economically justifiable.

Technology for LSD screening in the newborn population has been the focus of considerable research over the past few years. Lysosomal enzyme activities and protein are measurable in rehydrated dried blood spots. Fluorometric, radiometric, immunochemical (protein profiling) and electrospray ionization tandem mass spectrometry (ESI-MS/MS) assays have been developed. Protein profiling and ESI-MS/MS offer the capability of assaying the products of several enzymes simultaneously (multiplexing). There have been reports of using these two assay types to make direct measurements of both the amount of lysosomal protein and reaction velocities in rehydrated dried blood spots; the assays are readily adaptable to the process of newborn screening [38, 43, 44].

It is now technically possible to detect Fabry hemizygotes in the newborn period, but guidelines need to be developed to address the following issues before implementing general population screening programmes.
- What is the policy regarding the treatment of pre-symptomatic but affected patients?
- Should enzyme replacement therapy be initiated at the time of diagnosis?
- If therapy is initiated in asymptomatic patients, how should its effectiveness be monitored?

The X-linked inheritance and the potential detection of asymptomatic heterozygotes, who may or may not develop a clinical phenotype, will add a special significance to the debate.

Conclusions

Epidemiological data recording the prevalence and incidence of Fabry disease and other LSDs are limited as a result of differences between geographic regions and ethnic populations, and are likely to be underestimates due to missed diagnoses of these rare disorders. Diagnostic methods under development are addressing the problem of detection in high-risk populations, while the introduction of newborn screening for hemizygotes with Fabry disease and other LSDs will provide early and definitive diagnoses for these disorders. This will enable early intervention that, in many cases, is likely to provide substantial benefit to the newborn, as well as an opportunity for the parents to receive genetic counselling. Eventually, universal screening of the newborn population will provide accurate epidemiological data for all LSDs. Accurate data will be essential to understand the natural history of these diseases and the burden they place on individuals, families, societies and healthcare systems. These are important factors that will drive the development and introduction of new therapies for this group of rare disorders.

References

1. Meikle PJ, Fietz MJ, Hopwood JJ. Diagnosis of lysosomal storage disorders: current techniques and future directions. *Expert Rev Mol Diagn* 2004;4:677–91

2. Gelb BD, Shi GP, Chapman HA, Desnick RJ. Pycnodysostosis, a lysosomal disease caused by cathepsin K deficiency. *Science* 1996;273:1236–8

3. Vesa J, Hellsten E, Verkruyse LA, Camp LA, Rapola J, Santavuori P *et al.* Mutations in the palmitoyl protein thioesterase gene causing infantile neuronal ceroid lipofuscinosis. *Nature* 1995;376:584–7

4. Sleat DE, Donnelly RJ, Lackland H, Liu CG, Sohar I, Pullarkat RK *et al.* Association of mutations in a lysosomal protein with classical late-infantile neuronal ceroid lipofuscinosis. *Science* 1997;277:1802–5

5. Ezaki J, Kominami E. The intracellular location and function of proteins of neuronal ceroid lipofuscinoses. *Brain Pathol* 2004;14:77–85

6. Nishino I, Fu J, Tanji K, Yamada T, Shimojo S, Koori T *et al.* Primary LAMP-2 deficiency causes X-linked vacuolar cardiomyopathy and myopathy (Danon disease). *Nature* 2000;406:906–10

7. Hopwood J, Brooks D. An introduction to the basic science and biology of the lysosome and storage diseases. In: Applegarth D, Dimmick J, Hall J, editors. Organelle diseases. Clinical features, diagnosis, pathogenesis and management. London: Chapman and Hall Medical; 1997. p. 7–36

8. Meikle PJ, Hopwood JJ, Clague AE, Carey WF. Prevalence of lysosomal storage disorders. *JAMA* 1999;281:249–54

9. Rider J, Rider D. Batten disease: past, present, and future. *Am J Med Genet* 1988;Suppl 5:21–6

10. Poorthuis BJ, Wevers RA, Kleijer WJ, Groener JE, de Jong JG, van Weely S et al. The frequency of lysosomal storage diseases in The Netherlands. *Hum Genet* 1999;105:151–6

11. Dionisi-Vici C, Rizzo C, Burlina AB, Caruso U, Sabetta G, Uziel G et al. Inborn errors of metabolism in the Italian pediatric population: a national retrospective survey. *J Pediatr* 2002;140:321–7

12. Pinto R, Caseiro C, Lemos M, Lopes L, Fontes A, Ribeiro H et al. Prevalence of lysosomal storage diseases in Portugal. *Eur J Hum Genet* 2004; 12:87–92

13. Ozkara HA, Topcu M. Sphingolipidoses in Turkey. *Brain Dev* 2004;26:363–6

14. Baehner F, Schmiedeskamp C, Krummenauer F, Miebach E, Bajbouj M, Whybra C et al. Cumulative incidence rates of the mucopolysaccharidoses in Germany. *J Inherit Metab Dis.* 2005;28:1011–17

15. Arvio M, Autio S, Louhiala P. Early clinical symptoms and incidence of aspartylglucosaminuria in Finland. *Acta Paediatr* 1993;82:587–9

16. Petersen GM, Rotter JI, Cantor RM, Field LL, Greenwald S, Lim JS et al. The Tay-Sachs disease gene in North American Jewish populations: geographic variations and origin. *Am J Hum Genet* 1983;35:1258–69

17. MacDermot KD, Holmes A, Miners AH. Anderson–Fabry disease: clinical manifestations and impact of disease in a cohort of 60 obligate carrier females. *J Med Genet* 2001;38:769–75

18. Beutler E, Grabowski G. Gaucher disease. In: Scriver CR, Beaudet AL, Sly WS, Valle D, editors. The metabolic and molecular bases of inherited disease, 8th edn. New York: McGraw-Hill; 2001. p. 3635–68

19. Vallance H, Ford J. Carrier testing for autosomal-recessive disorders. *Crit Rev Clin Lab Sci* 2003; 40:473–97

20. Santavuori P. Neuronal ceroid-lipofuscinoses in childhood. *Brain Dev* 1988;10:80–3

21. Martiniuk F, Chen A, Mack A, Arvanitopoulos E, Chen Y, Rom WN et al. Carrier frequency for glycogen storage disease type II in New York and estimates of affected individuals born with the disease. *Am J Med Genet* 1998;79:69–72

22. Ausems MG, Verbiest J, Hermans MP, Kroos MA, Beemer FA, Wokke JH et al. Frequency of glycogen storage disease type II in The Netherlands: implications for diagnosis and genetic counselling. *Eur J Hum Genet* 1999,7.713–16

23. Linthorst GE, Hollak CE, Korevaar JC, Van Manen JG, Aerts JM, Boeschoten EW. α-Galactosidase A deficiency in Dutch patients on dialysis: a critical appraisal of screening for Fabry disease. *Nephrol Dial Transplant* 2003;18:1581–4

24. Branton MH, Schiffmann R, Sabnis SG, Murray GJ, Quirk JM, Altarescu G et al. Natural history of Fabry renal disease: influence of α-galactosidase A activity and genetic mutations on clinical course. *Medicine (Baltimore)* 2002;81:122–38

25. Bekri S, Enica A, Ghafari T, Plaza G, Champenois I, Choukroun G et al. Fabry disease in patients with end-stage renal failure: the potential benefits of screening. *Nephron Clin Pract* 2005;101:c33–8

26. Nakao S, Kodama C, Takenaka T, Tanaka A, Yasumoto Y, Yoshida A et al. Fabry disease: detection of undiagnosed hemodialysis patients and identification of a "renal variant" phenotype. *Kidney Int* 2003;64:801–7

27. Sachdev B, Takenaka T, Teraguchi H, Tei C, Lee P, McKenna WJ et al. Prevalence of Anderson–Fabry disease in male patients with late onset hypertrophic cardiomyopathy. *Circulation* 2002;105:1407–11

28. Nakao S, Takenaka T, Maeda M, Kodama C, Tanaka A, Tahara M et al. An atypical variant of Fabry's disease in men with left ventricular hypertrophy. *N Engl J Med* 1995;333:288–93

29. Chimenti C, Pieroni M, Morgante E, Antuzzi D, Russo A, Russo MA et al. Prevalence of Fabry disease in female patients with late-onset hypertrophic cardiomyopathy. *Circulation* 2004;110: 1047–53

30. Brady R, Grabowski G, Thadhani R. Fabry disease: review and new perspectives. *Synermed Communications* 2001:1–8

31. Rolfs A, Bottcher T, Zschiesche M, Morris P, Winchester B, Bauer P et al. Prevalence of Fabry disease in patients with cryptogenic stroke: a prospective study. *Lancet* 2005;366:1794–6

32. Owada M, Kitigawa T. [Lysosomal storage diseases]. *Nippon Rinsho* 2001;8:317–27

33. Tse KC, Chan KW, Tin VP, Yip PS, Tang S, Li FK et al. Clinical features and genetic analysis of a Chinese kindred with Fabry's disease. *Nephrol Dial Transplant* 2003;18:182–6

34. Chen CH, Shyu PW, Wu SJ, Sheu SS, Desnick RJ, Hsiao KJ. Identification of a novel point mutation (S65T) in α-galactosidase A gene in Chinese patients with Fabry disease. Mutations in brief no. 169. Online. *Hum Mutat* 1998;11:328–30

35. Ries M, Ramaswami U, Parini R, Lindblad B, Whybra C, Willers I et al. The early clinical phenotype of Fabry disease: a study on 35 European children and adolescents. *Eur J Pediatr* 2003;162:767–72

36. Wilcken B. Ethical issues in newborn screening and the impact of new technologies. *Eur J Pediatr* 2003; 162 (Suppl 1):S62–6

37. Meikle PJ, Dean CJ, Brooks DA, Hopwood JJ. Newborn screening for lysosomal storage disorders: ethical and technical considerations. *Italian J Pediatr* 2004;30:305–11

38. Li Y, Scott CR, Chamoles NA, Ghavami A, Pinto BM, Turecek F et al. Direct multiplex assay of lysosomal enzymes in dried blood spots for newborn screening. *Clin Chem* 2004;50:1785–96

39. Meikle PJ, Ranieri E, Simonsen H, Rozaklis T, Ramsay SL, Whitfield PD *et al.* Newborn screening for lysosomal storage disorders: clinical evaluation of a two-tier strategy. *Pediatrics* 2004;114:909–16

40. Chamoles NA, Blanco MB, Gaggioli D, Casentini C. Hurler-like phenotype: enzymatic diagnosis in dried blood spots on filter paper. *Clin Chem* 2001;47: 2098–102

41. Fuller M, Lovejoy M, Brooks DA, Harkin ML, Hopwood JJ, Meikle PJ. Immunoquantification of α-galactosidase: evaluation for the diagnosis of Fabry disease. *Clin Chem* 2004;50:1979–85

42. Fuller M, Sharp PC, Rozaklis T, Whitfield PD, Blacklock D, Hopwood JJ *et al.* Urinary lipid profiling for the identification of Fabry hemizygotes and heterozygotes. *Clin Chem* 2005;51:688–94

43. Umapathysivam K, Hopwood JJ, Meikle PJ. Determination of acid α-glucosidase activity in blood spots as a diagnostic test for Pompe disease. *Clin Chem* 2001;47:1378–83

44. Wang D, Eadala B, Sadilek M, Chamoles NA, Turecek F, Scott CR *et al.* Tandem mass spectrometric analysis of dried blood spots for screening of mucopolysaccharidosis I in newborns. *Clin Chem* 2005;51:898–900

3 Physiology of the lysosome

Paul Saftig

Biochemical Institute, Christian-Albrechts-University Kiel, Olshausenstrasse 40, D-24098 Kiel, Germany

Initially discovered by Christian de Duve in 1955, lysosomes are now known to contain more than 50 acid hydrolases (phosphatases, nucleases, glycosidases, proteases, peptidases, sulphatases and lipases) that can digest most macromolecules of the cell. The breakdown products, such as amino acids, monosaccharides, oligosaccharides and nucleotides, are transported back to the cytosol by specific transporter proteins in the lysosomal membrane. Functional deficiencies of both hydrolytic and non-hydrolytic polypeptides can result in lysosomal storage diseases, which are characterized by the intralysosomal deposition of macromolecules and a multisystemic phenotype. The detailed structure of the lysosome differs depending on the cell type. Most newly synthesized lysosomal hydrolases enter the lysosomal compartment directly via the biosynthetic route. After modification of one or several of their carbohydrates to mannose-6-phosphate moieties in the Golgi apparatus, the acid hydrolases bind mannose-6-phosphate receptors that deliver them to endosomes. As the vacuolar-type H^+-ATPase leads to acidification during the maturation of the endosomal compartment, the hydrolases dissociate from their receptors, which are then recycled back to the trans-Golgi network or to the cell surface. The sorting of most lysosomal membrane proteins depends on short sequence motifs within their cytoplasmic tails, which are necessary and sufficient to target them to lysosomes. Lysosomes can be involved in various cellular processes, such as cholesterol homeostasis, autophagy, membrane repair, bone and tissue remodelling, pathogen defence, cell signalling and death. These complex functions highlight the fact that the lysosome is a central organelle which is much more than just the wastebasket of the cell.

Introduction

Lysosomes are organelles that are found in all mammalian cells except red blood cells. They are acidic, hydrolase-rich organelles that are capable of degrading most biological macromolecules. Lysosomes receive input from both the endocytotic and biosynthetic pathways. It has been observed that these organelles can be morphologically heterogeneous due to variations in their content of internalized and degraded material. This led to a complex terminology for lysosomes, such as residual bodies, and primary and secondary lysosomes. In more recent studies, it has become clear that cells can also contain lysosome-like organelles, such as melanosomes, lytic granules, major histocompatibility complex (MHC) class II compartments, platelet-dense granules and synaptic-like microvesicles [1].

Lysosomes form part of a highly dynamic endocytotic system. The biogenesis of new lysosomes or lysosome-related organelles requires continuous substitution with newly synthesized components. Two mannose-6-

phosphate (M6P) receptors were identified because of their ability to bind M6P-containing soluble acid hydrolases in the Golgi apparatus and transport them to the endosomal/lysosomal system [2]. The acidification of endosomes, lysosomes and lysosome-related organelles facilitates the dissociation of the M6P–receptor–ligand complexes, and the proteolytic processing required for the enzymatic activation of several hydrolases. Acidification is also a prerequisite for the denaturation of proteins for lysosomal proteolysis [3]. Lysosomal proteases are also involved in processes such as antigen processing, degradation of matrix constituents in the extracellular space and initiation of apoptotic processes within the cytosol [4]. Alterations in the proteolytic machinery of the lysosomes or in the vesicular transport of the endosomal/lysosomal system, as well as deficiencies of lysosomal hydrolases, their activators or transporters, can occur as a consequence of mutations in the corresponding genes. These result in lysosomal storage diseases (LSDs), in which there is accumulation of specific substrates in the lysosomes [5]. Most therapies for LSDs attempt to supply deficient cells with the active counterpart of the defective protein. Such enzyme replacement therapies are distinct from substrate reduction therapies, which try to reduce the accumulated storage material by non-enzymatic means [6].

Lysosomes are surrounded by a limiting membrane. The lysosomal membrane has multiple functions including acidification of the lysosomal lumen, sequestration of lysosomal enzymes, mediation of fusion events and transport of degradation products to the cytoplasm. Lysosomal membrane proteins are usually highly glycosylated proteins decorating the luminal surface of lysosomal membranes [7]. The importance of the lysosomal membrane is highlighted in Niemann–Pick disease type C, in which a defect in lysosomal lipid efflux leads to lysosomal accumulation of cholesterol and glycolipids [8].

Lysosomes are also involved in processes such as membrane resealing in calcium-regulated exocytosis [9], and they can fuse with autophagic vacuoles to participate in the degradation of segregated cytoplasm [10]. Using specific chaperones, lysosomal membrane proteins can mediate the selective transport of cytosolic substrates into the lysosome [11]. Apart from such general central cellular functions, lysosomes are also involved in specific processes outside the cell, exemplified by the bone-degrading capacity of osteoclasts [12] or the secretion of lysosomal hydrolases by granulocytes to act as a first line of defence against bacterial pathogens.

This review highlights some of the physiological functions of the lysosomal compartment. It will also provide an overview of the current understanding of lysosomal protein transport and the central role of M6P receptors in these trafficking processes. Finally, some aspects of the presumed mechanisms underlying enzyme replacement, substrate reduction and chaperone therapies for the treatment of LSDs will be discussed.

Role of the lysosome in cell physiology

Microscopic identification of lysosomes is difficult due to heterogeneity in morphology, which arises as a consequence of their function as digestive organelles. The amount of space taken up by lysosomes varies in different cell types, ranging from 0.5% or less of the cytoplasmic volume in fibroblasts or hepatocytes, to a much larger proportion of the cytoplasmic volume in macrophages. The size and quantity of lysosomes can increase dramatically in any cell type when the lysosomes accumulate non-degraded material. Such conditions can either be induced by drugs that interfere with lysosomal digestion, or they are typically found in the inherited LSDs.

Today, approximately 50 lysosomal matrix proteins and 20 lysosomal membrane proteins have been identified. About 30 of the known lysosomal hydrolases are associated with LSDs. However, the *in vivo* function of many of these lysosomal proteins remains unknown. Studies using genetically engineered mouse mutants with deficiencies in single or multiple lysosomal proteins have helped to improve understanding of the (patho)physiological role, the substrate use and possible overlapping functions of some of these proteins.

Role of lysosomal enzymes and membrane proteins

Knockout mouse studies have provided insights into the functions of lysosomal enzymes (Table 1). They have also been useful in evaluating new therapies.

Cathepsins

Lysosomal proteases are expressed both ubiquitously and in a tissue- or cell-type-specific manner. These cathepsin proteases catalyse the hydrolysis of proteins within the endocytic pathway and sometimes also extracellularly. Only a few of these enzymes act as aminopeptidases or carboxypeptidases. Most of them are endopeptidases, preferentially cleaving peptide bonds within a polypeptide chain.

Cathepsin A has been shown to have a role in stabilizing lysosomal glycosidase by the formation of a multi-enzyme complex, and mice with a deficiency in this protease show a phenotype similar to human galactosialidosis

Table 1. *Selected examples of phenotypic alterations in knockout mice for lysosomal hydrolases and membrane proteins.*

Protein group	Protein	Phenotype of deficient mouse	Reference
Lysosomal proteases	Cathepsin A	Similar to galactosialidosis, e.g. bone and eye malformations, lysosomal storage	[13]
	Cathepsin D	Early postnatal death, neurodegeneration and impairment of immune system	[14, 15]
	Cathepsin B	No overt phenotype	[16, 17]
	Cathepsin K	Osteopetrosis, impaired lung function, atherosclerosis	[18–21]
	Cathepsin L	Loss of fur, impaired growth factor recycling	[22, 23]
Lysosomal phosphatases	Lysosomal acid phosphatase	Mild bone disorder, microglial activation, lysosomal storage in selected cells	[24]
	Lysosomal acid phosphatase/ TRAP	Bone disorder, hepatosplenomegaly, lysosomal storage in bone and macrophages	[25]
Lysosomal membrane proteins	LAMP-1	No overt phenotype, mild astrogliosis	[26]
	LAMP-2	Postnatal death, cardiomyopathy, accumulation of autophagic vacuoles, animal model for Danon disease	[27–29]
	LIMP-2/LGP-85	Deafness, hydronephrosis and peripheral neuropathy	[30]

LAMP, lysosome-associated membrane protein; LIMP-2/LGP-85, lysosomal integral membrane protein-2/lysosomal membrane glycoprotein-85; TRAP, tartrate-resistant acid phosphatase.

[13]. By contrast, the targeted deletion of the ubiquitously expressed cathepsin B did not result in an overt phenotype [14].

Cathepsin D [15] has proved to be essential for the survival of mice, as its deficiency leads to death due to anorexia about 3 weeks after birth. Recent observations suggest that mice deficient in cathepsin D present with a new form of LSD with a phenotype resembling neuronal ceroid lipofuscinosis [15]. Several lines of evidence suggested a direct role for cathepsin D in βA4-amyloid peptide generation, which is the major toxic agent in Alzheimer's disease; however, using primary cultures of hippocampal neurones derived from cathepsin D knockout mice, it was demonstrated that amyloid precursor protein processing and secretion of the toxic βA4-amyloid peptide was unaffected in the absence of cathepsin D. This result ruled out cathepsin D as a critical component of α-, β-, or γ-secretase, and therefore as a primary target for drugs aimed at decreasing the βA4-amyloid peptide burden in Alzheimer's disease [16].

Although cathepsin B and D were shown to be dispensable for MHC class II-mediated antigen processing [17], depending on the cell type, the two cysteine proteases cathepsin L and S are important for this process [31, 32]. Cathepsin L-deficient mice showed a couple of organ-specific phenotypes, demonstrating that cathespin L has important functions in neovascularization and growth factor recycling in the heart, skin, thymus and thyroid gland [4, 22, 23]. The importance of lysosomal enzymes in specialized tissues is exemplified by the phenotype of mice with a deficiency of the lysosomal cysteine protease, cathepsin K [18]. Mice deficient in cathepsin K represent an animal model for the rare human disorder pycnodysostosis, in which mutations within the cathepsin K gene lead to a non-functional cathepsin K, resulting in short stature, bone malformation and osteopetrosis. Osteoclasts derived from mice deficient in cathepsin K were unable to digest the bone matrix properly, leading to large areas of non-digested demineralized bone matrix [19]. Cathepsin K knockout mice were also used to show a function of this protease in the development of lung fibrosis [20] and in the progression of atherosclerosis [21]. Cathepsin K is a potential target for therapeutic intervention for the treatment of osteoporosis; however, the inhibition of cathepsin K function outside bone tissue – as indicated by the findings in mice deficient in cathepsin K – may cause unwanted side effects in such a therapeutic regimen.

Lysosomal acid phosphatases
The physiological role of the first lysosomal enzyme discovered by Christian de Duve, lysosomal acid phosphatase, remained unknown for a long time. Mice with a deficiency in lysosomal acid phosphatase displayed lysosomal storage in podocytes and tubular epithelial cells of the kidney. Within the CNS, lysosomal storage was detected in microglia, ependymal cells and astroglia, concomitant with the development of a progressive astrogliosis and microglial activation [24]. Deficiency of both known lysosomal acid phosphatases (lysosomal acid phosphatase and the tartrate-resistant acid phosphatase type 5) in mice leads to marked alterations in soft and mineralized tissues, with excessive lysosomal storage in the macrophages of the liver, spleen, bone marrow and kidney, and altered growth plates. Biochemical analyses revealed markedly reduced dephosphorylation of osteopontin, and accumulation of this bone protein in double-deficient mice suggests that osteopontin is a physiological substrate of both lysosomal phosphatases [25].

Lysosomal membrane proteins
In order to understand the possible contribution of the major components of the lysosomal membrane, mice were generated that were deficient in lysosome-associated membrane protein-1 (LAMP-1) and/or LAMP-2. Despite its abundance in the lysosomal

membrane, deficiency of LAMP-1 [26] was apparently well tolerated. LAMP-2-deficient mice [27] were more severely affected and about 50% died between 20 and 40 days of age. The major pathological feature was an extensive accumulation of autophagic vacuoles in the liver, pancreas, spleen, kidney, skeletal muscle, heart, capillary endothelium, intestinal wall, lymph nodes and neutrophilic leukocytes. Both skeletal and cardiac muscle cells showed an accumulation of autophagic vacuoles. The LAMP-2-deficient mice had large hearts with decreased contractility, and abnormal and degenerating myocytes. The physiological importance of LAMP-2 is supported by the finding that its deficiency is the primary defect in Danon disease, a lysosomal glycogen storage disease with normal acid maltase activity, fatal cardiomyopathy, variable mental retardation and mild skeletal myopathy [28]. Vacuoles in skeletal and cardiac muscle containing glycogen and cytoplasmic degradation products are the pathological hallmark of this disease. Autophagic vacuoles most likely accumulate due to an impaired capacity for lysosomal degradation [7, 29]. Surprisingly, in cells lacking both LAMP proteins, lysosomal cholesterol metabolism/trafficking was severely affected [29] in a similar manner to that seen in cells with a defect in the Niemann–Pick type C1 late endosomal membrane protein.

It has been shown that lysosomal integral membrane protein-2/lysosomal membrane glycoprotein-85 (LIMP-2/LGP-85) traverses the membrane twice and may be involved in endosome/lysosome biogenesis. LIMP-2-deficient mice [30] showed an increased postnatal mortality, which was associated with the development of unilateral or bilateral hydronephrosis caused by an obstruction of the ureteropelvic junction. Accumulation of lysosomes in the epithelial cells of the ureter adjacent to the ureteral lumen and a disturbed apical expression of uroplakin was observed, suggesting an impairment of membrane transport processes. Serious hearing deficiencies in LIMP-2-deficient mice and the development

of peripheral demyelinating neuropathy were further phenotypic hallmarks of these mice.

Trafficking of lysosomal enzymes
Role of the M6P receptor and post-translational glycosylation

Most soluble lysosomal enzymes are synthesized as N-glycosylated precursors, and the initial steps of biosynthesis are shared with secretory proteins (see Chapter 5). A summary of lysosomal enzyme trafficking is depicted in Figure 1. The diversion of the lysosomal enzymes from the secretory pathway is dependent on the acquisition of the M6P recognition marker [2, 3]. This marker is generated by the sequential action of two enzymes.

In the first step, GlcNAc-1-phosphate is added to the C6-hydroxyl group of selected mannoses on high-mannose-type oligosaccharides by the enzyme UDP-N-acetylglucosamine, known as lysosomal enzyme N-acetylglucosamine-1-phosphotransferase (phosphotransferase). The purified bovine phosphotransferase is a 540 kDa heterohexameric complex composed of two disulphide-linked homodimers of 166 and 51 kDa subunits and two non-covalently associated 56 kDa subunits ($\alpha2\beta2\gamma2$). It has been proposed that the α- and β-subunits harbour phosphotransferase activity and the γ-subunit has a function in the recognition of lysosomal enzymes. Mutations in the different phosphotransferase subunits cause mucolipidosis, also called I-cell disease, a fatal LSD.

In the second step, N-acetylglucosamine residues are removed by an uncovering enzyme (N-acetylglucosamine-1-phosphodiester α-N-acetylglucosaminidase) which exposes the M6P recognition marker. The human uncovering enzyme is a type I membrane-spanning glycoprotein of 515 amino acids with a transmembrane domain and a cytoplasmic tail of 41 amino acids. Following the uncovering of the M6P marker, lysosomal enzymes can be recognized by M6P receptors [2, 3]. Two M6P receptors – the

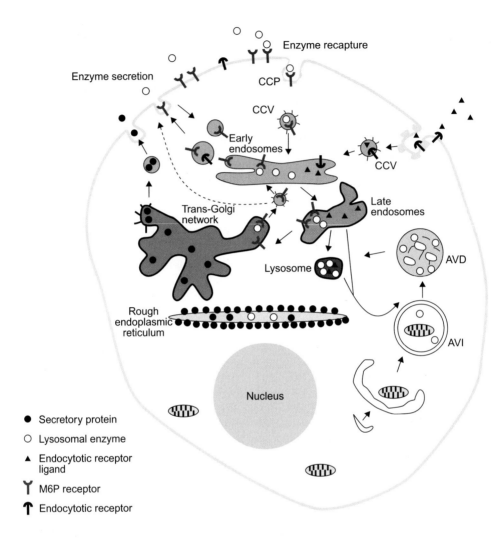

Figure 1. *Overview of lysosomal enzyme trafficking and model of intracellular transport of the mannose-6-phosphate (M6P) receptor. After synthesis in the rough endoplasmic reticulum and modification in the Golgi apparatus (not shown), precursors of soluble lysosomal enzymes decorated with M6P residues meet the M6P receptor in the trans-Golgi network, are packaged into clathrin-coated vesicles (CCV) and transported to late endosomes either directly or indirectly via early endosomes. The process of enzyme transfer from the late endosome to the lysosome is not yet fully elucidated; possibly, the late endosome matures to become the lysosome, or the late endosome and lysosome fuse to form a transient hybrid organelle. The M6P receptor is recycled from the late endosome to the trans-Golgi network. The lysosome is devoid of M6P receptors. A minor portion of the enzyme precursor enters the secretory pathway (dotted line) and is recaptured into clathrin-coated pits (CCP) by M6P receptors, which may be transferred from the early endosomes to the plasma membrane. Thus, the enzyme precursors can reach the lysosome via the endocytic pathway, as do endocytic tracer molecules whose receptors are recycled from the tubular extensions of the early endosome. Autophagic vacuoles and phagocytic vacuoles (not shown) acquire lysosomal enzymes by fusion with lysosomes and/or late endosomes. Late endosomes often resemble multivesicular bodies – i.e. they display invaginations of their membrane and internal vesicles budded off the invaginations. AVI, early, immature autophagic vacuoles; AVD, mature, degradative autophagic vacuoles. Adapted with permission from [55].*

46 kDa cation-dependent M6P receptor and the 300 kDa cation-independent M6P receptor/insulin-like growth factor II receptor–bind M6P-containing acid hydrolases in the Golgi apparatus and transport them to the endosomal/lysosomal system. This process involves binding of the hydrolases to the receptors, through their M6P-recognition moieties, and packaging of the ligand–receptor complexes into carriers that transport their cargo to target endosomes [2].

Ligand binding to M6P receptors is pH dependent

The binding of ligands to the extracellular domain of the cation-dependent M6P receptor is pH dependent. This receptor binds to lysosomal enzymes optimally in the Golgi apparatus (pH 6.5), releases its ligands in the acidic environment of the endosomal compartment (pH < 6.0), but fails to interact with lysosomal enzymes at the plasma membrane (pH 7.4) [2]. The lysosomal enzymes dissociate in the low pH of the endosomal compartment and are delivered to lysosomes, while the M6P receptors cycle back to the trans-Golgi network to mediate further transport. Small numbers of both types of M6P receptor are localized at the plasma membrane, but only the cation-independent M6P receptor is capable of binding and internalizing M6P-containing lysosomal enzymes from the extracellular space. Besides soluble lysosomal enzymes, the cation-independent M6P receptor binds other M6P-containing non-lysosomal proteins, such as transforming growth factor-β1 precursor, proliferin and granzyme B, as well as other classes of ligands like retinoic acid, the urokinase-type (plasminogen activator) receptor and plasminogen [33].

Localization of M6P receptors and signals for M6P receptor transport

The M6P receptors are localized in the trans-Golgi network, early endosomes, recycling endosomes, late endosomes and at the plasma membrane, but they are not found in lysosomes. Both receptors cycle constitutively

between these compartments, directed by signal structures located in their cytosolic tails [2, 8, 33]. The efficient sorting of lysosomal enzymes in the Golgi apparatus, mediated by the cation-independent M6P receptor, depends on an acidic cluster/dileucine-based sorting motif near the carboxyl terminus [34]. The rapid internalization of the cation-independent M6P receptor from the plasma membrane requires a tyrosine-based sorting motif. This retrieval mechanism ensures that transiently secreted lysosomal proteins will also end up in the lysosomes, provided that they contain M6P residues. The sorting signals in the cytoplasmic domains of M6P receptors are recognized by cytosolic adaptor proteins (AP) in distinct subcellular compartments mediating the packaging of the receptors in transport vesicles [35]. The anterograde transport of the M6P receptors is mediated by AP-1 and the Golgi-localized, γ-ear-containing, ARF-binding proteins, whereas the retrograde transport from early and late endosomes requires AP-1/phosphofurin acidic cluster sorting protein-1 and TIP47/Rab 9. The internalization of M6P receptors from the plasma membrane depends on AP-2 [35].

Studies in cells from M6P receptor-deficient mice and I-cell patients

Both M6P receptors are required to guarantee the targeting of all newly synthesized M6P-containing proteins to lysosomes [36]. Re-expression studies, either with cation-dependent or cation-independent M6P receptors in M6P receptor-deficient fibroblasts, have demonstrated that the two receptors exhibit complementary binding properties. Furthermore, each type of M6P receptor transports distinct subpopulations of lysosomal enzymes, presumably as a result of the heterogeneity of the M6P recognition marker [37]. A variable portion of newly synthesized lysosomal enzymes escapes binding to M6P receptors in the Golgi apparatus and is secreted. These M6P-containing enzymes can be partially internalized and transported to the lysosomes through cation-independent M6P receptor-mediated endocytosis. About 3–10% of the total cellular M6P receptors are localized at the plasma membrane at steady state and exchange with M6P receptors cycling in the bio-synthetic pathway. Studies of patients with I-cell disease and of mice lacking both M6P receptors, including several cell lines and primary cultured cells, have provided evidence for alternative, M6P-receptor-independent transport of newly synthesized lysosomal enzymes to lysosomes. Although all cells and tissues of patients with I-cell disease are deficient in phosphotransferase activity, and lysosomal enzymes lack the M6P recognition marker, in many cell types and organs, including the liver, spleen, kidney and brain, lysosomal enzyme levels were normal [2, 8, 33].

It has been shown that the sorting of LAMPs and lysosomal acid phosphatase is independent of M6P receptors, depending instead on short sequence motifs within the cytoplasmic tails, which are necessary and sufficient to target the protein to lysosomes. Newly synthesized LAMPs and LIMPs are transported from the trans-Golgi network to endosomes/lysosomes mainly via an intracellular route without appearing at the cell surface [29, 35, 38]. LAMP-1 and LAMP-2 molecules in the trans-Golgi network are packed into vesicles that are distinct from the clathrin-coated vesicles containing M6P receptors and AP-1 adaptors. Lysosomal targeting depends on either a tyrosine-based (LAMP-1, LAMP-2, LIMP-1) or a di-leucine-based (LIMP-2/LGP-85) sorting signal in the cytoplasmic tail. LAMP-1, LIMP-2/LGP-85 and LIMP-1/CD-63 are targeted from the trans-Golgi network to the lysosomes, dependent on the AP-3 adaptor complex [29, 35, 38].

Enzyme replacement and chaperone therapies

The many LSDs result from abnormal metabolism of substances such as glyco-sphingolipids, glygogen, mucopolysaccha-rides and glycoproteins. A genetic defect in an enzyme that is responsible for the step-wise lysosomal degradation of a particular substance is able to retard the entire cata-bolic process [39, 40]. Many LSDs develop progressively with age, and several involve the CNS and are associated with mental retardation. The severity of these diseases may correspond to the degree of residual enzyme activity, giving rise to phenotypes ranging from severe early-onset forms to milder late-onset forms. A small increase in residual enzyme activity could have a significant impact on disease development [41]. Enzyme replacement therapy (ERT), which compensates for the underlying enzyme defect by increasing the enzyme activity, and substrate reduction therapy, which reduces the synthesis of substrates, have been developed as clinical strategies for these disorders [6, 42]. Enhancing the residual activity of misfolded or unstable enzymes by using specific, small molecule ligands, known as pharmacological chaperones, may be clinically useful for many LSDs which affect the brain as, unlike therapeutic enzymes, low-molecular-weight chaperones might cross the blood–brain barrier [42, 43].

The uptake of exogeneous lysosomal enzymes into the lysosomal compartment of fibroblasts and other cells depends on receptor-mediated endocytosis via the 300 kDa M6P receptor. Exogenous lysosomal enzymes may also be taken up via additional carbohydrate recog-nition systems which bind, for example, terminal galactose (hepatocytes) or mannose residues (reticuloendothelial cells). ERT is a therapeutic option for deficiencies of soluble lysosomal polypeptides, but is generally not applicable to LSDs caused by lack of mem-brane-bound polypeptides. Studies of ERT in animal models of various LSDs, such as muco-polysaccharidosis (MPS) type I, MPS IIIB, MPS VI, MPS VII, Fabry disease, Niemann–Pick disease and Pompe disease [6], revealed that intravenously infused lysosomal enzymes are rapidly internalized by the liver, spleen and other peripheral tissues, but usually do not enter the brain parenchyma. Interestingly, two recent reports on ERT in animal models for α-mannosidosis and metachromatic leukodystrophy revealed improvement of CNS pathology and function. The molecular mechanisms for these unexpected results remain to be determined [44, 45].

The therapeutic efficacy of ERT in humans has been demonstrated by the successful treatment of patients suffering from type I (non-neuronopathic) Gaucher disease [46] and Fabry disease [47–49]. In Gaucher disease, the clinically available therapy makes use of mannose-terminated glucocerebrosidase, which is generated by the removal of terminal carbohydrates from the N-linked oligosaccharides by sequential exoglycosidase treatment, resulting in exposure of the core mannose residues. This modification targets the enzyme efficiently to cells of the monocyte–macrophage lineage, which are the main site of storage and mannose receptor expression. To date, ERT has been approved for use in patients with Gaucher disease, Fabry disease, Pompe disease, MPS I and VI, and clinical trials have been initiated for MPS II. Problems associated with the clinical use of ERT are: no improvement of CNS pathology, immune responses to the replacement protein, the need for life-long intervention and the high costs of treatment.

Enzyme enhancement therapy
Enzyme enhancement, or chaperone, therapy exploits the residual activity of the mutant endogenous polypeptide. Missense mutations that are distant from the active centre of the gene may cause thermodynamic instability of the polypeptide. As a consequence, only a few molecules adopt proper folding. The majority is misfolded and rapidly degraded through the ubiquitin–proteasome pathway and by lysosomal proteases. Chemical chaperones are specific small-molecule ligands that can bind to the catalytic site of an enzyme and then rescue mutant polypeptides by assisting their correct folding in a prelysosomal compartment [50]. It has been proposed that such compounds stabilize a folding intermediate, eventually leading to the formation of the correct tertiary structure. As a consequence of stabilization, a higher percentage of enzyme is properly folded, passes the quality-control system of the endoplasmic reticulum, and is targeted to the lysosome where its conformation might be stabilized by the acidic conditions. Clinical evidence for the feasibility of enzyme enhancement therapy in a human LSD has been demonstrated by the successful treatment of a patient suffering from a late-onset cardiac variant of Fabry disease [51].

Substrate reduction therapy
The rationale for the use of substrate reduction therapies is to reduce the de novo synthesis rate of an accumulating compound to a level at which the residual activity of the mutant catabolic enzyme is sufficient to prevent pathological storage. The glucose analogue N-butyldeoxynojirimycin (NB-DNJ) blocks glucosylceramide synthase, which catalyses the synthesis of glucocerebroside (glucosylceramide) by transferring a glucosyl moiety onto ceramide [52, 53]. To assess the potential of NB-DNJ in reducing visceral glycosphingolipid storage in humans, a clinical trial in type I Gaucher disease was initiated. Treatment resulted in a reduction in the volume of the spleen and liver, a slight improvement of haematological parameters, and a decrease in the number of Gaucher macrophages in the bone marrow [54]. To reduce or abrogate side effects that can be ascribed to the inhibition of non-specific enzymes, glucosylceramide synthase inhibitors with increased specificity are under investigation.

Conclusions
New insights into lysosomal functions have been possible through the use of combined

biochemical, morphological, cell biological and molecular methodologies. Numerous experiments have contributed to our understanding of the central role of the lysosome and lysosomal proteins in the homeostasis of the normal cell and in pathological processes.

Acknowledgements

I would like to thank Dr Eeva-Liisa Eskelinen, University of Helsinki, Finland and Jenny Schröder, University of Kiel, Germany for critically reading the manuscript. The author's work is supported by the Deutsche Forschungsgemeinschaft (DFG) and the European Union (HUE-MAN).

References

1. Dell'Angelica EC, Mullins C, Caplan S, Bonifacino JS. Lysosome-related organelles. *FASEB J* 2000;14: 1265–78

2. Ghosh P, Dahms NM, Kornfeld S. Mannose 6-phosphate receptors: new twists in the tale. *Nat Rev Mol Cell Biol* 2003;4:202–12

3. Storch S, Braulke T. Transport of lysosomal enzymes. In: Saftig P, editor. Lysosomes. New York: Springer Science, Landes Bioscience; 2005. p. 17–26

4. Brix K. Lysosomal proteases: revival of a sleeping beauty. In: Saftig P, editor. Lysosomes. New York: Springer Science, Landes Bioscience; 2005. p. 50–9

5. Greiner-Tollersrud OK, Berg T. Lysosomal storage disorders. In: Saftig P, editor. Lysosomes. New York: Springer Science, Landes Bioscience; 2005. p. 60–73

6. Matzner U. Therapy of lysosomal storage diseases. In: Saftig P, editor. Lysosomes. New York: Springer Science, Landes Bioscience; 2005. p. 112–30

7. Saftig P. Transport of lysosomal enzymes. In: Saftig P, editor. Lysosomes. New York: Springer Science, Landes Bioscience; 2005. p. 37–49

8. Storch S, Cheruku SR. Cholesterol transport in lysosomes. In: Saftig P, editor. Lysosomes. New York: Springer Science, Landes Bioscience; 2005. p. 100–11

9. Andrews NM. Membrane resealing mediated by lysosomal exocytosis. In: Saftig P, editor. Lysosomes. New York: Springer Science, Landes Bioscience; 2005. p. 156–65

10. Eskelinen EL. Macroautophagy in mammalian cells. In: Saftig P, editor. Lysosomes. New York: Springer Science, Landes Bioscience; 2005. p. 166–80

11. Knecht E. Chaperone-mediated autophagy. In: Saftig P, editor. Lysosomes. New York: Springer Science, Landes Bioscience; 2005. p. 181–94

12. Everts V, Beertsen W. External lysosomes: the osteoclast and its unique capacities to degrade mineralised tissues. In: Saftig P, editor. Lysosomes. New York: Springer Science, Landes Bioscience; 2005. p. 144–55

13. Hiraiwa M. Cathepsin A/protective protein: an unusual lysosomal multifunctional protein. *Cell Mol Life Sci* 1999;56:894–907

14. Saftig P, Hetman M, Schmahl W, Weber K, Heine L, Mossmann H et al. Mice deficient for the lysosomal proteinase cathepsin D exhibit progressive atrophy of the intestinal mucosa and profound destruction of lymphoid cells. *EMBO J* 1995;14:3599–608

15. Koike M, Nakanishi H, Saftig P, Ezaki J, Isahara K, Ohsawa Y et al. Cathepsin D deficiency induces lysosomal storage with ceroid lipofuscin in mouse CNS neurons. *J Neurosci* 2000;20:6898–906

16. Saftig P, Peters C, von Figura K, Craessaerts K, Van Leuven F, De Strooper B. Amyloidogenic processing of human amyloid precursor protein in hippocampal neurons devoid of cathepsin D. *J Biol Chem* 1996;271:27241–4

17. Deussing J, Roth W, Saftig P, Peters C, Ploegh HL, Villadangos JA. Cathepsins B and D are dispensable for major histocompatibility complex class II-mediated antigen presentation. *Proc Natl Acad Sci USA* 1998;95:4516–21

18. Saftig P, Hunziker E, Wehmeyer O, Jones S, Boyde A, Rommerskirch W et al. Impaired osteoclastic bone resorption leads to osteopetrosis in cathepsin-K-deficient mice. *Proc Natl Acad Sci USA* 1998; 95:13453–8

19. Saftig P, Hunziker E, Everts V, Jones S, Boyde A, Wehmeyer O et al. Functions of cathepsin K in bone resorption. Lessons from cathepsin K deficient mice. *Adv Exp Med Biol* 2000;477:293–303

20. Buhling F, Rocken C, Brasch F, Hartig R, Yasuda Y, Saftig P et al. Pivotal role of cathepsin K in lung fibrosis. *Am J Pathol* 2004;164:2203–16

21. Lutgens E, Lutgens SP, Faber BC, Heeneman S, Gijbels MM, de Winther MP et al. Disruption of the cathepsin K gene reduces atherosclerosis progression and induces plaque fibrosis but accelerates macrophage foam cell formation. *Circulation* 2006; 113:98–107

22. Roth W, Deussing J, Botchkarev VA, Pauly-Evers M, Saftig P, Hafner A et al. Cathepsin L deficiency as molecular defect of furless: hyperproliferation of keratinocytes and pertubation of hair follicle cycling. *FASEB J* 2000;14:2075–86

23. Urbich C, Heeschen C, Aicher A, Sasaki K, Bruhl T, Farhadi MR et al. Cathepsin L is required for endothelial progenitor cell-induced neovascularization. *Nat Med* 2005;11:206–13

24. Saftig P, Hartmann D, Lullmann-Rauch R, Wolff J, Evers M, Koster A et al. Mice deficient in lysosomal acid phosphatase develop lysosomal storage in the kidney and central nervous system. *J Biol Chem* 1997;272:18628–35

25. Suter A, Everts V, Boyde A, Jones SJ, Lullmann-Rauch R, Hartmann D et al. Overlapping functions of lysosomal acid phosphatase (LAP) and tartrate-

resistant acid phosphatase (Acp5) revealed by doubly deficient mice. *Development* 2001; 128:4899–910

26. Andrejewski N, Punnonen EL, Guhde G, Tanaka Y, Lullmann-Rauch R, Hartmann D *et al*. Normal lysosomal morphology and function in LAMP-1-deficient mice. *J Biol Chem* 1999;274:12692–701

27. Tanaka Y, Guhde G, Suter A, Eskelinen EL, Hartmann D, Lullmann-Rauch R *et al*. Accumulation of autophagic vacuoles and cardiomyopathy in LAMP-2-deficient mice. *Nature* 2000;406:902–6

28. Nishino I, Fu J, Tanji K, Yamada T, Shimojo S, Koori T *et al*. Primary LAMP-2 deficiency causes X-linked vacuolar cardiomyopathy and myopathy (Danon disease). *Nature* 2000;406:906–10

29. Eskelinen EL, Tanaka Y, Saftig P. At the acidic edge: emerging functions for lysosomal membrane proteins. *Trends Cell Biol* 2003;13:137–45

30. Gamp AC, Tanaka Y, Lullmann-Rauch R, Wittke D, D'Hooge R, De Deyn PP *et al*. LIMP-2/LGP85 deficiency causes ureteric pelvic junction obstruction, deafness and peripheral neuropathy in mice. *Hum Mol Genet* 2003;12:631–46

31. Reinheckel T, Deussing J, Roth W, Peters C. Towards specific functions of lysosomal cysteine peptidases: phenotypes of mice deficient for cathepsin B or cathepsin L. *Biol Chem* 2001;382:735–41

32. Chapman HA, Riese RJ, Shi GP. Emerging roles for cysteine proteases in human biology. *Annu Rev Physiol* 1997;59:63–88

33. Braulke T. Type-2 IGF receptor: a multi-ligand binding protein. *Horm Metab Res* 1999;31:242–6

34. Chen HJ, Yuan J, Lobel P. Systematic mutational analysis of the cation-independent mannose 6-phosphate/insulin-like growth factor II receptor cytoplasmic domain. An acidic cluster containing a key aspartate is important for function in lysosomal enzyme sorting. *J Biol Chem* 1997;272:7003–12

35. Schu P. Adaptor proteins in lysosomal biogenesis. In: Saftig P, editor. Lysosomes. New York: Springer Science, Landes Bioscience; 2005. p. 27–36

36. Ludwig T, Munier-Lehmann H, Bauer U, Hollinshead M, Ovitt C, Lobel P *et al*. Differential sorting of lysosomal enzymes in mannose 6-phosphate receptor-deficient fibroblasts. *EMBO J* 1994;13:3430–7

37. Kasper D, Dittmer F, von Figura K, Pohlmann R. Neither type of mannose 6-phosphate receptor is sufficient for targeting of lysosomal enzymes along intracellular routes. *J Cell Biol* 1996;134:615–23

38. Mullins C, Bonifacino JS. The molecular machinery for lysosome biogenesis. *Bioessays* 2001;23:333–43

39. Brady RO. Gaucher and Fabry diseases: from understanding pathophysiology to rational therapies. *Acta Paediatr Suppl* 2003;443:19–24

40. Brady RO. Heritable catabolic and anabolic disorders of lipid metabolism. *Metabolism* 1977;26:329–45

41. Desnick RJ, Schuchman EH. Enzyme replacement and enhancement therapies: lessons from lysosomal disorders. *Nat Rev Genet* 2002;3:954–66

42. Fan JQ. A contradictory treatment for lysosomal storage disorders: inhibitors enhance mutant enzyme activity. *Trends Pharmacol Sci* 2003;24:355–60

43. Eto Y, Ohashi T. Novel treatment for neuronopathic lysosomal storage diseases – cell therapy/gene therapy. *Curr Mol Med* 2002;2:83–9

44. Matzner U, Herbst E, Hedayati KK, Lullmann-Rauch R, Wessig C, Schroder S *et al*. Enzyme replacement improves nervous system pathology and function in a mouse model for metachromatic leukodystrophy. *Hum Mol Genet* 2005;14:1139–52

45. Roces DP, Lullmann-Rauch R, Peng J, Balducci C, Andersson C, Tollersrud O *et al*. Efficacy of enzyme replacement therapy in α-mannosidosis mice: a preclinical animal study. *Hum Mol Genet* 2004; 13:1979–88

46. Barton NW, Furbish FS, Murray GJ, Garfield M, Brady RO. Therapeutic response to intravenous infusions of glucocerebrosidase in a patient with Gaucher disease. *Proc Natl Acad Sci USA* 1990; 87:1913–16

47. Schiffmann R, Kopp JB, Austin HA 3rd, Sabnis S, Moore DF, Weibel T *et al*. Enzyme replacement therapy in Fabry disease: a randomized controlled trial. *JAMA* 2001;285:2743–9

48. Eng CM, Guffon N, Wilcox WR, Germain DP, Lee P, Waldek S *et al*. Safety and efficacy of recombinant human α-galactosidase A replacement therapy in Fabry's disease. *N Engl J Med* 2001;345:9–16

49. Beck M, Ricci R, Widmer U, Dehout F, de Lorenzo AG, Kampmann C *et al*. Fabry disease: overall effects of agalsidase alfa treatment. *Eur J Clin Invest* 2004; 34:838–44

50. Fan JQ, Ishii S, Asano N, Suzuki Y. Accelerated transport and maturation of lysosomal α-galactosidase A in Fabry lymphoblasts by an enzyme inhibitor. *Nat Med* 1999;5:112–15

51. Frustaci A, Chimenti C, Ricci R, Natale L, Russo MA, Pieroni M *et al*. Improvement in cardiac function in the cardiac variant of Fabry's disease with galactose-infusion therapy. *N Engl J Med* 2001;345:25–32

52. Jeyakumar M, Butters TD, Dwek RA, Platt FM. Glycosphingolipid lysosomal storage diseases: therapy and pathogenesis. *Neuropathol Appl Neurobiol* 2002;28:343–57

53. Alfonso P, Pampin S, Estrada J, Rodriguez-Rey JC, Giraldo P, Sancho J *et al*. Miglustat (NB-DNJ) works as a chaperone for mutated acid beta-glucosidase in cells transfected with several Gaucher disease mutations. *Blood Cells Mol Dis* 2005;35:268–76

54. Cox T, Lachmann R, Hollak C, Aerts J, van Weely S, Hrebicek M *et al*. Novel oral treatment of Gaucher's disease with N-butyldeoxynojirimycin (OGT 918) to decrease substrate biosynthesis. *Lancet* 2000; 355:1481–5

55. Lüllmann R. History and morphology of the lysosome. In: Saftig P, editor. Lysosomes. New York: Springer Science, Landes Bioscience; 2005. p. 1–16

4 Cellular pathophysiology of lysosomal storage diseases

Volkmar Gieselmann

Institut für Physiologische Chemie, Rheinische Friedrich-Wilhelms-Universität, Bonn 53115, Germany

The mutations responsible for most lysosomal storage diseases (LSDs) have been largely elucidated; however, the molecular pathways through which the storage material causes cellular and organ pathology are largely unknown. Recent studies have underlined the importance of inflammation, apoptosis, alteration in signal transduction and transport for some of the lysosomal disorders. Almost all LSDs show a broad clinical spectrum with respect to severity of symptoms, progression and age of onset. This can be explained, in part, by the residual enzyme activity associated with the particular alleles the patient carries. This correlation is loose, however, and does not allow prediction of the clinical course on an individual basis. Other as yet unknown genetic and epigenetic factors influence the disease phenotype substantially.

Introduction

Receiving the Nobel prize in 1974 for his discovery of lysosomes, Christian de Duve stated that "with more than 20 distinct congenital lysosomal enzyme deficiencies identified, this mysterious chapter of pathology has been largely elucidated" [1]. Although appropriate at that time, this statement does not reflect the current view of the pathophysiology of lysosomal storage diseases (LSDs). In all LSDs, the central pathophysiological question is how the storage material affects the metabolism of a cell and subsequently leads to organ pathology and clinical symptoms. The pathophysiology of a disorder is determined by the chemical nature of the storage compound, the extent of storage, the kinetics of accumulation and the type and spectrum of storage cells [2]. For example, the abundance of cerebrosides and gangliosides in the nervous system explains why sphingolipid storage disorders are characterized by severe neurological symptoms. Likewise, the glycogen content of muscle provides an explanation as to why myopathy dominates in the pathology of Pompe disease, in which glycogen breakdown is defective. The diversity of pathology and clinical phenotypes requires that different pathophysiological mechanisms must be elucidated for each specific disorder.

Cellular pathophysiology

In some related disorders, such as the sphingolipidoses, pathogenic mechanisms may, at least partially, be shared [3, 4]. In these disorders, inflammation, apoptosis and alterations in signal transduction and transport are all involved in pathogenesis. Mice deficient in the β-subunit of β-hexosaminidase are a model of the GM2-gangliosidosis, Sandhoff disease. The animals develop severe neurological symptoms at the age of 3–4 months. The development of symptoms correlates with the activation of microglia and an increased frequency of apoptotic neurones [4]. Transplantation of the affected mice with bone marrow from a normal donor leads to a substantial reduction in the number of apoptotic neurones, which is accompanied by an increased lifespan. Surprisingly, however, transplantation does not result in delivery of β-hexosaminidase to the brain or to a reduction in GM2-ganglioside storage, suggesting that neuronal storage, *per se*, is not responsible for apoptosis. However, bone marrow transplantation markedly reduces the activation of microglia and, consequently, the production of cytokines and tumour necrosis factor-α (TNFα). This suggests that the initial neuronal damage results in microglial phagocytosis. Subsequent accumulation of GM2-ganglioside in microglia causes activation accompanied by secretion of various cytokines, which promotes apoptosis. This example demonstrates that pathogenic mechanisms cannot simply be explained by cellular alterations of a single cell type but are rather the result of a complex interplay between different cells.

Microglial activation also occurs in a number of other LSDs, such as Krabbe disease [3], metachromatic leukodystrophy [5] and Gaucher disease [6]. In twitcher mice – a model of Krabbe disease – microglial activation and increased levels of interleukins and TNFα also correlate with the frequency of apoptotic cells. Thus, the role of microglial activation in the pathophysiology of the mouse model of Sandhoff disease may also apply to other lipidoses. Similarly, in Gaucher disease, the accumulation of glucosylceramide in macrophages results in their activation [6]. Interleukins 1β, 6 and 10 and TNFα are elevated in the serum of patients with Gaucher disease and have been implicated in the development of osteopenia and gammopathies in type I Gaucher disease [7, 8]. Interestingly, splenomegaly and hepatomegaly in patients with Gaucher disease cannot be explained by lipid accumulation, which accounts for only about 2% of the tissue mass in the up to 25-fold enlarged organs [9]. It is possible that secretion of mitogenic factors by activated macrophages is the dominant factor causing an increase in the number of cells in the liver and spleen.

In addition to Sandhoff disease, increased apoptosis has been demonstrated in a number of other LSDs, such as Krabbe, Gaucher, Niemann–Pick type C and Pompe diseases, mucopolysaccharidosis type VI and GM1-gangliosidosis [10–14]. Whether this is due to the activation of a common apoptotic pathway has not been elucidated. In contrast, apoptosis is inhibited in Niemann–Pick type A disease, which is caused by sphingomyelinase deficiency [15].

A pathological hallmark of GM2-gangliosidosis in humans, as well as in mice, is the development of meganeurites and additional spines on neurones, which is one reason for the severe neurological symptoms [16]. In the developing human brain, the appearance of GM2-ganglioside in the various layers of the cortex parallels dendritogenesis [17]. GM2-ganglioside is therefore considered to be part of the developmental programme involved in dendritogenesis. The accumulation of GM2-ganglioside in the brains of affected patients may result in an inability to terminate this developmental programme, leading to continued dendritogenesis and the development of meganeurites and spines. Contact of these spines with other dendrites can lead to abnormal spreading of signals within neuronal networks, which is likely to contribute to the neurological symptoms.

In some of the lysosomal disorders, toxic metabolites appear to play a major pathogenic role, rather than the storage material itself. Examples of these disorders are Krabbe disease, metachromatic leukodystrophy and Gaucher disease [18–20]. Besides galactosylceramide – which is the major storage compound in Krabbe disease and in its animal model, the twitcher mouse – patients and mice have substantially increased levels of the lysolipid galactosylsphingosine, also called psychosine. The structural difference between psychosine and galactosylceramide is the loss of the fatty acid chain attached to the amino group of the sphingosine backbone. Similarly, increased lysosulphatide and glucosylsphingosine concentrations have also been shown to occur in metachromatic leukodystrophy and Gaucher disease, respectively [19, 20]. Lysolipids are biologically very active compounds [21]. They are potent inhibitors of protein kinase C, interfere with the integrity of membranes and lead to activation of inducible nitric oxide synthase [21, 22]. Psychosine stimulates Ca^{2+} release from the endoplasmic reticulum [23] and binds with high affinity to a septahelical membrane receptor, termed TDAG 8 [24]. This receptor is coupled to G proteins, eliciting a cyclic AMP (cAMP) response. High concentrations of psychosine in the brains of patients with Krabbe disease may therefore produce constantly stimulated cAMP-dependent pathways, which is likely to be of pathophysiological relevance. Therefore, the interference of lysosphingolipids with protein kinase A, protein kinase C and Ca^{2+}-mediated signal transduction pathways suggests a major pathophysiological role for these lipids in various disorders. This is supported by the fact that glucosylsphingosine is found in higher levels in the brains of neurologically affected patients with type I and type II Gaucher disease [25].

Signal transduction

Storage compounds themselves also have effects on signal transduction. In Gaucher disease, cultured glucosylceramide-storing hippocampal neurones react to stimulation with glutamate or caffeine with a significantly increased release of Ca^{2+} from the endoplasmic reticulum by sensitizing the ryanodine receptor [26, 27]. This renders the cells more sensitive to glutamate, which contributes to neuronal damage in neuronopathic forms of Gaucher disease. Glucosylceramide is likely to act directly on the endoplasmic reticulum, as it was found to be elevated by about tenfold in microsomes

prepared from the brains of patients suffering from neuronopathic type II Gaucher disease. Thus, elevation of lipid levels is not restricted to the lysosomal compartment, but also influences the functions of other cellular membranes [27, 28], which must be considered in the pathophysiology of LSDs.

Cholesterol metabolism

Alterations in membrane trafficking and the distribution of cholesterol have been demonstrated in many sphingolipid storage diseases [29]. In normal cells, plasma membrane lactosylceramide is endocytosed and transported to the Golgi apparatus. In cells of patients affected with various lipidoses, the endocytosed lactosylceramide appears instead in the endosomal/lysosomal compartment. This phenomenon is accompanied by increased levels of cholesterol in many of these diseases [30]. Increased cholesterol levels are functionally linked to the missorting of lactosylceramide, as depletion of cholesterol in lipidosis cells corrects the sorting of lactosylceramide towards the Golgi apparatus [31]. The endocytosis of lactosylceramide occurs almost exclusively through a clathrin-independent, caveolae-mediated pathway. This pathway directs the lipids towards the Golgi apparatus and is sensitive to cholesterol levels [32]. Rab proteins, known to be important for membrane trafficking, are involved in this process [33]. Rab7 and Rab9 mediate the transport of lipids from the plasma membrane to the Golgi apparatus, and the activity of Rab4 can be influenced by cholesterol levels, which then affects membrane recycling [33]. In addition, trafficking of endocytic receptors is altered by lipid storage [34]. Thus, in sphingomyelin-storing macrophages isolated from a mouse model of Niemann–Pick type A disease, it was found that endocytosis of the mannose-6-phosphate (M6P) receptor was inhibited. Cells endocytosed much less lysosomal enzyme, despite the fact that the expression of the M6P receptor was enhanced in affected cells. Interestingly, the defect in endocytosis was specific for the M6P receptor and did not affect the mannose receptor. These findings are certainly interesting from the cell biological point of view, but their relevance for pathophysiology is unclear.

Effects of different mutations on pathophysiology

In the past two decades our knowledge about LSDs has grown considerably. Sequences of genes encoding lysosomal enzymes have been elucidated and resulted in the identification of many of the mutations responsible for the enzyme deficiencies in the various disorders. Today, from the genetic point of view, most LSDs are well understood; however, the biochemical mechanisms by which a mutation causes a deficiency have only partially been resolved. The molecular consequences of nonsense mutations, deletions, insertions and duplications that cause premature termination and/or frame shifts are mostly obvious, as they frequently lead to absent or truncated proteins, which results in a complete loss of functional enzyme. Several splice-site mutations have been identified in lysosomal disorders. In some instances, these mutations do not allow the generation of functional mRNA [35]. Frequently, however, the mutations are leaky, such that a small percentage of transcripts is still correctly spliced and translated, producing reduced amounts of normal enzyme. This kind of mutation, therefore, usually leads to attenuated forms of disease [36].

The effects of missense mutations or small in-frame deletions are less apparent and need molecular biological characterization to understand the cause of the enzyme deficiency. Compared with the large number of missense mutations identified in lysosomal disorders, however, only a limited number have been investigated to elucidate the biochemical consequences for the respective enzyme. The deleterious effect of a missense mutation is obvious if it affects amino acid residues that are involved in the active centre [37–39] or that are important for proper folding. Active-site mutations may lead to a complete loss of enzyme activity, but may also result in alterations of enzyme kinetics [39]. Substitution of cysteine residues or charged residues involved in formation of intramolecular disulphide bonds or salt bridges, respectively, is likely to interfere with proper folding of the enzyme [40, 41]. Mutations affecting the active centre or intramolecular bonds, however, are in the minority.

In spite of the fact that structural information [38, 40] was expected to shed more light on the molecular consequences of amino acid substitutions, the effects of most missense mutations are still not obvious. Thus, it is difficult to understand why even very conservative amino acid substitutions can severely affect a lysosomal enzyme [41]. In many cases, amino acid substitutions cause misfolding of the enzyme, which results in retention of the mutant polypeptide in the endoplasmic reticulum and its subsequent proteasomal degradation [42–44]. It has been estimated that degradation associated with the endoplasmic reticulum is responsible for about 50% of protein defects in all genetic diseases and thus represents the most frequent cause of deficiencies [45]. Although this proportion has never been specifically calculated for LSDs, it is reasonable to assume that comparable numbers apply [43]. In many cases, retention of the misfolded enzyme in the endoplasmic reticulum is complete, such that no functional enzyme reaches the Golgi apparatus to be phosphorylated and sorted into the lysosome [40–42]. Therefore, these mutations frequently lead to a complete deficiency of the enzyme. Even if these mutant enzymes still retain some activity they will not be functional, as they are mislocated [39]. As with splice-site mutations, however, the process of endoplasmic quality control can be leaky. There are examples in which the majority of misfolded enzyme is retained in the endoplasmic reticulum, with a small fraction bypassing the quality control and being sorted to the lysosomes (5, 12). If this enzyme still has residual activity, it can result in an attenuated disease phenotype [46, 47].

For therapeutic reasons, an escape from the endoplasmic reticulum may also be induced by 'molecular chaperones' – small molecules such as competitive enzyme inhibitors. In Fabry disease, the R301Q-substituted enzyme is usually retained in the endoplasmic reticulum. Treatment with a competitive inhibitor, however, improves folding and increases lysosomal delivery of the enzyme, which can be therapeutically exploited [48] (Figure 1).

Alternatively, amino acid substitutions allow for proper folding of the enzyme to pass the quality control of the endoplasmic reticulum. Arylsulphatase A deficiency causes metachromatic leukodystrophy, a lipid storage disease. The most frequent disease-associated allele in adult patients is characterized by a missense mutation causing substitution of proline 426 by leucine (P426L) [35]. The P426L substituted enzyme is active, reaches the Golgi apparatus, receives M6P residues and is correctly sorted to the lysosomes. Due to the amino acid substitution, however, the mutant protein is rapidly degraded by lysosomal proteases [49]. The half-life of the mutant enzyme, however, is still sufficient to provide a small amount of residual enzyme activity, explaining the juvenile or adult-onset forms of metachromatic leukodystrophy in patients carrying this allele. If the fibroblasts of patients expressing this mutant enzyme are treated with inhibitors of lysosomal proteases, the enzyme can be stabilized to

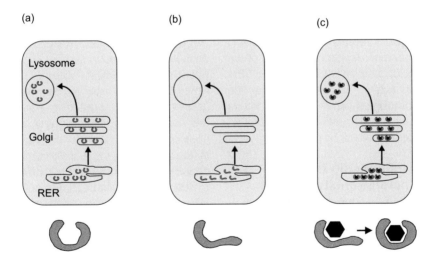

(a)   (b)   (c)

Figure 1. *Concept of treatment by molecular chaperones. All panels show schematically the rough endoplasmic reticulum (RER), the Golgi apparatus and a lysosome within a cell. A single lysosomal enzyme is represented below each cell. (a) A correctly folded enzyme is synthesized within the RER, passes to the Golgi apparatus and then reaches the lysosome. (b) The enzyme is misfolded due to a missense mutation. In many cases, newly synthesized defective enzymes do not pass RER quality control and are retained and degraded. No functional enzyme passes to the Golgi apparatus or reaches the lysosome. (c) Cells were fed with a competitive inhibitor of the misfolded enzyme. As has been shown for defective α-galactosidase A responsible for Fabry disease, this inhibitor, shown as a black hexagon, can induce correct folding and proper intracellular delivery of the defective enzyme. The inhibitor can be seen associated with the defective enzyme in the RER, the Golgi apparatus and the lysosome. This is hypothetical, as it is not known at which stage the inhibitor dissociates from the enzyme.*

yield low-normal activity values [49]. This demonstrates how a precise understanding of mutation effects can provide strategies for possible therapies.

To understand the molecular basis of enzyme deficiencies in even more detail requires not only the biochemical characterization but also the crystallization of mutant proteins. P426L-substituted arylsulphatase A is so far the only example of a lysosomal enzyme in which a mutant enzyme has been crystallized and the molecular consequences of the amino acid substitution revealed in detail [49]. A cleavage site for cathepsin L was found in close proximity to proline 426. In the normal enzyme, this cleavage site becomes inaccessible to cathepsin L, because arylsulphatase A octamerizes in the low pH environment of the lysosome. Thus, octamerization is a prerequisite for the intralysosomal stability of the enzyme.

The crystal structure of the P426L-substituted arylsulphatase A reveals that the amino acid substitution interferes with the capacity of the enzyme to octamerize at low pH [49]. The reason for enzyme deficiency due to the P426L subsitution is therefore the inability to octamerize intralysosomally and to protect the enzyme from attack by cathepsin L.

Factors influencing the clinical heterogeneity of LSDs

Most of the LSDs show a wide spectrum of clinical phenotypes (e.g. [50, 51]. In many disorders, severe early-onset forms of disease are distinguished from attenuated intermediate and late-onset forms. This classification suggests the existence of distinctive clinical entities. The clinical spectrum, however, represents a continuum with respect to severity, progression and age of onset. The identification of mutations in the various disorders was accompanied by a hope that clear genotype–phenotype correlations would be found, ideally allowing prediction of the clinical course of disease in

individual patients. Investigations of genotype–phenotype correlations, however, have only partially revealed the molecular basis of the clinical heterogeneity of disease [35, 52–54]. In many disorders, the clinical phenotype is loosely related to the amount of residual enzyme activity associated with the particular mutation.

One of the first diseases in which a genotype–phenotype correlation was identified was metachromatic leukodystrophy [35, 52]. In this disease, two defective alleles are particularly frequent, each representing about 25% of alleles among European patients. One allele is characterized by a splice donor-site mutation, which results in a complete loss of mRNA and, therefore, no enzyme is synthesized. This allele represents a null mutation. The other frequent allele is the above-mentioned P426L allele, which still allows for the expression of low enzyme activity. When the distribution of these alleles was investigated in patients with metachromatic leukodystrophy displaying clinical phenotypes of varying severity, a genotype–phenotype correlation became apparent. Homozygosity for null alleles was always associated with the most severe late-infantile form of disease; heterozygosity for a null allele and an allele with residual enzyme activity mitigated the course to the intermediate juvenile form; and homozygosity for alleles with residual enzyme activity was associated with the attenuated, mostly adult, form of metachromatic leukodystrophy [35].

Correlations with alleles allowing for the expression of low residual enzyme activity with attenuated clinical forms of disease are found in a number of lysosomal disorders, including Gaucher disease [53]. However, it must be emphasized that genotype–phenotype correlations become apparent only when large numbers of patients are studied [35, 54]. The variations between individual patients with an identical genotype can be enormous, even within the same family [54]. Therefore, in none of the LSDs does the genotype of a patient allow the prediction of the clinical course for the individual. The correlation between residual enzyme activity and attenuation of clinical phenotype has not only been found at the genetic level, but was also confirmed biochemically for metachromatic leukodystrophy and Tay–Sachs disease (52). The methods applied in this study were sophisticated and cannot be applied as routine diagnostic procedures. For this reason, it must be emphasized that enzyme activities that are determined for diagnostic purposes in, for example, leukocyte homogenates, do not enable even an approximate estimate of residual enzyme activity. Residual enzyme activities leading to attenuated forms of disease are in the range of 2–8% of normal activity. In routine assays, it is impossible to quantify enzyme activities reliably within this low range (Figure 2).

Residual enzyme activity is only one of the determinants of clinical outcome in many LSDs. The influence of other factors is substantial. These, so far unidentified factors, appear to be genetic as well as epigenetic. Clinical variability in Sandhoff and Pompe diseases suggests the existence of genetic factors [36, 55–57]. Sandhoff disease is caused by mutations in the gene for the β-subunit of β-hexosaminidase, which leads to the accumulation of GM2-ganglioside. Four siblings of a Canadian family were identified who were heterozygous for a null allele and an allele containing a mutation close to a splice acceptor site [36]. The latter is associated with low residual enzyme activity, as the normal splice site is used in a small percentage of transcripts. One of the siblings developed a very attenuated form of Sandhoff disease in his 50s, whereas the other siblings, aged 55–61 years, were still presymptomatic. A single copy of this splice-site allele allows for an attenuated form of disease or even an asymptomatic state in these individuals. The same mutation was independently found in a Japanese patient who suffered from a far more severe juvenile form of the disease [55]. Surprisingly, this patient was homozygous for the splice-site allele. A possible explanation could be that minor variations in genes coding for components of the splicing machinery lead to a more efficient use of the correct splicing site in the Canadian patients than in the Japanese patient. A similar situation occurs in Pompe disease, where a D645E missense mutation in the α-glucosidase gene causes divergent phenotypes in Chinese and African–American patients [56, 57]. This strongly suggests that differences in the genetic background account for the clinical outcome of the disease in patients from different ethnic groups.

The most frequent allele causing non-neuronopathic type I Gaucher disease is characterized by substitution of asparagine 370 by serine (N370S) in the glucocerebrosidase gene. This allele codes for an enzyme with 10–20% of normal activity [54]. When more than 200 patients homozygous for this allele were examined, an enormous heterogeneity became apparent [54]. The age of onset of disease in this group of patients varied between early childhood and senescence. In fact, calculation of allele frequencies and comparison with the prevalence of patients revealed that about two-thirds of the N370S homozygotes remain asymptomatic [58]. A particular case study of Gaucher disease revealed the importance of epigenetic factors for clinical variability in this disorder. N370S homozygous monozygotic twin sisters were recently identified [59]. They did not marry, lived together during their entire lives and both died at 84 years of age. Only one of the sisters, however, developed type I Gaucher disease, whereas the other twin remained asymptomatic. These monozygotic siblings demonstrate that epigenetic factors, perhaps infections, play a substantial role in the phenotypic variability of lysosomal disease.

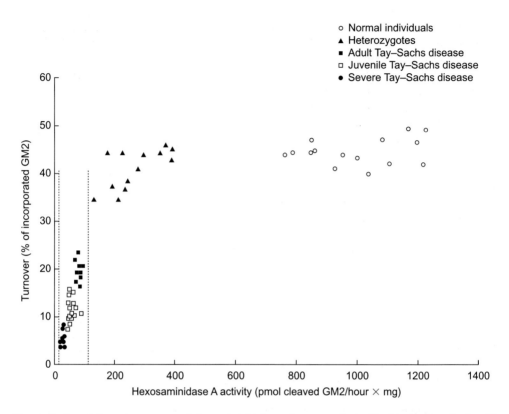

Figure 2. *Correlation of enzyme activity and lipid-degrading capacity in fibroblasts of patients with Tay–Sachs disease. Tay–Sachs disease is a lipid storage disorder caused by deficiency of hexosaminidase A. Patients store GM2-ganglioside and suffer primarily from neurological symptoms. As in many other lysosomal storage diseases the clinical spectrum encompasses severe early-onset to attenuated late-onset forms. Hexosaminidase A activities were determined in homogenates of fibroblasts from normal individuals, heterozygous parents and patients with severe, juvenile or adult forms of disease. These values do not necessarily reflect the in-vivo capacity of the cells to degrade GM2-ganglioside. To determine this, cultured cells were incubated with radioactively labelled GM2-ganglioside. After several hours of incubation, the percentage of GM2-ganglioside degraded by the various cultured cells was determined. Each of the symbols represents the values for one individual. The graph demonstrates that the capacity of cultured cells to degrade GM2-ganglioside is unaffected over a wide range of hexosaminidase A activity. Substrate degradation in the cultured cells is affected only if the enzyme activity falls below a threshold of about 10% of normal. The vertical dotted lines indicate the range of residual enzyme activity between which the entire clinical spectrum of disease develops. Adapted with permission from [52].*

Some diseases vary not only with respect to severity and age of onset but also with respect to organ involvement. Type I Gaucher disease is primarily a disease of macrophages, affecting the bone marrow, spleen, liver and lungs, but is not associated with CNS involvement [51]. In contrast, type II Gaucher disease has, in addition, severe nervous system involvement [51]. The degree of residual enzyme activity may explain these considerable differences in phenotype. The pool of glucosylceramide that must be degraded in a particular cell is derived from endogeneous synthesis and/or exogeneous sources. The latter are particularly important for phagocytosing macrophages. Thus, in the case of a severe enzyme deficiency, the amount of glucosylceramide synthesized in neurones is sufficient to cause storage in these cells. In the case of sufficiently high residual glucocerebrosidase activity, the endogenously synthesized lipid in neurones is degraded. The lipid load of macrophages, however, is much higher, as among other debris they phagocytose aged erythrocytes, which contain glucosylceramide. Storage in type I Gaucher disease therefore occurs in macrophages but not in neurones [53]. A comparable situation is also found in Niemann–Pick disease. Here, the Δ608 single amino acid deletion in the sphingomyelinase gene allows for the expression of some residual enzyme activity. The presence of at least one copy of this allele appears to prevent the development of the neurono-pathic Niemann–Pick type A disease, but attenuates the course to type B disease, with no or little neuronal involvement [60, 61].

Conclusions

The cellular pathophysiology of LSDs is a consequence of the underlying mutation and the toxic effects of the accumulating com-pounds. Mutations causing a complete loss of enzyme activity result mostly in severe disease of early onset. In contrast, alleles that still allow the expression of low amounts of residual enzyme activity are frequently associated with attentuated forms of disease. These forms, in particular, show substantial variability even among siblings. The factors causing this variability are unknown. Among the LSDs, lipidoses have been most intensively studied with respect to pathogenic mechanisms. In these disorders, microglial activation and/or apoptosis frequently play an important role in pathogenesis. In some disorders, toxic lysolipids accumulate. Cal-cium release from the endoplasmic retic-ulum is altered in some lipidoses and may account for alterations in calcium-mediated signal transduction. As the genetics of most disorders is now well understood, future research in the area of LSDs will focus on cellular pathophysiology and the development of therapies.

References

1. De Duve C. Exploring cells with a centrifuge; 1974 www.nobelprize.org/medicine/laureates/1974/duve-lecture.html

2. Futerman AH, van Meer G. The cell biology of lyso-somal storage disorders. *Nat Rev Mol Cell Biol* 2004; 5:554–65

3. Matsushima GK, Taniike M, Glimcher LH, Grusby MJ, Frelinger JA, Suzuki K et al. Absence of MHC class II molecules reduces CNS demyelination, microglial/macrophage infiltration, and twitching in murine globoid cell leukodystrophy. *Cell* 1994; 78:645–56

4. Wada R, Tifft CJ, Proia RL. Microglial activation precedes acute neurodegeneration in Sandhoff disease and is suppressed by bone marrow transplantation. *Proc Natl Acad Sci USA* 2000; 97:10954–9

5. Hess B, Saftig P, Hartmann D, Coenen R, Lullmann-Rauch R, Goebel HH et al. Phenotype of aryl-sulfatase A-deficient mice: relationship to human meta-chromatic leukodystrophy. *Proc Natl Acad Sci USA* 1996;93:14821–6

6. Barak V, Acker M, Nisman B, Kalickman I, Abrahamov A, Zimran A et al. Cytokines in Gaucher's disease. *Eur Cytokine Netw* 1999;10:205–10

7. Allen MJ, Myer BJ, Khokher AM, Rushton N, Cox TM. Pro-inflammatory cytokines and the pathogenesis of Gaucher's disease: increased release of interleukin-6 and interleukin-10. *QJM* 1997;90:19–25

8. Brautbar A, Elstein D, Pines G, Abrahamov A, Zimran A. Effect of enzyme replacement therapy on gammopathies in Gaucher disease. *Blood Cells Mol Dis* 2004;32:214–17

9. Cox TM. Gaucher disease: understanding the molecular pathogenesis of sphingolipidoses. *J Inherit Metab Dis* 2001;24 (Suppl 2):106–21; discussion 87–8

10. Zhou J, Cox NR, Ewald SJ, Morrison NE, Basker HJ. Evaluation of GM1 ganglioside-mediated apoptosis in feline thymocytes. *Vet Immunol Immunopathol* 1998;66:25–42

11. Finn LS, Zhang M, Chen SH, Scott CR. Severe type II Gaucher disease with ichthyosis, arthrogryposis and neuronal apoptosis: molecular and pathological analyses. *Am J Med Genet* 2000;91:222–6

12. Jatana M, Giri S, Singh AK. Apoptotic positive cells in Krabbe brain and induction of apoptosis in rat C6 glial cells by psychosine. *Neurosci Lett* 2002; 330:183–7

13. Erickson RP, Bernard O. Studies on neuronal death in the mouse model of Niemann–Pick C disease. *J Neurosci Res* 2002;68:738–44

14. Simonaro CM, Haskins ME, Schuchman EH. Articular chondrocytes from animals with a dermatan sulfate storage disease undergo a high rate of apoptosis and release nitric oxide and inflammatory cytokines: a possible mechanism underlying degenerative joint disease in the mucopolysaccharidoses. *Lab Invest* 2001;81:1319–28

15. Lozano J, Menendez S, Morales A, Ehleiter D, Liao WC, Wagman R et al. Cell autonomous apoptosis defects in acid sphingomyelinase knockout fibroblasts. *J Biol Chem* 2001;276:442–8

16. Purpura DP, Suzuki K. Distortion of neuronal geometry and formation of aberrant synapses in neuronal storage disease. *Brain Res* 1976;116:1–21

17. Walkley SU, Zervas M, Wiseman S. Gangliosides as modulators of dendritogenesis in normal and storage disease-affected pyramidal neurons. *Cereb Cortex* 2000;10:1028–37

18. Suzuki K. Globoid cell leukodystrophy (Krabbe's disease): update. *J Child Neurol* 2003;18:595–603

19. Toda K, Kobayashi T, Goto I, Ohno K, Eto Y, Inui K et al. Lysosulfatide (sulfogalactosylsphingosine) accumulation in tissues from patients with meta-chromatic leukodystrophy. *J Neurochem* 1990;55: 1585–91

20. Nilsson O, Svennerholm L. Accumulation of glucosyl-ceramide and glucosylsphingosine (psychosine) in cerebrum and cerebellum in infantile and juvenile Gaucher disease. *J Neurochem* 1982;39:709–18

21. Hannun YA, Bell RM. Lysosphingolipids inhibit protein kinase C: implications for the sphingolipidoses. *Science* 1987;235:670–4

22. Giri S, Jatana M, Rattan R, Won JS, Singh I, Singh AK. Galactosylsphingosine (psychosine)-induced expres-sion of cytokine-mediated inducible nitric oxide syn-thases via AP-1 and C/EBP: implications for Krabbe disease. *FASEB J* 2002;16:661–72

23. Lloyd-Evans E, Pelled D, Riebeling C, Futerman AH. Lyso-glycosphingolipids mobilize calcium from brain microsomes via multiple mechanisms. *Biochem J* 2003;375:561–5

24. Im DS, Heise CE, Nguyen T, O'Dowd BF, Lynch KR. Identification of a molecular target of psychosine and its role in globoid cell formation. *J Cell Biol* 2001; 153:429–34

25. Orvisky E, Park JK, LaMarca ME, Ginns EI, Martin BM, Tayebi N et al. Glucosylsphingosine accumulation in tissues from patients with Gaucher disease: correlation with phenotype and genotype. *Mol Genet Metab* 2002;76:262–70

26. Lloyd-Evans E, Pelled D, Riebeling C, Bodennec J, de-Morgan A, Waller H et al. Glucosylceramide and glucosylsphingosine modulate calcium mobilization from brain microsomes via different mechanisms. *J Biol Chem* 2003;278:23594–9

27. Korkotian E, Schwarz A, Pelled D, Schwarzmann G, Segal M, Futerman AH. Elevation of intracellular glucosylceramide levels results in an increase in endoplasmic reticulum density and in functional calcium stores in cultured neurons. *J Biol Chem* 1999;274:21673–8

28. Saravanan K, Schaeren-Wiemers N, Klein D, Sandhoff R, Schwarz A, Yaghootfam A et al. Specific downregulation and mistargeting of the lipid raft-associated protein MAL in a glycolipid storage disorder. *Neurobiol Dis* 2004;16:396–406

29. Pagano RE. Endocytic trafficking of glyco-sphingolipids in sphingolipid storage diseases. *Philos Trans R Soc Lond B Biol Sci* 2003;358:885–91

30. Puri V, Watanabe R, Dominguez M, Sun X, Wheatley CL, Marks DL et al. Cholesterol modulates membrane traffic along the endocytic pathway in sphingolipid-storage diseases. *Nat Cell Biol* 1999;1:386–8

31. Puri V, Watanabe R, Singh RD, Dominguez M, Brown JC, Wheatley CL et al. Clathrin-dependent and -independent internalization of plasma membrane sphingolipids initiates two Golgi targeting pathways. *J Cell Biol* 2001;154:535–47

32. Choudhury A, Dominguez M, Puri V, Sharma DK, Narita K, Wheatley CL et al. Rab proteins mediate Golgi transport of caveola-internalized glycosphingo-lipids and correct lipid trafficking in Niemann–Pick C cells. *J Clin Invest* 2002;109:1541–50

33. Choudhury A, Sharma DK, Marks DL, Pagano RE. Elevated endosomal cholesterol levels in Niemann–Pick cells inhibit rab4 and perturb membrane recycling. *Mol Biol Cell* 2004;15:4500–11

34. Dhami R, Schuchman EH. Mannose 6-phosphate receptor-mediated uptake is defective in acid sphingomyelinase-deficient macrophages: implica-tions for Niemann–Pick disease enzyme replacement therapy. *J Biol Chem* 2004;279:1526–32

35. Polten A, Fluharty AL, Fluharty CB, Kappler J, von Figura K, Gieselmann V. Molecular basis of different forms of metachromatic leukodystrophy. *N Engl J Med* 1991;324:18–22

36. McInnes B, Potier M, Wakamatsu N, Melancon SB, Klavins MH, Tsuji S et al. An unusual splicing mutation in the HEXB gene is associated with dramatically different phenotypes in patients from different racial backgrounds. *J Clin Invest* 1992;90:306–14

37. Huie ML, Hirschhorn R, Chen AS, Martiniuk F, Zhong N. Mutation at the catalytic site (M519V) in glycogen storage disease type II (Pompe disease). *Hum Mutat* 1994;4:291–3

38. Garman SC, Garboczi DN. The molecular defect leading to Fabry disease: structure of human α-galactosidase. *J Mol Biol* 2004;337:319–35

39. Zhang S, Bagshaw R, Hilson W, Oho Y, Hinek A, Clarke JT et al. Characterization of β-galactosidase mutations Asp332→Asn and Arg148→Ser, and a polymorphism, Ser532→Gly, in a case of GM1 gangliosidosis. *Biochem J* 2000;348 Pt 3:621–32

40. Saarela J, Laine M, Oinonen C, Schantz C, Jalanko A, Rouvinen J et al. Molecular pathogenesis of a disease: structural consequences of aspartylglucos-aminuria mutations. *Hum Mol Genet* 2001; 10:983–95

41. Hermann S, Schestag F, Polten A, Kafert S, Penzien J, Zlotogora J et al. Characterization of four arylsulfatase A missense mutations G86D, Y201C, D255H, and E312D causing metachromatic leukodystrophy. *Am J Med Genet* 2000;91:68–73

42. Schestag F, Yaghootfam A, Habetha M, Poeppel P, Dietz F, Klein RA et al. The functional consequences of mis-sense mutations affecting an intra-molecular

salt bridge in arylsulphatase A. *Biochem J* 2002; 367:499–504

43. Poeppel P, Habetha M, Marcao A, Bussow H, Berna L, Gieselmann V. Missense mutations as a cause of metachromatic leukodystrophy. Degradation of arylsulfatase A in the endoplasmic reticulum. *FEBS J* 2005;272:1179–88

44. Paw BH, Moskowitz SM, Uhrhammer N, Wright N, Kaback MM, Neufeld EF. Juvenile GM2 gangliosidosis caused by substitution of histidine for arginine at position 499 or 504 of the α-subunit of β-hexosaminidase. *J Biol Chem* 1990;265:9452–7

45. Carrell RW, Lomas DA. Conformational disease. *Lancet* 1997;350:134–8

46. Wicker G, Prill V, Brooks D, Gibson G, Hopwood J, von Figura K *et al*. Mucopolysaccharidosis VI (Maroteaux-Lamy syndrome). An intermediate clinical phenotype caused by substitution of valine for glycine at position 137 of arylsulfatase B. *J Biol Chem* 1991;266:21386–91

47. Marcao AM, Wiest R, Schindler K, Wiesmann U, Weis J, Schroth G *et al*. Adult onset metachromatic leukodystrophy without electroclinical peripheral nervous system involvement: a new mutation in the ARSA gene. *Arch Neurol* 2005;62:309–13

48. Fan JQ, Ishii S, Asano N, Suzuki Y. Accelerated transport and maturation of lysosomal α-galactosidase A in Fabry lymphoblasts by an enzyme inhibitor. *Nat Med* 1999;5:112–15

49. von Bulow R, Schmidt B, Dierks T, Schwabauer N, Schilling K, Weber E *et al*. Defective oligomerization of arylsulfatase A as a cause of its instability in lysosomes and metachromatic leukodystrophy. *J Biol Chem* 2002;277:9455–61

50. von Figura K, Gieselmann V, Jaeken J. Metachromatic leukodystrophy. In: Scriver C, Beaudet A, Sly W, Valle D, editors. The metabolic and molecular bases of inherited disease. 8th edn. New York: McGraw-Hill; 2001. p. 3695–724

51. Beutler E, Grabowski G. Gaucher disease. In: Scriver C, Beaudet A, Sly W, Valle D, editors. The metabolic and molecular bases of inherited disease. 8th edn. New York: McGraw-Hill; 2001. p. 3635–68

52. Leinekugel P, Michel S, Conzelmann E, Sandhoff K. Quantitative correlation between the residual activity of β-hexosaminidase A and arylsulfatase A and the severity of the resulting lysosomal storage disease. *Hum Genet* 1992;88:513–23

53. Zhao H, Bailey LA, Elsas LJ, 2nd, Grinzaid KA, Grabowski GA. Gaucher disease: *in vivo* evidence for allele dose leading to neuronopathic and nonneuronopathic phenotypes. *Am J Med Genet A* 2003;116:52–6

54. Zhao H, Grabowski GA. Gaucher disease: Perspectives on a prototype lysosomal disease. *Cell Mol Life Sci* 2002;59:694–707

55. Wakamatsu N, Kobayashi H, Miyatake T, Tsuji S. A novel exon mutation in the human β-hexosaminidase β subunit gene affects 3' splice site selection. *J Biol Chem* 1992;267:2406–13

56. Shieh JJ, Lin CY. Frequent mutation in Chinese patients with infantile type of GSD II in Taiwan: evidence for a founder effect. *Hum Mutat* 1998; 11:306–12

57. Hermans MM, de Graaff E, Kroos MA, Wisselaar HA, Willemsen R, Oostra BA *et al*. The conservative substitution Asp-645→Glu in lysosomal α-glucosidase affects transport and phosphorylation of the enzyme in an adult patient with glycogen-storage disease type II. *Biochem J* 1993;289 (Pt 3):687–93

58. Beutler E, Nguyen NJ, Henneberger MW, Smolec JM, McPherson RA, West C *et al*. Gaucher disease: gene frequencies in the Ashkenazi Jewish population. *Am J Hum Genet* 1993;52:85–8

59. Lachmann RH, Grant IR, Halsall D, Cox TM. Twin pairs showing discordance of phenotype in adult Gaucher's disease. *QJM* 2004;97:199–204

60. Simonaro CM, Desnick RJ, McGovern MM, Wasserstein MP, Schuchman EH. The demographics and distribution of type B Niemann–Pick disease: novel mutations lead to new genotype/phenotype correlations. *Am J Hum Genet* 2002;71:1413–19

61. Wasserstein MP, Desnick RJ, Schuchman EH, Hossain S, Wallenstein S, Lamm C *et al*. The natural history of type B Niemann–Pick disease: results from a 10-year longitudinal study. *Pediatrics* 2004; 114:e672–7

5 Importance of glycosylation in enzyme replacement therapy

Soumeya Bekri

Medical Biochemistry Laboratory, Rouen CHU, Hôpital Charles Nicolle, Anneau Central, 76031 Rouen, Cedex, France

Post-translational modification regulates the qualitative and quantitative control of a huge number of proteins in eukaryotes. Multiple sites may be targeted by a wide range of modifications, such as glycosylation, sulphation, methylation, sumoylation, citrullination, farnesylation, biotinylation, ubiquitination and proteolytic cleavage. These complex processes require a multitude of specific enzymes that are species and tissue specific. The subsequent changes modulate the physicochemical properties, folding, conformation, distribution, stability, activity and immunogenicity of the protein. This chapter discusses the post-translational changes of α-galactosidase A and the differences between agalsidase alfa, which is produced in a human cell line (fibroblasts), and agalsidase beta, which is produced in a non-human cell line (Chinese hamster ovary cells). The qualitative and quantitative differences in the post-translational modifications of these glycoproteins may have consequences for the biodistribution, activity and immunogenic potential of the enzyme.

Introduction

The recent availability of enzyme replacement therapy has changed the treatment of Fabry disease and should change the natural history of the disorder. There are currently two replacement enzymes available in Europe: agalsidase alfa (Replagal®; TKT Europe AB) and agalsidase beta (Fabrazyme®; Genzyme Corp.). Although the peptide sequence is identical to that of human α-galactosidase A in both cases, each of the enzyme preparations has a different and specific structure. This occurs as a result of the different production systems used: agalsidase beta is a recombinant protein synthesized in Chinese hamster ovary (CHO) cells, whereas agalsidase alfa is a human protein synthesized in a continuous line of human fibroblasts by a process of *in situ* activation of transcription of the *GLA* gene [1]. In order to better understand the differences between agalsidase alfa and agalsidase beta and the possible impact of these differences, this chapter will begin by briefly describing the structure and synthesis of α-galactosidase A.

Structure and synthesis of α-galactosidase A

The three-dimensional structure of α-galactosidase A was reported recently [2]. The enzyme is a homodimer; each monomer is composed of 398 amino acid residues and has an active site. Two aspartic acid residues in positions 170 and 231 determine the catalytic reaction that releases the galactose bound to the alpha component of the substrates of the enzyme.

After they have been synthesized in the endoplasmic reticulum, the monomers undergo post-translational modification in the Golgi apparatus. Each monomer of α-galactosidase A has three possible *N*-glycosylation sites (*N*139, *N*192 and *N*215). There are therefore several physiological glycoforms of α-galactosidase A. The *N*139 site links complex carbohydrates, whereas the *N*192 and *N*215 sites link oligosaccharides rich in mannose and are therefore involved in addressing the protein to the lysosome. After synthesis in the endoplasmic reticulum, the precursors of lysosomal enzymes are transferred to the Golgi apparatus. The post-translational modifications and, in particular, the addition of mannose-6-phosphate (M6P) residues, occur in the cis-Golgi. The M6P–enzyme complex binds to the M6P receptor and is released from the trans-Golgi network, from where it is transported to the prelysosomal/endosomal compartments. Once within the endosome

compartment, the acid pH causes the enzyme to dissociate from its receptor. It then undergoes dephosphorylation to produce the mature and functional enzyme. The receptor is then recycled to the trans-Golgi to recruit other enzymes, or moves to the plasma membrane where it can collect endogenous enzyme [3, 4] (Figure 1).

Post-translational modifications

The biological activity of the protein requires the integrity of the nucleotide sequence and, consequently, the polypeptide sequence; however, post-translational modifications are also important. These modifications include phosphorylation, glycosylation, sulphation, methylation, sumoylation, citrullination, farnesylation, biotinylation, ubiquitination and proteolytic

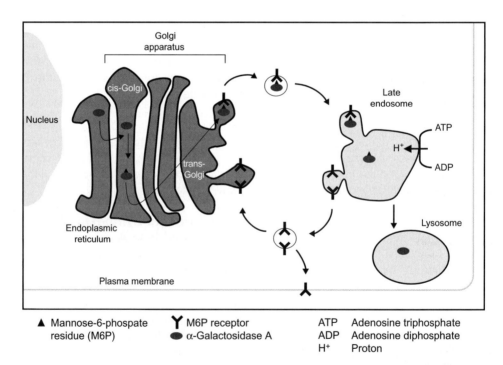

Figure 1. *Synthesis and trafficking of α-galactosidase A. After synthesis in the endoplasmic reticulum, α-galactosidase A undergoes post-translational modifications in the cis-Golgi, including the acquisition of mannose-6-phosphate (M6P) residues. The M6P–enzyme complex then progresses to the trans-Golgi where it binds to the M6P receptor. It is then released from the trans-Golgi network and transported to the prelysosomal/endosomal compartments. Here, the transport vesicles fuse with the endosomal compartment, and the acidic environment causes the M6P receptor to release the enzyme. The late endosome then matures to form the lysosome. The M6P receptor is now free to recycle to the trans-Golgi to recruit other enzymes or move towards the plasma membrane.*

cleavage. This complex process, with multi-site modifications, represents a new challenge in the postgenomic era and requires highly specialized, species-specific, enzymatic machinery.

The very large pool of targeted proteins is involved in a variety of key pathways, such as cell proliferation, control of gene expression, cellular response to DNA damage and enzyme activity. Post-translational modifications may result in alterations to the physicochemical properties, folding, conformation, intracellular and tissue distribution, stability, activity and immunogenicity of the protein. The elements that are added to the polypeptide can also serve as recognition tags, allowing interaction between the protein and a variety of other molecules. After initial modifications in the endoplasmic reticulum, these proteins move to the Golgi complex where the added elements may be subjected to further changes, such as additions, subtractions or more profound modifications. Starting with a basic polypeptide structure, several variants may therefore be obtained, and each variant may have a specific role. In fact, in certain cases, these forms are not intermediaries of synthesis but could play an independent role in the modulation of post-translational events (for review, see [5, 6]).

Glycosylation

The main class of post-translational modifications is represented by glycosylation, in which carbohydrates are linked to the protein component through either O-glycosidic bonds (to the hydroxyl of serine, threonine or hydroxylysine) or N-glycosidic bonds (to the amide group of asparagine). In O-linked glycoproteins, the carbohydrate directly attached to the protein is N-acetylgalactosamine, and in N-linked glycoproteins it is N-acetylglucosamine.

N-linked glycosylation is the most common covalent protein modification in eukaryotic cells. The process is highly conserved through evolution and is mandatory for viability. Almost all cell surface and secreted proteins undergo N-glycosylation, and several hundred specific enzymes, termed glycosyltransferases and glycosidases, are involved in the process. Variations in saccharide composition are observed, which depend on the cell type and state of differentiation. Glycosylation may also be influenced by other factors, such as environment and pathological processes (e.g. cancer). Terminal glycosylation – adding sialic acid residues to the end of the oligosaccharide chains – is essential for cellular and molecular interactions [7]. The pattern of sialylation is species specific and is highly regulated during embryonic development. Indeed, diversity in the structure (~40 species) and linkage (several sialyltransferases) of sialic acids contributes to glycoprotein specificity.

Glycosylation therefore appears to play a predominant part in the stability and three-dimensional configuration of the protein, as well as in its biodistribution and functional activity [8]. Moreover, a role has been demonstrated for post-translational modifications, such as glycosylation, in immunogenicity. Differences in glycosylation may increase the allergenic potential of the protein, most probably by increasing uptake and detection by the immune system [9]. In fact, the generation of a peptide that is recognized as an antigen by the immune system may require cleavage of the attached oligosaccharides; clearly, these oligosaccharides are involved in the presentation and thus the recognition of glycoproteins by the immune system [10].

The enzyme arsenal needed for post-translational modifications is very specific to a given cell type. The composition and the links of the saccharide residues in the oligosaccharide chains are therefore related to the cellular environment.

Role of glycosylation in α-galactosidase A

The importance of the process of glycosylation in the case of α-galactosidase A is illustrated by the fact that the substitution of a serine residue for the wild-type residue asparagine in position $N215$ causes impairment of enzyme trafficking to the lysosome [2, 11].

Genetically engineered cell lines are used to produce proteins of therapeutic value. Given the complexity of the post-translational events as described above, the nature and composition of the produced molecules are intimately dependent on the cellular environment of the source organisms. The CHO cell line is the most common host line used for the production of therapeutic enzyme preparations. When using such a non-human cell line, a major objective is to make the glycoproteins produced by the cells as similar to those produced in human cells as possible. To achieve this aim, metabolic engineering is used in non-human cell lines to produce protein modifications that are compatible with the required therapeutic application [12]. Two examples are given below to illustrate the differences between the α-galactosidase A glycoprotein produced from CHO and human cell lines.

First, the sialic acid N-glycolylneuraminic acid (NGNA) is widely expressed in the cells of most mammals, but is not naturally present in human tissues. The absence of this acid is due to the inactivation, in humans, of the enzyme cytidine monophosphate-NGNA hydroxylase, which is involved in the synthesis of NGNA [13]. Immune reactions linked to the introduction of this xenoantigen have been reported in humans. Moreover, NGNA is involved in the acute rejection of xenotransplantations [14]. NGNA is present in the CHO cell lines used in conventional industrial production of human recombinant glycoproteins [15] and was identified in α-galactosidase A preparations from CHO

cell lines [16]. The synthesis of proteins for therapeutic purposes in human fibroblasts guarantees the absence of NGNA from the oligosaccharide chains of the glycoprotein produced.

Secondly, sialylation of glycoproteins in CHO cells is incomplete, particularly under large-scale production conditions [17]. Incomplete sialylation leads to accelerated clearance of glycoproteins from the circulation via asialoglycoprotein receptors at the hepatocyte level [18] and, after internalization in the hepatocytes, these glycoproteins are catabolized. This has direct consequences on the circulating half-life of the glycoprotein and on its tissue biodistribution. A completely sialylated glycoprotein would have greater bioavailability for the target tissues. The M6P receptor is a transmembrane endocytic receptor expressed by several cell types, and its natural ligands include self and non-self glycoproteins [19]. The binding and internalization of lysosomal enzyme in cultured cells involves the M6P receptor [20]. It therefore appears that the internalization of replacement enzymes in the target cells takes place via the M6P receptor (Figure 2). The ratio of sialic residues to M6P is therefore important for optimal biodistribution. Moreover, natural human glycoproteins contain α2,3- and α2,6-linked sialic residues [21], whereas the glycoproteins synthesized in CHO cells contain only residues linked by α2,3 [22]. Indeed, CHO cells have no functional α2,6-sialyltransferase, and α-galactosidase A secreted by CHO cells harbours exclusively α2,3-linked sialic acid [16]. Studies have also shown differences in the degree of sialylation and phosphorylation of agalsidase alfa and agalsidase beta [23].

The qualitative and quantitative differences in the sialylation of glycoproteins produced in CHO cells in comparison with natural human glycoproteins have consequences for both the level of biodistribution and immunogenic potency. In fact, the presence of IgG

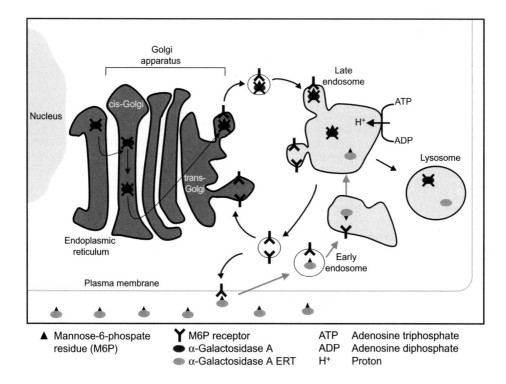

▲	Mannose-6-phospate residue (M6P)	Y	M6P receptor	ATP	Adenosine triphosphate
		●	α-Galactosidase A	ADP	Adenosine diphosphate
		●	α-Galactosidase A ERT	H⁺	Proton

Figure 2. *Transport of exogeneous enzyme to the lysosome. In patients with Fabry disease, the activity of α-galactosidase A is diminished. This may occur for several reasons: the enzyme may be absent, present but not addressed to the lysosome, or present but non-functional. Intravenous enzyme replacement therapy delivers functional enzyme to the cell; it enters by binding to mannose-6-phosphate receptors at the plasma membrane. Following internalization, the enzyme is transported in a vesicle to the prelysosomal/endosomal compartment, inside which it is released. ERT, enzyme replacement therapy.*

has been reported in 55% of patients treated with agalsidase alfa and in almost all patients treated with agalsidase beta [24, 25]. Clinical studies, however, have reported that both preparations produce a similar antibody reaction [26]. Moreover, in some cases, an allergic type reaction to treatment with agalsidase beta has been recorded, with the presence of IgE in the circulation and/or a positive intradermal reaction [27, 28].

Several studies are currently in progress that aim to modify CHO cells genetically to try to circumvent the problems mentioned above [29]. The use of human fibroblasts to obtain therapeutic glycoproteins offers a valuable alternative with potential benefits in terms of safety, bioavailability and biodistribution.

References

1. Schiffmann R, Kopp JB, Austin HA 3rd, Sabnis S, Moore DF, Weibel T *et al.* Enzyme replacement therapy in Fabry disease: a randomized controlled trial. *JAMA* 2001;285:2743–9

2. Garman SC, Garboczi DN. The molecular defect leading to Fabry disease: structure of human α-galactosidase. *J Mol Biol* 2004;337:319–35

3. Munier-Lehmann H, Mauxion F, Bauer U, Lobel P, Hoflack B. Re-expression of the mannose 6-phosphate receptors in receptor-deficient fibroblasts. Complementary function of the two mannose 6-phosphate receptors in lysosomal enzyme targeting. *J Biol Chem* 1996;271:15166–74

4. Sly WS, Fischer HD. The phosphomannosyl recognition system for intracellular and intercellular transport of lysosomal enzymes. *J Cell Biochem* 1982; 18:67–85

5. Helenius A, Aebi M. Roles of N-linked glycans in the endoplasmic reticulum. *Annu Rev Biochem* 2004; 73:1019–49

6. Rudd PM, Dwek RA. Glycosylation: heterogeneity and the 3D structure of proteins. *Crit Rev Biochem Mol Biol* 1997;32:1–100

7. Kelm S, Schauer R. Sialic acids in molecular and cellular interactions. *Int Rev Cytol* 1997;175:137–240

8. Nalivaeva NN, Turner AJ. Post-translational modifications of proteins: acetylcholinesterase as a model system. *Proteomics* 2001;1:735–47

9. Huby RD, Dearman RJ, Kimber I. Why are some proteins allergens? *Toxicol Sci* 2000;55:235–46

10. Rudd PM, Elliott T, Cresswell P, Wilson IA, Dwek RA. Glycosylation and the immune system. *Science* 2001;291:2370–6

11. Ioannou YA, Zeidner KM, Grace ME, Desnick RJ. Human α-galactosidase A: glycosylation site 3 is essential for enzyme solubility. *Biochem J* 1998; 332:789–97

12. Wildt S, Gerngross TU. The humanization of N-glycosylation pathways in yeast. *Nat Rev Microbiol* 2005; 3:119–28

13. Chou HH, Hayakawa T, Diaz S, Krings M, Indriati E, Leakey M *et al.* Inactivation of CMP-N-acetyl-neuraminic acid hydroxylase occurred prior to brain expansion during human evolution. *Proc Natl Acad Sci USA* 2002;99:11736–41

14. Zhu A, Hurst R. Anti-N-glycolylneuraminic acid antibodies identified in healthy human serum. *Xenotransplantation* 2002;9:376–81

15. Raju TS, Briggs JB, Borge SM, Jones AJ. Species-specific variation in glycosylation of IgG: evidence for the species-specific sialylation and branch-specific galactosylation and importance for engineering recombinant glycoprotein therapeutics. *Glycobiology* 2000;10:477–86

16. Matsuura F, Ohta M, Ioannou YA, Desnick RJ. Human α-galactosidase A: characterization of the *N*-linked oligosaccharides on the intracellular and secreted glycoforms overexpressed by Chinese hamster ovary cells. *Glycobiology* 1998;8:329–39

17. Santell L, Ryll T, Etcheverry T, Santoris M, Dutina G, Wang A *et al.* Aberrant metabolic sialylation of recombinant proteins expressed in Chinese hamster ovary cells in high productivity cultures. *Biochem Biophys Res Commun* 1999;258:132–7

18. Ashwell G, Harford J. Carbohydrate-specific receptors of the liver. *Annu Rev Biochem* 1982; 51:531–54

19. Allavena P, Chieppa M, Monti P, Piemonti L. From pattern recognition receptor to regulator of homeostasis: the double-faced macrophage mannose receptor. *Crit Rev Immunol* 2004; 24:179–92

20. Willingham MC, Pastan IH, Sahagian GG, Jourdian GW, Neufeld EF. Morphologic study of the internalization of a lysosomal enzyme by the mannose 6-phosphate receptor in cultured Chinese hamster ovary cells. *Proc Natl Acad Sci USA* 1981;78:6967–71

21. Takeuchi M, Takasaki S, Miyazaki H, Kato T, Hoshi S, Kochibe N *et al.* Comparative study of the asparagine-linked sugar chains of human erythropoietins purified from urine and the culture medium of recombinant Chinese hamster ovary cells. *J Biol Chem* 1988;263:3657–63

22. Bergwerff AA, van Oostrum J, Asselbergs FA, Burgi R, Hokke CH, Kamerling JP *et al.* Primary structure of *N*-linked carbohydrate chains of a human chimeric plasminogen activator K2tu-PA expressed in Chinese hamster ovary cells. *Eur J Biochem* 1993;212:639–56

23. Lee K, Jin X, Zhang K, Copertino L, Andrews L, Baker-Malcolm J *et al.* A biochemical and pharmacological comparison of enzyme replacement therapies for the glycolipid storage disorder Fabry disease. *Glycobiology* 2003;13:305–13

24. Fabrazyme, summary of product characteristics. August 2002

25. Replagal, summary of product characteristics. August 2001

26. Linthorst GE, Hollak CE, Donker-Koopman WE, Strijland A, Aerts JM. Enzyme therapy for Fabry disease: neutralizing antibodies toward agalsidase alpha and beta. *Kidney Int* 2004;66:1589–95

27. Germain DP. Fabry disease: recent advances in enzyme replacement therapy. *Expert Opin Investig Drugs* 2002;11:1467–76

28. Wilcox WR, Banikazemi M, Guffon N, Waldek S, Lee P, Linthorst GE *et al.* Long-term safety and efficacy of enzyme replacement therapy for Fabry disease. *Am J Hum Genet* 2004;75:65–74

29. Fukuta K, Yokomatsu T, Abe R, Asanagi M, Makino T. Genetic engineering of CHO cells producing human interferon-gamma by transfection of sialyltransferases. *Glycoconj J* 2000;17:895–904

6 Animal models of lysosomal storage diseases: their development and clinical relevance

Mark E Haskins, Urs Giger and Donald F Patterson

Laboratory of Pathology and Section of Medical Genetics, School of Veterinary Medicine, University of Pennsylvania, 3800 Spruce Street, Philadelphia, PA 19104-6051, USA

Progress in understanding how a particular genotype produces the phenotype of an inborn error of metabolism in human patients has been facilitated by the study of animals with mutations in the orthologous genes. These are not just animal 'models', but true orthologues of the human genetic disease, with defects involving the same evolutionarily conserved genes and the same molecular, biochemical and anatomical pathology as in human patients. Such animal orthologues are an important aid to the development of specific gene therapies for these disorders. The initial approach to finding suitable animals was to identify those with a naturally occurring disease. These animals were often domesticated species, because of the individual attention paid to such animals, particularly dogs and cats. In addition, naturally occurring mouse models have been found, and breeding lines established. Within the last several decades, advances in molecular biology and our understanding of murine reproductive physiology have combined to allow the production of knockout mouse models of human genetic disease expressed on various inbred backgrounds. Inbred strains of a small prolific species, such as the mouse, together with larger out-bred animals, discovered because of their disease phenotype, provide a powerful combination with which to elucidate the pathogenesis of human genetic disease and to investigate approaches to therapy. This has been true for inborn errors of metabolism and, in particular, the lysosomal storage diseases.

Introduction

Isolation of the genes involved in genetic disorders has paved the way to understanding the mechanisms underlying the molecular derangements associated with inherited diseases. There are encouraging new prospects for treating genetic diseases, including stem cell therapy and gene therapy. However, to understand fully and to treat human genetic diseases, authentic (gene-orthologous) animal models are required in studies that, for ethical and practical reasons, are not possible in humans. Mouse gene knockout technology has provided a valuable source of such models, but additional animal models are needed for studies that require larger and longer-lived species with clinical signs and underlying lesions more closely resembling those in humans.

As in humans, most of the lysosomal storage diseases (LSDs) known to occur in dogs and cats are inherited as autosomal recessive traits. Among humans, recessively inherited genetic diseases tend to aggregate in particular ethnic groups where consanguineous unions are likely to be more common. Similarly, many recessively inherited diseases in dogs and cats tend to aggregate

51

within particular breeds [1]. This follows from the requirement of the American Kennel Club (concerned with canine pedigrees), as well as pure-bred dog and cat registries, that, to be registered as a member of a particular breed, an animal must have parents that are both previously registered members of the same breed. Consanguineous matings are further promoted by the tendency for breeders to concentrate the genes from a sire famous for winning at shows by instituting matings between his descendants. Occurring as they do under the scrutiny of concerned breeders and their veterinarians, genetic diseases in dogs and cats, particularly those associated with specific breeds, are often well characterized.

The need for animal models

While much progress has been made in defining the molecular basis of genetic diseases in man, there are large gaps in our understanding of the complex chain of events between the underlying genetic defect and the phenotypic abnormalities at various levels – from cells, tissues and organs to the whole organism. As most of the studies necessary to unravel the pathogenic mechanisms involved cannot be performed in humans, animals with the same genetic disorders are an important source of knowledge. For example, while we know the genes and many of the mutations underlying the mucopolysaccharidoses (MPS), which constitute a particular class of LSD, and while the clinical and pathological features of the articular cartilage lesions in these diseases have been described, how sub-strate storage results in the cartilage lesions is only now beginning to be described and understood from investigations in cat, dog, and rat models of MPS (Figures 1 and 2) [2, 3].

For many lethal or debilitating genetic disorders in man, there are still no satisfactory means of treatment. One of the most exciting prospects for the use of animals with orthologous genetic diseases lies in testing

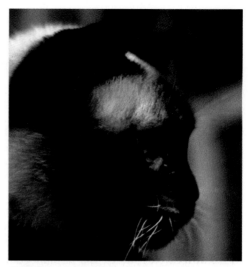

Figure 1. *The profile of a Siamese cat with muco-polysaccharidosis VI. Instead of the elongated face of a normal Siamese cat, affected cats have a shortened midface with a depressed nasal bridge, small ears and corneal clouding.*

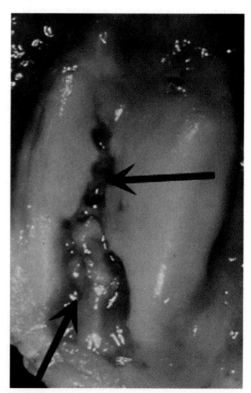

Figure 2. *Erosions (arrows) of the articular cartilage of the distal femur of a cat with muco-polysaccharidosis VI.*

new approaches to therapy. The monogenic inborn errors of metabolism are particularly attractive targets for gene and stem cell therapies because (i) they constitute a significant proportion of genetic diseases and (ii) they are usually autosomal recessive disorders involving the deficiency of a single specific protein gene product. Although simple in concept, examples of patients with inherited metabolic diseases being treated effectively using somatic cell gene therapy are limited [4], and not without complications, including insertional mutagenesis [5]. Currently, the major difficulties are obtaining adequate levels of gene product in the specific cell types in which they are needed (e.g. in the cells of the CNS), maintaining expression over long periods of time *in vivo*, and regulating the levels of gene expression.

The research necessary to improve this situation requires animal models that are true homologues of the human disease, with the same molecular, pathological and clinical phenotype as the human disease. Because the treatment of many different human disorders will eventually be attempted and the details of the approach will be specific to each genetic disease, many different animal models will be required.

Gene knockout technology

Gene knockout technology has been a powerful experimental approach that has contributed in a major way to the understanding of gene function in health and disease, and can be used in cases in which the gene of interest has been cloned. It is not always successful, however, in producing a model that accurately reproduces the human disease phenotype. Because large animal models are discovered through their clinical phenotype, they are more suitable than some knockout or point mutation mouse models that may have lesions but are lethal *in utero* or lack the full range of clinical disease, as has been the case in mice with Tay–Sachs disease, Fabry disease, cystinosis and

Gaucher disease [6–10]. In addition, in some knockout models, such as those with type II or type III Gaucher disease, animals die within a few days of birth, limiting their value for gene therapy research [10, 11]. Mice and other small laboratory animals will, however, continue to be a valuable source of disease models and have the advantages of being available in well-characterized inbred strains. In addition, it is easy to produce large numbers of affected as well as unaffected control animals with the same genetic background. For initial studies, naturally occurring and knockout mice with LSDs have proven extremely valuable.

Use of larger animal models

Clinical veterinary medicine provides a vast and sophisticated screening mechanism in which animals are examined individually and in detail by using diagnostic methods that have an accuracy and sensitivity approaching those used in humans. Furthermore, the naturally occurring disease models in dogs and cats exist in various genetic isolates (breeds) maintained by members of the public. Once identified, these models can be established in special research colonies, frequently associated with veterinary schools. Breeders have been eager to cooperate in these endeavours because the scientific knowledge gained aids in the understanding and control of the animal diseases as well as contributing to human health [12].

Larger species, such as the dog and cat, have the advantages of a heterogeneous genetic background more similar to humans, and a size and longevity more suitable for surgical manipulations, clinical evaluations, and assessment of the long-term consequences of therapy over many years. These advantages, along with the accumulated background of physiological and clinical veterinary knowledge in these species, make them extremely useful. Of course, not all genetic diseases have been found in large animals, and knockout mice have been essential to fill the gap. Nevertheless, domesticated animals have been a rich source of models for LSDs, perhaps due to the progressive nature and striking clinical signs of disease in these species. Some LSDs were recognized in veterinary medicine before the diseases were understood at the level of the specific enzymes involved. Because of the distinctive central and peripheral nervous system lesions, the first of these diseases to be described was globoid cell leukodystrophy in Cairn and West Highland white terriers in 1963 (Figures 3 and 4) [13]. These two breeds of dogs are now known to have the same mutation in the gene coding for galactosylceramidase [14]. This mutation apparently originated in the 19th century from an ancestor common to these two breeds, which diverged around the beginning of the 20th century. The first LSD in animals that was identified by its deficient enzyme (β-galactosidase) activity was GM1-gangliosidosis in a Siamese cat, in 1971 [15]. Since then, naturally occurring LSDs have been recognized in cats, cattle, dogs, guinea pigs, goats, mice, pigs, rats, sheep, quail, emus and horses [16, 17] (Table 1). Breeding colonies have been established and exist for a large number of LSDs in various species [80, 81].

These examples illustrate that it is important to continue to find and utilize genetic disease models that arise spontaneously in out-bred

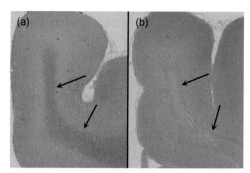

Figure 4. *Histological appearance of the cerebral cortex of (a) a normal dog and (b) a dog with globoid cell leukodystrophy. The sections were treated with luxol blue, which stains normal myelin blue, as can be seen in (a) [arrows]. The white matter in the affected dog [arrows] (b) is unstained, as the normal myelin is replaced with macrophages filled with ingested myelin breakdown products.*

animal populations, in addition to using knockout mouse models. In the Section of Medical Genetics at the University of Pennsylvania's School of Veterinary Medicine, dogs and cats with clinical signs suggestive of an inherited metabolic disease are routinely screened for the presence of abnormal metabolites in urine and blood, using methods similar to those used in paediatric hospitals. Urine screening has proven to be the most productive method, as the concentration of metabolites from many inborn errors of metabolism are highest in the urine. Defects in renal transport are also detected by these tests. Abnormalities detected by screening tests are further investigated by more definitive tests to determine the identity of abnormal metabolites, as indicated in Figure 5. If a disorder with tissue storage is suspected and urine and blood tests fail to reveal any abnormality, tissue biopsy material and other body fluids are examined. In addition, examinations of biopsy and post-mortem specimens from animals with congenital or genetic diseases are useful in identifying other inherited diseases with abnormalities of tissue and cell metabolism. From understanding the metabolic pathways, the genes involved in particularly promising animal models can be cloned from normal animals

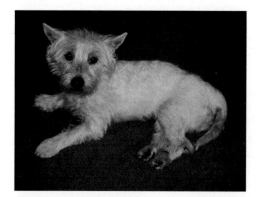

Figure 3. *A West Highland white terrier with globoid cell leukodystropy (Krabbe disease). The dog has early signs of posterior limb paresis.*

Table 1. *Naturally occurring mucopolysaccharidoses (MPS) and related diseases in animals.*

Disease	Deficient enzyme	Species and selected references
MPS I (Hurler, Scheie and Hurler/Scheie syndromes)	α-L-Iduronidase	Domestic cat [18–21] Plott hound dog [22–27] Rottweiler dog [unpublished] Boston terrier dog [unpublished]
MPS II (Hunter syndrome)	Iduronate sulphatase	Labrador retriever dog [28]
MPS IIIA (Sanfilippo A syndrome)	Heparan N-sulphatase	Wirehaired dachshund dog [29–30] Mouse [31] Huntaway dog [32, 33]
MPS IIIB (Sanfilippo B syndrome)	α-N-Acetylglucosaminidase	Emu [34] Schipperke dog [35]
MPS IIID (Sanfilippo D syndrome)	N-Acetylglucosamine-6-sulphatase	Nubian goat [36, 37]
MPS VI (Maroteaux–Lamy syndrome)	N-Acetylglucosamine-4-sulphatase (arylsulphatase B)	Siamese cat [38–40] Domestic short-haired cat [unpublished] Miniature pinscher dog [41, 42] Welsh corgi dog, Chesapeake Bay retriever dog [unpublished] Miniature schnauzer dog [43] Rat [44–46]
MPS VII (Sly disease)	β-Glucuronidase	German shepherd dog [47–50] GUS mouse [51–53] Cat [54, 55]
α-Mannosidosis	α-Mannosidosase	Persian cat [56–61] Angus and Murray grey cattle [62–66] Galloway cattle [67] Guinea pig [68]
β-Mannosidosis	β-Mannosidosase	Anglo-Nubian goat [69–72] Saler cattle [73–76]
Mucolipidosis II (I-cell disease)	N-Acetylglucosamine-1-phosphotransferase	Cat [77–79]

Adapted with permission from [80].

when the defective protein is known, providing the species-specific complementary DNA (cDNA) needed for therapy. Approaches for cloning include screening cDNA libraries and reverse transcriptase–polymerase chain reaction, taking advantage of the recently completed 7.6x canine genome sequence (where 7.6 times as many nucleotides of dog genome sequence were generated in the dog genome project) and an emerging feline genome sequence approved for 2x, which is currently more than half completed.

Clinical relevance to therapy

The basic approach to treating LSDs relies on the capacity of cells to take up exogenous normal enzyme and deliver it to the lysosome, usually by a mannose-6-phosphate receptor-

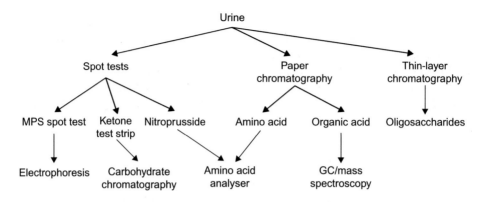

Figure 5. *The scheme used to evaluate urine from animals with clinical signs and history consistent with a genetic metabolic disease. The initial tests are relatively quick and inexpensive and are used to screen for abnormal metabolites present in urine; they can be followed up with more specific tests. Once a compound is identified, the metabolic pathway involved is reviewed to discover the possible location of the defect that produced the abnormal urinary excretion.*

mediated process [82]. Fortunately, the amount of enzyme needed in the lysosome for phenotypic correction of an individual cell is only a small percentage of normal. The three approaches to providing normal enzyme to a patient's cells are enzyme replacement therapy (ERT), bone marrow transplantation (BMT) and gene therapy. In general, the most difficult target tissue in the LSDs is the CNS. Approximately 60% of LSDs have a CNS component, for which systemic therapy is limited by the blood–brain barrier. Successful treatment of the neuronopathic LSDs will require direct therapy to, or systemic therapy that targets, the CNS. Animal models have been used extensively to evaluate these approaches to therapy.

ERT
The efficacy of the parenteral injection of purified recombinant enzyme has been tested in various animal models of LSDs, including MPS VII mice, MPS I dogs and cats, MPS VI cats, and glycogen storage disease in Japanese quail [80, 81]. In knockout mice, enzyme derived from rabbit milk or from Chinese hamster ovary cells has been used, including experiments in Fabry mice [83] (see below). Today, ERT is the standard

therapy for non-neuronopathic Gaucher disease and is available or under evaluation for the treatment of Fabry disease, Pompe disease, MPS I, MPS II and MPS VI.

BMT
Heterologous BMT as therapy for LSDs has been performed for decades (reviewed in [84–90]. This approach provides both normal bone marrow and bone-marrow-derived cells, which are available to release enzyme continuously for uptake by other cells. In addition, monocyte-derived cells can cross the blood–brain barrier, becoming microglia and secreting enzyme that can be available to neurones. BMT has been carried out in MPS VII mice, mannosidosis cats, GM2-gangliosidosis mice, MPS VI cats, and the MPS VII dog, among others [87]. A combination of neonatal ERT followed by BMT at 5 weeks of age in MPS VII mice has been shown to have long-term positive effects [91].

Gene therapy
The most striking clinical results of gene therapy involving an LSD have been those seen in a series of neonatal gene transfer studies conducted using viral vectors in the murine and canine models of MPS VII

[92–96]. Even for an LSD, MPS VII is a very rare condition, affecting fewer than 1/250 000 live births. In spite of the rarity of MPS VII, these models have become a paradigm for LSDs in general because of the ability to detect the normal enzyme (β-glucuronidase) activity directly by using a histochemical technique.

The α-galactosidase A knockout mouse

No large animal model for Fabry disease has been discovered, although a knockout mouse model has been developed [7]. The model displays a complete lack of α-galactosidase A activity, which in humans leads to impaired catabolism of α-galactosyl-terminal lipid (i.e. globotriaosylceramide). In this X-linked disease, humans develop painful neuropathy and vascular occlusions that progressively lead to cardiovascular, cerebrovascular and renal dysfunction, and early death. However, knockout Fabry mice appear clinically normal, with normal blood and urine analyses and a normal adult lifespan [7, 97]. The limitation imposed by a lack of clinical signs has not, however, prevented the use of these mice in therapy trials, as they do have lesions that can be evaluated for improvement. α-D-Galactosyl residues have been shown to accumulate progressively in the kidneys of Fabry mice until they are 20 weeks of age, and lipid analysis has shown a marked accumulation of ceramidetrihexoside in the liver and kidneys. However, there were no obvious histological lesions visible under light microscopy in haematoxylin–eosin-stained sections of the kidneys, liver, heart, spleen, lungs and brain. Typical lamellar inclusions have frequently been observed by electron microscopy in the lysosomes of Kupffer cells and, to a lesser degree, in hepatocytes from affected mice. In the brain, inclusions in the lysosomes were identified in vascular smooth muscle cells but not in neuronal or glial cells. In the kidney, compared with wild-type mice, there are increased numbers of lamellar bodies within proximal and distal tubular cells and, to a lesser extent, within glomerular epithelial cells and peritubular capillary endothelial cells.

Preclinical studies of ERT for Fabry disease have been performed in the knockout mouse model [83]. The pharmacokinetics and biodistribution of administered α-galactosidase A were evaluated. In spite of the lack of clinical signs, the reduction of substrate in various tissues and plasma was found to be dose dependent, and re-accumulation rates were determined for the liver, myocardium and spleen, providing an *in vivo* rationale for ERT in patients with Fabry disease [83].

Various gene therapy studies have been performed in the knockout Fabry mouse, including: *in vitro* transduction of bone marrow cells with a retroviral vector and transplantation into radiation-conditioned knockout mice [98, 99]; the intravenous or intramuscular injection of an adeno-associated virus vector [100–103]; and the pulmonary instillation [104] or intravenous injection of an adenovirus vector [105, 106]. Increased activity of α-galactosidase A was documented, with substrate reduction in various tissues, which was dependent upon the vector and mode of administration.

Conclusions

Domestic animals with spontaneous genetic diseases can be of great importance in understanding the pathogenesis of the condition and the development of therapy. Veterinary medicine provides an increasingly high degree of medical scrutiny of animals, particularly the dog and cat, and new orthologues of human genetic diseases are being recognized with increasing frequency. These models provide an opportunity to monitor therapeutic efficacy and the possible development of untoward side effects in out-bred, long-lived animals that can be monitored individually using the same methods that are applicable to humans. Finding spontaneous mouse models, as well as producing knockout mice with a disruption of the gene of interest, allows the evaluation of disease and therapy in a relatively large number of animals with a uniform genetic background. The ideal is to have a mouse model and a dog or cat model, together with an authentic primate model. This has so far been achieved only for globoid cell leukodystrophy (Krabbe disease), with the twitcher mouse [107], the dog [14] and the rhesus monkey [108] providing spontaneous models of the human disease.

Acknowledgements

The discovery and characterization of large animal models of human genetic disease have been supported by grants from the National Institutes of Health, currently P40-RR02512, DK25659 and DK54481.

References

1. Patterson DF. Companion animal medicine in the age of medical genetics. *J Vet Intern Med* 2000;14:1–9

2. Simonaro CM, Haskins ME, Schuchman EH. Articular chondrocytes from animals with a dermatan sulfate storage disease undergo a high rate of apoptosis and release nitric oxide and inflammatory cytokines: a possible mechanism underlying degenerative joint disease in the mucopolysaccharidoses. *Lab Invest* 2001;81:1319–28

3. Simonaro CM, D'Angelo M, Haskins ME, Schuchman EH. Joint and bone disease in mucopolysaccharidoses VI and VII: identification of new therapeutic targets and biomarkers using animal models. *Pediatr Res* 2005;57:701–7

4. Cavazzana-Calvo M, Hacein-Bey S, de Saint Basile G, Gross F, Yvon E, Nusbaum P *et al.* Gene therapy of human severe combined immunodeficiency (SCID)-X1 disease. *Science* 2000;288:669–72

5. Hacein-Bey-Abina S, von Kalle C, Schmidt M, Le Deist F, Wulffraat N, McIntyre E *et al.* A serious adverse event after successful gene therapy for X-linked severe combined immunodeficiency. *N Engl J Med* 2003;348:255–6

6. Phaneuf D, Wakamatsu N, Huang JQ, Borowski A, Peterson AC, Fortunato SR *et al.* Dramatically different phenotypes in mouse models of human Tay–Sachs and Sandhoff diseases. *Hum Mol Genet* 1996;5:1–14

7. Ohshima T, Murray GJ, Swaim WD, Longenecker G, Quirk JM, Cardarelli CO *et al.* α-Galactosidase A deficient mice: a model of Fabry disease. *Proc Natl Acad Sci USA* 1997;94:2540–4

8. Cohen-Tannoudji M, Marchand P, Akli S, Sheardown SA, Puech JP, Kress C *et al.* Disruption of murine Hexa gene leads to enzymatic deficiency and to neuronal lysosomal storage, similar to that observed in Tay–Sachs disease. *Mamm Genome* 1995;6:844–9

9. Cherqui S, Sevin C, Hamard G, Kalatzis V, Sich M, Pequignot MO *et al.* Intralysosomal cystine accumulation in mice lacking cystinosin, the protein defective in cystinosis. *Mol Cell Biol* 2002;22:7622–32

10. Xu YH, Quinn B, Witte D, Grabowski GA. Viable mouse models of acid β-glucosidase deficiency: the defect in Gaucher disease. *Am J Pathol* 2003;163:2093–101

11. Liu Y, Suzuki K, Reed JD, Grinberg A, Westphal H, Hoffmann A *et al.* Mice with type 2 and 3 Gaucher disease point mutations generated by a single insertion mutagenesis procedure. *Proc Natl Acad Sci USA* 1998;95:2503–8

12. Patterson DF, Haskins ME, Jezyk PF, Giger U, Meyers-Wallen VN, Aguirre G *et al.* Research on genetic diseases: reciprocal benefits to animals and man. *J Am Vet Med Assoc* 1988;193:1131–44

13. Frankhauser R, Luginbuhl H, Hartley W. Leukodystrophie vom Typus Krabbe Beim Hund. *Schweiz Arch Tierheilk* 1963;105:198–207

14. Victoria T, Rafi MA, Wenger DA. Cloning of the canine GALC cDNA and identification of the mutation causing globoid cell leukodystrophy in West Highland white and Cairn terriers. *Genomics* 1996;33:457–62

15. Baker HJ Jr, Lindsey JR, McKhann GM, Farrell DF. Neuronal GM1 gangliosidosis in a Siamese cat with β-galactosidase deficiency. *Science* 1971;174:838–9

16. Url A, Bauder B, Thalhammer J, Nowotny N, Kolodziejek J, Herout N *et al.* Equine neuronal ceroid lipofuscinosis. *Acta Neuropathol (Berl)* 2001;101:410–14

17. Haskins ME, Giger U. Lysosomal storage diseases. In: Kaneko JJ, Harvey JW, Bruss ML, editors. Clinical biochemistry of domestic animals, 5th edn. New York: Academic Press; 1997. p. 741–61

18. Haskins ME, Jezyk PF, Desnick RJ, McDonough SK, Patterson DF. Alpha-L-iduronidase deficiency in a cat: a model of mucopolysaccharidosis I. *Pediatr Res* 1979;13:1294–7

19. Haskins ME, Jezyk PF, Desnick RJ, McDonough SK, Patterson DF. Mucopolysaccharidosis in a domestic short-haired cat – a disease distinct from that seen in the Siamese cat. *J Am Vet Med Assoc* 1979;175:384–7

20. Haskins ME, McGrath JT. Meningiomas in young cats with mucopolysaccharidosis I. *J Neuropathol Exp Neurol* 1983;42:664–70

21. Haskins ME, Aguirre GD, Jezyk PF, Desnick RJ, Patterson DF. The pathology of the feline model of mucopolysaccharidosis I. *Am J Pathol* 1983;112:27–36

22. Shull RM, Munger RJ, Spellacy E, Hall CW, Constantopoulos G, Neufeld EF. Canine α-L-

iduronidase deficiency. A model of mucopolysaccharidosis I. *Am J Pathol* 1982;109:244–8

23. Shull RM, Helman RG, Spellacy E, Constantopoulos G, Munger RJ, Neufeld EF. Morphologic and biochemical studies of canine mucopolysaccharidosis I. *Am J Pathol* 1984;114:487–95

24. Shull RM, Hastings NE. Fluorometric assay of α-L-iduronidase in serum for detection of affected and carrier animals in a canine model of mucopolysaccharidosis I. *Clin Chem* 1985;31:826–7

25. Spellacy E, Shull RM, Constantopoulos G, Neufeld EF. A canine model of human α-L-iduronidase deficiency. *Proc Natl Acad Sci USA* 1983;80:6091–5

26. Stoltzfus LJ, Sosa-Pineda B, Moskowitz SM, Menon KP, Dlott B, Hooper L *et al.* Cloning and characterization of cDNA encoding canine α-L-iduronidase. mRNA deficiency in mucopolysaccharidosis I dog. *J Biol Chem* 1992;267:6570–5

27. Menon KP, Tieu PT, Neufeld EF. Architecture of the canine IDUA gene and mutation underlying canine mucopolysaccharidosis I. *Genomics* 1992;14:763–8

28. Wilkerson MJ, Lewis DC, Marks SL, Prieur DJ. Clinical and morphologic features of mucopolysaccharidosis type II in a dog: naturally occurring model of Hunter syndrome. *Vet Pathol* 1998;35:230–3

29. Fischer A, Carmichael KP, Munnell JF, Jhabvala P, Thompson JN, Matalon R *et al.* Sulfamidase deficiency in a family of dachshunds: a canine model of mucopolysaccharidosis IIIA (Sanfilippo A). *Pediatr Res* 1998;44:74–82

30. Aronovich EL, Carmichael KP, Morizono H, Koutlas IG, Deanching M, Hoganson G *et al.* Canine heparan sulfate sulfamidase and the molecular pathology underlying Sanfilippo syndrome type A in dachshunds. *Genomics* 2000;68:80–4

31. Bhaumik M, Muller VJ, Rozaklis T, Johnson L, Dobrenis K, Bhattacharyya R *et al.* A mouse model for mucopolysaccharidosis type III A (Sanfilippo syndrome). *Glycobiology* 1999;9:1389–96

32. Jolly RD, Allan FJ, Collett MG, Rozaklis T, Muller VJ, Hopwood JJ. Mucopolysaccharidosis IIIA (Sanfilippo syndrome) in a New Zealand Huntaway dog with ataxia. *N Z Vet J* 2000;48:144–8

33. Yogalingam G, Pollard T, Gliddon B, Jolly RD, Hopwood JJ. Identification of a mutation causing mucopolysaccharidosis type IIIA in New Zealand Huntaway dogs. *Genomics* 2002;79:150–3

34. Aronovich EL, Johnston JM, Wang P, Giger U, Whitley CB. Molecular basis of mucopolysaccharidosis type IIIB in emu (*Dromaius novaehollandiae*): an avian model of Sanfilippo syndrome type B. *Genomics* 2001;74:299–305

35. Ellinwood NM, Wang P, Skeen T, Sharp N, Cesta Bush W, Hardam E *et al.* Canine mucopolysaccharidosis IIIB: characterization of an inherited neuropathy recently identified in schipperkes. *Am J Hum Genet* 2001;69 (Suppl):482

36. Friderici K, Cavanagh KT, Leipprandt JR, Traviss CE, Anson DS, Hopwood JJ *et al.* Cloning and sequence analysis of caprine *N*-acetylgluco-

samine 6-sulfatase cDNA. *Biochim Biophys Acta* 1995;1271:369–73

37. Thompson JN, Jones MZ, Dawson G, Huffman PS. *N*-acetylglucosamine 6-sulphatase deficiency in a Nubian goat: a model of Sanfilippo syndrome type D (mucopolysaccharidosis IIID). *J Inherit Metab Dis* 1992;15:760–8

38. Cowell KR, Jezyk PF, Haskins ME, Patterson DF. Mucopolysaccharidosis in a cat. *J Am Vet Med Assoc* 1976;169:334–9

39. Haskins ME, Jezyk PF, Patterson DF. Mucopolysaccharide storage disease in three families of cats with arylsulfatase B deficiency: leukocyte studies and carrier identification. *Pediatr Res* 1979;13:1203–10

40. Haskins ME, Aguirre GD, Jezyk PF, Patterson DF. The pathology of the feline model of mucopolysaccharidosis VI. *Am J Pathol* 1980;101:657–74

41. Neer TM, Dial SM, Pechman R, Wang P, Giger U. Mucopolysaccharidosis VI (Maroteaux–Lamy syndrome) in a miniature pinscher. *J Vet Intern Med* 1992;6:124

42. Neer TM, Dial SM, Pechman R, Wang P, Oliver JL, Giger U. Clinical vignette. Mucopolysaccharidosis VI in a miniature pinscher. *J Vet Intern Med* 1995; 9:429–33

43. Berman L, Foureman P, Stieger K, van Hoeven M, Ellinwood N, Henthorn P *et al.* Mucopolysaccharidosis type VI caused by a point mutation in the miniature schnauzer. Proceedings of the 2nd International Conference: Advances in Canine and Feline Genomics. Utrecht, The Netherlands, 14–16 October 2004

44. Yoshida M, Tachibana M, Kobayashi E, Ikadai H, Kunieda T. The locus responsible for mucopolysaccharidosis VI (Maroteaux–Lamy syndrome) is located on rat chromosome 2. *Genomics* 1994;20:145–6

45. Yoshida M, Ikadai H, Maekawa A, Takahashi M, Nagase S. Pathological characteristics of mucopolysaccharidosis VI in the rat. *J Comp Pathol* 1993; 109:141–53

46. Yoshida M, Noguchi J, Ikadai H, Takahashi M, Nagase S. Arylsulfatase B-deficient mucopolysaccharidosis in rats. *J Clin Invest* 1993;91:1099–104

47. Haskins ME, Desnick RJ, DiFerrante N, Jezyk PF, Patterson DF. β-Glucuronidase deficiency in a dog: a model of human mucopolysaccharidosis VII. *Pediatr Res* 1984;18:980–4

48. Schuchman EH, Toroyan TK, Haskins ME, Desnick RJ. Characterization of the defective β-glucuronidase activity in canine mucopolysaccharidosis type VII. *Enzyme* 1989;42:174–80

49. Ray J, Bouvet A, DeSanto C, Fyfe JC, Xu D, Wolfe JH *et al.* Cloning of the canine β-glucuronidase cDNA, mutation identification in canine MPS VII, and retroviral vector-mediated correction of MPS VII cells. *Genomics* 1998;48:248–53

50. Silverstein Dombrowski DC, Carmichael KP, Wang P, O'Malley TM, Haskins ME, Giger U. Mucopolysaccharidosis type VII in a German shepherd dog. *J Am Vet Med Assoc* 2004;224:553–7, 532–3

51. Birkenmeier EH, Davisson MT, Beamer WG, Ganschow RE, Vogler CA, Gwynn B *et al.* Murine mucopolysaccharidosis type VII. Characterization of a mouse with β-glucuronidase deficiency. *J Clin Invest* 1989;83:1258–66

52. Vogler C, Birkenmeier EH, Sly WS, Levy B, Pegors C, Kyle JW *et al.* A murine model of mucopolysaccharidosis VII. Gross and microscopic findings in β-glucuronidase-deficient mice. *Am J Pathol* 1990;136:207–17

53. Sands MS, Birkenmeier EH. A single-base-pair deletion in the β-glucuronidase gene accounts for the phenotype of murine mucopolysaccharidosis type VII. *Proc Natl Acad Sci USA* 1993;90:6567–71

54. Gitzelmann R, Bosshard NU, Superti-Furga A, Spycher MA, Briner J, Wiesmann U *et al.* Feline mucopolysaccharidosis VII due to β-glucuronidase deficiency. *Vet Pathol* 1994;31:435–43

55. Fyfe JC, Kurzhals RL, Lassaline ME, Henthorn PS, Alur PR, Wang P *et al.* Molecular basis of feline β-glucuronidase deficiency: an animal model of mucopolysaccharidosis VII. *Genomics* 1999;58:121–8

56. Vandevelde M, Fankhauser R, Bichsel P, Wiesmann U, Herschkowitz N. Hereditary neurovisceral mannosidosis associated with α-mannosidase deficiency in a family of Persian cats. *Acta Neuropathol (Berl)* 1982;58:64–8

57. Jezyk PF, Haskins ME, Newman LR. α-Mannosidosis in a Persian cat. *J Am Vet Med Assoc* 1986; 189:1483–5

58. Raghavan S, Stuer G, Riviere L, Alroy J, Kolodny EH. Characterization of α-mannosidase in feline mannosidosis. *J Inherit Metab Dis* 1988;11:3–16

59. Maenhout T, Kint JA, Dacremont G, Ducatelle R, Leroy JG, Hoorens JK. Mannosidosis in a litter of Persian cats. *Vet Rec* 1988;122:351–4

60. Cummings JF, Wood PA, de Lahunta A, Walkley SU, Le Boeuf L. The clinical and pathologic heterogeneity of feline α-mannosidosis. *J Vet Intern Med* 1988; 2:163–70

61. Castagnaro M. Lectin histochemistry of the central nervous system in a case of feline α-mannosidosis. *Res Vet Sci* 1990;49:375–7

62. Hocking JD, Jolly RD, Batt RD. Deficiency of α-mannosidase in Angus cattle. An inherited lysosomal storage disease. *Biochem J* 1972;128:69–78

63. Jolly RD. Animal model of human disease: mannosidosis of children, other inherited lysosomal storage diseases. *Am J Pathol* 1974;74:211–14

64. Jolly RD, Thompson KG, Winchester BG. Bovine mannosidosis – a model lysosomal storage disease. *Birth Defects Orig Artic Ser* 1975;11:273–8

65. Jolly RD, Thompson KG. The pathology of bovine mannosidosis. *Vet Pathol* 1978;15:141–52

66. Phillips NC, Robinson D, Winchester BG, Jolly RD. Mannosidosis in Angus cattle. The enzymic defect. *Biochem J* 1974;137:363–71

67. Embury DH, Jerrett IV. Mannosidosis in Galloway calves. *Vet Pathol* 1985;22:548–51

68. Crawley AC, Jones MZ, Bonning LE, Finnie JW, Hopwood JJ. α-Mannosidosis in the guinea pig: a new animal model for lysosomal storage disorders. *Pediatr Res* 1999;46:501–9

69. Jones MZ, Dawson G. Caprine β-mannosidosis. Inherited deficiency of β-D-mannosidase. *J Biol Chem* 1981;256:5185–8

70. Kumar K, Jones MZ, Cunningham JG, Kelley JA, Lovell KL. Caprine β-mannosidosis: phenotypic features. *Vet Rec* 1986;118:325–7

71. Lovell KL, Jones MZ. Distribution of central nervous system lesions in β-mannosidosis. *Acta Neuropathol (Berl)* 1983;62:121–6

72. Jones MZ, Cunningham JG, Dade AW, Alessi DM, Mostosky UV, Vorro JR *et al.* Caprine β-mannosidosis: clinical and pathological features. *J Neuropathol Exp Neurol* 1983;42:268–85

73. Abbitt B, Jones MZ, Kasari TR, Storts RW, Templeton JW, Holland PS *et al.* β-Mannosidosis in twelve Salers calves. *J Am Vet Med Assoc* 1991;198:109–13

74. Bryan L, Schmutz S, Hodges SD, Snyder FF. Bovine β-mannosidosis: pathologic and genetic findings in Salers calves. *Vet Pathol* 1993;30:130–9

75. Healy PJ, Kidd GN, Reuter RE, Bunce C, Hosie I, Stapleton T. β-Mannosidosis in Salers calves in Australia. *Aust Vet J* 1992;69:145

76. Patterson JS, Jones MZ, Lovell KL, Abbitt B. Neuropathology of bovine β-mannosidosis. *J Neuropathol Exp Neurol* 1991;50:538–46

77. Bosshard NU, Hubler M, Arnold S, Briner J, Spycher MA, Sommerlade HJ *et al.* Spontaneous mucolipidosis in a cat: an animal model of human I-cell disease. *Vet Pathol* 1996;33:1–13

78. Hubler M, Haskins ME, Arnold S, Kaser-Hotz B, Bosshard NU, Briner J *et al.* Mucolipidosis type II in a domestic shorthair cat. *J Small Anim Pract* 1996;37:435–41

79. Mazrier H, Van Hoeven M, Wang P, Knox VW, Aguirre GD, Holt E *et al.* Inheritance, biochemical abnormalities, and clinical features of feline mucolipidosis II: the first animal model of human I-cell disease. *J Heredity* 2003;94:353–73

80. Haskins M, Casal M, Ellinwood NM, Melniczek J, Mazrier H, Giger U. Animal models for mucopolysaccharidoses and their clinical relevance. *Acta Paediatr Suppl* 2002;439:88–97

81. Ellinwood NM, Vite CH, Haskins ME. Gene therapy for lysosomal storage diseases: the lessons and promise of animal models. *J Gene Med* 2004;6:481–506

82. Fratantoni JC, Hall CW, Neufeld EF. Hurler and Hunter syndromes: mutual correction of the defect in cultured fibroblasts. *Science* 1968;162:570–2

83. Ioannou YA, Zeidner KM, Gordon RE, Desnick RJ. Fabry disease: preclinical studies demonstrate the effectiveness of α-galactosidase A replacement in enzyme-deficient mice. *Am J Hum Genet* 2001; 68:14–25

84. Krivit W, Aubourg P, Shapiro E, Peters C. Bone marrow transplantation for globoid cell leukodystrophy,

adrenoleukodystrophy, metachromatic leukodystrophy, and Hurler syndrome. *Curr Opin Hematol* 1999;6:377–82

85. Brochstein JA. Bone marrow transplantation for genetic disorders. *Oncology* (Williston Park) 1992; 6:51–8; discussion 58, 63–6

86. Haskins M, Abkowitz J, Aguirre G, Casal M, Evans SM, Hasson C et al. Bone marrow transplantation in animal models of lysosomal storage diseases. In: Ringden O, Hobbs JR, Stewards C, editors. Correction of genetic diseases. Middlesex: COGENT press; 1977. p. 1–11

87. Haskins M. Bone marrow transplantation therapy for metabolic disease: animal models as predictors of success and *in utero* approaches. *Bone Marrow Transplant* 1996;18 (Suppl 3):S25–7

88. Hoogerbrugge PM, Valerio D. Bone marrow transplantation and gene therapy for lysosomal storage diseases. *Bone Marrow Transplant* 1998;21 (Suppl 2):S34–6

89. O'Marcaigh AS, Cowan MJ. Bone marrow transplantation for inherited diseases. *Curr Opin Oncol* 1997;9:126–30

90. Wraith JE. Enzyme replacement therapy in mucopolysaccharidosis type I: progress and emerging difficulties. *J Inherit Metab Dis* 2001;24:245–50

91. Sands MS, Vogler C, Torrey A, Levy B, Gwynn B, Grubb J et al. Murine mucopolysaccharidosis type VII: long-term therapeutic effects of enzyme replacement and enzyme replacement followed by bone marrow transplantation. *J Clin Invest* 1997; 99:1596–605

92. Daly TM, Vogler C, Levy B, Haskins ME, Sands MS. Neonatal gene transfer leads to widespread correction of pathology in a murine model of lysosomal storage disease. *Proc Natl Acad Sci USA* 1999;96:2296–300

93. Daly TM, Ohlemiller KK, Roberts MS, Vogler CA, Sands MS. Prevention of systemic clinical disease in MPS VII mice following AAV-mediated neonatal gene transfer. *Gene Ther* 2001;8:1291–8

94. Ponder KP, Melniczek JR, Xu L, Weil MA, O'Malley TM, O'Donnell PA et al. Therapeutic neonatal hepatic gene therapy in mucopolysaccharidosis VII dogs. *Proc Natl Acad Sci USA* 2002;99:13102–7

95. Xu L, Haskins ME, Melniczek JR, Gao C, Weil MA, O'Malley TM et al. Transduction of hepatocytes after neonatal delivery of a Moloney murine leukemia virus based retroviral vector results in long-term expression of β-glucuronidase in mucopolysaccharidosis VII dogs. *Mol Ther* 2002;5:141–53

96. Xu L, Mango RL, Sands MS, Haskins ME, Ellinwood NM, Ponder KP. Evaluation of pathological manifestations of disease in mucopolysaccharidosis VII mice after neonatal hepatic gene therapy. *Mol Ther* 2002; 6:745–58

97. Ohshima T, Schiffmann R, Murray GJ, Kopp J, Quirk JM, Stahl S et al. Aging accentuates and bone marrow

transplantation ameliorates metabolic defects in Fabry disease mice. *Proc Natl Acad Sci USA* 1999;96:6423–7

98. Takenaka T, Murray GJ, Qin G, Quirk JM, Ohshima T, Qasba P et al. Long-term enzyme correction and lipid reduction in multiple organs of primary and secondary transplanted Fabry mice receiving transduced bone marrow cells. *Proc Natl Acad Sci USA* 2000;97:7515–20

99. Qin G, Takenaka T, Telsch K, Kelley L, Howard T, Levade T et al. Preselective gene therapy for Fabry disease. *Proc Natl Acad Sci USA* 2001;98:3428–33

100. Jung SC, Han IP, Limaye A, Xu R, Gelderman MP, Zerfas P et al. Adeno-associated viral vector-mediated gene transfer results in long-term enzymatic and functional correction in multiple organs of Fabry mice. *Proc Natl Acad Sci USA* 2001;98:2676–81

101. Takahashi H, Hirai Y, Migita M, Seino Y, Fukuda Y, Sakuraba H et al. Long-term systemic therapy of Fabry disease in a knockout mouse by adeno-associated virus-mediated muscle-directed gene transfer. *Proc Natl Acad Sci USA* 2002;99:13777–82

102. Park J, Murray GJ, Limaye A, Quirk JM, Gelderman MP, Brady RO et al. Long-term correction of globotriaosylceramide storage in Fabry mice by recombinant adeno-associated virus-mediated gene transfer. *Proc Natl Acad Sci USA* 2003;100:3450–4

103. Shimada T, Zenri K, Ogawa K, Takahashi H, Hirai Y, Seino Y et al. AAV vector mediated gene therapy of Fabry knockout mice. *Am J Hum Genet* 2003; 73:S626

104. Li C, Ziegler RJ, Cherry M, Lukason M, Desnick RJ, Yew NS et al. Adenovirus-transduced lung as a portal for delivering α-galactosidase A into systemic circulation for Fabry disease. *Mol Ther* 2002;5:745–54

105. Ziegler RJ, Yew NS, Li C, Cherry M, Berthelette P, Romanczuk H et al. Correction of enzymatic and lysosomal storage defects in Fabry mice by adenovirus-mediated gene transfer. *Hum Gene Ther* 1999;10:1667–82

106. Ziegler RJ, Li C, Cherry M, Zhu Y, Hempel D, van Rooijen N et al. Correction of the nonlinear dose response improves the viability of adenoviral vectors for gene therapy of Fabry disease. *Hum Gene Ther* 2002;13:935–45

107. Kobayashi T, Yamanaka T, Jacobs JM, Teixeira F, Suzuki K. The Twitcher mouse: an enzymatically authentic model of human globoid cell leukodystrophy (Krabbe disease). *Brain Res* 1980;202:479–83

108. Luzi P, Rafi MA, Victoria T, Baskin GB, Wenger DA. Characterization of the rhesus monkey galactocerebrosidase (GALC) cDNA and gene and identification of the mutation causing globoid cell leukodystrophy (Krabbe disease) in this primate. *Genomics* 1997; 42:319–24

7 General aspects of X-linked diseases

Dominique P Germain
Assistance Publique – Hôpitaux de Paris, Paris, France

Concepts of dominance and recessiveness were initially used for autosomal traits, and then applied to 'sex'-linked traits to distinguish X-linked recessive and X-linked dominant inheritance. The former was defined as vertical transmission in which carrier females pass the trait to affected sons, while the latter was defined as vertical transmission in which daughters of affected males are always affected; hence the trait can be transmitted to offspring of both sexes. However, X-linked disorders do not always fit these rules. In many of these disorders, the penetrance and severity index of the phenotype are high in males, while the severity index is low in females. However, in contrast with standard presentations of X-linked inheritance, penetrance appears highly variable in females and can be classified as high, intermediate or low. Classic definitions of X-linked recessive and dominant inheritance neither reflect the variable expressivity of X-linked disorders, nor take into account the multiple mechanisms that can lead to disease expression in females. The use of the terms X-linked recessive and dominant should probably be abandoned and all such traits simply described as following X-linked inheritance.

Introduction

More than 100 X-linked inherited human disorders or traits have now been identified (Table 1). Most of them are classified as recessive [1], a much smaller number as dominant [2] and a few as dominant and lethal in hemizygotes [3, 4]. Due to their particular mode of inheritance, X-linked diseases have a more significant place in genetic counselling than would be thought from the relative contribution of the X chromosome to the human genome. In this chapter, the issues associated with X-linked disease inheritance are discussed.

Random X-chromosome inactivation

The words 'dominant' and 'recessive' should be used cautiously to describe X-linked disorders [5], as a much higher degree of variability in heterozygotes is observed than is the case with autosomal traits. Figure 1 shows left ventricular hypertrophy in a female patient with Fabry disease, exemplifying that high penetrance of the disease is possible in heterozygotes. This is largely due to random X-chromosome inactivation [6], which affects almost an entire X chromosome in human females. In a process known as Lyonization, one of the two X chromosomes is randomly inactivated during early embryonic stages and becomes visible as the Barr body under the nuclear membrane. As the descendants of each cell keep the same pattern of inactivation, a heterozygote for an X-linked disease will be a mosaic, with two cell populations, one of which will express the normal and the other the abnormal X chromosome. As a consequence, some disorders demonstrate 'mosaic' or 'patchy' symptoms in heterozygous females [4]. More often, variability in X inactivation can lead to a milder and more variable clinical and biochemical phenotype in females than in males [2].

Table 1. *Principal Mendelian disorders following X-linked inheritance.*

Disorder	OMIM number	Locus	Gene
Addison's disease with cerebral sclerosis	300100	Xq28	ABCD1
Adrenal hypoplasia	300200	XP21.3–p21.2	DAX1
Agammaglobulinaemia, Bruton type	300300	Xq21.3–q22	BTK
Albinism, ocular	300500	Xp22.3	OA1
Albinism–deafness syndrome	300700	Xq26.3–q27.1	ADFN
Aldrich syndrome	301000	Xp11.23–p11.22	WAS
Alport syndrome	301050	Xq22.3	COL4A5
Anaemia, hereditary hypochromic	301300	Xp11.21	ALAS2
Cataract, congenital	302200	Xp	CCT
Charcot–Marie–Tooth, peroneal	302800	Xq13.1	GJB1
Choroidaemia	300390	Xq21.2	CHM
Choroidoretinal degeneration	300389	Xp21.1	RPGR
Coffin–Lowry syndrome	309580	Xq13	ATRX
Colour blindness	303800	Xq28	OPN1MW
Diabetes insipidus, nephrogenic	304800	Xq28	AVPR2
Dyskeratosis congenita	305000	Xq28	DKC1
Ectodermal dysplasia, anhidrotic	305100	Xq12–q13.1	ED1
Fabry disease	301500	Xq22	GLA
Faciogenital dysplasia (Aarskog syndrome)	305400	Xp11.21	FGD1
Focal dermal hypoplasia*	305600	Unknown	Unknown
Glucose-6-phosphate dehydrogenase deficiency	305900	Xq28	G6PD
Glycogen storage disease type VIII	306000	Xp22.2–p22.1	PHKA2
Gonadal dysgenesis (XY female type)	306100	Xp22.11–p21.2	GDXY
Granulomatous disease (chronic)	306400	Xp21.1	CYBB
Haemophilia A	306700	Xq28	F8
Haemophilia B	306900	Xq27.1–q27.2	F9
Hydrocephalus (aqueduct stenosis)	307000	Xq28	L1CAM
Hypophosphataemic rickets	307800	Xp22.2–p22.1	PHEX
Incontinentia pigmenti*	308300	Xq28	IKBKG
Kallmann syndrome	308700	Xp22.3	KAL1
Keratosis follicularis spinulosa	308800	Xp22.1	SAT
Lesch–Nyhan syndrome (hypoxanthine-guanine-phosphoribosyl transferase deficiency)	308000	Xq26–q27.2	HPRT1
Lowe (oculocerebrorenal) syndrome	309000	Xq26.1	OCRL
Menkes syndrome	309400	Xq12–q13	ATP7A
Mental retardation, with or without fragile site (numerous specific types)	309530	Xp11.3–q21.1	MRX1
Microphthalmia with multiple anomalies (Lenz syndrome)	309800	Xq27–q28	MAA
Muscular atrophy	313200	Xq11–q12	AR
Muscular dystrophy (Becker, Duchenne and Emery–Dreifuss types)	310300	Xq28	EMD
Myotubular myopathy	310400	Xq28	MTM1
Night blindness, congenital stationary	310500	Xp11.4	CSNB1

continued

Table 1. *Principal Mendelian disorders following X-linked inheritance (continued).*

Disorder	OMIM number	Locus	Gene
Norrie's disease (pseudoglioma)	310600	Xp11.4	*NDP*
Nystagmus, oculomotor or 'jerky'	310700	Xq26–q27	*NYS1*
Ornithine transcarbamylase deficiency (type I hyperammonaemia)	311250	Xp21.1	*OTC*
Orofaciodigital syndrome (type I)	311200	Xp22.3–p22.2	*OFD1*
Phosphoglycerate kinase deficiency	311800	Xq13	*PGK1*
Phosphoribosylpyrophosphate synthetase deficiency	311850	Xq22–q24	*PRPS1*
Retinitis pigmentosa	312610	Xp21.1	*RPGR*
Retinoschisis	312700	Xp22.2–p22.1	*RS1*
Rett syndrome*	312750	Xq28, Xp22	*MECP2*
Spastic paraplegia	303350	Xq28	*L1CAM*
Spinal muscular atrophy	313200	Xq11–q12	*AR*
Spondyloepiphyseal dysplasia tarda	313400	Xp22.2–p22.1	*SEDL*
Testicular feminization syndrome	300068	Xq11–q12	*AR*
Thrombocytopenia, hereditary	313900	Xp11.23–p11.22	*WAS*
Thyroxine-binding globulin, absence	314200	Xq22.2	*TBG*

*X-linked lethality in the male.

Although inactivation applies to almost the entire human X chromosome, there are a few loci that escape inactivation. The short arm of the X chromosome is homologous, in its terminal region, with part of the Y chromosome [7]. This allows pairing between the sex chromosomes during meiosis. A different region of the X chromosome, the X-inactivation centre, located on the proximal long arm, is involved in the control of the X inactivation process [8].

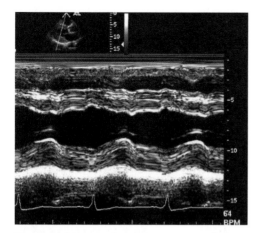

Figure 1. *Echocardiogram (TM mode) showing left ventricular hypertrophy (cardiac mass, 310 g) with increased septum (14 mm) and posterior wall (14 mm) thickness in a 60-year-old female heterozygote with Fabry disease. BPM, beats per minute.*

Identification of X-linked inheritance

In X-linked inheritance, the following simple rules apply to most genetic counselling issues [2].

- Male-to-male transmission does not exist, as a man never passes his X chromosome to his sons.
- All daughters of an affected man will inherit the mutant gene.
- Women who are carriers have a 50% chance of passing the mutant gene to their sons.
- Similarly, 50% of the daughters of heterozygous women will themselves be heterozygous for the disorder.
- Affected homozygous females are exceptionally rare in X-linked recessive disorders [9].

- Unaffected males do not transmit the disease to offspring of either gender. The only exception to this is fragile-X mental retardation [10], where normal transmitting males can carry a premutation [11].

The possibility of non-paternity or occurrence of the disorder in a female affected with Turner syndrome should be considered in cases of discrepancy with these rules.

Classic X-linked recessive pattern of inheritance

Recessive genes on the X chromosome have different consequences in males and females. A mutated recessive gene on the X chromosome tends to have little impact in a female because there is a second, normal, copy of the gene on the other X chromosome. By contrast, a mutated recessive X-linked gene will have an impact in a male because the genes on the Y chromosome are different from those on the X chromosome, and no second copy of the gene exists. The male must therefore pass the mutated X-linked gene to all of his daughters, but does not pass it to his sons, who all receive his Y chromosome.

Disorders where affected males do not reproduce

In cases of X-linked disorders in which the affected males do not survive to reproduce, the absence of male-to-male transmission cannot be tested. One-third of isolated cases of affected males are due to new mutations, whereas the mutation is inherited from a heterozygous mother in the remaining two-thirds of cases [12]. These proportions, however, may vary in disorders in which the mutation rate is different in the paternal and maternal lineages [2].

X-linked dominant inheritance

Classic X-linked dominant inheritance may be mistaken for autosomal dominant inheritance, but if descendants of affected males are considered, all sons are healthy while all daughters are affected. The excess of affected female heterozygotes may also be indicative of X-linked dominant inheritance.

X-linked dominant inheritance with lethality in the male

X-linked dominant disorders that are lethal in males *in utero* are, by definition, seen only in female heterozygotes, the affected (hemizygous) males appearing as an excess of spontaneous abortions. This situation is well known for several disorders, including incontinentia pigmenti [13] and Rett syndrome [14]. With regard to genetic counselling, it should be kept in mind that, leaving aside spontaneous abortions, one-third of the offspring of an affected woman will be affected; all the live-born males will be unaffected, as will half of the females. Two-thirds of all live offspring will be females.

Frequent X-linked mutations

If an X-linked mutation is frequent in a given population, misleading family trees may occur. For example, in European populations, it is not uncommon for both parents to carry the mutant gene leading to colour blindness (i.e. an affected male and a heterozygous female). In such cases, all female offspring will carry the mutant allele on one or both X chromosomes. In turn, the sons of the homozygous female offspring will all be affected [2]. Such a pedigree pattern can also be observed with rarer traits in cases of consanguinity or endogamy [15].

Identification of individuals heterozygous for X-linked diseases
The risk of being a carrier

In inherited disorders, a carrier is often defined as an individual who is heterozygous for the gene responsible for an inherited disorder and who has no signs or symptoms of the disease at the time of investigation (but see Chapter 34). It is important to estimate by pedigree analysis the *a priori* genetic risk that a female relative of an affected individual is a carrier, in order to interpret correctly the information obtained from laboratory carrier testing.

X-linked recessive disorders are the most important diseases in terms of detecting carriers. Indeed, in X-linked disorders, carriers are usually healthy and will consequently be likely to reproduce, with the risk of giving birth to affected male offspring. In this context, the detection of women at high risk of being heterozygous for an X-linked disorder forms such an integral part of genetic counselling that it is often unwise to give a definitive risk estimate until information from testing is available [2].

In classic X-linked recessive diseases, a few heterozygous females may occasionally be clinically detectable, probably as a consequence of skewed X-chromosome inactivation, which results in a higher percentage of the X chromosomes bearing the mutant gene being expressed in the particular tissue of importance. In contrast, skewed inactivation can also result in carriers in whom a higher percentage of the X chromosomes bearing the normal gene are expressed. Such variability in symptom severity is characteristic of X-linked heterozygotes [5] and should be kept in mind when assessing and diagnosing potential patients. The most widely used phenotypic test for carrier detection in Fabry disease is an enzymatic assay that detects decreases in levels of α-galactosidase A in leukocytes. However, the enzymatic assay demonstrates a large overlap in values between normal individuals and heterozygotes, which makes it almost impossible to classify at-risk females dependably without genotyping [16]. DNA-based tests are not influenced by X inactivation, which is a key reason for their wide use in detecting X-linked heterozygotes.

Detection of female heterozygotes is feasible in some X-linked disorders. The spectrum of methods is wide and may be morphological, functional, biochemical or molecular. As a group, X-linked disorders are probably the most interesting in terms of our ability to identify the carrier state and, consequently, to prevent recurrence of the genetic disease in subsequent generations [2].

Isolated cases of an X-linked disorder
Any isolated case of an X-linked disease is a source of additional difficulty in detection of heterozygotes. There is huge uncertainty as to the percentage of cases that are due to *de-novo* mutations and, correspondingly, the proportions of mothers who are heterozygotes. It is probable that this varies from one disease to another.

Conclusions

Standard definitions of X-linked recessive and dominant inheritance do not capture the variable expressivity of X-linked disorders or take into account the multiple mechanisms that can result in disease expression in females. These include skewed X inactivation [17, 18], clonal expansion [19] and somatic mosaicism [20, 21]. Use of the terms X-linked recessive and dominant should probably be discontinued and all such disorders simply described as following X-linked inheritance [5].

References

1. McKusick V. Mendelian inheritance in man. 12th edn. Baltimore: John Hopkins University Press; 1998

2. Harper PS. Practical genetic counselling. 6th edn. London: Arnold; 2004

3. Wettke-Schafer R, Kantner G. X-linked dominant inherited diseases with lethality in hemizygous males. *Hum Genet* 1983;64:1–23

4. Happle R. Lyonization and the lines of Blaschko. *Hum Genet* 1985;70:200–6

5. Dobyns WB, Filauro A, Tomson BN, Chan AS, Ho AW, Ting NT et al. Inheritance of most X-linked traits is not dominant or recessive, just X-linked. *Am J Med Genet A* 2004;129:136–43

6. Lyon MF. Gene action in the X-chromosome of the mouse (*Mus musculus* L.). *Nature* 1961;190:372–3

7. Ellis N, Goodfellow PN. The mammalian pseudo-autosomal region. *Trends Genet* 1989;5:406–10

8. Herzing LB, Romer JT, Horn JM, Ashworth A. Xist has properties of the X-chromosome inactivation centre. *Nature* 1997;386:272–5

9. Rodriguez-Mari A, Coll MJ, Chabas A. Molecular analysis in Fabry disease in Spain: fifteen novel GLA mutations and identification of a homozygous female. *Hum Mutat* 2003;22:258

10. Sherman SL, Jacobs PA, Morton NE, Froster-Iskenius U, Howard-Peebles PN, Nielsen KB *et al*. Further segregation analysis of the fragile X syndrome with special reference to transmitting males. *Hum Genet* 1985;69:289–99

11. Fu YH, Kuhl DP, Pizzuti A, Pieretti M, Sutcliffe JS, Richards S *et al*. Variation of the CGG repeat at the fragile X site results in genetic instability: resolution of the Sherman paradox. *Cell* 1991;67:1047–58

12. Haldane JB. The rate of spontaneous mutation of a human gene. 1935. *J Genet* 2004;83:235–44

13. Smahi A, Courtois G, Rabia SH, Doffinger R, Bodemer C, Munnich A *et al*. The NF-kappaB signalling pathway in human diseases: from incontinentia pigmenti to ectodermal dysplasias and immune-deficiency syndromes. *Hum Mol Genet* 2002;11:2371–5

14. Amir RE, Van den Veyver IB, Wan M, Tran CQ, Francke U, Zoghbi HY. Rett syndrome is caused by mutations in X-linked MECP2, encoding methyl-CpG-binding protein 2. *Nat Genet* 1999;23:185–8

15. Zlotogora J. Problems in diagnosis and delineation of inherited disorders in highly inbred populations. *Am J Med Genet* 1991;41:451–3

16. Germain DP, Poenaru L. Fabry disease: identification of novel α-galactosidase A mutations and molecular carrier detection by use of fluorescent chemical cleavage of mismatches. *Biochem Biophys Res Commun* 1999;257:708–13

17. Maier EM, Kammerer S, Muntau AC, Wichers M, Braun A, Roscher AA. Symptoms in carriers of adreno-leukodystrophy relate to skewed X inactivation. *Ann Neurol* 2002;52:683–8

18. Plenge RM, Stevenson RA, Lubs HA, Schwartz CE, Willard HF. Skewed X-chromosome inactivation is a common feature of X-linked mental retardation disorders. *Am J Hum Genet* 2002;71:168–73

19. Rosti V. The molecular basis of paroxysmal nocturnal hemoglobinuria. *Haematologica* 2000;85:82–7

20. Gleeson JG, Minnerath S, Kuzniecky RI, Dobyns WB, Young ID, Ross ME *et al*. Somatic and germline mosaic mutations in the doublecortin gene are associated with variable phenotypes. *Am J Hum Genet* 2000;67:574–81

21. Wolach B, Scharf Y, Gavrieli R, de Boer M, Roos D. Unusual late presentation of X-linked chronic granulomatous disease in an adult female with a somatic mosaic for a novel mutation in CYBB. *Blood* 2005;105:61–6

8 Laboratory diagnosis of lysosomal storage diseases

Soumeya Bekri

Medical Biochemistry Laboratory, Rouen CHU, Hôpital Charles Nicolle, Anneau Central, 76031 Rouen, Cedex, France

Sophisticated laboratory biochemical and molecular genetic techniques are often necessary to establish a definitive diagnosis of lysosomal storage diseases (LSDs). Measurements of the accumulated primary substrate or lysosomal enzyme activities in blood, urine, amniotic fluid and cultured skin fibroblasts are the usual initial approaches to laboratory diagnosis and screening. Secondary biochemical changes, however, may also occur and may be sufficiently disease specific to be used in the diagnosis of LSDs and the subsequent monitoring of disease progression and response to treatment.

Introduction

Lysosomal storage diseases (LSDs) represent a heterogeneous group of disorders that all have one feature in common: progressive and massive accumulation of a variety of non-metabolized macromolecular substrates within lysosomes. This chapter provides insights into the general approach and the tools used for the diagnosis of LSDs, together with a brief description of lysosomal function, biogenesis and the heterogeneity of LSDs.

Lysosomal enzyme function

The lysosome is an intracellular organelle that is responsible for the degradation of intra-cellular and extracellular macromolecules into monomers that can be reutilized by the cell or eliminated. Thus, numerous lysosomal acid hydrolases catabolize a wide variety of sub-strates, such as proteins, carbohydrates, lipids and sulphates. Some of these lysosomal en-zymes require a specific intracellular environ-ment to be functionally active (Table 1).

Activator proteins

The function of some hydrolases, involved in the catabolism of glycosphingolipids,

requires the presence of activator proteins. The following two types of activator proteins have been identified.

Sphingolipid activator proteins
Four sphingolipid activator proteins (sapo-sins) originate from a single precursor – prosaposin. These saposins, designated A, B, C and D, act as cofactors for the hydro-lases involved in the catabolism of different glycosphingolipids and thus control glyco-sphingolipid flux within the lysosome [1, 2] (Table 1).

GM2-activator protein
The GM2-activator protein is a small protein (16 kDa) associated with β-hexosaminidases A and B [3].

Multi-enzyme complexes

The catalytic activity of some lysosomal pro-teins is exhibited only when the proteins are incorporated into multi-enzyme complexes. Thus, α-neuraminidase and β-galactosidase are functional when associated together with protective protein/cathepsin A (PPCA) in a single complex.

Table 1. *Proteins required for the functional activity of some hydrolases.*

Protein	Enzyme		Associated disease
	Name	**Number**	
Prosaposin			Complex sphingolipidosis
Saposin A	Galactocerebrosidase	EC 3.2.1.46	Krabbe disease
Saposin B	α-Galactosidase A	EC 3.2.1.22	
	Arylsulphatase A	EC 3.1.6.8	Metachromatic leukodystrophy
	β-Galactosidase	EC 3.2.1.23	
Saposin C	Glucocerebrosidase	EC 3.2.1.45	Gaucher disease
	Galactocerebrosidase	EC 3.2.1.46	Gaucher disease
Saposin D	Ceramidase	EC 3.5.1.23	
GM2-activator	β-Hexosaminidase	EC 3.2.1.52	GM2-gangliosidosis
PPCA	β-Galactosidase	EC 3.2.1.23	Galactosialidosis
	α-Neuraminidase	EC 3.2.1.18	
SUMF1	Sulphatases		Multiple sulphatase deficiency

PPCA, protective protein/cathepsin A; SUMF1, sulphatase-modifying factor 1.

Chemical modification

Other enzymes, such as sulphatases, require chemical modification of a cysteine residue to Cα-formylglycine at the catalytic site in order to exert their activity. This modification is catalysed by sulphatase-modifying factor 1 (SUMF1) [4].

Lysosome biogenesis

Biogenesis of the lysosome is complex. The lysosome is one component of the endo-somal–lysosomal system [5]. A finely balanced dynamic links these different compartments, and the system is also tightly linked to the trans-Golgi network (TGN). Mannose-6-phosphate (M6P) receptors – the 46 kDa cation-dependent M6P receptor and the 300 kDa cation-independent M6P receptor – bind newly synthesized lysosomal enzymes in the TGN and transport them to the endosomal–lysosomal system. This trafficking is responsible for endocytosis, autophagy and exocytosis [6].

In addition to its macromolecule-degrading function, this system has recently been found to have other specific functions associated with its major membrane proteins. These proteins are highly glycosylated and have been termed lysosome-associated membrane proteins (LAMPs), lysosomal glyco-proteins or lysosomal integral membrane proteins (LIMPs) [7–10]. The function of these membrane proteins is discussed in Chapter 3.

Heterogeneity of LSDs

Given the multiple steps and numerous pathways involved in lysosomal biogenesis, it is not surprising that there are many points at which changes can produce adverse metabolic effects. Indeed, some 50 disorders have been described as a result of alterations in specific genes (see Chapter 2), with a combined prevalence of approximately 1 in 5000 births [11]. The primary consequence of abnormal processing of substrates or altered transport of metabolites through the lysosomal membrane is the accumulation of these molecules in the lysosome. The occurrence of different subtypes of the same disorder and the large spectrum of phenotypes in these disorders make recognition and diagnosis difficult. Storage may begin during early embryonic development, and the clinical presentation for a particular disease can vary from an early and very severe phenotype to late-onset mild disease.

Laboratory diagnosis of LSDs

Biochemical and genetic diagnosis of LSDs should be performed in specialized laboratories. Various clinical samples can be used for analysis, such as blood, urine, amniotic fluid, skin fibroblasts and tissue biopsies.

Measurement of the accumulated substrate is often the first approach when an LSD is suspected or in screening programmes. Specific secondary changes may also occur in cells associated with a lysosomal deficiency. Such changes may result in the modification of other proteins or cellular components that may be useful as markers of specific diseases, or for following disease progression. Identification of the molecular basis of a disorder may enable the use of more specific testing, such as the assessment of lysosomal enzymes and molecular analyses.

The tests performed for diagnosis can be divided into the six categories outlined below.

Commonly used screening tests

Urinary oligosaccharides
Urinary oligosaccharide screening is performed by high-performance thin-layer chromatography (HPTLC), using the technique first described by Humbel and colleagues [12]. This method, however, has severe limitations. Metabolite quantification is not possible, and the identification of metabolites is assumed on the basis of migration rates. Definitive

identification of specific metabolites is therefore not possible. Furthermore, several medications or physiological situations can produce an abnormal profile. Despite these limitations, this screening technique can provide an initial indication of a possible diagnosis, although further investigations are needed to confirm the diagnosis. Examples of disorders that present with an abnormal HPTLC profile are aspartylglucosaminuria, GM1-gangliosidosis, GM2-gangliosidosis, sialidosis, galactosialidosis, fucosidosis, α-mannosidosis and glycogen storage disease type II.

Urinary glycosaminoglycans
Mucopolysaccharidoses (MPS) may be suspected from measurements of urinary glycosaminoglycans (GAGs). After purification by repeated precipitation with cetylpyridinium chloride, GAGs are isolated by centrifugation and quantified by a colorimetric assay, often using harmine [13, 14]. This method assesses the amount of hexuronic acid contained in the extracted GAGs and can give false-negative results when the accumulated GAG is keratin sulphate, which contains galactose instead of hexuronic acid; in this case the diagnosis of Morquio disease may be missed.

The second pitfall when quantifying GAGs is linked to the progressive decrease of urinary GAG levels that occurs with age. In the case of MPS, the normal age-related decline in urinary GAGs should be taken into account when diagnosis is suspected in older individuals.

One-dimensional electrophoresis is used to separate the main classes of GAGs: chondroitin sulphate, keratan sulphate, dermatan sulphate and heparan sulphate [14]. In the normal physiological situation, only chondroitin sulphate is detectable, except in the urine of newborns, where a band corresponding to heparan sulphate may be present. Although urinary GAG levels may be affected by nutrient

Table 2. Biochemical classification of the mucopolysaccharidoses (MPS).

Disease	Enzyme/protein deficiency	GAGs detected
MPS type I (Hurler/Sheie syndrome)	α-L-Iduronidase	Dermatan sulphate/ heparan sulphate
MPS type II (Hunter syndrome)	Idurate-2-sulphatase	Dermatan sulphate/ heparan sulphate
MPS type IIIA (Sanfilippo syndrome)	Heparan-N-sulphatase	Heparan sulphate
MPS type IIIB (Sanfilippo syndrome)	α-N-Acetylglucosaminidase	Heparan sulphate
MPS type IIIC (Sanfilippo syndrome)	AcetylCoA:N-acetyltransferase	Heparan sulphate
MPS type IIID (Sanfilippo syndrome)	N-Acetylglucosamine-6-sulphatase	Heparan sulphate
MPS type IVA (Morquio syndrome)	Galactose-6-sulphatase	Keratan sulphate
MPS type IVB (Morquio syndrome)	β-Galactosidase	Keratan sulphate/ chondroitin sulphate
MPS type VI (Maroteaux– Lamy syndrome)	N-Acetylgalactosamine-4-sulphatase	Dermatan sulphate
MPS type VII (Sly syndrome)	β-Glucuronidase	Dermatan sulphate/ chondroitin sulphate
MPS type IX	Hyaluronidase	Hyaluran

GAGs, glycosaminoglycans.

levels and drugs, the detection of keratan sulphate, dermatan sulphate and heparan sulphate may suggest the possibility of an MPS. The individual diseases and the specific products that accumulate in each condition are reported in Table 2.

Global tests

Recognition of the high combined pre-valence of LSDs and the increasing avail-ability of specific therapies have encouraged the search for reliable biomarkers that can be used to identify LSDs in newborns or in high-risk populations. It has been suggested that LAMP-1 [15], LAMP-2 [16], saposins [17] and GM2-ganglioside [18] are elevated in almost all LSDs. However, further studies measuring LAMP-1 and saposin C, along with quantification of specific substrates, in blood spots from newborn infants [11] and in amniotic fluid [19] failed to show consistent changes in these putative biomarkers, even within the same disorder.

Assessment of specific substrates

The development of tandem mass spectro-metry for the identification and quantification of lysosomal substrates and metabolites has been a significant advance in the diagnosis of LSDs [11, 19]. In almost all cases, glyco-sphingolipids and oligosaccharides analysed by this method have been shown to differ significantly in controls and affected patients: 12 diseases were identified in 47 patients, with only two cases not presenting with an elevation of the corresponding substrate [11].

Assessment of lysosomal enzyme activities

Lysosomal enzyme activities are usually determined by a fluorometric assay in cultured fibroblasts, leukocytes or sera, using a 4-methylumbelliferyl-containing fluorescent substrate. The activity of another lysosomal enzyme should also be assayed as a control for cell integrity.

LSDs can be associated with either low or undetectable enzyme activity. In some diseases, a correlation has been found between the level of residual enzyme activity and phenotypic severity [20].

A direct multiplex assay of lysosomal enzyme activity has been proposed for screening newborn infants. This assay uses specific substrates involved in five LSDs (Fabry, Gaucher, Niemann–Pick types A and B, Krabbe and Pompe diseases) and tandem mass spectrometry to analyse the obtained metabolites [21].

It is noteworthy that, in some cases, lysosomal enzyme activity *in vitro* can be low in samples taken from individuals who do not have an LSD, a condition termed pseudodeficiency. Such pseudodeficiency has been reported for β-galactocerebrosidase, β-glucuronidase, β-glucosidase, β-hexosaminidase A and arylsulphatase A, and is linked to specific mutations [22].

Indirect biomarkers

Indirect biomarkers may be useful for the identification of LSDs and for monitoring the effects of treatment. For example, increased plasma levels of two molecules, chitotriosidase and CCL-18/pulmonary and activation-regulated chemokine (PARC), have been reported in patients with Gaucher disease (see Chapter 9).

Molecular genetics

LSDs are monogenic diseases, the majority of which have an autosomal recessive mode of inheritance. To date, X-linked inheritance has been observed in Hunter disease, Fabry disease and Danon disease. Identification of the mutations responsible for the LSDs has facilitated understanding of the pathophysiology of these diseases. It also enables prenatal and postnatal testing and allows the provision of genetic counselling.

Non-immune hydrops fetalis

The use of laboratory diagnosis can be illustrated in the case of non-immune hydrops fetalis. This is a relatively common and recurrent antenatal presentation in several LSDs, including MPS VII, MPS IVA, sialic storage disease, sialidosis type II, galactosialidosis, mucolipidosis type II, GM1-gangliosidosis, Gaucher disease type II, Niemann–Pick disease type C and Farber lipogranulomatosis [23]. Isolated neonatal ascites has also been described [24], in which urinary excretion of storage metabolites occurred at approximately 12 weeks when the fetal kidneys became functional. The metabolites then appeared in the amniotic fluid. Specific lysosomal investigations are therefore recommended when non-immune hydrops fetalis is identified. These should include screening for the abnormal presence of GAGs, oligosaccharides and sialic acid, and assessment of hydrolase activities in amniotic fluid supernatant. Additionally, enzymatic studies should be conducted on cultured amniotic fluid cells.

Conclusions

The phenotypic heterogeneity of LSDs can be partially related to variations in residual enzyme activity; however, the correlation is not reliable and other conditions may modulate the clinical presentation, such as modifiying genes and epigenetic factors. Thus, although understanding of the molecular basis of the known LSDs is increasing, several aspects remain unclear. In addition, some patients may present with clinical features of LSDs in the absence of a definitive diagnosis, possibly due to deficiencies in previously unidentified or newly identified lysosomal proteins [25]. The complexity of the metabolic and cellular transport pathways associated with the lysosome, and the phenotypic variability of individual LSDs, underline the importance of appropriate biological investigations for patient identification and management.

References

1. Leonova T, Qi X, Bencosme A, Ponce E, Sun Y, Grabowski GA. Proteolytic processing patterns of prosaposin in insect and mammalian cells. *J Biol Chem* 1996;271:17312–20

2. O'Brien JS, Kishimoto Y. Saposin proteins: structure, function, and role in human lysosomal storage disorders. *FASEB J* 1991;5:301–8

3. Conzelmann E, Sandhoff K, Nehrkorn H, Geiger B, Arnon R. Purification, biochemical and immunological characterisation of hexosaminidase A from variant AB of infantile GM2 gangliosidosis. *Eur J Biochem* 1978;84:27–33

4. Dierks T, Schmidt B, Borissenko LV, Peng J, Preusser A, Mariappan M et al. Multiple sulfatase deficiency is caused by mutations in the gene encoding the human C(α)-formylglycine generating enzyme. *Cell* 2003; 113:435–44

5. de Duve C, Wattiaux R. Functions of lysosomes. *Annu Rev Physiol* 1966;28:435–92

6. Reddy A, Caler EV, Andrews NW. Plasma membrane repair is mediated by Ca(2^+)-regulated exocytosis of lysosomes. *Cell* 2001;106:157–69

7. Andrejewski N, Punnonen EL, Guhde G, Tanaka Y, Lullmann-Rauch R, Hartmann D et al. Normal lysosomal morphology and function in LAMP-1-deficient mice. *J Biol Chem* 1999;274:12692–701

8. Gamp AC, Tanaka Y, Lullmann-Rauch R, Wittke D, D'Hooge R, De Deyn PP et al. LIMP-2/LGP85 deficiency causes ureteric pelvic junction obstruction, deafness and peripheral neuropathy in mice. *Hum Mol Genet* 2003;12:631–46

9. Eskelinen EL, Illert AL, Tanaka Y, Schwarzmann G, Blanz J, Von Figura K et al. Role of LAMP-2 in lysosome biogenesis and autophagy. *Mol Biol Cell* 2002;13:3355–68

10. Kuronita T, Eskelinen EL, Fujita H, Saftig P, Himeno M, Tanaka Y. A role for the lysosomal membrane protein LGP85 in the biogenesis and maintenance of endosomal and lysosomal morphology. *J Cell Sci* 2002; 115:4117–31

11. Meikle PJ, Ranieri E, Simonsen H, Rozaklis T, Ramsay SL, Whitfield PD et al. Newborn screening for lysosomal storage disorders: clinical evaluation of a two-tier strategy. *Pediatrics* 2004;114:909–16

12. Humbel R, Collart M. Oligosaccharides in urine of patients with glycoprotein storage diseases. I. Rapid detection by thin-layer chromatography. *Clin Chim Acta* 1975;60:143–5

13. Pennock CA, Barnes IC. The mucopolysaccharidoses. *J Med Genet* 1976;13:169–81

14. Piraud M, Boyer S, Mathieu M, Maire I. Diagnosis of mucopolysaccharidoses in a clinically selected population by urinary glycosaminoglycan analysis: a study of 2,000 urine samples. Clin Chim Acta 1993; 221:171–81

15. Meikle PJ, Brooks DA, Ravenscroft EM, Yan M, Williams RE, Jaunzems AE et al. Diagnosis of lysosomal storage disorders: evaluation of lysosome-associated membrane protein LAMP-1 as a diagnostic marker. *Clin Chem* 1997;43:1325–35

16. Hua CT, Hopwood JJ, Carlsson SR, Harris RJ, Meikle PJ. Evaluation of the lysosome-associated membrane protein LAMP-2 as a marker for lysosomal storage disorders. *Clin Chem* 1998;44:2094–102

17. Chang MH, Bindloss CA, Grabowski GA, Qi X, Winchester B, Hopwood JJ et al. Saposins A, B, C, and D in plasma of patients with lysosomal storage disorders. *Clin Chem* 2000;46:167–74

18. Walkley SU. Secondary accumulation of gangliosides in lysosomal storage disorders. *Semin Cell Dev Biol* 2004;15:433–44

19. Ramsay SL, Maire I, Bindloss C, Fuller M, Whitfield PD, Piraud M et al. Determination of oligosaccharides and glycolipids in amniotic fluid by electrospray ionisation tandem mass spectrometry: *in utero* indicators of lysosomal storage diseases. *Mol Genet Metab* 2004;83:231–8

20. Conzelmann E, Sandhoff K. Partial enzyme deficiencies: residual activities and the development of neurological disorders. *Dev Neurosci* 1983;6:58–71

21. Li Y, Scott CR, Chamoles NA, Ghavami A, Pinto BM, Turecek F et al. Direct multiplex assay of lysosomal enzymes in dried blood spots for newborn screening. *Clin Chem* 2004;50:1785–96

22. Zlotogora J, Bach G. Deficiency of lysosomal hydrolases in apparently healthy individuals. *Am J Med Genet* 1983;14:73–80

23. Palladini G, Venturini G, Conforti A, Medolago-Albani L, Zelazek S, Pistone A et al. [Copper and nervous system. An experimental study (author's transl)]. *Pathol Biol* (Paris) 1977;25:299–306

24. Saxonhouse MA, Behnke M, Williams JL, Richards D, Weiss MD. Mucopolysaccharidosis type VII presenting with isolated neonatal ascites. *J Perinatol* 2003;23:73–5

25. Kubo Y, Sekiya S, Ohigashi M, Takenaka C, Tamura K, Nada S et al. ABCA5 resides in lysosomes, and ABCA5 knockout mice develop lysosomal disease-like symptoms. *Mol Cell Biol* 2005;25:4138–49

9 Biomarkers in lysosomal storage diseases

Timothy M Cox

Department of Medicine, University of Cambridge, Addenbrooke's Hospital, Cambridge CB2 2QQ, UK

Biomarkers have long been used to reflect the presence of a given disease (diagnostic biomarkers) or the activity of a given condition either during its natural course or in response to therapeutic intervention. Biomarkers may also have prognostic significance for disease outcome, and emphasis is placed on those quantitative biomarkers which correlate with the clinical manifestations of the disease that affect quality of life, risk of complications or survival (surrogate biomarkers). Surrogate biomarkers have a critical role in the pharmaceutical licensing process and the monitoring of disease after the introduction of approved treatments. Surrogate biomarkers have special significance in the monitoring of treatments for rare diseases, where the small number of patients and heterogeneous expression of their underlying pathology pose formidable difficulties for direct study and where costly treatment must be justified in terms of efficacy.

Enzyme replacement therapy and other treatments, including substrate reduction therapy and the use of molecular chaperones, are being introduced for lysosomal storage diseases (LSDs). However, apart from in Gaucher disease, there are currently very few biomarkers detectable in the blood that are available to monitor LSDs and which are in clinical use. Hence, improved biomarkers are being sought for Fabry disease, Hunter syndrome, Hurler syndrome, Maroteaux–Lamy disease and Pompe disease. Once a new candidate biomarker is identified, rigorous operational evaluation will be required to authenticate its application in the clinical setting.

The pre-eminent importance of biomarkers in the field of LSDs is considered not only with reference to their utility, but also for the insights they may offer into the true nature and cause of the different storage diseases. Biomarkers are important factors in decisions concerning pharmaceutical regulation and licensing issues; the discovery of biomarker molecules also presents rich opportunities for contemporary clinical and basic biological research.

Introduction

A biomarker is generally an analyte that indicates the presence and/or extent of a biological process, which is itself usually directly linked to the clinical manifestations and outcome of a particular disease. The biomarker serves as an indirect but ongoing and specific correlate of disease 'activity' – a surrogate biomarker. The surrogate biomarkers of greatest use are those that facilitate the non-invasive and repeated monitoring of a given condition and have implications for understanding disease processes. Biomarkers can be used to monitor the natural course of the condition and to evaluate the efficacy of treatments; they may also contribute to the development of agreed therapeutic goals, thus providing benchmarks by which the success of chronic disease management may be judged.

Biomarkers have particular relevance in the field of the lysosomal storage diseases (LSDs), where spectacular therapeutic initiatives have been achieved, most notably with the introduction of enzyme replacement therapy (ERT). Novel biological treatments for rare diseases in the so-called 'orphan' class (where the frequency is variously defined, but always less than 1 in 1000 of the population) are subject to the same constraints as conventional therapeutic agents licensed by normal regulatory procedures. Patients with orphan diseases are entitled to treatment with drugs of the same quality, safety and efficacy as those with more common diseases; hence, there is a need for rigorous evaluation of any new agent [1]. With only small cohorts of patients available to participate in clinical trials, the development of an orphan drug, particularly a therapeutic protein, is a very expensive and high-risk investment for biotechnology companies [2]. The need for trials that are sufficiently powered to demonstrate unambiguous clinical benefits thus places particular limitations on the demonstration of therapeutic efficacy.

To compensate for the limited numbers and to obviate the need for biopsy procedures in patients already stricken by severe multi-system pathology, valid indicators for monitoring therapeutic responses are needed. Clearly, such biomarkers should be readily quantifiable in accessible tissues or fluids and provide an authentic reflection of the extent of disease in all the participants of a given therapeutic trial. In rare diseases, analytes that may be quantified specifically to reflect the presence of a given pathological process are also used for diagnosis. In addition, bio-markers have a clear application in routine clinical monitoring after the licensing of new drugs – and at the same time may provide opportunities for a better understanding of molecular pathogenesis.

Categories of biomarker used in LSDs
Direct and indirect biomarkers

There are two main types of biomarker for the LSDs. The first group is comprised of those molecules whose accumulation is directly enhanced as a result of defective lysosomal function. These molecules represent the storage of the principal macro-molecular substrate(s) of a specific enzyme or protein, the function of which is deficient in the given disease. The elevation of blood glucose and of the fraction of glycosylated haemoglobin (HbA_{1c}) or albumin, are excellent examples of direct biomarkers of the frequent disease, diabetes mellitus. These biomarkers are in widespread use for diagnosis and management of this disorder and have been used to develop therapeutic goals. Biomarkers in this category usually, but not always, reflect pathological storage of a substrate or substrates at the site where tissue injury occurs; however, on occasion, this material is also to be found in the plasma, urine or other body fluids. Once the underlying biochemical defect of a given LSD is known, it is generally relatively straightforward to search for increased abundance of this class of macromolecular substrate.

In the second category of biomarker, the relationship between the lysosomal defect and the biomarker is indirect; such biomarkers pose considerable intellectual challenges for scientific discovery. In this group, the biomarker reflects the effects of the primary lysosomal defect on cell, tissue or organ function. Such biomarkers include molecules whose concentrations in biological samples are increased as a consequence of ill-understood pathophysiological effects. These pathophysiological effects may reflect injurious changes resulting from cellular storage as well as the activation of compensatory processes used by the cell to contain or limit injury. As these effects may be experienced at numerous sites, indirect biomarkers may prove to be more informative than direct markers, providing greater information about total burden of storage and disruption of function, as their presence is amplified by the effect of cascade mechanisms peculiar to the condition.

Examples of biomarkers for LSDs in the first category would include plasma, tissue or urinary concentrations of globotriaosylceramide (Gb_3) in Fabry disease or glycosaminoglycans in the mucopolysaccharidosis (MPS) syndromes. An example of the second category of indirect biomarkers is chitotriosidase (a chitinase secreted by activated macrophages as they become engorged with glucocerebroside) in Gaucher disease [3]. The release of this chitinase is a property of the storage cell and an indirect consequence of the disease process, just as the increased volume of the spleen, with its clinical effects on the formed elements of the blood, might similarly be regarded as an operationally informative parameter for Gaucher disease as it affects the viscera [4].

Discovery of biomarkers

It must be admitted that many of the biomarkers in current use, especially those for LSDs, have been discovered either by chance or by the application of elementary reasoning with knowledge of the underlying biochemical defect [5–7]. In this respect, blood glucose and HbA_{1c} monitoring are excellent examples in the metabolic disease, diabetes mellitus; these biomarkers set the standard for routine clinical monitoring. However, the emergence of contemporary molecular methods with systematic application to altered patterns of gene expression and protein modification will have increasing power to identify many more candidate biomarkers. With the growing importance of therapeutic evaluation as new drugs are developed, there will be an ever stronger drive for the use of emerging laboratory techniques to meet the challenges of biomarker research.

Mass spectrometry methods for polypeptide identification and complementary DNA (cDNA) microarray techniques have already borne fruit in this field [8–13]. A cautionary note is needed, however, both to temper the current commercial enthusiasm for the sale of expensive machines for the identification and quantitative analysis of non-abundant biological molecules – and to highlight the formidable challenges in demonstrating a causal relationship between lysosomal storage, its tissue effects and the ultimate outcome of a given disease. Nowhere is the gap in our molecular understanding of pathogenesis more acutely felt than in the field of lysosomal diseases, where the presence of minute quantities of a storage material in association with difficult-to-understand disruption of cell function leads to far-reaching inflammatory effects, tissue injury and human disability [14].

Characteristics of ideal biomarkers for LSDs

Ideal biomarkers should have certain characteristics, some of which are summarized in Table 1. They should be easy to quantify reliably in accessible clinical samples. Many biomarkers for LSDs, including those utilized recently, require tissue biopsies (e.g. of the liver and the heart) and are clearly far from ideal. While it may be claimed that such biomarkers provide more direct evidence of the effects of storage in a given tissue, the occurrence of sampling error and the limited size of tissue obtained by biopsy render their use open to the criticism that these are unacceptably invasive methods which often demonstrate poor reproducibility.

Table 1. *Characteristics of an ideal biomarker.*

- Quick, reliable and inexpensive measurement
- Readily quantifiable in accessible clinical samples (e.g. plasma, urine)
- Expression greatly increased specifically in the relevant disease
- No overlap in biomarker levels between untreated patients and healthy control subjects
- Biomarker levels not subject to wide variation in the general population
- Biomarker levels correlate with the total burden of disease at all sites, but are unaffected by unrelated conditions and associated comorbid factors
- Biomarker levels correlate closely with the established clinicopathological parameters of disease that influence quality of life and survival
- Biomarker levels vary rapidly in response to specific treatments
- Large deviations of the biomarker from the reference values in the control population have predictive power for disease severity and prognosis

Technical considerations

Ideally, quantification of a biomarker should be simple, rapid, inexpensive and, above all, reliable. Plasma chitotriosidase is elevated several hundred-fold in Gaucher disease and has widespread use for diagnosis and for monitoring the response to specific treatments. It is notable that determination of plasma activity of chitotriosidase, an established biomarker of Gaucher disease, is subject to considerable methodological difficulty. This arises because the enzyme has both hydrolytic and transglycosidase activities towards its substrate, chitotrioside. Thus, it is not possible to assay the chitinolytic function of the enzyme under V_{max} conditions, and several dilutions are required to ensure reproducibility. The imaginative development of a novel desoxy substrate that cannot participate in the transglycosidase reaction avoids this pitfall but, as yet, is not generally available for routine use in the clinical laboratory setting. At present, there are no internationally agreed criteria for validation of chitotriosidase measurement in routine biochemical laboratories.

Genetic variation

Another operational characteristic of the ideal biomarker is that its abundance or activity should not be subject to wide variation in subjects within the general population. Again, chitotriosidase, which is subject to polymorphic genetic variation, has disadvantages: 6% of the general population, as well as patients with Gaucher disease, are completely deficient in chitotriosidase activity. This occurs because of the presence of null alleles of the human chitotriosidase gene that have arisen as a result of a DNA insertional event (iatrogenic partial gene implication). Approximately 30% of the population, whether healthy or suffering from Gaucher disease, are heterozygous for this null allele, and their chitotriosidase activity is therefore approximately one-half that of individuals expressing two functional chitotriosidase genes. In most populations, homozygosity for null alleles of chitotriosidase affects approximately 6% of individuals, rendering the use of this biomarker impossible [15].

Technical sources of variation

There are other potential sources of variation in enzyme activities and the activities of other biomarkers related to storage material. This variation may arise from non-genetic sources, including stability of the analyte within biological tissues and the presence of inhibitors in tissue samples (including the influence of chelators such as ethylenediamine tetraacetic acid or citrate and the effect of altered charge in the presence of heparin), as well as other effects related to the sample (e.g. frothing of the fluid or irregular fixation of tissue specimens). Clearly, it is of paramount importance for the biomarker to be stable within the fluid or tissue upon storage, thus allowing transport to the laboratory and an opportunity for analysis within a reasonable time-frame. It is also advantageous for a given analyte to be reproducibly quantifiable, for example after repeated freeze–thaw cycles.

Specificity

The specificity of the biomarker is an important characteristic and, ideally, its expression should be increased only in the relevant disease in which it is to be analysed. For example, chitotriosidase activity is elevated not only in patients with Gaucher disease, but also in those with the macrophage disorders Niemann–Pick disease types A and B, and other conditions, including iron-overload syndromes such as β-thalassaemia. However, the greatest increase in chitotriosidase activity compared with healthy control subjects is seen in Gaucher disease, where the increase in activity is often as much as 1000-fold in untreated subjects while it is generally increased by only about one order of magnitude in patients with other macrophage storage disorders when measured under appropriate assay conditions that allow for activity comparisons in parallel [3]. Spectacular elevation of a biomarker, specifically in relation to a given disease, has enormous advantages for clinical diagnosis as well as for monitoring disease activity. The magnitude of the increased expression of a biomarker in groups of patients suffering from disease should not only be great compared with healthy control subjects but, for statistical purposes, ideally there should also be no overlap between untreated patients with the condition and healthy control subjects. It is also of value to show consonance between subjects with a disease and those with other comorbid conditions occurring in the context of the particular disease for which the biomarker is to be investigated.

Validity

Biomarkers as surrogate measures of disease

Rigorous consideration should be given to the use of a particular analyte as a surrogate biomarker of disease. The ideal biomarker should reflect the total burden of the disease at all sites at which the disease is manifest, including sites that are not readily accessible to clinical examination. For example, one manifestation of Gaucher disease is thrombocytopenia, which is related to functional hypersplenism (due to splenomegaly) as well as to infiltration of the bone marrow. Thrombocytopenia reflects the impact of Gaucher disease on quality of life because of bleeding (or the risk of bleeding); however, patients with Gaucher disease who have hypersplenism may also have anaemia, neutropenia and infarction crises in the bone as independent clinical manifestations [12]. The ideal biomarker should be similarly elevated as a result of storage-related inflammatory changes and infiltration occurring, for example, in the liver, spleen, bone marrow and lungs, so that its elevation gives an overall view of the generalized effect of the disease rather than its manifestation at a single site or in a single organ [12, 16].

Predictive aspects of biomarkers

Ideally, the level of a surrogate biomarker would also change rapidly in response to interventions known to be specific for the condition. In the LSDs, one would expect ERT to reduce the expression of the chosen analyte, resulting in clearance of storage and correction of the effects of that storage within the affected tissues. However, clearance of storage may have only slow or, indeed, no effect on established disease parameters, and the extent of variability and reversal of the expression of the biomarker may vary. For example, in Gaucher disease, one would not expect that established avascular necrosis of the bone – a sporadic event in the long-term course of disease – would be reflected directly in the expression of a tissue molecule originating from the engorged macrophages or Gaucher cells in the bone marrow. Similarly, in Fabry disease, it would not necessarily be expected that a surrogate biomarker, for example urinary or plasma Gb_3, would predict or reflect sporadic events such as stroke. It may be that the frequency of cerebrovascular events and neurovascular manifestations is most elevated in those patients with the greatest degree of storage within the body, but in general the occurrence of any individual secondary event of whatever severity could not reasonably be expected to be predicted by the activity of a given biomarker, such as Gb_3.

It would be ideal if the abundance of a biomarker varied rapidly in response to treatment and showed a clear correlation with the extent of disease as reflected by independently established clinicopathological parameters. In practice this can rarely be achieved. Although 'the stage' of the condition may be set as a result of cellular storage consequent upon the lysosomal defect, many clinical manifestations represent complex sequelae, and their occurrence at any given time cannot be predicted. Nevertheless, one expectation of science is that it should be predictive; thus, the extent to which surrogate biomarkers can be utilized to allow confident forecasting of disease outcome lies at the heart of their application to medicine and, more prosaically, in the context of clinical trials. In essence, it is the author's view that while the use of biomarkers may prove to be crucial for the evaluation of a given condition, they can never be used in isolation either to predict disease manifestations or to fully appraise a therapeutic response.

Disease burden

The emerging canon of published work concerned with biomarkers in medicine frequently makes reference to the concept of the 'burden of disease'. Despite the apparently persuasive and emotive tone, the idea of a 'mass' of disease, tumour 'bulk' or – as applied to the lysosomal diseases – 'storage load', is simplistic beyond belief. Even when one considers the more straightforward case of, for example, an α-fetoprotein-secreting hepatocellular carcinoma, the concentration of α-fetoprotein in blood cannot reflect the severity of disease, the stage of 'advancement' of the cancer, or the true effects of the hepatocellular carcinoma on its host.

It is probably unnecessary to remind ourselves here that the human consequences of an hepatocellular carcinoma, possessing as it does a useful diagnostic biomarker (serum α-fetoprotein), cannot ever be measured in terms of this biomarker alone, tumour mass or any factor other than the extent to which the tumour affects the current life and the expectation of life of the patient who has the misfortune to harbour it. The tumour itself may be large or small; it may or may not invade locally or distantly metastasize to the lungs; it may cause fever, anorexia, weight loss, pain, a sustained acute-phase response, anaemia and mood changes. In short, it may impair the entity we have now designated semi-quantitatively as 'quality of life'.

Two main forces at work in the evaluative perception of healthcare outcomes and the practice of medicine, despite their bias towards the preoccupation with 'self' that characterizes occidental societies, have enlarged and fleshed-out the concept of 'disease burden'. These are (1) the general societal move towards higher personal expectations of life, health and well-being, and (2) measures, however faulted, of 'quality of life'. It is not difficult to realize that there remains an immense gulf between the measurable burden of disease, even a disease as frankly declared as a tumour with all the provisos about 'tumour mass', and its effects on life quality, expectation of life quality and the variably anxious personal world of the sufferer, their family and friends. A small localized tumour associated with fear in an anxious person cannot be compared with a medium-sized tumour invading retroperitoneal nerves in the coeliac region or a large tumour with pulmonary metastases in a solitary cachectic individual using the coping strategy of denial. Simply put: this disease cannot be comprehensively measured by objective criteria.

The Emperor has no clothes: the concept of disease burden, that absolute quantity by which any surrogate biomarker of disease must be judged in the clinical forum, has no basis in reality. So it is – but science is also a matter of compromises and contingency. To conclude optimistically, the author would make the familiar plea for more data, more time and more evaluation; but in truth we must recognize that many biological facts are established by the coming together of several unknown variables at one time. Biomarkers, at their base, reflect the operation of biological processes and it would be a poor thing for rational scientists not to expect greater understanding of a disease once the essential mechanism was understood and its biological parameters were measurable.

New biomarkers for LSDs

Newly identified biomarkers of use in clinical practice are most often biological molecules, such as proteins, polypeptides, lipoproteins, glycoconjugates or lipids, which are present in blood and other readily accessible body fluids or tissues. In the LSDs, these may either be molecules that accumulate directly as a result of the hereditary defect in lysosomal function (e.g. Gb_3 in Fabry disease) or molecules whose expression is modified in the affected tissues as a result of the storage

process (e.g. chitotriosidase or angiotensin-converting enzyme [ACE], which are secreted principally by the pathological macrophages of Gaucher disease). Modern techniques of immunoassay lend themselves to the analysis of protein and peptide biomarkers and, because they frequently include an enzymatic amplification step, are often highly sensitive. Thus, immunoassays allow detection of very small amounts of a given analyte in biological fluids and samples. Enzymes are also good candidates as biomarkers because they can be detected specifically by sensitive assays that are amplified by the catalytic process. In general, however, enzyme activities are subject to difficulties associated with lability, and the loss of enzymatic activity often long precedes the loss of the antigenic recognition properties on which modern immunoassay techniques depend.

Those lysosomal diseases in which there are prominent systemic features more readily lend themselves to the search for biomarkers that reflect disease manifestations and activity. In contrast, disorders that principally affect the CNS are less tractable because the effect of disease and inflammation within the brain may not be readily detected through sampling of tissues and body fluids at distant sites [17]. Thus, in the field of biomarker discovery, the most challenging lysosomal diseases are those that affect the CNS, such as the glycosphingolipidoses. Hitherto, the most frequently used biomarker for these disorders has been the presence of excess protein in the cerebrospinal fluid, but even this crude measure is not informative in all such diseases.

Biomarkers in current use

Several biomarkers are already in use as surrogate indicators of the presence of lysosomal diseases. They are of principal value in diagnosis, but are also used as an adjunct to the monitoring of therapy. Most of the biomarkers in this class are molecules that accumulate directly as a result of the primary genetic defect, such as Gb_3 in Fabry disease, which accumulates due to a deficiency of α-galactosidase A, and the glycosaminoglycans present in the urine of many, but not all, patients suffering from a group of diseases known as the MPS syndromes.

Fabry disease

In Fabry disease, deposits of the principal storage product, Gb_3, accumulate in lysosomes. Plasma and urine concentrations of this glycosphingolipid are of value in the diagnosis of Fabry disease, particularly in affected hemizygote males, and may also be of value in following its course and response to therapy [18–20]. Clearance of Gb_3 deposits in the renal interstitial capillary endothelial cells was an agreed endpoint in at least one of the pivotal trials of ERT for Fabry disease [19]. Early evidence suggests that, in those patients who show a 'good' clinical response to ERT, elevated Gb_3 concentrations fall progressively after initiation of therapy. However, the recent report of autopsy findings in a patient with Fabry disease who died as a result of myocardial infarction, and who had received ERT for 2.5 years prior to death, is informative [21]. Extensive clearance of endothelial cell storage of Gb_3 was observed, but widespread pathological storage of glycosphingolipid was found to persist in numerous sites and organs throughout the body.

In classic Fabry disease, Gb_3 can be reliably measured in the plasma and urine using the technique of tandem mass spectrometry. However, there is wide variation in the concentrations detected and it seems that some affected patients harbouring so-called mild mutations in the human α-galactosidase gene, which are not associated with an absolute deficiency of the enzyme, may show normal concentrations of Gb_3 in these body fluids. In female heterozygotes, plasma

concentrations of Gb_3 may be normal, but there is evidence that the concentration of Gb_3 is usually elevated in the urine of females heterozygous for Fabry disease (see Chapter 18).

Several studies have reported the effects of recombinant α-galactosidase A in patients with Fabry disease. Urinary glycolipid concentrations are reported to decrease impressively in hemizygote patients and in the absence of renal transplantation; in heterozygotes and in recipients of a renal allograft, the elevation in urinary glycolipid concentration and the changes following the introduction of ERT appear to be less pronounced [22]. A cause–effect relationship between the introduction of ERT and the decrease in urinary Gb_3 is emphasized by the elevation in Gb_3 concentrations (to pretreatment levels) that accompanies the development of antibodies to the therapeutic protein [23]. Use of Gb_3 as a potential marker of disease severity, as well as of responses to treatment, therefore deserves further investigation. Unlike the great majority of heterozygous females in families affected by MPS II (Hunter syndrome), most Fabry heterozygotes manifest signs and symptoms of the disease [24, 25]. Fabry heterozygotes may, as a result of uncomplemented mosaicism, experience many disabling effects of Fabry disease but at the same time will not necessarily have marked or even any abnormalities in Gb_3 metabolism.

The MPS syndromes

In patients with MPS types I, II and VI, introduction of the respective recombinant human ERT has been associated with decreased urinary glycosaminoglycan concentrations. It should be noted, however, that the MPS syndromes are complex systemic disorders commonly associated with neurological impairment and brain disease. They are also associated with breathing difficulties, heart disease, and musculoskeletal and connective tissue injury. This renders the simple quantification of glycosaminoglycans inadequate for judging therapeutic outcomes in response to enzyme therapy [26]. In these disorders, improvement in quality of life is more likely to be due to improved mobility of the joints, ventilatory capacity and altered structures in the upper airways and sinuses, rather than solely to reduction in the glycosaminoglycan content of the urine – itself more likely to reflect visceral disease, principally in the liver and spleen. However, a comprehensive international survey of patients with MPS VI (Maroteaux–Lamy syndrome) indicated that very high urinary concentrations of glycosaminoglycans (> 200 µg/mg creatinine) are associated with an accelerated clinical course of the disease in its untreated state [27]. It has yet to be shown whether this applies to other MPS syndromes.

Gaucher disease

The other frequently used biomarkers of lysosomal disease activity are encountered most convincingly in Gaucher disease and, to some extent, in the rare and analogous macrophage disorder, Niemann–Pick disease type B. In these disorders, it is the elevation of proteins, principally in the plasma, that reflects the influence of cellular storage. The source of these proteins appears in all cases to be the pathological macrophage that serves as the principal focus of the storage disorder and in which altered morphology and function leads, in a manner as yet illunderstood, to the over-production and secretion of various enzymatic biomarkers and other proteins [28]. In Gaucher disease, serendipitous biochemical determinations identified the elevation of plasma β-hexosaminidase as well as elevated tartrateresistant acid phosphatase (TRAP). These proteins both derive from the pathological storage cell and have been used diagnostically and to monitor the effects of ERT. Knowledge that the Gaucher cell is a pathological macrophage led to investigation of other macrophage proteins, such as the lysozyme chitotetrasidase and, latterly,

chitotriosidase, as potential enzymatic biomarkers for the disease [3, 5–7].

Chitotriosidase has become the most commonly used enzymatic biomarker for Gaucher disease since it was first fully reported in 1994. Chitotriosidase is in effect a chitolytic enzyme secreted by activated human macrophages as well as polymorphonuclear leukocytes. Chitotriosidase is elevated several hundred-fold in the plasma of the majority of individuals with Gaucher disease, but 5–6% of the population lack the enzyme as the result of a genetic deficiency due to an expressional mutation in the human chitotriosidase gene that occurs with high polymorphic frequency in European populations [15, 28]. Approximately one-third of patients with Gaucher disease (and a similar fraction of the general population) are heterozygous for this null allele and thus the extent to which Gaucher disease may increase the activity of chitotriosidase in the plasma is reduced in these individuals.

Chitotriosidase is difficult to measure under steady-state conditions, as it has a transglycosidase activity that precludes measurement of its hydrolytic activity at optimal saturating concentrations of substrate. However, the recent ingenious development of a substrate that cannot serve as a partner in the transglycosidase reaction has greatly assisted the reliable determination of chitotriosidase activity in the plasma of patients with Gaucher disease [29]. Plasma chitotriosidase is not only of diagnostic use in the majority of patients with suspected Gaucher disease, it also falls rapidly on introduction of definitive therapies, including substrate reduction therapy with the iminosugar, miglustat, and ERT using imiglucerase.

TRAP is neither specific for Gaucher disease nor greatly elevated in patients with this condition. Furthermore, the protein appears to be unstable in the blood, as well as being subject to marked analytical variability. Mice lacking TRAP (type 5 acid phosphatase, an iron-containing enzyme [30]) have mild osteopetrosis and various endochondral skeletal defects) but the role of TRAP as a biomarker of Gaucher disease remains ill-understood. TRAP activity decreases after splenectomy and in the pivotal trial of ERT decreased significantly in response to enzyme supplementation [31]. ACE activity is also subject to variable expression, principally as a result of the presence of a common genetic polymorphism in the population; moreover, in older patients, co-administration of frequently used ACE inhibitors invalidates its measurement [12].

Thus, in most European patients with Gaucher disease, plasma chitotriosidase is the biomarker in current use. The intro-duction of the novel fluorogenic substrate, 4-methylumbelliferyldeoxychitotrioside, pro-vides a convenient, highly sensitive and accurate method for the determination of chitotriosidase. Chitotriosidase activity is greatly elevated in patients with Gaucher disease and is also elevated in patients with other diseases of the macrophage, including Niemann–Pick disease types A and B [32].

Use of biomarkers in screening for LSDs

There are few exceptions to the axiom, now a mantra for frequent recitation in clinical medicine: namely, that early diagnosis gives rise to a better outcome (than a missed, wrong or delayed diagnosis). Moreover, for most disorders – and the LSDs are no exception – there is abundant evidence to support this contention. With the emergence of specific innovative medicinal products licensed for the treatment of LSDs, the prompt detection of these diseases is ever more desirable. This has generated much interest in the devel-opment of presymptomatic mass screening methods for the newborn population [13].

So far, beyond the introduction of sensitive micro-methods to detect specific deficien-cies of lysosomal enzyme activities in at-risk populations, neonatal screening for lysosomal diseases remains a formidable technological challenge – and a challenge to those charged with translating discoveries rapidly into the clinical forum. Key questions need to be answered about the means by which diagnostic information should be processed and the general utility of an enzymatic diagnosis for disorders whose clinical expression is subject to enormous variability. With a birth frequency of approxi-mately 1 in 5000, there is clearly potential for the use of diagnostic biomarkers for the detection of LSDs in neonatal screening programmes [13].

Meikle and colleagues in Australia have shown that expansion of the lysosomal compartment in many storage disorders is associated with elevated concentrations of lysosome-associated membrane protein-1 (LAMP-1), which is readily quantified by immunoassay [33]. Studies have indicated that about 70% of patients known to have LSDs have significantly raised concen-trations of immunoreactive LAMP-1 antigen in their plasma. Pilot studies quantifying this putative biomarker in blood spot samples on Guthrie cards obtained in the neonatal period have shown some promise for mass diagnostic screening. This procedure alone, however, was not found to be sufficiently sensitive to confidently identify patients with LSDs when tested in clinical practice. More-over, with the current level of technological development, the combined use of lysosomal protein marker immunoassays and quantifi-cation of related metabolites using tandem mass spectroscopy was not satisfactory for the detection of the broad range of LSDs [34]. Given the ability of existing methods to identify several LSDs at birth, and the need to make effective treatments available to patients at the earliest phase of their disease, further investment in biomarker development in this field is clearly justified [13].

Discovery of new biomarkers for LSDs

Hitherto, most surrogate biomarkers for use in the LSDs have been developed as a result of fortuitous investigations based on clinical biochemistry measurements. Discovery of new biomarkers requires application of innovative laboratory methods for the systematic analysis of biological molecules, and great hope is placed in the use of techniques that will systematically detect increased or altered expression of genes. Similarly, it is the use of systematic identification procedures, combined with highly sensitive methods for the isolation of proteins, that have allowed the application of modern proteomic technology to the study of human diseases, including LSDs.

Differentially expressed genes encoding potential biomarkers can be identified from disease tissues subjected to cDNA microarray analysis; other methods to identify genes whose expression is increased in diseased tissues include the generation of subtractive libraries by, for example, the suppression subtractive hybridization technique [10].

In the identification of proteins whose expression is altered in biological fluids and tissues, it has been the introduction of mass spectrometric techniques into the arena of biology that has proved to be the most profitable [8, 9, 11]. At the least, this strategy provides the greatest hope of identifying proteins that can be utilized as biomarkers of disease. In this connection, high-resolution two-dimensional gel electrophoresis combined with matrix-assisted laser desorption ionization and surface-enhanced laser desorption ionization (SELDI) are the methods used for isolation of proteins. These procedures may then be linked to time-of-flight mass spectrometry, thus allowing identification of minute amounts of proteins, variably expressed in the complex biological mixtures present, for example, in plasma or urine [11, 32].

The introduction of the chemokine biomarker, PARC (pulmonary and activation-regulated chemokine), also known as CCL-18, as a biomarker for Gaucher disease was the result of simultaneous research by two collaborative groups [10–12]. On the one hand, SELDI mass spectrometry proteomic methods were used to identify proteins present in the plasma of patients with Gaucher disease that altered during the course of ERT [11]; on the other hand, a method that examined the differential expression of genes in the splenic tissue of patients with Gaucher disease and control splenic tissue was used to identify Gaucher-specific mRNA sequences in a Gaucher-specific cDNA expression library – the suppression subtractive hybridization technique [10].

The systematic combination of these methods to facilitate the identification of expressed genes in Gaucher disease that can serve as biomarkers led to the identification of PARC/CCL-18, a 7.8 kDa polypeptide, which was known to be chemotactic for naive resting T cells [35]. This chemokine does not occur in rodents, and appears to be unique to humans and higher primates. Indeed, its cognate receptor has yet to be characterized, although increased expression of the protein has been identified in the tissues of patients with sarcoidosis and other immune/allergic disorders.

Moran and co-workers identified increased expression of PARC mRNA in splenic tissue from a patient with Gaucher disease using the technique of suppressive subtractive hybridization cDNA, and greatly increased concentrations of the 7.8 kDa polypeptide was identified in the plasma of patients with Gaucher disease before ERT was introduced [11]. A comparison of the information from these two sources allowed the confident identification of PARC as the biomarker of interest in these samples.

PARC – like ACE, TRAP and hexosaminidase – is produced by macrophages and dendritic cells, but may represent a unique by-product of alternative activation. CCL-18/PARC has been implicated in chronic inflammation and fibrotic scarring in other disorders [36]. CCL-18/PARC is stable on storage in plasma and resistant to multiple freeze–thaw cycles [11, 12]. PARC can be readily measured by an enzyme-linked immunoassay procedure with reasonable reproducibility and is increased 15- to 20-fold in the serum of patients with Gaucher disease; at least two studies have identified that there is no overlap in PARC levels between untreated patients with Gaucher disease and control subjects. Preliminary studies indicate that serum PARC is increased in Niemann–Pick disease types A and B and, in two patients with α-mannosidosis, serum concentrations were also increased [10]. A useful characteristic of PARC has been its elevation in Gaucher patients harbouring null chitotriosidase alleles; and no patient with a genetic deficiency of PARC expression has yet been identified [12].

In many respects, Gaucher's disease serves as the exemplar of LSDs: it is not only the most common but is also the one that appears to be most successfully treated by ERT directed at the pathological macrophage. It remains to be seen whether secondary markers of lysosomal disease activity can be developed by the application of proteomic and/or systematic genomic expression studies, as outlined above, to yield markers that can be used in diagnosis and therapeutic monitoring of LSDs. At present, there are no readily apparent biomarkers that can be studied beyond the primary storage molecules in Fabry disease and the MPS syndromes. The identification of useful surrogate biomarkers in these diseases thus poses a challenge to the technology that is now available for the systematic identification of biological molecules of interest that are present in diseased tissues and complex mixtures, such as plasma [8, 9].

It would be chastening and appropriate at this juncture to examine the history of the surrogate biomarkers that have been developed in the LSDs and other conditions. Most of these putative biomarkers have been discovered as a result of inspired experimentation and investigation, or serendipitously as a result of random biochemical testing of samples obtained from patients suffering from the disease in question. In this regard, there are parallels with the field of toxicology. Here, those involved in the diagnosis and monitoring of at-risk subjects (e.g. industrial workers) can determine the concentrations of the primary toxic chemical, (e.g. lead, arsenic or cadmium), or the effects of poisoning (e.g. of porphyrin metabolism), [37], or the effects on the kidney through the determination of urinary proteins and enzymes such as N-acetyl glucosaminidase or β_2-microglobulin [38]. In these disorders, a knowledge of metabolism and inspired guesswork has allowed the development of biomarkers of disease or toxic injury – as hitherto has been the case in the LSDs and in diabetes with determination of blood glucose measurements and HbA_{1c} concentrations or the quantification of micro-albuminuria [39, 40]. It remains to be seen whether the new biomarkers of use will arise principally from the rational application of technology or the imaginative concepts of broadly based investigators.

In this connection, it will be interesting to see whether the newly emerging biomarker glucose tetrasaccharide, which is elevated in the urine of patients with glycogen storage disease type II (acid maltase deficiency, Pompe disease), will cross the boundary between old and new technologies. It has long been known that patients with glycogen storage disease type II excrete increased amounts of this glycogen-derived tetrasaccharide, but its accurate measurement in dried urine spot samples and other easily accessible sources has depended on the development of robust procedures based on electrospray ionization tandem mass spectrometry for biological samples [41]. It has been the use of sensitive contemporary procedures for the specific analysis of oligosaccharides in complex biological fluids that offers the hope of introducing an informative biomarker for this challenging disease. Pompe disease principally affects cardiac and skeletal muscles and can now be treated with recombinant human acid α-glucosidase. Hence, the combination of fortuitous biochemical analysis, inspired chemical judgement and the application of the latest methods of molecular analysis to complex mixtures in biological fluids may yield an effective biomarker for patients with a highly challenging and truly crippling lysosomal disease.

Clinical evaluation of biomarkers

Once any candidate biomarker has been identified and quantified in patients suffering from a given disease, the utility of the marker for diagnostic or monitoring purposes will need to be determined in the clinical context [8, 12, 16]. The rarity of LSDs has led to the introduction of specific treatments of great expense. Physicians are therefore obliged to justify the expense of administering these treatments by ensuring that the therapeutic responses they observe can be monitored objectively. It is thus mandatory that any analyte that serves as a putative surrogate biomarker of any given LSD undergoes extensive evaluation to establish its ability to predict disease outcome and prognosis accurately.

Earlier in this chapter, the ideal characteristics of a surrogate biomarker in a disease were set out. It is worth emphasizing here that any given biomarker will be required to reflect disease in different organs of the body and the response of that disease to specific treatment in a manner that corresponds to significant clinical endpoints. Ultimately, all biomarkers will be required to satisfy tests of their ability to reflect key aspects of a disease that are agreed to

influence outcome and quality of life for the individual patient in whom they are determined [12, 26].

Clearly, no single biomarker is likely to be the sole determinant of outcome and prognosis in a given disease. Moreover, most biomarkers will serve simply as a guide to the severity of the condition and to its ultimate outcome in the treated or untreated state. If a given biomarker that reflects the burden of a disease continues to be expressed in abundance when therapy is given, this probably indicates that that treatment is suboptimal and also provides a guide to increasing either the amount or quality of a given therapy. At the same time, it should be accepted that even if the activity of a surrogate biomarker is brought within the reference range of healthy subjects, this does not necessarily absolve the treating physician from the responsibility of vigilant follow-up and monitoring. Thus, quantification of any useful biomarker should provide material assistance in the indications for treatment and justify the appropriate reimbursement of the healthcare costs consequent upon delivering such treatment. In this context, it is worth emphasizing that LSDs are multisystem disorders and that many are subject to sporadic clinical events that usually occur on a background of indolent progression. In Gaucher disease, for example, there is usually progressive enlargement of the liver and spleen after onset in childhood, but this may be accompanied by sporadic crises (e.g. bone infarction events). These crises resolve in a matter of weeks, but often lead to considerable long-term disability and impaired quality of life. It would be surprising if any association between the surrogate biomarker and Gaucher disease or another related lysosomal disorder provided anything but the most general indication of disease activity. Much work will be needed to show any convincing relationship between the activity of biomarkers and survival or the prognosis for disability-free years.

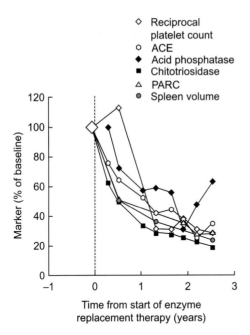

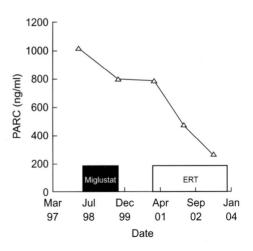

Figure 1. *Correlation between pulmonary and activation-regulated chemokine (PARC) and other markers of disease activity in a patient with Gaucher disease receiving enzyme replacement therapy (ERT) with imiglucerase. The start of ERT is represented by the dotted vertical line. The large diamond represents the baseline value (100%) for each parameter just prior to the start of ERT. ACE, angiotensin-converting enzyme. Reproduced with permission from [42].*

Figure 2. *Changes in the serum concentration of pulmonary and activation-regulated chemokine (PARC) during treatment with the substrate inhibitor, miglustat, and enzyme replacement therapy (ERT), with imiglucerase, in a patient with Gaucher disease. Adapted with permission from [42].*

We have evaluated the application of several well-established enzymatic biomarkers of Gaucher disease, as well as the use of serum CCL-18/PARC concentrations, to predict responses to therapy (Figures 1 and 2). The serum concentration of immunoreactive CCL-18/PARC was found to be associated with the risk of infarction in the liver and spleen, although this association was indirect and probably dependent on total organ volume [12].

It is generally agreed by experienced clinicians that spleen volume and platelet count in patients with Gaucher disease are of value in reflecting relevant outcomes, as hypersplenism due to massive splenomegaly may require splenectomy, and the platelet

count itself is a determinant of the need for splenectomy, as well as a risk factor for life-threatening haemorrhage. However, clinical and biochemical markers that include spleen size, platelet count and chitotriosidase activity have not been applicable in all groups of patients [42]. We have found that CCL-18/PARC is of value in splenectomized patients where spleen size and platelet count are not informative for the activity of the disease. We have also shown that serum CCL-18/PARC reflects disease activity in patients homozygous for the null variant of chitotriosidase and that serum PARC more closely reflects spleen volume and platelet count during treatment than does chitotriosidase. In a practical appraisal, we have also shown that, unlike the measurement of chitotriosidase and acid phosphatase activity, enzyme-linked immuno-absorbent assay of serum CCL-18/PARC concentrations is straightforward and readily amenable to standardization in the routine laboratory assessment. On the other hand, our evaluation of all these markers has shown no significant correlation between any of the blood markers and the clinical severity score published by Zimran and co-workers [12, 42, 43]. Others have also failed to demonstrate an association between serum CCL-18/PARC and this index. The clinical index has been subject to considerable discussion in the literature; it appears not to distinguish between some severe prognostic aspects of Gaucher disease and is not designed to reflect any improvement achieved by ERT. We believe that the lack of association between CCL-18/PARC and the clinical severity score index results from the light weighting given to visceral bulk. Although changes in chitotriosidase activity give a biased account of the response of splenic volume and platelet count to ERT, changes in PARC levels did accurately reflect salutary changes in organ volume and platelet count without bias.

Conclusions

Each lysosomal disorder is unique, with singular pathology and manifestations in different tissues. Each disease is moreover a consequence of different pathological mechanisms causing disruption of membrane flow and molecular storage in the lysosomal system and related membrane compartments within the cell. Only now are we aware that the effects of pathological storage lead to compensating reactions of containment with their own catalogue of actions, just as they induce disturbed cell membrane trafficking and inflammatory reactions to storage cells and molecules.

Operationally, however, and in the real world of therapeutic orphans, the author considers that Gaucher disease illustrates the paradigm for evaluating clinical biomarkers systematically in a given disease. For each candidate biomarker in other LSDs, a similar clinical evaluation will be required that is modified according to the clinical features and natural history of each condition. Much work will be needed to discover putative biomarkers and develop them for clinical use. More work generally will be needed across the fields of medicine to understand

lysosomal diseases and their critical consequences on the whole perception of life quality by those who suffer from them. At the time of writing, the development of valid clinical instruments for appraising each LSD and its effects on key life outcomes is but a science in the earliest period of embryonic development.

References

1. European Commission Review of Orphan Drug Legislation. Inventory of Community and National Incentive 2002. Available from http://pharmacos. eudra.org/F2/orphanmp/index.htm

2. Haffner ME. Developing treatments for inborn errors: incentives available to the clinician. *Mol Genet Metab* 2004;81 (Suppl 1):S63–6

3. Hollak CE, van Weely S, van Oers MH, Aerts JM. Marked elevation of plasma chitotriosidase activity. A novel hallmark of Gaucher disease. *J Clin Invest* 1994;93:1288–92

4. Renkema GH, Boot RG, Muijsers AO, Donker-Koopman WE, Aerts JM. Purification and characterization of human chitotriosidase, a novel member of the chitinase family of proteins. *J Biol Chem* 1995;270:2198–202

5. Tuchman LR, Suna H, Carr JJ. Elevation of serum acid phosphatase in Gaucher's disease. *J Mt Sinai Hosp NY* 1956;23:227–9

6. Beutler E, Kuhl W, Matsumoto F, Pangalis G. Acid hydrolases in leukocytes and platelets of normal subjects and in patients with Gaucher's and Fabry's disease. *J Exp Med* 1976;143:975–80

7. Silverstein E, Friedland J. Elevated serum and spleen angiotensin converting enzyme and serum lysozyme in Gaucher's disease. *Clin Chim Acta* 1977;74:21–5

8. MacGregor JT. Biomarkers of cancer risk and therapeutic benefit: new technologies, new opportunities, and some challenges. *Toxicol Pathol* 2004;32 (Suppl 1):99–105

9. Zolg JW, Langen H. How industry is approaching the search for new diagnostic markers and biomarkers. *Mol Cell Proteomics* 2004;3:345–54

10. Moran MT, Schofield JP, Hayman AR, Shi GP, Young E, Cox TM. Pathologic gene expression in Gaucher disease: up-regulation of cysteine proteinases including osteoclastic cathepsin K. *Blood* 2000; 96:1969–78

11. Boot RG, Verhoek M, de Fost M, Hollak CE, Maas M, Bleijlevens B *et al*. Marked elevation of the chemokine CCL18/PARC in Gaucher disease: a novel surrogate marker for assessing therapeutic intervention. *Blood* 2004;103:33–9

12. Deegan PB, Moran MT, McFarlane I, Schofield JP, Boot RG, Aerts JM *et al*. Clinical evaluation of chemokine and enzymatic biomarkers of Gaucher disease. *Blood Cells Mol Dis* 2005;35:259–67

13. Meikle PJ, Hopwood JJ. Lysosomal storage disorders: emerging therapeutic options require early diagnosis. *Eur J Pediatr* 2003;162 (Suppl 1):S34–7

14. Cox TM. Gaucher disease: understanding the molecular pathogenesis of sphingolipidoses. *J Inherit Metab Dis* 2001;24 (Suppl 2):106–21

15. Boot RG, Renkema GH, Verhoek M, Strijland A, Bliek J, de Meulemeester TM *et al*. The human chitotriosidase gene. Nature of inherited enzyme deficiency. *J Biol Chem* 1998;273:25680–5

16. Colburn WA. Optimizing the use of biomarkers, surrogate endpoints, and clinical endpoints for more efficient drug development. *J Clin Pharmacol* 2000;40:1419–27

17. Lachmann RH, te Vruchte D, Lloyd-Evans E, Reinkensmeier G, Sillence DJ, Fernandez-Guillen L *et al*. Treatment with miglustat reverses the lipid-trafficking defect in Niemann–Pick disease type C. *Neurobiol Dis* 2004;16:654–8

18. Boscaro F, Pieraccini G, la Marca G, Bartolucci G, Luceri C, Luceri F *et al*. Rapid quantitation of globotriaosylceramide in human plasma and urine: a potential application for monitoring enzyme replacement therapy in Anderson–Fabry disease. *Rapid Commun Mass Spectrom* 2002;16:1507–14

19. Eng CM, Banikazemi M, Gordon RE, Goldman M, Phelps R, Kim L *et al*. A phase 1/2 clinical trial of enzyme replacement in Fabry disease: pharma-cokinetic, substrate clearance, and safety studies. *Am J Hum Genet* 2001;68:711–22

20. Schiffmann R, Murray GJ, Treco D, Daniel P, Sellos-Moura M, Myers M *et al*. Infusion of α-galactosidase A reduces tissue globotriaosylceramide storage in patients with Fabry disease. *Proc Natl Acad Sci USA* 2000;97:365–70

21. Schiffmann R, Rapkiewicz A, Abu-Asab M, Ries M, Askari H, Tsokos M *et al*. Pathological findings in a patient with Fabry disease who died after 2.5 years of enzyme replacement. *Virchows Arch* 2005:1–7

22. Young E, Mills K, Morris P, Vellodi A, Lee P, Waldek S *et al*. Is globotriaosylceramide a useful biomarker in Fabry disease? *Acta Paediatr Suppl* 2005;447:51–4

23. Whitfield PD, Calvin J, Hogg S, O'Driscoll E, Halsall D, Burling K *et al*. Monitoring enzyme replacement therapy in Fabry disease – role of urine globotriao-sylceramide. *J Inherit Metab Dis* 2005;28:21–33

24. MacDermot KD, Holmes A, Miners AH. Anderson–Fabry disease: clinical manifestations and impact of disease in a cohort of 60 obligate carrier females. *J Med Genet* 2001;38:769–75

25. Chase DS, Morris AH, Ballabio A, Pepper S, Giannelli F, Adinolfi M. Genetics of Hunter syndrome: carrier detection, new mutations, segregation and link-age analysis. *Ann Hum Genet* 1986;50 (Pt 4):349–60

26. Wraith JE. The first 5 years of clinical experience with laronidase enzyme replacement therapy for mucopolysaccharidosis I. *Expert Opin Pharmacother* 2005;6:489–506

27. Swiedler SJ, Beck M, Bajbouj M, Giugliani R, Schwartz I, Harmatz P *et al*. Threshold effect of urinary glycosaminoglycans and the walk test as indicators of disease progression in a survey of subjects with mucopolysaccharidosis VI (Maroteaux–Lamy syndrome). *Am J Med Genet A* 2005;134:144–50

28. Aerts JM, Hollak CE. Plasma and metabolic abnormalities in Gaucher's disease. *Baillieres Clin Haematol* 1997;10:691–709

29. Aguilera B, Ghauharali-van der Vlugt K, Helmond MT, Out JM, Donker-Koopman WE, Groener JE *et al*. Transglycosidase activity of chitotriosidase: improved enzymatic assay for the human macrophage chitinase. *J Biol Chem* 2003;278:40911–16

30. Hayman AR, Jones SJ, Boyde A, Foster D, Colledge WH, Carlton MB *et al*. Mice lacking tartrate-resistant acid phosphatase (Acp 5) have disrupted endochondral ossification and mild osteopetrosis. *Development* 1996;122:3151–62

31. Barton NW, Brady RO, Dambrosia JM, Di Bisceglie AM, Doppelt SH, Hill SC *et al*. Replacement therapy for inherited enzyme deficiency–macrophage-targeted glucocerebrosidase for Gaucher's disease. *N Engl J Med* 1991;324:1464–70

32. Aerts JM, Hollak C, Boot R, Groener A. Biochemistry of glycosphingolipid storage disorders: implications for therapeutic intervention. *Philos Trans R Soc Lond B Biol Sci* 2003;358:905–14

33. Ranierri E, Gerace RL, Ravenscroft EM, Hopwood JJ, Meikle PJ. Pilot neonatal screening program for lysosomal storage disorders, using LAMP-1. *Southeast Asian J Trop Med Public Health* 1999;30 (Suppl 2):111–13

34. Meikle PJ, Ranieri E, Simonsen H, Rozaklis T, Ramsay SL, Whitfield PD *et al*. Newborn screening for lysosomal storage disorders: clinical evaluation of a two-tier strategy. *Pediatrics* 2004;114:909–16

35. Hieshima K, Imai T, Baba M, Shoudai K, Ishizuka K, Nakagawa T *et al*. A novel human CC chemokine PARC that is most homologous to macrophage-inflammatory protein-1 alpha/LD78 alpha and chemo-tactic for T lymphocytes, but not for monocytes. *J Immunol* 1997;159:1140–9

36. Mrazek F, Sekerova V, Drabek J, Kolek V, du Bois RM, Petrek M. Expression of the chemokine PARC mRNA in bronchoalveolar cells of patients with sarcoidosis. *Immunol Lett* 2002;84:17–22

37. Wang JP, Qi L, Zheng B, Lui F, Moore MR, Ng JC. Porphyrias as early biomarkers for arsenic exposure in animals and humans. *Cell Mol Biol (Noisy-le-Grand)* 2002;48:835–43

38. Nordberg GF, Jin T, Hong F, Zhang A, Buchet JP, Bernard A. Biomarkers of cadmium and arsenic interactions. *Toxicol Appl Pharmacol* 2005;206:191–7

39. The Diabetes Control and Complications Trial Research Group. The effect of intensive treatment of diabetes on the development and progression of long-term complications in insulin-dependent diabetes mellitus. *N Engl J Med* 1993;329:977–86

40. Mogensen CE. Microalbuminuria, blood pressure and diabetic renal disease: origin and development of ideas. *Diabetologia* 1999;42:263–85

41. Young SP, Stevens RD, An Y, Chen YT, Millington DS. Analysis of a glucose tetrasaccharide elevated in Pompe disease by stable isotope dilution-electrospray ionization tandem mass spectrometry. *Anal Biochem* 2003;316:175–80

42. Deegan PB, Cox TM. Clinical evaluation of biomarkers in Gaucher disease. *Acta Paediatr Suppl* 2005;447:47–50

43. Zimran A, Kay A, Gelbart T, Garver P, Thurston D, Saven A *et al*. Gaucher disease. Clinical, laboratory, radiologic, and genetic features of 53 patients. *Medicine (Baltimore)* 1992;71:337–53

10 Enzyme replacement therapy – a brief history

Elizabeth F Neufeld

Department of Biological Chemistry, David Geffen School of Medicine at UCLA, Los Angeles, California 90095-1737, USA

The concept of enzyme replacement therapy for lysosomal storage diseases was enunciated by de Duve in 1964. However, much cell biology had to be learned before lysosomal enzymes could be developed into pharmaceuticals. A model system, consisting of cultured skin fibroblasts from patients with mucopolysaccharidoses (MPS), showed that their defective glycosaminoglycan catabolism could be corrected by factors derived from cells of a different genotype. The corrective factors were identified as lysosomal enzymes with a special feature, or recognition signal, that would permit efficient uptake. As the recognition signal was absent from a number of lysosomal enzymes secreted by fibroblasts from patients with I-cell disease (a monogenic disorder), it was postulated to be a post-translational modification of the lysosomal enzymes. It was subsequently shown to be a carbohydrate and identified as mannose-6-phosphate (M6P), which was recognized by ubiquitous M6P receptors. A second model system was the clearance, in vivo, of lysosomal enzymes from plasma. The recognition signal for this system was identified as mannose, and clearance was shown to be mediated by the mannose receptor of the reticuloendothelial system. This second system was immediately put to use for the treatment of Gaucher disease type I, in which macrophages are the affected cells. Native, and later recombinant, glucocerebrosidase was modified to expose terminal mannose residues; it became the first successful pharmaceutical for a lysosomal storage disease. Recombinant lysosomal enzymes containing the M6P signal have been developed (or are in the advanced stages of development) into pharmaceuticals for the treatment of Fabry disease, MPS I, MPS II, MPS VI and Pompe disease.

Introduction

The concept of enzyme replacement therapy for lysosomal storage diseases was introduced four decades ago by Christian de Duve, with the following brief explanation: "In our pathogenic speculations and in our therapeutic attempts, it may be well to keep in mind that any substance which is taken up intracellularly in an endocytic process is likely to end up within lysosomes. This obviously opens up many possibilities for interaction, including replacement therapy" [1]. The connection between endocytosis and lysosomes was already well established [2] but the concept of lysosomal storage diseases was new at the time, having just been proposed by Hers and collaborators after the discovery of acid maltase deficiency as the basis of Pompe disease [3]. Experimental support for enzyme replacement came from the effectiveness of administering invertase to hydrolyse sucrose in liver lysosomes *in vivo* [2] or in lysosomes of cultured macrophages *in vitro* [4]. However, immediate attempts to apply the concept to the treatment of patients with Pompe disease were not successful [3, 5].

Corrective factors and recognition signals

A model system for enzyme replacement therapy arose from studies of cultured skin fibroblasts derived from patients with muco-polysaccharide storage diseases (MPS). Such fibroblasts showed excessive accu-mulation of [35S]glycosaminoglycans, which was interpreted as being due to inadequate degradation of these macromolecules [6]. It was discovered serendipitously that a mixture of fibroblasts derived from patients with MPS I (Hurler syndrome) and MPS II (Hunter syn-drome) had a normal pattern of [35S]glycos-aminoglycan metabolism (Figure 1) [7]. The two diseases were known to be genetically distinct [8], MPS I being inherited in an auto-somal recessive fashion and MPS II being an X-linked disorder, leading Fratantoni et al. [7] to hypothesize that the fibroblasts of dif-ferent genotypes were providing each other

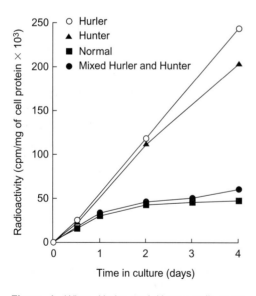

Figure 1. *When Hurler and Hunter cells were mixed in culture, an essentially normal pattern of [35S]mucopolysaccharide accumulation was obtained; that is, cells of the two different genotypes had corrected each other in culture. Adapted with permission from [7].*

with the missing gene product. Further studies showed that it was not necessary to have the genetically distinct cells in contact with each other for such cross-correction, as medium conditioned by one could be corrective to the other [9]. The strategy of cross-correction could be extended to related diseases – cells that corrected each other would have a different genotype, whereas cells that didn't cross-correct would have the same genotype (but see the important exception below).

As Hurler syndrome had been postulated to be a lysosomal storage disease based on observation of the dramatically swollen liver lysosomes in affected patients [10], Fratantoni et al. [9] hypothesized that the 'corrective factors' in conditioned medium might be lysosomal enzymes that were secreted by one cell line and endocytosed by the other. However, the corrective factors did not correspond to any lysosomal enzyme known at the time (this situation changed a couple of years later, when a β-glucuronidase deficiency MPS was discovered [11, 12]). Purification of the Hurler and Hunter cor-rective factors was undertaken, not from conditioned medium but from urine, a body fluid relatively rich in lysosomal enzymes. Function was assigned to the purified factors by using a variety of biochemical methods, resulting in the Hurler and Hunter corrective factors being named α-L-iduronidase and iduronate sulfatase respectively [13, 14].

Cells that required Hurler corrective factor to normalize their [35S]glycosaminoglycan meta-bolism (from patients with Hurler syndrome and with Scheie syndrome [15]) were also deficient in α-L-iduronidase activity [13, 14]). Correction of Hurler fibroblasts was accom-panied by uptake of α-L-iduronidase. As good portents for enzyme replacement therapy, uptake was remarkably efficient and only a very small amount of α-L-iduronidase had to be internalized in order to provide complete correction.

This might have been the end of the story, except for a small discrepancy in the elution pattern of the enzymatic activity and the corrective activity from a hydroxyapatite column [13], suggesting that the two activities of the Hurler corrective factor were not precisely identical. Following up on this discrepancy, Shapiro et al. [16] separated α-L-iduronidase into corrective and non-corrective fractions on a column of heparin-Sepharose, indicating that the corrective factor had some feature that was not needed for catalytic activity but was needed for uptake. Similarly, multiple forms of β-glucuronidase were found, differing in uptake and corrective activity [17, 18].

The existence of a specific signal for uptake of a lysosomal enzyme had been suggested by the results of a study into a newly discovered disorder resembling the MPS – named inclusion-cell disease (I-cell disease) because of the prominent phase-dense inclusions in cultured fibroblasts [19]. While these fibroblasts had multiple lysosomal enzyme deficiencies, the medium surrounding them contained a large excess of lysosomal enzymes [20, 21]. However, the enzymes secreted by I-cell disease fibroblasts were not endocytosed by other cells and were not corrective; presumably, they lacked the signal for uptake into lysosomes [22]. Because a number of lysosomal enzymes were affected by this single gene defect (I-cell disease is inherited in an autosomal recessive manner), the signal was postulated to be a post-translational modification of the enzyme proteins. It was further postulated to be carbohydrate in nature, as it could be destroyed by mild periodate treatment [23]. The concept of a recognition system based on carbohydrates was strongly influenced by the discoveries of Ashwell and colleagues regarding the role of carbohydrates in the uptake of circulating glycoproteins by the liver [24, 25].

The presence of a specific recognizable signal implied a saturable, receptor-mediated

process, and suggested that uptake of lysosomal enzymes would follow Michaelis–Menten kinetics. It was expected that analogues of the recognition signals would behave as competitive inhibitors of uptake. This expectation was investigated via the uptake of α-L-iduronidase [26] and of β-glucuronidase [27] by the corresponding deficient fibroblasts. The discovery by Kaplan et al. [27] that the best inhibitor of β-glucuronidase uptake was mannose-6-phosphate (M6P), and their suggestion that M6P was (or was part of) the long-sought recognition signal, was startling, as no phosphorylated carbohydrate had previously been reported to exist on mammalian glycoproteins [27]. It was immediately confirmed for the uptake of α-L-iduronidase [26] and other lysosomal enzymes, using a variety of biochemical methods [28–30]; the ultimate proof came from structural analysis of the phosphorylated carbohydrate groups [31]. The signal discovered through endocytosis proved also to be the signal for targeting nascent hydrolases to lysosomes [32].

The defect in I-cell disease, which prevents the cells from synthesizing the M6P recognition signal, was shown to be a deficiency of the first of two enzymes involved in the synthesis of the M6P signal [33, 34]. Two receptors for M6P were discovered; the chemistry and biology of the M6P receptors and their role in cell trafficking became a broad and very active field of cell biology [35]. These topics are the subjects of many reviews, including Chapters 3 and 5 of this volume. The significance of the M6P system for enzyme replacement therapy will be discussed below.

Concurrent with these studies in cultured fibroblasts, an in-vivo system led to the finding of another signal for uptake of lysosomal enzymes. Several lysosomal enzymes, injected intravenously into rats, were found to be rapidly cleared from the circulation; however, they persisted much longer if pretreated with periodate or if co-injected with an agalactoglycoprotein [36, 37]. Again, carbohydrates were postulated to provide signals for specific recognition. In this case, the key sugar for recognition was mannose [38], and uptake was into reticuloendothelial cells of the liver [39, 40]. The mannose receptor, which recognizes *N*-acetylglucosamine and L-fucose as well as mannose, was shown to occur on the surface of macrophages [41, 42]. It is of some historic interest that the invertase uptake experiments, which featured prominently in the original proposal of enzyme replacement therapy (see above [2, 4]), were successful because invertase is a glycoprotein with mannan chains that are recognized by the mannose receptor [43].

Development of enzyme replacement therapy

Realization that uptake of lysosomal enzymes was receptor-mediated had obvious implications for therapy. To be safe and therapeutically useful, not only would a lysosomal enzyme have to be of human origin, highly purified and available in adequate quantity, but it would also have to carry the recognition signal for the target cells. Such an enzyme was first developed by Brady and colleagues for type 1 Gaucher disease. In this disorder, the target cells are macrophages, cells that have surface receptors recognizing mannose residues. Highly purified placental glucocerebrosidase was sequentially treated with exoglycosidases to remove the sialic acid, galactose and *N*-acetylglucosamine residues from its complex oligosaccharides; uptake into non-parenchymal cells was highest when all three glycosidases were used [44]. In contrast to native enzyme, which gave limited results when administered to patients, glucocerebrosidase with exposed mannose residues was remarkably successful in reversing clinical manifestations of type I Gaucher disease [45, 46] and was approved by the Food and Drug Administration. It was soon replaced with recombinant glucocerebrosidase secreted

by over-expressing Chinese hamster ovary (CHO) cells, which was as effective clinically as the placental enzyme but was preferable because it could be made available in unlimited amounts and was free of pathogens. The recombinant enzyme was also trimmed with the three exo-glycosidases to expose mannose residues [47].

Producing lysosomal enzymes with the M6P signal for targeting to other cells was more difficult because it was not possible to use enzyme purified from tissue. The phosphate group is necessary to target the enzyme to lysosomes, but is not needed for the activity of the enzyme once it resides within the organelle; thus, tissue enzyme is generally dephosphorylated, in whole or in part, by acid phosphatase present in lysosomes. However, CHO cells and other cultured cells over-expressing a soluble recombinant lysosomal enzyme can secrete a highly phosphorylated form, as first demonstrated for α-galactosidase [48]. Such secretion by over-expressing CHO cells has also been demonstrated for a number of other lysosomal enzymes, including α-L-iduronidase [49] and α-glucosidase [50]. The cell biology underlying this secretion is not well understood, but its usefulness is undeniable and forms the basis of commercial production of several therapeutic lysosomal enzymes. Human cells may be used in a similar way, and therapeutic recombinant enzymes made by CHO cells and by human fibroblasts have been produced for Fabry disease. The development of enzyme replacement therapy for Fabry disease is the subject of Chapter 36 in this volume.

The story of enzyme replacement therapy would not be complete without some mention of animal models in the development process. Although therapeutic glucocerebrosidase was developed without pre-testing in an animal model (none would be available for another 8 years [51]), subsequent preclinical studies all included trials on animal models of the deficiency. Dogs [52], cats [53], quail [54] and mice [55] have been used to show a therapeutic effect of the lysosomal enzyme prior to initiation of clinical trials.

It took nearly three decades to progress from the concept of enzyme replacement to commercial development of glucocerebrosidase as a pharmaceutical for Gaucher disease, and an additional decade for the commercial development of α-L-iduronidase, α-galactosidase, α-glucosidase, N-acetylgalactosamine 4-sulfatase and iduronate sulfatase as pharmaceuticals for their respective deficiency diseases (MPS I, Fabry disease, Pompe disease, MPS VI and MPS II). Much of that delay was time needed for understanding the basic science underlying receptor-mediated endocytosis and trafficking of these enzymes. Perhaps this holds a lesson for other forms of therapy that are currently under development, such as gene therapy or stem cell therapy.

References

1. de Duve C. From cytases to lysosomes. *Fed Proc* 1964;23:1045–9

2. de Duve C, Wattiaux R. Functions of lysosomes. *Annu Rev Physiol* 1966;28:435–92

3. Baudhuin P, Hers HG, Loeb H. An electron microscopic and biochemical study of type II glycogenosis. *Lab Invest* 1964;13:1139–52

4. Cohn ZA, Ehrenreich BA. The uptake, storage, and intracellular hydrolysis of carbohydrates by macrophages. *J Exp Med* 1969;129:201–25

5. de Barsy T, Jacquemin P, Van Hoof F, Hers HG. Enzyme replacement in Pompe disease: an attempt with purified human acid α-glucosidase. *Birth Defects Orig Artic Ser* 1973;9:184–90

6. Fratantoni JC, Hall CW, Neufeld EF. The defect in Hurler's and Hunter's syndromes: faulty degradation of mucopolysaccharide. *Proc Natl Acad Sci USA* 1968;60:699–706

7. Fratantoni JC, Hall CW, Neufeld EF. Hurler and Hunter syndromes: mutual correction of the defect in cultured fibroblasts. *Science* 1968;162:570–2

8. McKusick VA, Kaplan D, Wise D, Hanley WB, Suddarth SB, Sevick ME *et al*. The genetic mucopolysaccharidoses. *Medicine (Baltimore)* 1965; 44:445–83

9. Fratantoni JC, Hall CW, Neufeld EF. The defect in Hurler and Hunter syndromes. II. Deficiency of specific factors involved in mucopolysaccharide degradation. *Proc Natl Acad Sci USA* 1969;64:360–6

10. Van Hoof F, Hers HG. L'ultrastructure des cellules hepatiques dans la maladie de Hurler (gargoylisme). [Ultrastructure of hepatic cells in Hurler syndrome (gargoylism)] *C R Acad Sci* 1964;259:1281–3

11. Sly WS, Quinton BA, McAlister WH, Rimoin DL. Beta glucuronidase deficiency: report of clinical, radiologic, and biochemical features of a new mucopolysaccharidosis. *J Pediatr* 1973;82:249–57

12. Hall CW, Cantz M, Neufeld EF. A β-glucuronidase deficiency mucopolysaccharidosis: studies in cultured fibroblasts. *Arch Biochem Biophys* 1973; 155:32–8

13. Bach G, Friedman R, Weissmann B, Neufeld EF. The defect in the Hurler and Scheie syndromes: deficiency of α-L-iduronidase. *Proc Natl Acad Sci USA* 1972;69:2048–51

14. Bach G, Eisenberg F Jr, Cantz M, Neufeld EF. The defect in the Hunter syndrome: deficiency of sulfoiduronate sulfatase. *Proc Natl Acad Sci USA* 1973;70:2134–8

15. Wiesmann U, Neufeld EF. Scheie and Hurler syndromes: apparent identity of the biochemical defect. *Science* 1970;169:72–4

16. Shapiro LJ, Hall CW, Leder IG, Neufeld EF. The relationship of α-L-iduronidase and Hurler corrective factor. *Arch Biochem Biophys* 1976;172: 156–61

17. Brot FE, Glaser JH, Roozen KJ, Sly WS, Stahl PD. *In vitro* correction of deficient human fibroblasts by β-glucuronidase from different human sources. *Biochem Biophys Res Commun* 1974;57:1–8

18. Glaser JH, Roozen KJ, Brot FE, Sly WS. Multiple isoelectric and recognition forms of human β-glucuronidase activity. *Arch Biochem Biophys* 1975; 166:536–42

19. Hanai J, Leroy J, O'Brien JS. Ultrastructure of cultured fibroblasts in I-cell disease. *Am J Dis Child* 1971;122:34–8

20. Lightbody J, Wiesmann U, Hadorn B, Herschkowitz N. I-cell disease: multiple lysosomal-enzyme defect. *Lancet* 1971;i:451

21. Wiesmann UN, Lightbody J, Vassella F, Herschkowitz NN. Multiple lysosomal deficiency due to enzyme leakage? *N Engl J Med* 1971;284:109–10

22. Hickman S, Neufeld EF. A hypothesis for I-cell disease: defective hydrolases that do not enter lysosomes. *Biochem Biophys Res Commun* 1972; 49:992–9

23. Hickman S, Shapiro LJ, Neufeld EF. A recognition marker required for uptake of a lysosomal enzyme by cultured fibroblasts. *Biochem Biophys Res Commun* 1974;57:55–61

24. Morell AG, Gregoriadis G, Scheinberg IH, Hickman J, Ashwell G. The role of sialic acid in determining the survival of glycoproteins in the circulation. *J Biol Chem* 1971;246:1461–7

25. Ashwell G, Morell AG. The role of surface carbohydrates in the hepatic recognition and transport of circulating glycoproteins. *Adv Enzymol Relat Areas Mol Biol* 1974;41:99–128

26. Sando GN, Neufeld EF. Recognition and receptor-mediated uptake of a lysosomal enzyme, α-L-iduronidase, by cultured human fibroblasts. *Cell* 1977;12:619–27

27. Kaplan A, Achord DT, Sly WS. Phosphohexosyl components of a lysosomal enzyme are recognized by pinocytosis receptors on human fibroblasts. *Proc Natl Acad Sci USA* 1977;74:2026–30

28. Kaplan A, Fischer D, Achord D, Sly W. Phospho-hexosyl recognition is a general characteristic of pinocytosis of lysosomal glycosidases by human fibroblasts. *J Clin Invest* 1977;60:1088–93

29. Ullrich K, Mersmann G, Weber E, Von Figura K. Evidence for lysosomal enzyme recognition by human fibroblasts via a phosphorylated carbohydrate moiety. *Biochem J* 1978;170:643–50

30. Hasilik A, Neufeld EF. Biosynthesis of lysosomal enzymes in fibroblasts. Phosphorylation of mannose residues. *J Biol Chem* 1980;255:4946–50

31. Varki A, Kornfeld S. Structural studies of phosphorylated high mannose-type oligosaccharides. *J Biol Chem* 1980;255:10847–58

32. Fischer HD, Gonzalez-Noriega A, Sly WS, Morre DJ. Phosphomannosyl-enzyme receptors in rat liver. Subcellular distribution and role in intracellular transport of lysosomal enzymes. *J Biol Chem* 1980; 255:9608–15

33. Reitman ML, Varki A, Kornfeld S. Fibroblasts from patients with I-cell disease and pseudo-Hurler polydystrophy are deficient in uridine 5'-diphosphate-*N*-acetylglucosamine: glycoprotein *N*-acetylglucosaminylphosphotransferase activity. *J Clin Invest* 1981;67:1574–9

34. Hasilik A, Waheed A, von Figura K. Enzymatic phosphorylation of lysosomal enzymes in the presence of UDP-*N*-acetylglucosamine. Absence of the activity in I-cell fibroblasts. *Biochem Biophys Res Commun* 1981;98:761–7

35. Dahms NM, Lobel P, Kornfeld S. Mannose 6-phosphate receptors and lysosomal enzyme targeting. *J Biol Chem* 1989;264:12115–18

36. Stahl P, Six H, Rodman JS, Schlesinger P, Tulsiani DR, Touster O. Evidence for specific recognition sites mediating clearance of lysosomal enzymes *in vivo*. *Proc Natl Acad Sci USA* 1976;73:4045–9

37. Stahl P, Schlesinger PH, Rodman JS, Doebber T. Recognition of lysosomal glycosidases *in vivo* inhibitied by modified glycoproteins. *Nature* 1976; 264:86–8

38. Achord DT, Brot FE, Sly WS. Inhibition of the rat clearance system for agalacto-orosomucoid by yeast mannans and by mannose. *Biochem Biophys Res Commun* 1977;77:409–15

39. Achord DT, Brot FE, Bell CE, Sly WS. Human β-glucuronidase: *in vivo* clearance and *in vitro* uptake by a glycoprotein recognition system on reticulo-endothelial cells. *Cell* 1978;15:269–78

40. Schlesinger PH, Doebber TW, Mandell BF, White R, DeSchryver C, Rodman JS *et al*. Plasma clearance of glycoproteins with terminal mannose and *N*-acetylglucosamine by liver non-parenchymal cells. Studies with β-glucuronidase, *N*-acetyl-β-D-glucosaminidase, ribonuclease B and agalacto-orosomucoid. *Biochem J* 1978;176:103–9

41. Stahl PD, Rodman JS, Miller MJ, Schlesinger PH. Evidence for receptor-mediated binding of glycoproteins, glycoconjugates, and lysosomal glycosidases by alveolar macrophages. *Proc Natl Acad Sci USA* 1978;75:1399–403

42. Pontow SE, Kery V, Stahl PD. Mannose receptor. *Int Rev Cytol* 1992;137B:221–44

43. Rodman JS, Schlesinger P, Stahl P. Rat plasma clearance of horseradish peroxidase and yeast invertase is mediated by specific recognition. *FEBS Lett* 1978;85:345–8

44. Furbish FS, Steer CJ, Krett NL, Barranger JA. Uptake and distribution of placental glucocerebrosidase in rat hepatic cells and effects of sequential deglycosylation. *Biochim Biophys Acta* 1981;673:425–34

45. Barton NW, Furbish FS, Murray GJ, Garfield M, Brady RO. Therapeutic response to intravenous infusions of glucocerebrosidase in a patient with Gaucher disease. *Proc Natl Acad Sci USA* 1990;87:1913–16

46. Barton NW, Brady RO, Dambrosia JM, Di Bisceglie AM, Doppelt SH, Hill SC *et al*. Replacement therapy for inherited enzyme deficiency – macrophage-targeted glucocerebrosidase for Gaucher's disease. *N Engl J Med* 1991;324:1464–70

47. Grabowski GA, Barton NW, Pastores G, Dambrosia JM, Banerjee TK, McKee MA *et al*. Enzyme therapy in type 1 Gaucher disease: comparative efficacy of mannose-terminated glucocerebrosidase from natural and recombinant sources. *Ann Intern Med* 1995;122:33–9

48. Ioannou YA, Bishop DF, Desnick RJ. Overexpression of human α-galactosidase A results in its intracellular aggregation, crystallization in lysosomes, and selective secretion. *J Cell Biol* 1992;119:1137–50

49. Kakkis ED, Matynia A, Jonas AJ, Neufeld EF. Overexpression of the human lysosomal enzyme α-L-iduronidase in Chinese hamster ovary cells. *Protein Expr Purif* 1994;5:225–32

50. Van Hove JL, Yang HW, Wu JY, Brady RO, Chen YT. High-level production of recombinant human lysosomal acid α-glucosidase in Chinese hamster ovary cells which targets to heart muscle and corrects glycogen accumulation in fibroblasts from patients with Pompe disease. *Proc Natl Acad Sci USA* 1996;93:65–70

51. Liu Y, Suzuki K, Reed JD, Grinberg A, Westphal H, Hoffmann A *et al*. Mice with type 2 and 3 Gaucher disease point mutations generated by a single insertion mutagenesis procedure. *Proc Natl Acad Sci USA* 1998;95:2503–8

52. Shull RM, Kakkis ED, McEntee MF, Kania SA, Jonas AJ, Neufeld EF. Enzyme replacement in a canine model of Hurler syndrome. *Proc Natl Acad Sci USA* 1994;91:12937–41

53. Byers S, Crawley AC, Brumfield LK, Nuttall JD, Hopwood JJ. Enzyme replacement therapy in a feline model of MPS VI: modification of enzyme structure and dose frequency. *Pediatr Res* 2000;47:743–9

54. Kikuchi T, Yang HW, Pennybacker M, Ichihara N, Mizutani M, Van Hove JL *et al.* Clinical and metabolic correction of Pompe disease by enzyme therapy in acid maltase-deficient quail. *J Clin Invest* 1998; 101:827–33

55. Ioannou YA, Zeidner KM, Gordon RE, Desnick RJ. Fabry disease: preclinical studies demonstrate the effectiveness of α-galactosidase A replacement in enzyme-deficient mice. *Am J Hum Genet* 2001; 68:14–25

11 Regulatory framework for the treatment of orphan diseases

Rashmi R Shah*

Gerrards Cross, Buckinghamshire, SL9 7JA, UK

Pharmaceutical Consultant, former Senior Clinical Assessor, Medicines and Healthcare products Regulatory Agency, London, and former UK Member of the Committee for Orphan Medicinal Products

Orphan diseases are typically those that are sufficiently rare that there are no commercial incentives to research and develop effective therapies. In order to encourage pharmaceutical companies to invest in orphan drug development, various countries, beginning with the USA, have introduced legislation to provide suitable incentives. Although the definition of what constitutes a 'rare' disease varies from one region to another, there is a remarkable degree of similarity in the incentives provided. These range from market exclusivity for the product in its proposed indication (the most important incentive) to tax credits and reduction or waivers of fees. The USA and Japan also provide sizeable research grants. There is little denying that these measures have had a remarkable effect in meeting the expectations of patients with rare diseases. Among the major pharmaceutical markets, the European Union has most recently enacted orphan drug legislation, in 2000. The success of this legislation has been spectacular and compares well with the first 5 years following the introduction of US legislation. However, scientific advances have outstripped healthcare budgets. Pricing and access seem to vary widely across the globe and are intricately linked with reimbursement. There are inequalities and, in some regions, patients are often faced with having to make difficult choices. There is no doubt, however, that there is greater societal recognition now than ever before that patients with rare diseases are entitled to medicines and, importantly, medicines developed to the same high standard as those for other, more common, conditions.

Introduction

The estimated average cost of developing a new drug has increased progressively and currently ranges from €500 million to €895 million depending on the therapeutic class of drug [1, 2]. Commercially, such costs are not conducive to developing therapies for diseases that are rare, because the expected returns would be too low.

Consequently, orphan diseases are typically those that are sufficiently rare that there are no commercial incentives to research and develop effective therapies for them. In 1983, the USA became the first country to introduce orphan drug legislation. Following its success, a number of other countries introduced similar legislation (Singapore in 1991, Japan in 1993 and Australia in 1998).

---

*The views expressed in this chapter are those of the author and do not necessarily reflect the views or opinions of the European Medicines Agency, Medicines and Healthcare products Regulatory Agency, other regulatory authorities or any of their advisory bodies.

In 2000, the European Union (EU) also adopted regulations relating to this important area of drug development and public health. Other countries have either introduced (Taiwan in 2000) or are preparing (Switzerland) similar legislation. In order to encourage pharmaceutical companies to invest in orphan drug development, almost all legislation provides a number of incentives.

There are approximately 30 000 recognized diseases, 6000–8000 of which can be regarded as rare. Of these rare diseases, about 70% are genetic in origin. The definition of what constitutes a 'rare' disease varies from one region to another. The prevalence figure accepted in the EU is no more than five individuals per 10 000 of the population. In the USA, the proposed prevalence is less than 200 000 individuals out of the entire population, which currently equates to approximately 7.5 per 10 000 of the population (see later). Similarly, the prevalence thresholds stipulated in Japan and Australia are no more than 50 000 and 2000 patients, respectively, which equate to no more than 4.2 and 1.1 individuals, respectively, per 10 000 of the corresponding populations.

This chapter summarizes the current legislation and regulatory framework for the development of treatment for orphan diseases, with a special focus on the EU. The chapter concludes with a summary of pricing and reimbursement of, and access to, orphan medicinal products across the EU and other regions.

Orphan drug legislation in the EU

In the EU, there are two primary pieces of orphan drug legislation – both of which are Regulations and, therefore, directly applicable in all Member States. These Regulations were modelled on the US legislation with careful attention to the experience gained by the Office of Orphan Products Development (OOPD) of the Food and Drug Administration (FDA). The first is the Regulation (EC) No 141/2000, which is concerned with the purpose, definitions and criteria for designation, and the procedures for and provision of protocol assistance (scientific advice), as well as establishing the Committee for Orphan Medicinal Products (COMP), access to centralized procedure without further justification for community marketing authorization, market exclusivity and other incentives. The other is the Commission Regulation (EC) No 847/2000, which lays down the provisions for implementation of the criteria for designation, as well as defining the concepts of 'similar medicinal product' and 'clinical superiority'.

The incentives offered in the EU are summarized in Table 1, together with a comparison of those offered in the USA and Japan. They include market exclusivity and fee reductions. The period of market exclusivity in the EU is 10 years from authorization of the product. A Member State must not accept another application for a marketing authorization or grant a marketing authorization or accept an application to extend an existing marketing authorization for the same therapeutic indication in respect of a similar medicinal product. However, exclusivity may be lost by the first applicant consenting to a second application from another applicant, if the first applicant is unable to meet demand, if a similar product is found to be clinically superior, if the criteria are no longer met or if, at the end of the first 5 years, a Member State can show that the product is (highly) profitable.

Fee reductions apply to fees for preauthorization activities, such as protocol assistance (scientific advice), and the application for marketing authorization, inspections and post-authorization activities, such as variations, annual fees etc. Since 2002, protocol assistance is provided with 100% reduction in the fees applicable to provision of scientific advice, and all other fees are reduced by 50%. From 2006, however, the inspection fees will also attract a 100% reduction, whereas the reduction in

Table 1. *Incentives for the development of orphan drugs.*

Incentive	EU	USA	Japan
Market exclusivity	10 years normally (6 years if product is highly profitable)	7 years	10 years
Research grants	Available in some Member States Also central funding available from the EC	Funded by Office of Orphan Products Development	Funded by government
Tax reductions on development costs	Available in some Member States	50%	15%
Waiver of fees	Yes (variable)	100%	Yes (variable)
Protocol assistance	Yes	Yes	Yes
Access to centralized procedure	Yes	–	–
Access to continuous regulatory assistance	–	Yes	–
Accelerated or fast-track review	Possible	Possible	Possible

fees for post-authorization activities will be limited to the first year (unless the sponsor is a small- or medium-sized enterprise).

Over the 5 years to April 2005, the fee reduction granted to orphan medicinal products totalled just under €12.5 million. The funds made available by the Community for fee exemptions for orphan medicinal products amounted to €3 700 000 in 2005. As of April 2005, 48% of this fund had already been utilized and it was estimated that up to €6 000 000 would be needed in 2005 to cover the higher than expected level of activities. For the year 2006, the Community has been able to provide funds amounting to €4 000 000 for fee exemptions for orphan medicinal products.

There is also a central EU fund to support research generally. In the first three calls of the 6th Framework Programme, which supports research in key areas targeted by the European Commission (EC), a total of €93 million has already been awarded by the EC to 26 projects dealing with rare diseases or medicinal products. In addition, some Member States (including the UK) provide tax credits and research grants.

The sponsor proposing to develop a drug for an orphan indication is required to submit to the European Medicines Agency (EMEA) an application for the designation of a drug as orphan for a defined clinical entity. To meet the criteria for a successful orphan designation, the applicant should establish that:

- the prevalence of the condition in the EU is no more than 5 in 10 000 or that the product is unlikely to generate sufficient return on investment
- the condition applied for is life threatening or debilitating
- no satisfactory methods exist for the treatment of the condition or, if there is a product already authorized in the EU, the medicinal product that is the subject of the application will be of significant benefit.

All three criteria must be satisfied and all claims require supporting data or should be substantiated by references. Although 'medical plausibility' is not an explicit criterion, the COMP view is that the text of the Regulation implies a scientific need to consider 'medical plausibility' in the context of an application for orphan designation. This view is consistent with views on orphan designation in the USA and Japan. Over the years, sponsors have put forward a variety of different arguments for significant benefit, some deemed acceptable by COMP and others not. In the interest of clarity and transparency, the EC issued a communication in July 2003 and the COMP has also released for consultation a draft guideline on the elements required to support the medical plausibility and the assumption of significant benefit for an orphan designation. Both provide further information in this regard, together with examples.

Regulatory framework and processes in the EU

Orphan diseases affect approximately 30 million patients in the EU, out of a population of approximately 450 million [3]. At the regulatory level, the process of developing and marketing orphan drugs can be divided into three discrete steps:

- application for designation (a process based on assumption)
- application for protocol assistance (a science-driven process for optimal use of resources and conducting clinical trials)
- application for marketing authorization (a process based on demonstration of evidence).

The EMEA and COMP

The EMEA, based in London since 1995, is an executive agency of the EC and has the functions of a professional secretariat. It works in very close liaison with the national authorities of the Member States of the EU and includes the COMP, the Committee for Medicinal Products for Human Use (CHMP), the Committee for Herbal Medicinal Products and the Committee for Medicinal Products for Veterinary Use, in addition to the various Working Parties of these committees.

The COMP held its inaugural meeting in April 2000 and meets 11 times per year. Until May 2004, it was constituted of one member from each of the 15 Member States, three nominated by the EC to liaise with the CHMP and three from patient organizations, making a total of 21 members. It is the first decision-making committee in the EU to include direct patient representation. Following the accession of the ten new Member States (Cyprus, Czech Republic, Estonia, Hungary, Latvia, Lithuania, Malta, Poland, Slovak Republic and Slovenia) to the EU on 1 May 2004, the membership has now increased to 31. In addition, the Committee also includes one member appointed by each of the states of the EEA–EFTA (European Economic Area–European Free Trade Association).

The COMP has access to the expertise of all the Working Parties set up by the EMEA and the CHMP. These are the Efficacy Working Party, Safety Working Party, Quality Working Party, Pharmacogenetics Working Party, Pharmacovigilance Working Party, Biotechnology Working Party, Blood and Plasma Products Working Party, Gene Therapy Working Party, Vaccine Working Party, Scientific Advice Working Party and Paediatric Working Party. In addition, it has at its disposal a network of approximately

350 rare disease experts in a wide range of therapeutic areas. The COMP is highly proactive in promoting the development of orphan drugs and in interacting with academia, industry and patient groups.

Applications for designation

The applicants are generally advised to have a pre-submission meeting with the EMEA Secretariat. On receipt of a valid application, the COMP appoints one of its members and a professional staff member of the EMEA Secretariat to act as the two coordinators (day 0). The two coordinators prepare a joint assessment report for discussion at the following COMP meeting (day 30). If the COMP is satisfied that the criteria are met, a positive opinion is issued. More often, there are issues that require clarification and a list of questions or issues to be addressed is sent to the applicant. The responses are assessed by the two coordinators and discussed at the next meeting (day 60). If there are still any outstanding issues, these can be dealt with during an oral hearing on day 90, when an opinion is issued. In the case of a negative opinion, the applicant has full appeal rights.

Whenever possible, scientific opinions, decisions or recommendations of the Committee are taken by consensus. If a consensus cannot be reached, the scientific opinion is adopted if supported by at least two-thirds of the total number of Committee members eligible to vote (i.e. 21 or more). In the absence of a two-thirds majority in favour of designation, the Committee's opinion is deemed to be negative. Members representing the EEA–EFTA states do not have formal voting rights, but they participate in the discussions and their views are recorded separately.

Following its consideration of an application, the COMP adopts an opinion. This is transmitted to the EC, which is responsible for issuing a binding decision on the orphan designation status of the product for the indication concerned. The product is then entered in the EC register of orphan products. The EC decision is binding on all the Member States. However, designation of a product as orphan is not sacrosanct. The product may be removed from the register (i) at the request of the sponsor, (ii) if it is established before the marketing authorization is granted that the designation criteria are no longer met or (iii) at the end of the period of market exclusivity. In accordance with the Regulation, sponsors are required to submit annual reports to the EMEA to update the status of the development of the orphan medicinal product.

Applications for protocol assistance

The approval of any medicinal product for a marketing authorization requires robust data on its quality, safety and efficacy. The data on safety and efficacy can be generated only from well-designed and executed clinical trials. In order to optimize drug development and the use of resources, it is often necessary to obtain scientific views ('scientific advice') from the regulatory authorities. Scientific advice may concern issues that are not regulatory in nature and that are not covered by existing guidelines or when the applicant is proposing to deviate from these guidelines. It is particularly important to seek this advice before embarking on expensive and resource-intensive phase III studies. Conduct of well-designed and executed clinical trials is a critical step in the development of orphan drugs. 'Protocol assistance' is the term used for scientific advice in the context of the development of orphan medicinal products.

Regulations require the EMEA to provide the Member States and the institutions of the Community with the best possible scientific advice on any question relating to the evaluation of a medicinal product for human or veterinary use with regard to its quality, safety and efficacy. For this purpose, the

EMEA and the CHMP have set up a Scientific Advice Working Party (SAWP). The SAWP is a multidisciplinary expert group consisting of 21 members, including three from the COMP. The chairpersons of the Efficacy Working Party and Safety Working Party are invited members. The mandate of the SAWP requires it to include members who have expertise in methodology and statistics, especially with regard to studies in small populations and pharmacoepidemiology. The SAWP brings forward to the CHMP an integrated view of all the Member States on scientific matters. Clearly, development of a drug in line with the scientific advice also facilitates the evaluation of the dossier, as there are no ambiguities or inconsistencies between Member States.

Protocol assistance for orphan drugs is essential and probably the most important step in their development in view of the unique challenges associated with developing these products. These challenges are related to small sample sizes, a widely distributed patient population, choice of the right study design with the appropriate endpoints, selection of comparators and/or placebo, and making sure that all the criteria on which the designation was granted are likely to be addressed. It is important to ensure that the clinical development will demonstrate significant benefit over authorized products if the orphan designation was based on this assumption. The number of protocol assistances requested and delivered by the SAWP reflects the pharmaceutical activity resulting from the EU orphan drug legislation and the number of products designated by the COMP.

On receipt of a request for protocol assistance, the SAWP appoints two co-ordinators, to whom the applicant should submit the full documentation. These two coordinators circulate to all the members their individual initial reports on draft CHMP advice. Following a well-structured and interactive process, the procedure is completed by day 100 at the latest, and the final scientific advice is prepared for approval by the CHMP. If required during the process, an expert meeting may be set up and the applicant has the opportunity of providing an oral explanation. Issues that are relevant to orphan drug designation also require approval by the COMP.

Effective from January 2005, there is an initiative for a Pilot Scheme for Parallel Scientific Advice Meetings between the SAWP and the FDA. The goal of this 1-year pilot is to provide a mechanism for EMEA and FDA assessors and sponsors to exchange their views on scientific issues during the development phase of new medicinal products. It is envisaged that the prime candidates for parallel scientific advice will be important or breakthrough medicinal products, especially if the product is being developed for indications for which development guidelines do not exist or, when guidelines do exist, if those from the EMEA and the FDA differ significantly. The experience to date has been most rewarding for all concerned. Products for orphan indications or paediatric populations would clearly benefit from this initiative. Each agency will provide their independent advice to the sponsor on the questions posed during the Parallel Scientific Advice Meetings, according to their usual procedures. The advice of each agency may still differ after the joint discussion.

Applications for marketing authorization

Under new pharmaceutical legislation effective from November 2005, an application for marketing authorization of an orphan medicinal product will be required to be submitted to the EMEA via the central route for evaluation by CHMP, with the same scientific rigour as other drugs. A successful application results in a single marketing authorization (a single document from the EC) for the medicinal product valid throughout the EU under a single trade name and a common Summary of Product Characteristics (known as the 'label' in the USA).

The CHMP is the scientific advisory body responsible for formulating an opinion on the granting, variation, suspension or withdrawal of an authorization to place a medicinal product for human use on the EU market. The current CHMP consists of one member and one alternate member appointed by each of the 25 Member States. In broad terms, the alternate member deputizes for the corresponding principal member from a Member State who is unable to attend the CHMP. In order to complement its expertise, the CHMP has also co-opted five members chosen on the basis of their specific scientific competence. The scientific opinion or recommendation is adopted if supported by an absolute majority of the members of the Committee (i.e. favourable votes by at least half of the total number of Committee members eligible to vote plus one, which is 16).

Briefly, a rapporteur and a co-rapporteur, selected from among the members of the CHMP, primarily evaluate each application for marketing authorization for a new drug. The two assessment reports are considered at the plenary meeting of the CHMP. Issues of quality, safety and efficacy that are a matter of concern or require clarification are identified and communicated to the applicant. Following responses by the applicant, there is a secondary assessment of, and plenary discussion on, the responses. The applicant has ample opportunities to respond to any remaining issues. The process is concluded with an opinion by the CHMP; if negative, the applicant has full appeal rights. Finally, the opinion is communicated to the EC for a binding decision.

The EMEA ensures that the opinion of the CHMP is given within 210 days of receipt of a valid application for marketing authorization submitted through the centralized route. For medicinal products that are of major interest with regard to public health and/or therapeutic innovation, the applicant may request an accelerated assessment procedure. If the request is substantiated and the CHMP accepts the request, the time limit is reduced to 150 days.

Directive 2003/63/EC describes the data required in support of a marketing authorization application. A typical dossier for a non-orphan new drug includes data on 2000–4000 patients. This is, of course, not usually possible with diseases that are rare. Not surprisingly, the datasets for orphan drugs already approved by the CHMP have varied widely. The applications that have been approved by the CHMP as of April 2005 have included datasets ranging from as few as 12 to as many as 1064 patients for efficacy analysis and from as few as 20 to as many as just over 4600 patients for safety analysis.

The normal standards of quality, safety and efficacy that prevail for non-orphan medicinal products have not been compromised in a rush to approve these orphan products. This is an important point to emphasize, as patients with rare diseases are just as entitled to medicines that have been tested to the highest standards. However, like other medicinal products, designated orphan medicinal products may be granted a marketing authorization under exceptional circumstances, subject to annual re-assessment and certain specific post-approval obligations or commitments for additional data. In particular, such authorizations may be granted when the indications for which the product is intended are encountered so rarely that the applicant cannot reasonably be expected to provide comprehensive evidence at the outset. An accelerated review might also be initiated by the CHMP in exceptional circumstances when a medicinal product is intended to meet a major public health need, defined by the seriousness of the condition, lack of or inadequate alternative therapeutic approaches and anticipated high therapeutic benefits.

Article 83 of Regulation (EC) No 726/2004 also provides for making a medicinal product available for compassionate reasons to a group of patients with a chronically or seriously debilitating disease or whose disease is considered to be life threatening, and who cannot be treated satisfactorily by an (already) authorized medicinal product. The medicinal product concerned must either be the subject of an application for a marketing authorization or must be undergoing clinical trials. When compassionate use is envisaged, the CHMP, after consulting the manufacturer or the applicant, may adopt opinions on the conditions for use, the conditions for distribution and the patients targeted.

Five-year experience and achievements in the EU

The EU experience in the first 5 years following the implementation of the orphan drug legislation has been most rewarding.

Activities of the COMP

In the first 5 years of its operation, 458 applications for orphan designation were submitted to the EMEA and the COMP had determined 431 applications. Of these, 287 (67%) were given a positive opinion and 144 (33%) were either withdrawn or were

given a negative opinion (Table 2) [4]. The average time from the start of the procedure to the opinion was 67 days for the 296 applications given an opinion. The average time for the EC then to issue the decision was about 45 days. As of April 2005, 268 of the 287 products given a positive opinion by the COMP were officially designated as orphan by the EC.

Of the products given a positive opinion, the main therapeutic categories were oncology (36%), metabolic (11%), immunology (11%), cardiovascular or respiratory (10%), musculoskeletal or neurology (8%) and infections (4%). Miscellaneous therapeutic categories accounted for the remaining 20% of the products designated. For 69% of the products, the positive opinion has been based on the criterion of significant benefit (improved efficacy in 78.8%, potential improvement in safety in 5.2%, contribution to patient care in 5.7% and a combination of any of these in the remainder).

Of the 458 applications submitted to the EMEA, all except two had been based on the prevalence criterion. The prevalence of the condition was less than 1 per 10 000 for 43%, 1–3 per 10 000 for 47% and more than 3 per 10 000 for the remaining 10% of the products designated. The target populations of the 287 designated products were adults (46%), children (11%) or both (43%).

Table 2. *Committee for Orphan Medicinal Products opinions from April 2000 to April 2005.*

Year	Positive opinion	Withdrawn	Negative opinion	Total
2000	26	6	0	32
2001	64	27	1	92
2002	43	30	3	76
2003	54	41	1	96
2004	75	22	4	101
2005	25	9	0	34
Total	287	135	9	431

Of the two applications submitted on the basis of insufficient return on investment, one was withdrawn by the sponsor prior to COMP opinion while the other was given a positive opinion in September 2005.

Activities of the CHMP

Of the 268 EC-designated orphan medicinal products, 44 had filed an application for a marketing authorization through the centralized route as of April 2005. The CHMP had given a positive opinion in the case of 20 applications for marketing authorization. These products are listed in Table 3. Two applications were given a negative opinion, the sponsors had withdrawn seven, and the remaining 15 were still under evaluation. Eight of the 20 products were authorized for conditions for which there were no satisfactory treatment options, whereas the other 12 were authorized in expectation of significant benefit to patients. The 20 products are estimated to potentially benefit more than 1 million patients suffering from orphan diseases in the Community.

Of the centrally authorized orphan medicinal products, 35% have been approved on the basis of phase III, double-blind, randomized, placebo-controlled or phase III, single-blind, randomized, active controlled, multicentre clinical trials, whereas 40% were based on phase II studies (two of them double-blind, randomized and placebo-controlled). Compassionate use data and bibliographic data

Table 3. *Orphan medicinal products given a positive opinion by the Committee for Medicinal Products for Human Use (to April 2005).*

Product	Active ingredient	Route of administration	Summary indication
Fabrazyme	Agalsidase beta	i.v. infusion	Fabry disease
Replagal	Agalsidase alfa	i.v. infusion	Fabry disease
Glivec CML	Imatinib mesilate	Oral	Chronic myeloid leukaemia
Trisenox	Arsenic trioxide	i.v. infusion	Acute promyelocytic leukaemia
Tracleer	Bosentan monohydrate	Oral	Pulmonary arterial hypertension
Zavesca	Miglustat	Oral	Gaucher disease
Somavert	Pegvisomant	s.c. injection	Acromegaly
Carbaglu	Carglumic acid	Oral	Hyperammonaemia due to *N*-acetylglutamate synthase deficiency
Busilvex	Busulfan	i.v. infusion	Haematopoietic progenitor cell transplantation
Aldurazyme	Laronidase	i.v. infusion	Mucopolysaccharidosis
Ventavis	Iloprost	Inhalation	Pulmonary arterial hypertension
Xagrid	Anagrelide hydrochloride	Oral	Essential thrombocythaemia
Onsenal	Celecoxib	Oral	Familial adenomatous polyposis
Litak	Cladribine	s.c. injection	Hairy cell leukaemia
Photobarr	Porfimer sodium	i.v. infusion	Barrett's oesophagus
Lysodren	Mitotane	Oral	Adrenal cortical carcinoma
Pedea	Ibuprofen	i.v. infusion	Patent ductus arteriosus
Wilzin	Zinc acetate dihydrate	Oral	Treatment of Wilson's disease
Prialt	Ziconotide	Intraspinal	Treatment of chronic pain requiring intraspinal analgesia
Orfadin	Nitisinone	Oral	Treatment of tyrosinaemia type I

i.v., intravenous; s.c., subcutaneous.

provided the basis for successful applications in four cases. Sixty-five per cent of the marketing authorizations were granted under 'exceptional circumstances', which means that at the time of the evaluation it was deemed that the applicant could not reasonably be expected to provide comprehensive evidence on the safety and efficacy of the medicinal product.

During the same period, five applications were submitted through the mutual recognition route (i.e. a national authorization in any one Member State followed by its mutual recognition by the remainder). Of these, two received positive opinions for marketing authorizations. These two products are Dudopa (levodopa/carbidopa) for advanced idiopathic Parkinson's disease with severe motor fluctuations not responding to oral treatment, and Impavido (miltefosine) for the treatment of visceral leishmaniasis. Of the remainder, two were still under evaluation and one was withdrawn.

With regard specifically to Fabry disease, the FDA has designated a number of drugs for its treatment. These have included 1,5-(butylimino)-1,5-dideoxy-D-glucitol in May 1998 and 1-deoxygalactonojirimycin in February 2004. The first company to be granted orphan drug designation for recombinant α-galactosidase A (ceramide-trihexosidase) for the treatment of Fabry disease was Genzyme Corporation, in January 1988. Various other sponsors were also granted designation for recombinant α-galactosidase A in July 1990, June 1991, June 1998 and January 2003, for the same indication. Designated as orphan on 8 August 2000 in the EU, two products containing agalsidase were approved on 3 August 2001 for marketing in the EU: agalsidase alfa (Replagal®, TKT Europe AB; produced in a human cell line) and agalsidase beta (Fabrazyme®, Genzyme Europe BV; produced in Chinese hamster ovary cells). The applications for these two

products had been submitted simultaneously and were therefore evaluated and determined simultaneously. Since August 2001, it has been estimated that a total of approximately 1000 patients in the Community have received either Fabrazyme or Replagal. Fabrazyme was also approved for marketing in the USA in April 2003 and in Japan in January 2004.

Orphan drug legislation in the USA and Japan
Orphan drugs in the USA
The US Orphan Products Act, amending the US Federal Food, Drug and Cosmetic Act, was enacted on 4 January 1983. The Act, administered by the OOPD of the FDA, did not initially include a prevalence figure to determine the eligibility of a drug as orphan. It did, however, include many incentives and defined a product for a rare disease as one that would not be profitable for 7 years following FDA approval. The US Internal Revenue Service, which determined profitability, had difficulty with this concept, and the original definition of a 'rare disease or condition' in the Orphan Drug Act was therefore amended in October 1984 by PL 98-551 to add a numeric prevalence threshold: "…the term rare disease or condition means any disease or condition which (a) affects less than 200 000 persons in the US or (b) affects more than 200 000 persons in the US but for which there is no reasonable expectation that the cost of developing and making available in the US a drug for such disease or condition will be recovered from sales in the US of such drug".

The definition of orphan products also includes products other than drugs; in particular, biological products, medical devices and medical foods. Examples of orphan medical foods might include special foods for diseases such as phenylketonuria. PL 100-290 further amended the Orphan Drug Act in April 1988 to require that the application for designation be made prior to the submission of an application for marketing approval (instead of at any time prior to FDA approval to market the product).

In order for a product to be designated as orphan, the sponsor submits to the OOPD documentation that they are developing a product that is rational for use in a specific disease and has a reasonable scientific basis, and that the disease has a prevalence of fewer than 200 000 patients in the USA. The documentation should include some key information. First, there should be a description of the disease for which use of the drug is claimed and the intended conditions of use. Secondly, the sponsor should provide the size and other chief characteristics of the population likely to be treated in the USA. Thirdly, the documentation should include a description of the drug and its known risk:benefit ratio. A summary of the principal preclinical and clinical data concerning use of the product in the claimed indication, as well as basic documentation, should be provided, and all available information, published or otherwise, must be supplied. Finally, if the product is claimed not to be profitable for 7 years following its approval for marketing, an estimate must be given of the cost of development and distribution of the drug, as well as an assessment of potential sales in the USA, confirming the absence of commercial viability of marketing the drug in specific cases. Scientific staff at the OOPD review the application and determine whether the drug qualifies as an orphan product. If the OOPD is satisfied, the product is designated as orphan and incentives provided for by the Act begin.

The incentives offered in the USA include (i) 7-year market exclusivity for the drug for the indication, (ii) availability of orphan product development grants, (iii) tax credits equal to 50% of the expenses for clinical (not preclinical) development costs, (iv) protocol assistance and (v), from 1997, an exemption from charges related to the review of the pre-market approval dossier, called the 'user fees'. Section 1205 of PL 104-188 reinstated the tax credits for clinical testing expenses of orphan drugs and allowed these credits to be carried forward 20 years and back 1 year – similar to some other business tax credits.

Of all the incentives, the most important is the market exclusivity for the product for the indication. Although more than one sponsor can receive designation for the same drug for the same use, the 7-year period of exclusive marketing is granted only to the first sponsor who obtains marketing approval for a designated orphan drug or biological product. Exclusivity begins on the date that the marketing application is approved by the FDA and applies only to the indication for which the drug has been designated and approved. The FDA could approve a second application for the same drug for a different use. If a second product is approved for the same indication because of its improved safety profile, greater efficacy or its major contribution to patient care, then it is considered to be a different product that is clinically superior. In such an event, the exclusivity of the first product will most likely be compromised.

The Orphan Drug Act provides for formal protocol assistance when requested by the sponsors of orphan drugs. The formal review of a request for protocol assistance is the direct responsibility of the Center for Drug Evaluation and Research or the Center for Biologics Evaluation and Research, depending on which Center has authority for review of the product concerned. However, the OOPD is responsible for ensuring that the request qualifies for consideration. This includes determining "whether there is reason to believe the sponsor's drug is a drug for a disease or condition that is rare in the United States". A sponsor need not have obtained orphan drug designation to receive protocol assistance. Interaction between OOPD reviewers, orphan product sponsors and FDA review divisions is common; however, protocol assistance is rarely used in the USA because of several major changes in the FDA's regulations and philosophy governing the Investigational New Drug, and New Drug Application processes.

The research grants programme has also been instrumental in stimulating the development of orphan products. Applications are reviewed by panels of outside experts and are funded by priority score. The US government allocates a large fund annually to support clinical trials – approximately $15 million in 2005. Grants ranging from $200 000 to $350 000 have been provided in 2005, primarily to academic/university-based researchers, for clinical study. When it is difficult to find a sponsor for a very rare disease (despite the incentives), the availability of positive data from clinical trials supported by the OOPD provides a significant additional incentive that the product will work and is worthy of further development.

These incentives have clearly worked. In the 10 years prior to the Act, an estimated ten products came on to the US market that could have been designated as orphan products. Since the passage of the Act, 1449 products have been designated as orphan and, of these, 269 have received FDA approval as of April 2005. In total, these products could treat more than 13 million patients in the USA.

Devices are supported in the orphan products grants programme if they treat an orphan population of less than 200 000 in the USA. Additionally, the FDA Medical Device law contains a provision that creates Humanitarian Device Exemptions (HUD) for devices that will be used fewer than 4000 times in a year. The OOPD is involved in ascertaining the population that would make use of the device. The devices receive FDA approval and are exempt from much of the efficacy documentation needed for a Pre-market Approval of a Device – the standard approval. More than 70 HUDs have been approved since the passing of that part of the Medical Device Act.

Orphan drugs in Japan

In 1985, the Japanese Ministry of Health, Labour and Welfare (MHLW) announced preferential measures for facilitating the approval of orphan drugs, focusing mainly on tropical diseases. In 1990, the Science Council of Japan emphasized the importance of orphan drugs, and the basic drug research programme was restructured in 1993 to target orphan drugs exclusively. This culminated in Notification No 725, published in August 1993, amending the Pharmaceutical Affairs Law, and in October 1993 the orphan drug regulation came into force. In April 2004, the newly created Pharmaceutical and Medical Devices Agency (PMDA), under the supervision of MHLW, took over the operation of orphan product promotion from the Ministry's Organization for Pharmaceutical Safety and Research, also known as 'KIKO'.

Article 77-2 of the Japanese Medicines Act stipulates three criteria for orphan designation. These are (i) the number of patients affected must be less than 50 000 within the Japanese territories, (ii) there must be a medical need with no suitable alternatives or the efficacy and safety of the drug to be designated must be better than available drugs or interventions and (iii) there must be a high potential for actual development (the existence of a theoretical basis for the use of the drug and a feasible development plan). Although not explicitly stated in the criteria, the disease must be life threatening. Applicants are advised not to subcategorize a disease more than necessary with the intention of making the number of affected patients below 50 000.

As in the EU and USA, orphan drug designation is granted to a combination of an applicant, a product and an indication.

Apart from a reduced fee for Japanese marketing authorization application, other incentives offered include (i) consultation and advice for development, (ii) an orphan products development grant (up to 50% of the research and development cost per year for a maximum of 3 years after designation), (iii) authorization for tax deduction, (iv) fast-track review for approval and (v) extension of the re-examination period from a normal 5-year period to a 10-year period for orphan drugs and a 7-year period for orphan devices. In Japan, although patent issues are important, the period before a generic drug can enter the market is related to the re-examination period. A downside of the extended re-examination period is that the sponsor has to pay the additional postmarketing surveillance costs, which could be substantial.

The average amount per grant (and the number of grants awarded) for development of orphan products was 30.07 million yen ($n = 23$) during the year 2000, 26.68 million yen ($n = 26$) during 2001 and 38.53 million yen ($n = 18$) during 2002. The cumulative amount awarded from 1993 to 2002 was 5.101 billion yen divided among 278 grants. Sponsors are entitled to tax deductions of 15% of the authorized expenses for preclinical and clinical studies. Companies making profits on sales of orphan drugs must return a proportion of the subsidy granted as a contribution to these funds. The threshold for repayment of grants is annual sales exceeding 100 million yen and the rate of repayment is 1% of the excess sales. This requirement can continue for up to 10 years as long as the repayment does not exceed the amount of the grant received.

The MHLW receives and determines an application for designation of a drug as orphan, and it is also the MHLW that receives and determines an application for approval of an orphan medicinal product for marketing. The responsibilities for various activities are shared among a number of organizations within the MHLW. The Evaluation and Licensing Division of the MHLW is responsible for consultation concerning designation and application, the National Institute of Biomedical Innovation is responsible for the grant-awarding programme, the tax credit authorization programme and for consultation on testing and research after designation (fees are not chargeable), and the Centre for Product Evaluation of the PMDA is responsible for specialist consultation and advice (fees are chargeable).

The procedure for designation involves an application (may be made by telephone or facsimile) for a pre-designation hearing. The Evaluation and Licensing Division of the MHLW accepts the application and a contact person is appointed who arranges a date for the pre-designation consultation. The pre-designation hearing usually lasts for 30 minutes. Following this, if there are no particular problems, the applicant submits a formal application for designation to the Evaluation and Licensing Division. The PMDA evaluates the application and, if the product is determined appropriate for designation, the MHLW asks the opinion of the Pharmaceutical Affairs and Food Sanitation Council. When the Council determines that the criteria for designation are met, the MHLW designates the product as an orphan product and the applicant is notified accordingly. The public is informed of the newly designated orphan product by notification from the Director of Evaluation and Licensing Division in the government gazette.

As of April 2004, 168 orphan products were designated and, of these, 96 have been approved for marketing. The corresponding figures for orphan devices were ten and four, respectively. Among the four devices are implantable defibrillation cardioverter and implantable left ventricular assist systems.

Access and reimbursement

Access and reimbursement of orphan products are contentious issues and have given rise to much debate. The system in every country, including within the Member States of the EU, is different.

When discussing 'price' there are two values to be considered. First, there is the manufacturer's price before taxes (MPBT). This is the pharmaceutical company's price to its customers (distributors, wholesalers, pharmacies, hospitals), which is the price when considering margins (or profit for the manufacturer). The other is the public price including taxes (PPIT), which, in addition to the MPBT, includes middleman mark-ups and taxes, such as VAT and taxes on advertising. The PPIT is the relevant price when considering healthcare expenditures or patient access to orphan drugs.

Pricing and access in the EU

In November 2004, the EC published an independent study on the price of orphan drugs in the EU. The study, conducted by Alcimed, looked at the price of ten orphan drugs authorized in the EU and how these prices were determined. The findings from this study should be interpreted with caution. Apart from the small sample of orphan drugs studied, the prevalence of the conditions for which they are indicated varied widely. The following is a summary of findings from this study, the full report of which can be accessed on the EC website [5].

Among the 15 countries of the former EU, the MPBT is the highest in Germany and France, followed by Austria, Finland and Luxembourg, The Netherlands and Sweden and then Belgium, Denmark, Greece, Ireland and Italy. The three countries with the lowest MPBT are Spain, Portugal and the UK. For PPIT, the ranking of countries is very different from the MPBT. Austria had the highest annual cost per patient, followed by Germany and Denmark, then Finland, France and Ireland and, finally, Spain, Portugal, the UK and Sweden.

The average ratio of the highest to the lowest prices among the countries was 1.7 for PPIT in contrast to 1.2 for MPBT. This suggests that the price differences between countries do not arise from the desire of sponsors, who try to harmonize their prices to limit parallel imports. The maximal variations of MPBT between countries are, in fact, not very different, being on average 122% of the lowest price, and with the two extremes being 105% and 173%.

The PPIT:MPBT ratio can approach 1 in countries that do not require taxes on these medicines and that do not permit commercial transactions between hospital pharmacies and patients. This is the case for Luxembourg, The Netherlands and Sweden. In other countries this ratio can range from 1.4 to 1.6. These are countries in which orphan drugs are often distributed via retail pharmacies, or where taxes on medicines are high (Austria and Denmark). It should also be noted that in some countries, such as France, even if medicines are available only in hospitals and are exempt from taxes, the PPIT:MPBT ratio is not 1, as hospital pharmacies can include profit margins (15% in France) for medicines sold to outpatients.

The potential revenues from some of the ten orphan drugs studied were estimated using current sales figures, the potential market in terms of patient numbers and current market penetration. The analysis concluded that the estimated potential annual turnover is between €100 million and €1.5 billion, depending on the medicine. Thus, even if some orphan drugs could become 'blockbusters', the maximal sales of these medicines would remain below the top ten medicines whose individual sales are in the range of €2 billion and €7 billion.

The study conducted by Alcimed also looked at access to the orphan drugs authorized in the EU. Access is clearly linked to reimbursement. The best indicator of accessibility to a medicine is the proportion of patients who are effectively treated and reimbursed. At the European level, there are very few data available on accessibility of orphan drugs, and no thorough study has been conducted.

The main factor that determines access to an orphan drug is the reimbursement by national health insurance systems. The annual cost of these treatments (€6000 to €300 000) is beyond the budget of average households. Another factor that correlates with access to orphan drugs is the time taken to assess and determine the applications for price and reimbursement. These are different in different countries of the EU. National systems of drug pricing and reimbursement of orphan drugs are linked to accessibility and are the same as those applied to non-orphan medicines. However, for orphan drugs, Member States have little negotiating leverage, as these medicines have no therapeutic alternative and are often still investigational new drugs. The Alcimed analysis did reveal two facts. First, more than half of the orphan drugs studied were marketed in the 15 countries of the EU. Secondly, the countries with a maximum number of orphan drugs on their reimbursement list were France, Germany, Spain, The Netherlands and Sweden. Orphan drugs were less fully reimbursed in some EU Member States whose health budgets might be considerably lower than those of the others.

Pricing and access in the UK
Although EC regulations and directives govern much of the pharmaceutical regulation in the EU, four major activities still remain entirely within the remit of national competent authorities. Among these is the pricing policy. Each Member State of the EU operates its own policy regarding the pricing of pharmaceutical products. In the UK, the primary tool is the Pharmaceutical Price Regulation Scheme, which is better described as a profit-regulating scheme.

The National Institute for Health and Clinical Excellence (NICE) plays a pivotal role in influencing access to medicines in the UK. NICE recognizes that it has to make two kinds of judgements: scientific, based on evidence, and social values, based on societal aspirations, preferences and ethical principles. To this end, it has established a 30-member Citizens Council to help provide the necessary societal input. During their meeting in October 2004, the Citizens Council was asked to advise on whether the UK National Health Service (NHS) should be prepared to pay premium prices for drugs to treat patients with very rare diseases. Just over half ($n = 16$) of the Council members thought that, with certain conditions, the NHS should consider paying premium prices for drugs to treat patients with very rare diseases. A further four people thought that the NHS should pay whatever premium price is required for drugs to treat patients with very rare diseases. The main criteria that the Citizens Council thinks the NHS should take into account when deciding to pay premium prices for ultra-orphan drugs are, in descending order of importance:
- the degree of severity of the disease
- whether the treatment will provide health gain, rather than just stabilization of the condition
- whether the disease or condition is life threatening.

The interested reader is advised to read the full report published in November 2004 [6].

In terms of reimbursement and access in England, there are some 300 Primary Care Trusts (PCTs) that are funded directly by the Department of Health. Since April 2002, PCTs have had the responsibility for providing health services or securing access to services, while 28 Strategic Health Authorities monitor performance and standards. In a Department of Health document entitled 'Primary care prescribing and budget-setting', PCT finance directors and prescribing advisors are required to consider and agree the advice to be provided to their PCT Boards about the resources to underpin prescribing in primary care. Additional factors to consider include:

- NICE recommendations – PCTs are reminded that they are under a statutory obligation to provide funding for clinical decisions within recommendations from NICE contained in Technology Appraisal Guidance reports
- newly licensed drugs – most significant new drugs will be referred to NICE for appraisal, but plans should recognize the scope for prescribing during the interim period between the reference and NICE providing its guidance; underlying trends for new drugs are picked up in the drugs bill forecast but any large spends may need to be factored in.

By devolving decision making to a local level, it is possible for neighbouring PCTs to adopt different policies, which can give rise to patients in one part of the country having access to a therapy that is denied to patients living only a few miles away. Clearly, tensions and a sense of unfairness may also arise if one PCT were to be responsible for a number of patients with orphan diseases whereas another may be responsible for none. This is not an unlikely scenario, given that many orphan diseases are genetic and, therefore, familial in nature and there may be a cluster of patients within a PCT. Consequently, the presence of patients with an orphan disease requiring expensive treatment in the population of a PCT has a disproportionate effect on the ability of that PCT to fund services for the rest of its population. The development of a risk-sharing model across PCTs enables that impact to be smoothed out across a number of organizations, thus limiting the impact on any one PCT. There are now several different risk-sharing models in operation across the NHS. The simplest are based on a pooling of

the total drug costs and the distribution of that cost across PCTs in proportion to their share of the patient population.

Of course, one way out of this is for such treatments to be funded centrally. The UK Department of Health has taken an important first step in this direction. In October 2004, the Department wrote to the Chief Executives of all the PCTs and other relevant bodies to inform them that for a period of 2 years, from April 2005 to March 2007, six centres will be nationally designated and funded by the Department of Health, under the auspices of the National Specialised Commissioning Advisory Group, to provide a service for patients with lysosomal storage disorders. The service will include diagnostic, assessment and treatment services. This means that the cost of drug treatments, including enzyme replacement therapies, will be funded on a national basis. What is important as a matter of principle with regard to access to treatment of other orphan diseases is that the announcement also made clear that "In the interim period between now and April 2005 when national funding commences, PCTs will be expected to respond in a timely fashion to consideration of requests from clinicians at the designated centres for funding for enzyme replacement therapies or equivalent treatments".

Access in the USA and Japan

Orphan drugs are reimbursed like all drug products in the USA. The government is not responsible for providing drugs to patients except in the case of parenteral medications to the Medicare (over 65 years of age) population. People must pay for their own drug prescriptions or their insurance may pay all or a proportion of the costs for the product. Consequently, access can be a problem. If an individual does not have sufficient funds to pay for their drugs, they may have to make some very difficult choices. However, virtually all the pharmaceutical companies have 'give-away' programmes for truly needy individuals. These programmes are administered via a means test. The National Organization for Rare Disorders, Inc. administers some of these needs programmes.

In Japan, the cost of orphan drugs is usually covered by medical insurance, as for other drugs. Thus, the patient pays 20–30% of the cost and insurance companies pay the rest. However, in some cases, the amount to be paid by patients is limited by regulation to a certain amount, and the government pays the rest. In some other cases, the drug cost is fully covered by the government and medical insurance.

Conclusions

Following the introduction of the Orphan Drugs Act in the USA in 1983, the number of active substances designated orphan as of 2005 is 1449, with an average of 66 designations per year. Of these, 269 (18.6%) have received marketing authorizations (12.2 per year). The average number for the EU is 57 designations per year and 20 (7%) of the 287 designations have received marketing authorizations. These figures have to be seen in the context of differences between the USA and the EU in threshold and other criteria for designation. There is little doubt that the Community Regulation on orphan medicines has the potential to be a spectacular success. As of April 2005, the COMP had designated 287 drugs as orphan. Of these, 20 have been given a positive opinion by the CHMP for marketing authorization. These first 5-year numbers compare well with those in the first 5 years of the US Orphan Drug Act (1983–1987) that included 181 designations and 27 marketing authorizations. Of the sponsors surveyed by the EMEA, 67% plan to submit an application for marketing authorization by 2008 (9% in 2005, 15% in 2006, 26% in 2007 and 17% in 2008). Based on the current EMEA experience and this survey, it is anticipated that the number of orphan products reaching

the market will escalate quite dramatically in the next 3–4 years.

The number of applications for designation received and determined by the COMP has far exceeded initial expectations. This unexpected surge of applications enabled the COMP to identify rapidly a number of complex issues that were not fully elaborated upon in the Regulation. Article 10 of Regulation (EC) No 141/2000 requires that before 22 January 2006, the Commission shall publish a general report on the experience acquired as a result of the application of this regulation, together with an account of the public health benefits that have been obtained. Commensurate with its policy advisory functions, in July 2005 the COMP published a report that reviews the entire designation process, difficulties with some aspects of the legislation and its activities over the first 5 years to April 2005, as well as making a number of recommendations to stimulate and foster EU policy on orphan medicinal products. This report, available on the EMEA website [4], is highly informative, as well as being a source of valuable statistics and identifying areas requiring greater regulatory clarity.

Indeed, the EC communication issued in July 2003 is a step in this direction. This communication (2003/C178/02) sets out the EC's position on certain matters relating to the implementation of the designation and market exclusivity provisions of Regulation (EC) No 141/2000. Among other issues, it considers those in relation to criteria for designation, procedure for designation, Community marketing authorization and market exclusivity. It also provides guidance to the EMEA, the Member States, the pharmaceutical industry and other interested parties, and clarification in several areas in order to avoid a departure from the spirit of the regulation. A more complete discussion of this clarification is beyond the scope of this chapter, but the interested reader should refer to the full text of the communication for further details. Needless to add that as a result of these changes, the COMP should be able to promote the development of a wide range of orphan medicines even more effectively and with greater equity.

Acknowledgements

I wish to record my appreciation to the Secretariat of COMP, especially Dr Melanie Carr and Professor Spiros Vamvakas, for their unfailing support, and to my COMP colleagues for their friendship during my membership of the Committee. I am also grateful to Dr Marlene Haffner, Director, Office of Orphan Products Development, Food and Drug Administration, USA, Dr Keiji Ueda, Senior Adviser, Pharmaceutical and Medical Devices Agency, Japan, and Mr Steve Sparks, Assistant Director, Specialist Commissioning, Kent, Surrey & Sussex Specialist Commissioning Group, UK for their valuable and constructive comments and advice during the preparation of this chapter. Any shortcomings, however, are entirely my own responsibility.

References

1. DiMasi JA, Hansen RW, Grabowski HG. The price of innovation: new estimates of drug development costs. *J Health Econ* 2003;22:151–85
2. DiMasi JA, Grabowski HG, Vernon J. R & D costs and returns by therapeutic category. *Drug Inf J.* 2004;38: 211–23
3. Rare Diseases: understanding this Public Health Priority. European Organisation for Rare Diseases (EURORDIS), Paris. http://www.eurordis.org/IMG/pdf/eurordis_princeps_july05draft.pdf (Accessed on 20 October 2005)
4. COMP Report to the Commission in Relation to Article 10 of Regulation 141/2000 on Orphan Medicinal Products (25 July 2005) http://www.emea.eu.int/pdfs/human/comp/3521805en.pdf
5. ALCIMED study on the price of orphan drugs http://pharmacos.eudra.org/F2/orphanmp/doc/pricestudy/Final%20final%20report%20part%201%20web.pdf
6. Citizens Council report: Ultra Orphan drugs http://www.nice.org.uk/page.aspx?o=243905

Useful websites for further information

Orphan Drug Regulation (EC) No 141/2000
http://pharmacos.eudra.org/F2/orphanmp/doc/141_2000/141_2000_en.pdf

Orphan Drug Regulation (EC) No 847/2000
http://pharmacos.eudra.org/F2/eudralex/vol-1/REG_2000_847/REG_2000_847_EN.pdf

Commission Communication Regulation (EC) No 141/2000 on orphan medicinal products
http://pharmacos.eudra.org/F2/orphanmp/doc/com_0703/com_orphan_en.pdf

COMP Report to the Commission in Relation to Article 10 of Regulation 141/2000 on Orphan Medicinal Products (25 July 2005)
http://www.emea.eu.int/pdfs/human/comp/3521805en.pdf

US Orphan Drug Act, 1983 (as amended)
http://www.fda.gov/orphan/lawsregs.html

Other information with regard to orphan medicines:
http://pharmacos.eudra.org/F2/orphanmp/index.htm.

The rules of procedure for CHMP
http://www.emea.eu.int/pdfs/human/regaffair/11148104en.pdf

The rules of procedure for COMP
http://www.emea.eu.int/pdfs/human/comp/821200en.pdf

Details about orphan drug legislation, its application, and associated procedures and guidance notes
http://www.emea.eu.int/sitemap.htm.

Draft guideline on elements required to support the medical plausibility and the assumption of significant benefit for an orphan designation
http://www.emea.eu.int/pdfs/human/comp/6697204en.pdf

The rules of procedure of SAWP
http://www.emea.eu.int/pdfs/human/sciadvice/6968604en.pdf

Details of guidance for companies requesting scientific advice and protocol assistance
http://www.emea.eu.int/pdfs/human/sciadvice/426001en.pdf

Clinical Trial Directive 2001/20/EEC
http://pharmacos.eudra.org/F2/eudralex/vol-1/DIR_2001_20/DIR_2001_20_EN.pdf

Clinical Trials in the UK
http://medicines.mhra.gov.uk/ourwork/licensingmeds/types/clintrialdir.htm

Centralized procedur
http://pharmacos.eudra.org/F2/pharmacos/docs.htm.

Directive 2001/83/E
http://pharmacos.eudra.org/F2/eudralex/vol-1/DIR_2001_83/DIR_2001_83_EN.pdf

Regulation EEC/2309/93
http://pharmacos.eudra.org/F2/eudralex/vol-5/pdfs-en/932309en.pdf

Directive 2004/27/EC
http://pharmacos.eudra.org/F2/review/doc/final_publ/Dir_2004_27_20040430_EN.pdf

Regulation (EC) No 726/2004
http://pharmacos.eudra.org/F2/review/doc/final_publ/Reg_2004_726_20040430_EN.pdf

Directive 2003/63/EC
http://pharmacos.eudra.org/F2/eudralex/vol-1/DIR_2003_63/DIR_2003_63_EN.pdf

Information regarding each of the products approved through the centralized procedure (European Public

Assessment Report – EPAR)
http://www.emea.eu.int/htms/human/epar/epar.htm

Report from Round Table meeting on drugs for paediatric use
http://www.emea.eu.int/pdfs/human/regaffair/
2716498en.pdf

Commission consultation paper on 'Better Medicines for Children – proposed regulatory actions in paediatric medicinal products'
http://pharmacos.eudra.org/F2/pharmacos/docs/
Doc2002/feb/cd_pediatrics_en.pdf

Regulation on Medicinal Products for Paediatric Use together with an explanatory memorandum, the Extended Impact Assessment and questions and answers document
http://pharmacos.eudra.org/F2/Paediatrics/index.htm

Work plan for Paediatric Expert Group (PEG) for 2004–2005
http://www.emea.eu.int/pdfs/human/peg/2289603en.pdf

ALCIMED study on the price of orphan drugs
http://pharmacos.eudra.org/F2/orphanmp/doc/pricestudy
/Final%20final%20report%20part%201%20web.pdf

Primary care trusts
http://www.dh.gov.uk/PolicyAndGuidance/
OrganisationPolicy/PrimaryCare/PrimaryCareTrusts/fs/en

Citizens Council report: Ultra Orphan drugs
http://www.nice.org.uk/page.aspx?o=243905

Orphan drugs register of the FDA
http://www.fda.gov/orphan/designat/list.htm

Orphan drugs register of the EU
http://pharmacos.eudra.org/F2/register/alforphreg.htm

12 Role of patient support groups in lysosomal storage diseases

Christine Lavery MBE

Society for Mucopolysaccharide and Related Diseases, MPS House, White Lion Road, Amersham, Bucks HP7 9LP, UK

Patient support groups provide patients and their families with information on the various lysosomal storage diseases (LSDs), encourage and fund research, treatment and education, and act as advocates for those affected by LSDs. The advocacy role is important in ensuring that the obligations of healthcare and other authorities are fulfilled, particularly with respect to provision of enzyme replacement therapy. In addition to their invaluable role in educating those directly affected by LSDs and also healthcare workers, patient support groups facilitate the sharing of information through regular national and international conferences. Through such activities, patient support groups have had a considerable positive impact on the lives of individuals affected by these rare diseases.

In the beginning

Although the first lysosomal storage diseases (LSDs) were described in the late 19th and early 20th centuries – Fabry disease in 1898, Gaucher disease in 1882 and mucopolysaccharidosis (MPS) type I (Hurler disease) in 1919 – the founding of patient support organizations is principally a phenomenon of the second half of the 20th century and, in particular, the past 25 years.

The first charities dedicated to the support of children and adults with specific medical conditions – such as epilepsy and Raynaud disease – were founded in the UK in 1852. By 1973, 57 patient organizations for specific diseases had become active. By 2005, the number had grown to nearly 300, perhaps reflecting greater awareness of different diseases in the period since the 1980s. A better educated population, not content that patients should be seen and not heard, has also played a part. The creation of LSD support groups is being replicated in other

countries in Europe and in most of the rest of the world, largely through initiatives taken by patients and their parents and, in some cases, by leading paediatricians and clinicians pioneering research into – and treatment for – specific rare conditions. Disturbed by the lack of remedial treatments for rare conditions and the paucity of advice on the daily management of their affected children, parents have, generally speaking, taken the lead in creating support groups, setting the terms of reference, and managing and finding funding for their activities and programmes. Since 2000, some groups, such as those representing patients with Fabry and Gaucher diseases, have been stimulated into greater purpose by the prospects of enzyme replacement therapies developed by the pharmaceutical industry.

In the 1980s, patient organizations were, on the whole, viewed with scepticism by many health professionals. An approach in May 1982 to the *British Medical Journal (BMJ)* by the Society for Mucopolysaccharide

Diseases (MPS Society) was met with the response "the editorial board at the BMJ does not enter into correspondence with lay people". Fortunately, however, attitudes are changing and, in 2003, the *BMJ* published an editorial on the treatment of LSDs from both the clinician and patient organization perspective [1].

Due to confidentiality issues, it was often difficult to obtain from a paediatrician the name and address of another family with an affected child with whom experience might be shared. Generic or umbrella patient organizations were occasionally able to help with family introductions. Initially, however, many groups were hampered by the reluctance of healthcare professionals to inform patients and their families of appropriate patient/ parent support groups. Clearly, there was concern that information acquired by a support group might be mismanaged or be too overwhelming. Sometimes, there was arrogance. At the first MPS Society family conference in 1983, one professional referred to those present as "middle-class activists". Little did this person know that the majority of the 50 families attending were not middle class, had never stayed a night in a good hotel, and that some were struggling to make ends meet, but all had gone out of their way to live up to the occasion. They were a proud first generation of individuals determined to make a difference for those suffering from one group of LSDs.

Making a difference

The aims of patient organizations for LSDs have not changed over the passage of time and are common to groups worldwide:

- to offer support to those affected
- to provide an educational role
- to encourage and fund research and treatment.

Differences between the various LSD patient organizations lie in the detail of their objectives and how those objectives meet the needs of patients and their families. In the early development of a patient organization, the focus is generally on encouraging membership and public awareness through the organization of meetings and conferences, publication of newsletters and information on specific disorders, and the development of a website. Support for patients with LSDs and their families is extremely important, but differs widely between patient organizations and between countries. Success in raising additional finance for research, from general fundraising activities or by obtaining grants restricted to specific research projects and programmes, is usually dependent on the growing maturity and competence of the patient organization, demonstrated to potential donors by its track record of reliability, achievement, probity and management abilities.

Advocacy and support

Advocacy and support available for adult and paediatric patients and their families varies considerably between patient organizations and the countries in which they operate. Advocating individuals' and families' needs and rights is often achieved by telephone, letter or e-mail to service providers and other professional workers. When these methods are not adequate, home visits may be made, and support from the relevant local professionals may be offered at patients' meetings. Specific medical information should not be given by patient organizations. However, patients and their families can often benefit from guidance on the various medical or non-medical questions or issues they might raise with medical specialists or service providers. Common questions include those concerning medical management of the disease, carrier status and prenatal diagnosis.

Some patient organizations facilitate valuable specialized regional clinics for LSDs at which a leading paediatrician or clinician will meet affected patients. (A lay organization will not give medical advice, but will defer to the specialists and provide them with the necessary administrative support, which makes regional clinics so effective and worthwhile for individual patients.) Depending on the resources, skill and knowledge of a particular patient organization's 'workforce' (volunteers or salaried employees), other areas of support may involve providing information or advice and individual advocacy on:

- disability benefit applications
- special educational needs
- grants for equipment and holidays
- independent living
- respite care
- home adaptations
- sibling support
- bereavement.

Nearly all patient organizations offer a telephone listening service to enable patients, parents or other family members to discuss their issues and concerns.

Whatever the range of services offered, the principles underpinning individual advocacy are confidentiality, equity of service and the right for the service to be needs-led, with an emphasis on enabling individuals and families to help themselves. Occasionally, however, support groups will intercede with providers on behalf of patients and parents or accompany patients and parents to providers' hearings or tribunals. In extreme cases, when statutory obligations are not being met by central or local government, societies will advise on appropriate legal representation.

Fulfilling an educational role

In recent years, the LSD patient organizations have become the authors of the most informative booklets and pamphlets on specific LSDs. The range of available written information varies for different diseases and in different countries. The publications may be aimed at patients and families, non-specialized paediatricians, clinicians and nurses, as well as social workers, occupational therapists, teachers and dieticians. Before publication, patient organizations should adopt best practice and have drafts checked for the accuracy of clinical and treatment information by leading experts in the field of LSDs.

Publications produced by patient organizations commonly include disorder-specific clinical management booklets and disease-progression booklets. The latter are aimed at health and social care professionals and have a series of photographs showing year-by-year disease progression. These booklets are invaluable when advocating a long-term care plan to social care professionals. Such professionals often have little concept of an affected child's long-term needs, perhaps seeing the child as currently mobile and hyperactive and recognizing only their present needs. Parents and advocates, on the other hand, are also concerned with patient care in future years, when lack of mobility and the need for full-time nursing care may become important issues. Well-presented and accurate patient-led information empowers those affected and their families with strong and inarguable grounds for the provision of much-needed resources. For example, it is not always easy to demonstrate the medium- and long-term care needs of a hyperactive 3-year-old child with Sanfilippo disease, who is displaying challenging behaviour and severe sleep disturbance, without pictorial evidence of disease progression. Some patient organizations have also developed specialist booklets appropriately written for the benefit of affected children and their siblings.

Education extends well beyond written materials. Patient organizations are able to convey eloquently their first-hand experiences of living with a person who suffers from an LSD. They are able to put patients and their families in touch with others in a similar situation, facilitating the provision of mutual support and information. Patients and their families have also proved to be valuable speakers to a range of audiences for public awareness and educational purposes.

In recent years, the Internet has come to play a vital educational role for patient organizations, but is also a challenge. The management of a vibrant, informative and up-to-date website needs constant attention. Given the speed with which new information relating to LSDs is becoming available, it is a major administrative task to maintain awareness of new developments and transfer information to the patient organization website. The initial enthusiasm of some patient organizations to host interactive chat rooms is diminishing due to the inherent responsibilities in their policing, with the care and safety of children and young adults in mind.

Data collection

Patient organizations clearly have the potential to collect valuable data on their membership. For the smaller or less-established organizations, information collection may extend only to identifying minimum incidence data, including names, addresses, dates of birth and disease type. Even these limited data are useful for the rarer LSDs, particularly when the natural history of the disease is uncertain and there is no treatment or therapy available. At the other end of the scale, a few patient organizations have developed sophisticated disease registries. In the case of the MPS Society, the registry is nearly 25 years old and has comprehensive incidence and epidemiological data on over 1200 UK patients with MPS and related diseases. This registry also has more limited data on over 4000 MPS sufferers from mainland Europe. The UK incidence and epidemiological data are highly reliable and, in their anonymous form, the MPS Society shares them with government departments, statutory agencies and pharmaceutical companies researching and developing new therapies.

Lobbying and campaigning

In the 21st century, lobbying and campaigning have also become an absolute necessity for LSD patient organizations. Campaign themes regularly include the need

for improved clinical management and patient choice. Since 2001, the difficulty of achieving funded enzyme replacement therapy (ERT) for Fabry disease and, more recently, MPS I has concentrated the minds of patient organizations around the world. Whilst most central and western European countries accepted the need to fund ERT for Gaucher disease in the 1990s, it was considerably more difficult achieving government-funded ERT for Fabry disease when this therapy was approved by the Food and Drug Administration and the European Agency for the Evaluation of Medicinal Products in 2001. Indeed, funding approval for the treatment of Fabry disease has only recently been achieved in Australia, and campaigning for equality of treatment across Canada continues.

All lobbying and campaigning needs a long-term strategy to have any chance of success. The strategy must be well defined, as must the arguments. There needs to be consistency, and effort must be maintained over many months and, sometimes, years. The MPS Society adopted a two-pronged approach in its campaign for ERT for MPS I in the UK. At the political level, the Society engaged with patients' Members of Parliament, resulting in a meeting with the Minister for Health. This was followed by regular contact with the Minister and Department of Health officials to remind them of our expectations of a favourable outcome. In parallel, the MPS Society worked with a law firm specializing in human rights and medical negligence to develop the arguments to be used if patients were denied ERT by their Primary Care Trusts. Twelve families whose children had been denied ERT for MPS I sought the support of the MPS Society who, with the backing of expert paediatric consultants, drafted appeals and, in the case of flawed due process, worked with lawyers to take out judicial reviews funded by the public purse. The outcome was the award of funded ERT for the 12 patients, and the Department of

Health's approval of dedicated funding through the National Specialised Commission Advisory Group, taking away funding responsibility from the local funding bodies – the Primary Care Trusts.

Working in partnership

From the early stages in their development, patient organizations need to work in partnership with a wide range of other professionals. Developing an honest and trusting dialogue with the key experts in LSDs should be mutually beneficial and should open channels of communication, especially over sensitive issues. Those who serve or work in a patient organization are increasingly, and through necessity, responsible for running an organization that upholds the rights of patients, their families, their carers and the professionals who manage their care. Equally, patient organizations should reasonably expect to be respected by their professional partners.

Lay-directed patient organizations must win this respect by being professional themselves in sharing and using information appropriately and safely, by respecting medical and research confidentialities and by not giving medical advice themselves, by providing a reliable service and by facilitating the work of professional health carers. That is not to say that patient organizations should not be determined in pursuit of their aims, within the accepted rules of engagement: well, nearly always.

International collaboration

International networking has been important in the rapid gain in knowledge of patient organizations regarding all aspects of diagnosis, clinical management and provision of new therapies. Some patient organizations have been leaders in the field, whilst others have benefited from those who went before them.

In the case of the ultra-rare LSDs, for example Sly disease, sialidosis and multiple sulphatase deficiency, where there are only one or two affected patients in many countries, international links are vital in providing support to these patients and their families.

The decision by politicians in Europe and other parts of the world to fund ERT for Fabry disease and MPS I has helped some patient organizations to make a case for government funding in their own countries. Furthermore, those organizations fortunate enough to have overcome the challenges of achieving funded ERT have been able to support other patient organizations in a less enviable position.

Such is the importance of dialogue at an international level that several of the LSD patient associations have official organizers' networks that meet in order to learn from each other.

Conclusions

The medical, clinical and scientific knowledge about LSDs has been growing rapidly over the past 5 years. There are large numbers of people throughout the world – professionals, patients and parents – with a direct interest in these diseases. In contrast to 25 years ago, it is of great comfort to know, at least for those affected and their families, that there is now such a focus of interest in the LSDs.

We must occasionally, however, remind ourselves that the LSDs are rare. It is very likely that a general practitioner will not see a patient with an LSD during the whole of his or her career. Even hospital-based general paediatricians and non-specialist clinicians will rarely meet undiagnosed children with an LSD, and when they do they will have to make considerable efforts to diagnose the condition correctly. This is particularly true for Fabry disease and the rarest mucopolysaccharide and oligosaccharide storage diseases.

Besides this book, there are many opportunities to learn about the LSDs. Hardly a month goes by when there is not a specialist medical and clinical symposium or family conference somewhere in the world. Nearly all of these welcome participants from other countries. If you are seeking first-hand knowledge of the LSDs, you can do no better than sign up for a patient organization's family conference, where you will have the opportunity to meet patients with a range of LSDs, witness their differences and abilities, and learn about the 24-hour care needed by some of those affected and given unconditionally by parents, partners and carers. Some of the knowledge they impart can be rather surprising. For example, boys with Hunter disease like car keys, and children with Sanfilippo and Hunter diseases are often fearful of people dressed as Father Christmas or in other guises, such as clowns or animals. These are not scientifically proven observations, and are unlikely to be noticed by paediatricians who meet MPS patients for perhaps an hour once or twice a year. Such traits are rarely discussed. By exposure to many contacts with a range of LSD sufferers, those working in patient organizations learn a great deal about the disorders they represent and are a very important resource for physicians, as well as patients and their carers.

Reference

1. Mehta AB, Lewis S, Lavery C. Treatment of lysosomal storage diseases (editorial). *BMJ* 2003;327:462–3

Patient support groups

Australia
Australian MPS Society
PO Box 623
Hornsby
NSW 1630

Tel: +61 2 9476 8411
Fax: +61 2 9476 8422
Email: info@mpssociety.org.au
www.mpssociety.org.au

Fabry's Support Group
PO Box 269
Willoughby
NSW 2068

Tel: +61 2 9967 4395
Email: fookesy@au.gateway.net

Austria
Austrian MPS Society
Finklham 90
4075 Breitenaich

Tel: +43 7249 47795
Fax: +43 7249 47752
Email: office@mps-austria.at
www.mps-austria.at

Belgium
Belgische Organisatie voor Kinderen
en volwasserien mit een Stofwisselingsziekte vzw
Floralaan 35A
9120 Beveren

Email: info@boks.be
www.boks.be

Brazil
Sociedade Brasileira de
Mucopolissacaridoses (SBMPS)
R Dra Maria Luiza Azevedo
15 Jardim Eldorado
IAPI
Salvador 40310-110

Tel/Fax: +55 71 9947 4111
Email: presidente@mpsbrasil.org.br
www.mpsbrasil.org.br

Canada
Canadian Society for Mucopolysaccharide
and Related Diseases
PO Box 30034
RPO Parkgate
North Vancouver
British Columbia V7H 2Y8

Tel: +1 604 924 5130
Fax: +1 604 924 5131
Email: kirsten@mpssociety.ca
www.mpssociety.ca

Fabry Society of Canada
9011–142 Street NW
Edmonton
Alberta T5R OM6

Tel/Fax: +1 780 489 0012
Email: koning@compusmart.ab.ca
www.fabrysociety.org

Czech Republic
Společnost pro Mukopolysacharidosu
Chaloupky 35
772 00 Olomouc

Tel/Fax: +420 585 315 787
Email: spmps@seznam.cz
www.mukopoly.cz

Finland
Finnish Fabry Association
Uurrekuja 9 A
01650 Vantaa

Email: tuula.meriluato@kolumbas.fi
Email: heikki_lehtinen@suomi24.fi

France
Vaincre les Maladies Lysosomales
2 Ter avenue de France
91300 Massy

Tel: +33 1 69 75 40 30
Fax: +33 1 60 11 15 83
Email: vml@vml-asso.org
www.vml-asso.org

Germany
Gesellschaft fur Mukopolysaccharidosen e.v
Rupert Mayer Str 13
63741 Aschaffenburg

Tel: +49 6 021 858 373
Fax: +49 6 021 858 372
Email: info@mps-ev.de
www.mps-ev.de/index.php

Morbus Fabry Selbsthilfegruppe (MFSH) e.v
Guilleaumester. 13
51065 Cologne

Tel/Fax: +49 221 222 73 93
Email: info@fabry-selbsthilfegruppe.de
www.fabry-selbsthilfegruppe.de

Hungary
Mucopolysaccharidozis Tarsasag
Rath Gyorgy u.27
1122 Budapest

Tel: +36 1 3554 553
Fax: +36 1 3637 256
Email: hegybiro@elgi.hu

Hong Kong
Hong Kong Mucopolysaccharidoses
Rare Genetic Diseases Mutual Aid Group

Email: mps@hk-mps.com
www.hk-mps.com

Ireland
Irish Society for Mucopolysaccharide Diseases
Ballymacreese
Ballyneety
Co Limerick

Tel: +353 61 351778
Fax: +353 61 319099
Email: mps@mpssociety.ie
www.mpssociety.ie

Israel
Fabry Patient Association
Menahem Begin Str. 3/6
Ramat Hasharon

Email: asimo@cellcom.co.il

Italy
Associazione Italiana Mucopolysaccaridosi per
le Malatie Affini
Via Savona
13-20144 Milan

Tel: +39 2 832 41 292
Fax: +30 2 894 25 180
Email: info@mucopolisaccaridosi.it
www.mucopolisaccaridosi.it

Associazione Italiana Pazienti Anderson–Fabry
(A.I.P.A.F. Onlus)
Via Tino Corzani, 3
47026 – San Piero in Bagno
Forlí/Cesana

Tel/Fax:+39 543 901260
Email: info@aipaf.org
www.aipaf.org

Japan
Japanese Society of Patients and Families with
Mucopolysaccharidosis
2-13-17
Nan-youdai
Yoshii-machi
Tano-gun
Gunma-ken
370-2101

Email: ginchann@ann.hi-ho.ne.jp

Korea
Association of MPS in Korea
Department of Paediatrics
Sumsung Medical Centre
50 Ilwan-dong Kangnam-ku
Seoul
135-710

Tel: +82 2 3410 3539
Fax: +82 2 3410 0043
Email: mps_kr@yahoo.co.kr
www.mps.or.kr

The Netherlands
VKS
Postbus 664
8000 AR
Zwolle

Tel: +31 38 420 1764
Fax: +31 38 420 1447
Email: info@stofwisselingsziekten.nl
www.stofwisselingsziekten.nl/vks

Fabry Support & Informatie Groep Nederland
Boelenkamp 10
8431 BL Oosterwolde

Tel: +31 516 523773
Email: FSIGN@fabry.nl
www.fabry.nl

New Zealand
Lysosomal Diseases New Zealand
PO Box 38-58
125 Cuba Street
Petone

Tel: +64 4 566 7707
Fax:+64 4 566 7717
Email: john.forman@xtra.co.nz
www.ldnz.org.nz

Norway
FRAMBU
Centre for Rare Disorders
Sandbakkvn 18
1404 Siggerud

Tel: +47 64 85 60 00
Fax: +47 64 85 60 99
Email: info@frambu.no
www.frambu.no

Fabry Patients Organisation – Norway
DnB-IT Leveranse
Sandslimarka 55
Postboks 7100
5020 Bergen

Tel: +47 552 19148
Fax: +47 552 19172
E-mail: rune.sedal@dnb.no
www.fabry.dk

Poland
Society of Friends and Family of Children with
Mucopolysaccharidosis and Related Diseases
05-503 Gloskow ul.
Radnych 9A

Tel: +48 22 715 33 19
Fax: +48 22 715 33 11
Email: tmatulka@wp.pl
www.mps.sart.pl

Polish Fabry Patients Association
Ul. Slowicza 10
53-320 Wroclaw

Email: romekmichalik@pooztaonet.pl

Romania
Fundatia Roman Pentru Boli Lisosomale
Str. Ardealului nr 17
Campina
Cod 2150

Tel: +40 44 333753
Fax: +40 44 333936
Email: teo.tit@usa.net

Slovenia
Slovenian MPS Society
Maistrova 5
2230 Lenart
Tel: +38 662 726 751

Spain
Alteraciones de Crecimiento/Desarrollo y
Enfermedades Lisosomales (ADAC)
Enrique Marco 6
41 018 Sevilla

Tel: +34 954 989 889
Fax: +34 954 989 790
Email: a.d.a.c@telefonica.net

Asociación para las Deficienciasque Afectan al
Crecimiento y al Desarrollo (ADAC)

Tel: +34 954 989 889
Fax: +34 954 989 790
Email: a.d.a.c@telefonica.net
www.adac-es.net

Sweden
Swedish MPS Society
Email: veronica_rasmus@hotmail.com

Swedish Fabry Association
Vallmovägen 16
SE-66341 Hammarö

Email: chr-pol@hotmail.com

Switzerland
Fabrysuisse

Email: willikon@goldnet.ch
www.fabrysuisse.ch

Fabrysuisse
Willikon 58
8618 Oetwil am See

Tel/Fax: +41 1 929 05 74
Email: willikon@goldnet.ch

Taiwan
Taiwan MPS Society
357 Jin-Zhou St
Taipei

Tel: +886 2 2503 2125
Fax: +886 2 2503 9435
Email: ttmps@ms32.hinet.net
www.tacocity.com.tw.cks49

UK
Society for Mucopolysaccharide and Related Diseases
MPS House
Repton Place
White Lion Road
Amersham
Bucks HP7 9LP

Tel: +44 845 389 9901
Fax: +44 845 389 9902
Email: mps@mpssociety.co.uk
www.mpssociety.co.uk

USA
National MPS Society
PO Box 736
Bangor
ME 04402-0736

Tel: +1 207 947 1445
Fax: +1 207 990 3074
Email: info@mpssociety.org
www.mpssociety.org

Fabry Support & Information Group (FSIG)
108 NE 2nd St, Suite C
PO Box 510
Concordia
MO 64020

Tel: +1 660 463 1355
Fax: +1 660 463 1356
Email: info@fabry.org
www.fabry.org

13 The patient's perspective of Fabry disease – a report from the German Fabry Patient Support Group

Ditmar Basalla

Morbus Fabry Selbsthilfegruppe e.V. (MFSH), Cologne, Germany

The Morbus Fabry Selbsthilfegruppe e.V. (MFSH) is a German-based support group for patients with Fabry disease. The aims of the MFSH are manifold and include raising awareness of Fabry disease within the medical profession and in general, offering support to patients and the families of those affected by Fabry disease, and campaigning for prompt diagnosis and widespread treatment for all affected. The MFSH, together with other Fabry patient support groups within Europe, is actively involved in disseminating information to patients with Fabry disease through newsletters, information booklets and conferences. Between 2002 and 2005, patient support groups successfully organized four International Fabry Patient Meetings, and the number of registered members continues to increase. They operate a much-needed and well-utilized patient support network and are campaigning for the screening and treatment of Fabry disease to become standard practice in all appropriate medical settings.

Introduction

Fabry disease was first described independently by Professor Johannes Fabry and Dr William Anderson in 1898 [1, 2]. On 16 March 2002, almost 104 years after the first description of Fabry disease, seven male and three female patients met in Frankfurt, Germany to establish a patient support group. Until the establishment of this first support group, awareness of Fabry disease was not widespread, even amongst doctors. One of the problems with treating patients with Fabry disease effectively is that it is not always easy to diagnose, as it is characterized by many different symptoms that do not necessarily occur in all patients. Moreover, the onset of characteristic symptoms is not uniform between patients. Thus, symptoms that appear early in some patients may appear later or not at all in others. For diagnosis in male patients, it is sufficient to detect a deficiency of α-galactosidase A in blood, whereas genetic analysis is required for diagnosis in female patients.

For many years it was the case that there were no satisfactory therapies available for treating Fabry disease. Analgesics were administered for severe pain, and dialysis was offered to patients with renal impairment. In those days, Fabry patient groups did not exist, probably because patients had never met or been aware of each other's existence. It was not until the introduction of enzyme replacement therapy for Fabry disease that patients began to meet each other. The focus of activity for clinical trials meant that patients found themselves together in one place for the first time. For patients in Germany, it was the University Hospital in Mainz, and from here the German Fabry Patient Support Group (Morbus Fabry Selbsthilfegruppe e.V.; MFSH) was born.

Initially, only a few patients were actively involved in the group but, with time, the group gained more recognition and the number of members has increased encouragingly in the past few years (Figure 1). The MFSH is proud to have Hermann Fabry as an honorary member of the group. Hermann Fabry is the nephew of Professor Johannes Fabry, who published the first description of the disease over a century ago (Figure 2).

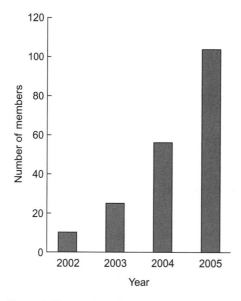

Figure 1. *The number of members in the German Fabry Support Group has increased rapidly since its start in 2002.*

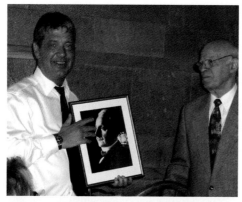

Figure 2. *The author (left) with Professor Hermann Fabry, the nephew of Johannes Fabry (pictured) – who described a patient with Fabry disease in 1898.*

The MFSH believes that only a minority of individuals with Fabry disease have been identified and correctly diagnosed. This is supported by many personal communications with people seeking help for their symptoms. It is the aim of the MFSH to assist fellow sufferers and guide them to a correct and early diagnosis.

Information from patients for patients

One of the first aims of the MSFH was to make information about Fabry disease available to other patients and to individuals seeking advice about a disease they did not understand or of which may not have been aware. The following activities were therefore initiated.

- Development of a website at www.fabry-selbsthilfegruppe.de, which includes a forum that continues to be widely used by patients and provides up-to-date subjects for discussion.
- Organization of national meetings for patients – in most cases, in connection with a treatment centre. Such meetings serve to strengthen and expand contact among patients with Fabry disease and between patients and medical experts.
- Distribution of a regular patients' newsletter that summarizes the latest news from medical research in an impartial, easy-to-understand format.
- Production of patient information booklets, which have been developed in cooperation with leading experts in the field.
- Telephone counselling for patients, and the provision of information to individuals seeking help.
- Extensive public-relations activities, aimed at local and national media, to raise awareness of Fabry disease and the MFSH.

Despite these efforts, it soon became apparent that additional activities were required in order to satisfy the enormous interest in Fabry disease and the growing demand for information by patients and their relatives. These included:

- patient counselling, and assistance in dealing with the authorities, such as applications for severe disability status
- provision of support for patients in connection with health insurance and in the workplace
- organization of patient-related events, such as Fabry Forums
- counselling for relatives of patients, including the compilation of family pedigrees
- contact with other national support groups, such as the Gaucher Disease Society and the Society for Mucopolysaccharide and Related Diseases and associated organizations.

Between 2003 and 2005, the MFSH has organized three Fabry Forums. These local events took place in cooperation with medical centres specializing in the treatment of this rare disease. The meetings had three main objectives. First, to allow experts in the field of Fabry disease to explain clearly and simply the causes of the disease to patients and their relatives. Secondly, to provide patients and their families with the opportunity to receive genetic counselling, individual heart examinations and demonstration of how lymph drainage treatment is performed. Thirdly, to enable even the most introverted of patients to participate actively and to share their concerns within small groups. These meetings are very instructive and valuable for all participants.

In 2005, as a result of the growing demand for information and answers to complex medical questions, the MFSH established a medical board for its members, their families and anyone seeking advice. The medical board comprises experts in the fields of genetics, internal medicine/nephrology and paediatrics, and is available to answer any questions regarding Fabry disease.

Information for physicians and specialized medical staff

Another aim of the MFSH is to increase awareness concerning Fabry disease and its support groups amongst physicians and specialized medical staff. Representatives from the MFSH have regularly been invited to national and international congresses, symposia and workshops in order to learn about the latest findings concerning Fabry disease and its treatment. The MFSH has also been actively involved in these events and is particularly pleased to see its contributions published in the specialist medical press [3–5].

There is still a great unmet need to increase awareness of Fabry disease within the medical profession. The large numbers of regional and national specialist medical conferences held every year provide good opportunities for publicizing Fabry disease. Indeed, in 2005, the MFSH participated in several such congresses with its own information stand. The MFSH is also represented at national and international congresses, attended by dermatologists, cardiologists, nephrologists, paediatricians, neurologists and other specialists. The numerous contacts we have established with physicians, journalists and other support groups at these congresses attests to the usefulness of such activities.

Working at an international level

After several meetings between Fabry disease patient groups in Europe, many of them by chance, it was decided that combined meetings should be organized for patients and their families in Europe. The MFSH assumed responsibility for this, organizing the first International Fabry Patient Meeting in Barcelona, Spain, in November 2002. The significance of the meeting was demonstrated by the fact that we successfully assembled more than 170 male and female adult and paediatric patients with Fabry disease from 18 countries – the largest number of Fabry patients ever to convene in one place.

The second International Fabry Patient Meeting was organized in Sitges, Spain by the Swiss

Fabry patient organization (2003), the third in Rome, Italy by the Italian organization (2004), and the fourth in Paris, France by the Spanish organization (2005). The success of these meetings is illustrated by the increasing numbers of participants every year (Figure 3).

At these meetings, physicians present the latest developments in the field of Fabry disease, such as the beneficial effects of enzyme replacement therapy on the heart, kidneys, psychological state and quality of life, and recent discoveries on the genetics of Fabry disease. Contributions from patients and their relatives are also regular features of the International Fabry Patient Meetings. These have included personal accounts of the impact of Fabry disease on school, work and family life, and the possible advantages of home treatment. From these accounts, it is clear that patients often feel excluded by society, with the result that Fabry disease causes emotional suffering besides the physical symptoms. Moreover, the parents of patients with Fabry disease often feel an overwhelming sense of guilt for transmitting the condition to their offspring.

The highlights of these meetings are summarized in several publications after the event. They include patient newsletters, which are available in English, German, French, Italian and Spanish, and are distributed across Europe. These newsletters are useful resources for those people unable to attend the meetings and are convenient memory aids to those who were present.

The International Fabry Patient Meetings have become established regular events for Fabry disease support groups and patients. In many informal discussions with patients at these international meetings, the MFSH has learnt that the quality of life of patients with Fabry disease has improved considerably during the past few years. Through these meetings, patients have not only learnt to cope with their condition, but have also gained new hope that their disease can be specifically and successfully treated. As a result of these meetings, an unofficial international support network for patients with Fabry disease has emerged and continues to grow.

Outlook

With the help of physicians in many specialized fields, awareness of Fabry disease is increasing; however, there is still a long way to go. The MFSH will continue to pursue its aims and to offer help to people affected by Fabry disease. The number of recurring misdiagnoses, such as rheumatism, Bechterew's disease, multiple sclerosis, heart defects and renal insufficiency, in patients now known to have Fabry disease reveals the scale of the problem. The labelling of patients as malingerers must stop, and proper and prompt treatment must be available to all.

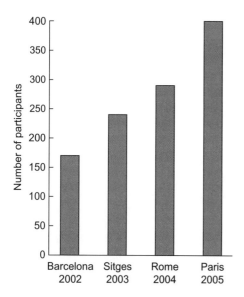

Figure 3. *Numbers of participants attending the previous four International Fabry Patient Meetings.*

References

1. Anderson W. A case of "angeio-keratoma". *Br J Dermatol* 1898;10:113–17

2. Fabry J. Ein Beitrag zur Kenntniss der Purpura haemorrhagica nodularis (Purpura papulosa haemorrhagica Hebrae). *Archiv für Dermatologie und Syphilis* 1898;43:187–200

3. Whybra C, Ramaswami U, Barba M, Parini R, Ricci R,

Basalla D. Fabry disease: patients' perspectives (First International Fabry Patient Group meeting, Barcelona, November 2002). *Acta Paediatr* 2003;92:103

4. Hoffmann B, Basalla D, Walther A, on behalf of the Morbus Fabry Selbsthilfegruppe e. V. and Fabrysuisse.

The patient's perspective of pain in Fabry disease. *Acta Paediatr* 2005;94:118

5. Basalla D, Hilliger M, Vohwinkel D. The German Patient Support Group for Fabry Disease: philosophy, aims and highlights. *Acta Paediatr* 2005;94:119

Section 2:

Development of FOS – the Fabry Outcome Survey

14 Formal trials versus observational studies

Ravi Thadhani

Harvard Medical School, Boston, Massachusetts, USA

Randomized, placebo-controlled clinical trials are the 'gold standard' for assessing the safety and effectiveness of therapy. They are designed to answer very specific questions about a particular treatment strategy. In contrast, observational studies are often considered inferior to randomized trials as, in some cases, they have been shown to overestimate treatment effects. Despite this, observational studies, if well designed and conducted appropriately, can be a valuable and effective approach to determining associations between specific exposures and outcomes, and are the method of choice when it is not possible to conduct randomized trials. FOS – the Fabry Outcome Survey – is a multinational, multicentre, observational database that, as of October 2005, contains data from 752 patients with Fabry disease who are receiving, or who are candidates for, enzyme replacement therapy (ERT) with agalsidase alfa. The large amount of data within the database allows sequential assessment of clinical outcomes to assess the efficacy of ERT and the reporting of adverse events. Databases such as FOS are of great value in providing long-term follow-up data and a high degree of patient ascertainment for Fabry disease and other orphan diseases.

Introduction

Clinical studies can be divided into two broad categories: trials, in which the investigator intervenes to prevent or treat a disease, and observational studies, in which the investigator makes no intervention and patients are allocated treatment based on clinical decisions. There are several types of observational study. Case series are the simplest form and follow the clinical course of a particular condition in a group of individuals. Cross-sectional studies, such as surveys and chart reviews, are studies in which exposures and outcomes are ascertained simultaneously. Case–control studies are those in which the frequency of specific exposures are compared between cases and matched controls. In cohort studies, the presence of specific exposures are ascertained within a group of individuals who are free of the outcome of interest, and incident events are evaluated from that point forward. Database studies involve the analysis of the relationship between exposures and outcomes based on patient data from a registry. Cross-sectional, case–control and cohort studies constitute the bulk of observational studies in the medical literature.

FOS – the Fabry Outcome Survey – is a database for all patients with Fabry disease who are receiving, or are candidates for, enzyme replacement therapy (ERT) with agalsidase alfa [1]. With 752 patients now enrolled, it is more than five times larger than the total number of patients enrolled in any clinical trial of this disease to date. Data from FOS can be used in cross-sectional, case–control and cohort studies. Here, an overview is presented of the strengths and weaknesses of randomized placebo-controlled and observational studies, with specific reference to FOS.

Randomized clinical trials

In the first half of the 20th century, investigators setting up clinical trials commonly used a selection process known as alternation to try to achieve unbiased results: patients received treatment according to the order in which they presented. Although this method is unbiased in principle, in some cases it led to imbalances in the characteristics of patients in the treatment and control groups, as foreknowledge of the treatment affected the decision to enter the patient into the trial. For this reason, randomization was introduced into medicine in the 1940s [2]. Randomization has the advantage that the allocation of treatment is unbiased because of easier concealment of the allocation scheme [3–5].

Studies are now classified using a hierarchical ranking system on the basis of study design (Table 1) [6], with the highest grade being "evidence obtained from at least one properly randomized controlled trial". The first randomized controlled trials evaluated the efficacy of the antibiotic streptomycin in the treatment of pulmonary tuberculosis [7]. This trial was initiated after it was recognized that, due to the variable and unpredictable natural course of pulmonary tuberculosis, evidence of improvement or cure following the use of a

new drug in a few individuals was not proof of the efficacy of the drug. Subsequently, this type of study design became established as the gold standard for assessing the safety and effectiveness of therapy [8].

Limitations of randomized controlled clinical trials

Clinical trials are research studies, often with formal, controlled protocols, designed to test ways to prevent, diagnose or treat a disease. Their purpose is to assess the effectiveness of new treatments and answer very specific questions about a particular treatment strategy. However, despite being the method of choice for assessing the efficacy of therapy, it should be kept in mind that randomized clinical trials do have limitations. Inaccuracies may derive from limitations in principle (i.e., limitations in the inherent nature of the method), or from limitations in procedure (i.e., limitations in the way in which the trial is conducted) [9]. While limitations in principle are difficult to resolve, it should be possible to overcome limitations in procedure.

An example of a limitation in procedure of a randomized trial comes from an assessment in which perioperative mortality in patients who had undergone carotid endarterectomy in clinical trials was compared with that in patients in hospitals that did not participate in the trials. The clinical trial results indicated that 30-day mortality was 1.4%; however,

Table 1. *Grades of evidence for assessing the quality of design of a clinical study. Information taken from [6].*

I	Evidence obtained from at least one properly randomized controlled trial
II-1	Evidence obtained from well-designed controlled trials without randomization
II-2	Evidence obtained from well-designed cohort or case–control analytical studies, preferably from more than one centre or research group
II-3	Evidence obtained from multiple time series with or without the intervention. Dramatic results in uncontrolled experiments could also be regarded as this type of evidence
III	Opinions of respected authorities, based on clinical experience, descriptive studies and case reports or reports of expert committees

perioperative mortality in non-trial hospitals was higher, and was nearly twice as high in those non-trial hospitals that carried out a low volume of these procedures ($p < 0.001$). In fact, patients undergoing carotid endarterectomy at trial hospitals had a mortality risk that was 15% lower than that in non-trial hospitals that carried out a high volume of these procedures, 25% lower than in non-trial hospitals that carried out an average volume, and 43% lower than in non-trial hospitals that carried out a low volume (p for trend < 0.001). These discrepancies may be due to differences in the characteristics of patients enrolled in the trials and those in non-trial hospitals. For example, randomized patients were younger and healthier than those in non-trial hospitals. While the clinical trials demonstrated that carotid endarterectomy was effective, the uses and outcomes of the procedure in more representative settings (i.e., in the non-trial hospitals) had not been established. This assessment has shown, therefore, that results of clinical trials may be inaccurate if the study population is not representative of the patient population as a whole, or if the setting in which therapies are usually administered differ significantly from the settings of the clinical trial [10, 11].

There are several reasons why randomized clinical trials may not be conducted [9]. First, it may be impossible to conduct a randomized trial, due to cultural, political or social obstacles. For example, when investigating the relationship between moderate alcohol consumption and hypertension in women in the USA [12], data were collected prospectively because it is considered unethical to randomly expose individuals to long-term alcohol consumption in a controlled trial. Secondly, a randomized placebo-controlled trial may be unnecessary; for example, in diseases where treatment can lead to a huge decrease in mortality. It may also be unethical where sufficient data can be obtained from observational studies using

historical cohorts [8]. Thirdly, there are circumstances under which it is difficult or inappropriate to conduct a placebo-controlled study, such as when the number of patients required to obtain definitive results is prohibitive or when the disorder under investigation is an orphan disease (defined in the European Union as a disease with a prevalence < 5 per 10 000 of the general population), such as Fabry disease. Finally, experimentation may be inadequate in cases where the outcome of intervention is determined by activities of the care provider, such as surgery or physiotherapy (an example of a limitation in principle). In these cases, observational studies are often preferable.

Need for observational studies to evaluate healthcare

The great value of observational studies is that they are much easier to complete and less expensive to conduct than clinical trials. When recruitment of a sufficient number of patients into a long-term, placebo-controlled trial is difficult, which is often the case for orphan diseases, databases such as FOS are invaluable as they provide a large amount of patient data over a long period of follow-up. Additionally, the inclusion criteria are often broader and there are wider spectra of coexisting illnesses, disease severity and concomitant treatments. Results from database studies may often, therefore, be applied more generally to the population as a whole.

Limitations of observational studies

The largest drawback of non-experimental studies is selection bias, as to enter into a database or study, an individual generally must already have been diagnosed and/or be showing signs and symptoms of the disease to be studied. Selection bias occurs when the study participants are not representative of the broader population at risk of the outcome. In contrast, the purpose of randomization in a clinical trial is to balance variation and unknown confounders.

Cohort studies may be historical or contemporaneous. In historical cohort studies, individuals are identified based on a common feature that was determined previously. The ascertainment of exposures antedates the development of the outcome and, hence, the temporal sequence of events is preserved. The advantage of using historical cohorts is that they are efficient, relatively inexpensive and data are immediately available. They can also provide valuable information when there is a dramatic difference in outcome between treated and untreated individuals (i.e., when non-treatment results in a severe outcome). However, as exposure data were not collected specifically for the cohort study, datasets are likely to be incomplete and the risk of confounding is high. When the results of treatment are not so dramatic, historical controls seem to exaggerate the beneficial effects of treatment, as outcome of controls in these individuals tends to be worse than that of controls in randomized trials [13]. This may be due to selection bias [8]. The possibility of bias relating to multiple comparisons means that conclusions drawn from cohort studies should be hypothesis driven and biologically plausible [14]. Nevertheless, both historical and contemporaneous cohort studies are well suited to examine rare exposures and multiple potential effects of a single exposure.

Careful patient selection and design are required for the results of observational studies to be considered reliable. Grodstein et al. [15] examined the results of randomized clinical trials and observational studies of the effects of hormone replacement therapy (HRT) in women. Both the randomized and observational studies reported a higher risk of breast cancer and a lower risk of colon cancer and hip fracture in women receiving HRT than in control women; however, while the randomized trials reported a higher risk of coronary heart disease in the treated patients, the observational studies

reported that HRT protects against coronary heart disease. This significant difference in the findings could be due to a number of factors: methodological differences, such as incomplete capture of early clinical events in the observational studies and confounding and compliance bias; or biological differences, such as the hormone regimen that patients were receiving and the characteristics of the study populations. This demonstrates that careful design of observational studies is necessary in order for the results to be interpreted correctly.

Advantages of observational studies

Despite possible drawbacks, data from observational research can be as valid as those from randomized trials [16]. For example, the average randomized drug trial is too small and the follow-up period is too short to detect adverse events that occur less than once per 200 patients per year. However, provided that the risk of an adverse event in a patient is unknown, selection of patients into a study cannot be made on the basis of this risk; therefore, in terms of the outcome (the occurrence of adverse events), the selection process is effectively random. In these cases, case–control or large observational follow-up studies are ideal for the study of adverse events [16].

Observational studies can also provide important data on treatment efficacy. In order to reduce selection bias, it is important that entry criteria into observational studies should be similar for both historical and contemporaneous controls. Concato et al. [13] compared results from published randomized clinical trials and observational studies of the same clinical topics and found that the average results of observational studies were remarkably similar to those of the trials. This analysis demonstrated that well-designed observational studies do not systematically overestimate the magnitude of the effects of treatment, when compared with randomized clinical trials.

Importance of outcomes databases

There are three types of clinical database [17], as follows.

- Protocol-oriented research databases, used in large randomized controlled clinical trials.
- Practice-oriented medical record databases, such as electronic medical record systems, which are more informal.
- Databases that combine features of protocol-oriented and practice-oriented databases. The goal of these databases is to create a large and diverse source of prospective longitudinal patient data. FOS is an example of this type of database.

Databases that fall into the third category are usually multinational and multicentre, and record data over several years of clinical practice. While randomized clinical trials are designed to answer very specific questions, outcomes databases can collate a broad range of information from a large number and a wide variety of patients, and therefore may provide the answers to several questions simultaneously. Data from large outcomes databases such as FOS can be used in several types of observational study, including cross-sectional, case–control and cohort studies. The evidence contained within these outcomes databases may contribute to clinical decision-making and allows the natural history of a disease and the efficacy and safety of therapy over several years to be assessed.

Evidence of the value of large multinational, multicentre databases comes from the success of KIGS (Pfizer International Growth Database) and KIMS (Pfizer International Metabolic Database), two international research outcomes databases designed to collect data on growth hormone (GH) therapy in children [18]. KIGS was established in 1987 and now contains data from approximately 60 000 patients from over 45 countries. KIMS began in 1994 and, to date, contains information on about 9300 patients,

equating to approximately 30 000 patient-years. Data from KIGS and KIMS can be used to answer questions about specific groups of patients or particular issues. They provide important information on mortality and morbidity outcomes and quality of life, and allow continued surveillance of the safety of GH therapy. Furthermore, analyses of data within KIGS and KIMS have led to the identification of new areas of research.

Importance of outcomes databases for studying orphan diseases

One of the particular strengths of FOS is that it provides a large amount of long-term follow-up data on patients with Fabry disease. It is difficult to obtain such a large amount of data from randomized trials, due to problems in recruiting a sufficient number of patients. Data from FOS allow sequential measurement of clinical outcomes, such as kidney function and quality of life. As centres located throughout Europe participate in FOS, the database allows comparison of information from different countries, to determine whether there are differences in the delivery and efficacy of treatment. Additionally, it contains data from both treated and untreated patients; therefore, in the future, FOS researchers will be able to follow untreated and treated patients from the same time point and under similar conditions, allowing accurate assessment of the efficacy of treatment in the absence of possible confounding variables. It should be acknowledged, however, that it is likely that untreated patients in FOS who are from countries in which therapy is available will have less severe disease. It is certainly possible to assess the consistency of results across many centres, which indicates the accuracy of the objective measures of the efficacy of ERT. Finally, the design of FOS encourages the reporting of adverse events, with benefits for both post-marketing surveillance and the clinical management of patients with Fabry disease. FOS has great potential and, as experience of the database grows, it will continue to provide valuable data on the safety and efficacy of ERT with agalsidase alfa.

Conclusions

Randomized controlled clinical trials remain the gold standard for assessing the effectiveness of healthcare; however, despite their many strengths, they have some limitations. Observational studies are a relatively inexpensive complement to randomized trials and are especially useful in the study of adverse events. In particular, multinational databases such as FOS provide large amounts of data on a broad spectrum of patients, which can be used in cross-sectional, case–control and cohort studies, and are therefore of great value for studying orphan diseases such as Fabry disease. Whatever method is used to assess healthcare interventions, the results of single studies should be interpreted cautiously, because the reproducibility of findings is essential as a protection against false-positive results.

Acknowledgements

The author wishes to thank Dr Charlotte Hanson at Oxford PharmaGenesis™ for support in producing this manuscript.

Dr Thadhani is a consultant for Shire Pharmaceuticals.

References

1. Mehta A, Ricci R, Widmer U, Dehout F, Garcia de Lorenzo A, Kampmann C et al. Fabry disease defined: baseline clinical manifestations of 366 patients in the Fabry Outcome Survey. Eur J Clin Invest 2004;34:236–42

2. D'Arcy Hart P. A change in scientific approach: from alternation to randomised allocation in clinical trials in the 1940s. BMJ 1999;319:572–3

3. Schulz KF, Grimes DA. Allocation concealment in randomised trials: defending against deciphering. Lancet 2002;359:614–18

4. Chalmers I. Why transition from alternation to randomisation in clinical trials was made. BMJ 1999;319:1372

5. Altman DG, Bland JM. Statistics notes. Treatment allocation in controlled trials: why randomise? BMJ 1999;318:1209

6. Preventive Services Task Force. Guide to clinical preventive services: report of the U.S. Preventive Services Task Force. Baltimore: Williams and Wilkins; 1997

7. Streptomycin treatment of pulmonary tuberculosis: a Medical Research Council investigation. BMJ 1948;2:769–82

8. Sacks H, Chalmers TC, Smith H, Jr. Randomized versus historical controls for clinical trials. Am J Med 1982;72:233–40

9. Black N. What observational studies can offer decision makers. Horm Res 1999;51 (Suppl 1):44–9

10. Wennberg DE, Lucas FL, Birkmeyer JD, Bredenberg CE, Fisher ES. Variation in carotid endarterectomy mortality in the Medicare population: trial hospitals, volume, and patient characteristics. JAMA 1998; 279:1278–81

11. Cebul RD, Snow RJ, Pine R, Hertzer NR, Norris DG. Indications, outcomes, and provider volumes for carotid endarterectomy. JAMA 1998;279:1282–87

12. Thadhani R, Camargo CA, Jr, Stampfer MJ, Curhan GC, Willett WC, Rimm EB. Prospective study of moderate alcohol consumption and risk of hypertension in young women. Arch Intern Med 2002;162:569–74

13. Concato J, Shah N, Horwitz RI. Randomized, controlled trials, observational studies, and the hierarchy of research designs. N Engl J Med 2000;342:1887–92

14. Rothman KJ, Green S. Modern epidemiology. Boston: Little Brown; 1998

15. Grodstein F, Clarkson TB, Manson JE. Understanding the divergent data on postmenopausal hormone therapy. N Engl J Med 2003;348:645–50

16. Vandenbroucke JP. When are observational studies as credible as randomised trials? Lancet 2004; 363:1728–31

17. Kahn MG. Clinical research databases and clinical decision making in chronic diseases. Horm Res 1999;51 (Suppl 1):50–7

18. Ranke MB, Dowie J. KIGS and KIMS as tools for evidence-based medicine. Horm Res 1999;51 (Suppl 1):83–6

15 Organization and technical aspects of FOS – the Fabry Outcome Survey

Elizabeth Hernberg-Ståhl

Fabry Outcome Survey, TKT Europe AB, Rinkebyvägen 11B, SE-182 36, Danderyd, Sweden

As a comprehensive database on the efficacy and safety of enzyme replacement therapy with agalsidase alfa, FOS – the Fabry Outcome Survey – is providing important insights into treatment outcomes, in addition to increasing our understanding of the natural history of Fabry disease. The success of FOS not only depends on the quantity of information collected, but also on the quality control processes that ensure the relevance and accuracy of the data submitted. Importantly, decision making concerning data collection, hypothesis testing and dissemination of information based on data analyses is controlled by participating physicians who are elected to the various National and International Boards and to specific scientific Working Groups. Hence, FOS is designed for the ultimate benefit of patients whilst remaining a practical tool for physicians and other health workers involved in caring for affected individuals and their families.

History and aims

FOS – the Fabry Outcome Survey – was initiated in 2001 to gain further understanding of the nature of Fabry disease and to improve the clinical management of patients with this disorder. FOS is an outcomes database for all patients with Fabry disease, including women and children, who are receiving, or are candidates for, enzyme replacement therapy (ERT) with agalsidase alfa (Replagal®; TKT Europe AB, Danderyd, Sweden).

The type of data collected in FOS has been recommended by international experts on Fabry disease. The principal aims of FOS are to document the efficacy and safety of ERT with agalsidase alfa in patients with Fabry disease and to drive improvements in clinical management, with the goal of making treatment as effective, simple and convenient as possible.

As of October 2005, FOS contains data on 752 patients from 11 countries and is the world's most comprehensive database on patients with Fabry disease. Information from FOS complements and extends the results of earlier placebo-controlled clinical trials and has the advantages of its longer duration, larger number of unselected patients and broader range of variables available for analysis. For a rare disorder such as Fabry disease, optimal use of pooled data from hundreds of patients with a wide range of disease severity and different treatment modalities is of great clinical value.

Organization of FOS

The organization of FOS (Figure 1) ensures that the scientific, ethical and policy decisions regarding the use and publication of FOS data are made by the National and International Boards. The members of these boards are participating physicians who have been elected by medical colleagues who are also involved in FOS. The National Boards govern all national activities, including

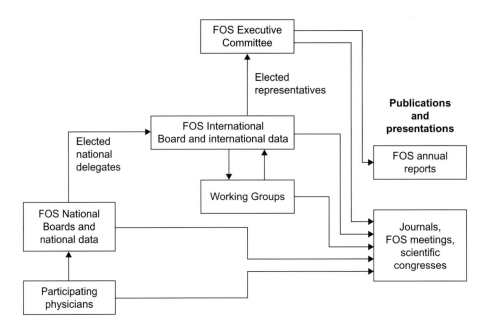

Figure 1. *Overview of the organization of FOS – the Fabry Outcome Survey.*

meetings and publications based on national data. The National Boards are organized to reflect the particular healthcare systems applied to the management of patients with Fabry disease in individual countries. National Boards provide important networks between a wide range of specialists, reflecting the multi-systemic nature of Fabry disease and the number of different specialties that are required to manage patients effectively.

Each National Board appoints one representative or, in some cases, several – depending on the number of patients from that country – to the International Board. The International Board governs international activities, such as meetings and publications, and also elects the members of the Executive Committee, which is responsible for the strategic and scientific long-term planning of FOS. The International Board meets twice a year and the Executive Committee four times a year. The Executive Committee or the International Board can appoint special Working Groups for specific scientific tasks. As of October 2005, Working Groups have

been established in the following areas: renal, cardiac, CNS, paediatric, female, eye, ear and gastrointestinal. The aim of the Working Groups is to improve collection and analysis of data and, ultimately, to optimize disease management in specific patient groups.

Data capture

The number of groups contributing data to FOS has expanded to include many centres throughout Europe. The size of the patient cohorts varies significantly between centres, and the services and facilities available differ according to the healthcare system in the various countries. Furthermore, some centres are based in regional or district general hospitals, while others are local centres within specialist clinics or operate as satellites. Each centre has access to FOS via a dedicated central server and is supported by a data manager.

At entry into FOS, each patient's medical history is documented, including the year of diagnosis of Fabry disease, details of Fabry-related signs and symptoms, and a record of previous treatment.

Each clinical centre should then follow the patients over time, recording the results of general physical examinations and standard laboratory investigations as well as information from additional investigations, such as echocardiography. Guidelines are available on how different measurements should be carried out. These help to ensure that the various investigations and evaluations are performed in a similar manner in all participating clinics. The different FOS Working Groups continually review and update these guidelines as necessary.

Data are obtained from both treated and untreated patients. Patients receiving ERT are reviewed at least every 6 months to assess their response to treatment. Untreated patients are reviewed annually in order to monitor disease progression.

FOS has been approved by the Ethics Committee/Institution Review Board of all participating centres.

Patient questionnaires

Patient questionnaires are a valuable tool for evaluating a patient's perception of their disease and its management. Within FOS, several questionnaires are available to participating patients in their respective languages. Efforts have been made to harmonize these questionnaires so that answers can be interpreted in international analyses. The following paragraphs provide an overview of the questionnaires and their intended use.

For adults
Brief Pain Inventory (BPI)
The BPI contains questions that measure both the intensity of pain and the effects of pain on a patient's life [1].

EQ-5D questionnaire
The EQ-5D questionnaire covers five dimensions: mobility, pain/discomfort, self-care, anxiety/depression and usual activities. Each dimension comprises three levels (no problems, some/moderate problems, extreme problems). The questionnaire is designed for self-completion and has been validated for use in different countries within Europe, as well as in the USA and in other countries worldwide. The questionnaire produces an overall single score as an index of health status. Patients can also assess their current health-related quality of life by rating their perceived health status on a visual analogue scale [2].

General FOS questionnaire
The general FOS questionnaire asks patients about the level of different Fabry-related problems that they experience, as well as collecting socioeconomic information.

Female FOS questionnaire
The FOS Female Working Group has developed a questionnaire for women with Fabry disease. The questionnaire aims to identify potential early predictive factors for disease progression and severity in this patient group. Questions include the amount of time taken off school, problems with reduced sweating, levels of physical activity, and number and timing of hospital admissions.

For children
FOS Paediatric Health and
Pain questionnaire
The FOS Paediatric Health and Pain questionnaire is an adaptation of the BPI and FOS questionnaire and covers health and social problems that are relevant to children. It is available for three age groups: 4–7 years, 8–12 years and 13–16 years.

KINDL questionnaire
The KINDL questionnaire contains 24 items to assess health-related quality of life in children [3]. It is available for three age groups: 4–7 years, 8–12 years and 13–16 years, and has also been used in other diseases for comparative purposes.

The FOS system

Data are entered into FOS electronically, directly from each participating clinic. This is achieved through use of the FOS application, a comprehensive software tool for recording and reviewing data on patients with Fabry disease. The FOS program connects to a central database managed by an independent external service provider in order to ensure the highest possible level of security and confidentiality during recording, transfer and storage of data.

Technology

The FOS application uses 'Smart Client' technology whereby a standard Windows application is installed in the clinic. The FOS application holds most of the screens and programming locally and can therefore react quickly to user input and actions. The client application uses a secure channel over the Internet to connect to the application server and the central FOS database. Once connected, only the FOS data are transferred across the Internet, which reduces the strain on bandwidth and minimizes the actual connection time. After initial installation, the application will automatically upgrade itself when new versions become available.

The relevant clinic staff are assigned individual user names and passwords that give them access to data from their own clinic. In addition, users within a clinic can be assigned specific user rights to grant or refuse certain functionality, enabling the system to be tailored to the needs of the clinic. Data managers have access to an application with individual log-in but no editing capabilities, so that they can monitor the data submitted by the clinics.

Protecting patient privacy

The processing of information in the FOS database conforms to the requirements of the Swedish Personal Data Act (1998:204) and the EU Directive 2002/58/EC (July 12, 2002) on the processing of personal data and the protection of privacy in the electronic communication sector.

Although the clinics can record the name of the patient (optional information), this is available only to the clinics and intended solely for their use. Instead of a name, a unique identification code, the FOS code, is generated automatically by the system upon first data entry for a new patient. This FOS code is derived from the country and clinic codes as well as a numerical value.

Usability

The FOS application was designed and built by a team of developers with experience from several other outcome surveys. Dedicated Fabry experts contributed with their feedback throughout the development phase. For the project group, usability was a high priority in order to minimize the time and effort needed to enter data, resulting in an intuitive user application closely adapted to the specific needs of FOS.

The application was built using the PC PAL Application Framework, which is a configurable foundation for outcome surveys and patient registries. It has a number of specifically enhanced components to produce a highly customized application to suit the specific needs of FOS. Screens are laid out clearly, and are self-explanatory and user friendly. Many options are available from drop-down lists and sometimes from more comprehensive listings, such as those containing all known published Fabry mutations or all commonly used concomitant medications. Some screens present data in a graphical form, whereas others assist the recording of data with easy-to-use clickable images, such as those used to record the location and severity of pain.

As Fabry disease is a multisystemic disorder, it is common for several different physicians to be involved in patient care, each performing various specialist investigations. In

Technical architecture

- The FOS system uses the Secure Socket Layer (SSL) protocol to carry data between the database and the Smart Client application installed on each user's personal computer.
- The SSL protocol provides a secure way to transfer data over the Internet using the RSA encryption standard.
- FOS data have to pass several layers of firewalls between the database and the client application. The following figure shows a typical configuration that, in principle, is identical to any other connection to a secure website (such as an Internet bank or when making online purchases), except that the FOS application runs outside of a web browser.

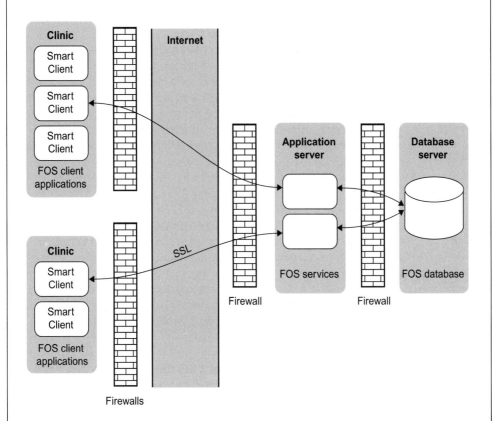

Technical architecture of the FOS system. Smart Client refers to the application installed on each user's personal computer. SSL, Secure Socket Layer.

- To prevent unauthorized use, an individual's password is transferred and stored in such a way that it is unavailable even to system and database administrators.
- On the server side, users are assigned individual and unique sessions once logged in, preventing malicious access by hackers to the database.
- Access to the data is logged – both in terms of activity and changes to the data – through audit logs, which are available to administrators and authorities should the need arise.

order to secure data capture and recording of these investigations in FOS, specific forms can be printed from the application. These forms can then be used for recording the data from the specialist investigation and can be returned to the person responsible for data entry in the FOS clinic.

Data quality

Obtaining quality data remains one of the key objectives of FOS. The FOS application helps to ensure quality data by making a number of checks on the data as they are entered, in order to assure their accuracy and completeness.

Data are automatically checked at entry into the FOS database by verifying logical relationships set within the program. Additional controls are implemented once data have been signed and submitted. Clarification requests may be generated by the data managers to obtain additional information or to question the recorded data. These requests are made available electronically to the FOS centres. Resolutions may include data changes, which are again signed and submitted, or be limited to explanations made available to the data managers. All requests and their resolutions are stored within the database, as is a complete audit log of every change to the FOS data.

Patient management

The FOS application also serves as an advanced patient management tool for the clinics' own Fabry patients entered into FOS. Data entered can be displayed graphically for each patient, allowing physicians to follow patient development visually over time with respect to clinical examinations and laboratory data. Detailed and configurable reports can be produced for patient monitoring.

Patient diaries can be printed from the system to make it easy for patients to record significant events, such as visits to other clinics or hospitals, missed infusions, changes in medication and other medications taken. This will help the patient to remember to report these events at the next visit to the FOS clinic and hence ensures that relevant information is reported to FOS.

A query facility with which to interrogate the clinic's own patient data is also available. Users can extract data from the database by selecting the appropriate variables and applying criteria for selection of patients.

Role of FOS in pharmacovigilance

Clinical trials usually involve relatively few patients for a relatively short period of time. As ERT with agalsidase alfa is intended as a life-long treatment, it is important to continue to report data on adverse events over the total period of treatment, as rare adverse events can only be detected in this way. Also, speculation about possible events can be investigated only if all physicians treating patients with ERT continue to report adverse events on a regular basis, whether or not they are considered to be related to treatment. All adverse events should therefore be reported, even those that physicians are convinced are not related to treatment. Efforts have been made to facilitate adverse event reporting as much as possible in the FOS application.

Publications arising from FOS

Regular analyses are performed on the FOS database, and findings are communicated to the participating physicians at a variety of FOS meetings, such as FOS Investigators' meetings and FOS Forums. In addition, FOS information is disseminated via the FOS newsletter and annual reports, as well as by presentations at congresses and publications in peer-reviewed journals (Table 1) [4–9]. The FOS Working Groups also provide guidelines to physicians on how to manage patients with Fabry disease.

Table 1. *Peer-reviewed publications arising from analyses of the FOS – Fabry Outcome Survey – database.*

Year	Authors	Subject area	Reference
2004	Mehta *et al.*	Baseline clinical characteristics of Fabry disease	*Eur J Clin Invest* [4]
2004	Beck *et al.*	Overall effects of agalsidase alfa treatment	*Eur J Clin Invest* [5]
2005	Hoffmann *et al.*	Effects of agalsidase alfa on pain and quality of life	*J Med Genet* [6]
2005	Kleinert *et al.*	Anaemia as a new complication of Fabry disease	*Kidney Int* [7]
2005	Deegan *et al.*	Fabry disease in females	*J Med Genet* [8]
2006	Ramaswami *et al.*	Fabry disease in children	*Acta Paediatr* [9]

Conclusions

After 5 years of follow-up of patients in FOS, the data collected have provided new insights into Fabry disease, as well as confirming and significantly expanding efficacy and safety data on treatment with agalsidase alfa. With increasing patient numbers and treatment duration, FOS will be instrumental in optimizing the management of individuals with Fabry disease.

References

1. Cleeland CS, Ryan KM. Pain assessment: global use of the Brief Pain Inventory. *Ann Acad Med Singapore* 1994;23:129–38

2. The EuroQol Group. EuroQol – a new facility for the measurement of health-related quality of life. *Health Policy* 1990;16:199–208

3. Ravens-Sieberer U, Bullinger M. Assessing health-related quality of life in chronically ill children with the German KINDL: first psychometric and content analytical results. *Qual Life Res* 1998;7:399–407

4. Mehta A, Ricci R, Widmer U, Dehout F, García de Lorenzo A, Kampmann C *et al.* Fabry disease defined: baseline clinical manifestations of 366 patients in the Fabry Outcome Survey. *Eur J Clin Invest* 2004;34:236–42

5. Beck M, Ricci R, Widmer U, Dehout F, García de Lorenzo A, Kampman C *et al.* Fabry disease: overall effects of agalsidase alfa treatment. *Eur J Clin Invest* 2004;34:838–44

6. Hoffmann B, García de Lorenzo A, Mehta A, Beck M, Widmer U, Ricci R *et al.* Effects of enzyme replacement therapy on pain and health related quality of life in patients with Fabry disease: data from FOS (Fabry Outcome Survey). *J Med Genetic* 2005;42:247–52

7. Kleinert J, Dehout F, Schwarting A, de Lorenzo AG, Ricci R, Kampmann C *et al.* Anemia is a new complication in Fabry disease: data from the Fabry Outcome Survey. *Kidney Int* 2005;67:1955–60

8. Deegan P, Bähner AF, Barba-Romero MA, Hughes D, Kampmann C, Beck M. Natural history of Fabry disease in females in the Fabry Outcome Survey. *J Med Genet* 2006;43:347–52

9. Ramaswami U, Whybra C, Parini R, Pintos-Morell G, Mehta A, Sunder-Plassmann G *et al.* Clinical manifestations of Fabry disease in children: data from the Fabry Outcome Survey. *Acta Paediatr* 2006;95:86–92

Section 3:

Fabry disease: clinical features and natural course

16 Demographics of FOS – the Fabry Outcome Survey

Michael Beck

Universitäts-Kinderklinik, Langenbeckstrasse 1, D-55101 Mainz, Germany

Baseline data from a cohort of 815 patients (48% males and 52% females) with Fabry disease from 87 centres in 13 European countries who were enrolled in FOS – the Fabry Outcome Survey – were analysed in terms of demography and clinical manifestations of Fabry disease. From this database, it can be seen that there is a significant period of time between the onset of symptoms and diagnosis, with an average delay of 12.4 ± 15.0 years in females and 12.2 ± 13.0 years in males. The database also confirms that heterozygous females should be considered as patients rather than carriers and that children with Fabry disease are symptomatic. Furthermore, data are now available from 483 patients (60% males and 40% females) who are receiving enzyme replacement therapy (ERT), with 224 patients having received ERT for more than 3 years.

FOS – the Fabry Outcome Survey – is a European outcomes database for patients with Fabry disease who are receiving, or are candidates for, enzyme replacement therapy (ERT) with agalsidase alfa. FOS is the world's most comprehensive database of patients with Fabry disease. Data from all consenting patients are entered into the database following a structured clinical assessment by a physician or a nurse specialist. By pooling data from different specialist centres, FOS enables the natural history of this rare disease to be studied in a large group of patients, including men, women and children, and provides baseline data against which the effects of treatment with agalsidase alfa can be measured.

Patient demographics

Since the start of FOS in 2001 there has been a continuous increase in the number of patients who are included in the database (Figure 1). At the end of 2005, data on 815 patients, who were recruited from 87 centres in 13 European countries, had been entered. So far, the largest groups of patients come from Germany (22%) and the UK (15%), whereas most other countries each contribute less than 10% of the patient population.

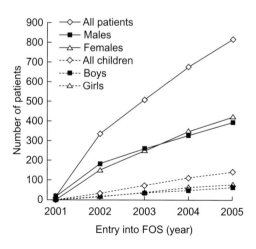

Figure 1. *Number of patients with Fabry disease enrolled in FOS – the Fabry Outcome Survey – over time. Data shown include all patients enrolled by the end of each year.*

In the first few years of FOS, there were more males than females in the database [1]; however, in the last quarter of 2004, for the first time, the number of heterozygotes exceeded the number of hemizygotes (348 females, 328 males) (Figure 1). At entry into FOS, males were significantly younger than females ($p = 0.0045$) and they were diagnosed at an earlier age ($p < 0.0001$) (Table 1). In many cases (35%), the diagnosis of Fabry disease was suspected by other affected family members; however, a range of different medical specialists were involved in diagnosis, including nephrologists (14%), geneticists (10%), paediatricians (8%), dermatologists (7%), general practitioners (5%), cardiologists (5%) and a range of other physicians. Data show that there is no difference in the severity of Fabry disease in patients diagnosed as a result of examinations following the suspicions of relatives or geneticists and those diagnosed by other physicians (FOS-Mainz Severity Score Index, 14.7 versus 15.2, respectively, adjusted for gender and age).

Delay in diagnosis

Previous studies have reported a significant delay in diagnosis and a wide range of prior misdiagnoses [1, 2]. However, early diag-nosis is essential to enable optimal symptomatic management which, in combination with ERT, may improve quality of life and prevent late complications.

Although awareness of the clinical manifestations of Fabry disease has been increased dramatically by publications and scientific presentations, the latest analysis of FOS data shows that there is still a noteworthy time delay between the onset of symptoms and diagnosis (Table 1). The mean time ($\pm$ SD) between the onset of symptoms and diagnosis was 12.4 ± 15.0 years in females and 12.2 ± 13.0 years in males.

Reported signs and symptoms in male and female patients

The main signs and symptoms in male and female patients, according to age at entry into FOS, are shown in Tables 2 and 3. Multiple organ systems were involved in the majority of patients with Fabry disease. Only 36 of the patients in FOS (5 males, 31 females) had no reported signs and symptoms of Fabry disease at their latest visit. These patients were generally young (males, 20.8 ± 14.1 years; females, 26.0 ± 18.6 years).

Table 1. *Characteristics of 815 patients with Fabry disease at entry into FOS – the Fabry Outcome Survey – (data until end of 2005). Values are expressed as means $\pm$ SD.*

	Males	Females
Age at entry (years)	34.1 ± 15.1	37.4 ± 18.4**
	($n = 394$)	($n = 421$)
Age at diagnosis (years)	25.7 ± 15.3	31.3 ± 17.4*
	($n = 362$)	($n = 374$)
Number of symptomatic patients	389	390
Age at onset of symptoms (years)	12.7 ± 11.1	19.4 ± 15.2*
	($n = 301$)	($n = 239$)
Time from onset of symptoms to diagnosis (years)	12.2 ± 13.0	12.4 ± 15.0
	($n = 295$)	($n = 229$)
Number of asymptomatic patients	5	31
Age of asymptomatic patients (years)	20.8 ± 14.1	26.0 ± 18.6
	($n = 5$)	($n = 31$)

*$p = 0.0045$, **$p < 0.0001$ versus males.

Table 2. *Frequency and age at onset of specific signs and symptoms of Fabry disease in male patients (n = 375) enrolled in FOS – the Fabry Outcome Survey.*

	Frequency		Age at symptom onset (years)	
	Proportion of population (%)	**Number of patients**	**Mean ± SD**	**Number of patients**
Cerebrovascular	20.0	75	33.5 ± 14.5	52
Stroke	8.5	32	39.4 ± 12.1	26
TIA	8.8	33	32.4 ± 14.5	23
Neurological	82.9	311	16.3 ± 15.7	180
Pain attacks	69.3	260	13.6 ± 13.6	188
Chronic pain	49.9	187	17.2 ± 15.9	128
Cardiac	61.1	229	32.9 ± 14.5	141
Chest pain	19.5	73	38.4 ± 12.4	59
Palpitations	20.3	76	35.7 ± 12.8	51
LV hypertrophy	40.3	151	39.4 ± 11.5	92
Renal/urinary	57.3	215	33.9 ± 13.1	143
Proteinuria	45.9	172	33.2 ± 12.4	113
Haemodialysis	9.6	36	39.6 ± 13.2	32
Peritoneal dialysis	2.7	10	42.7 ± 7.1	8
Transplantation	8.8	33	37.2 ± 11.6	28
Gastrointestinal	56.3	211	23.3 ± 16.2	138
Diarrhoea	36.3	136	23.9 ± 16.9	89
Abdominal pain	41.1	154	22.4 ± 15.5	117
Constipation	13.6	51	23.3 ± 17.5	38
Auditory	56.3	211	29.9 ± 14.6	129
Tinnitus	31.7	119	28.1 ± 13.7	87
Vertigo	29.1	109	29.6 ± 14.4	77
Sudden deafness	6.1	23	30.8 ± 14.5	15
Ophthalmological	62.1	233	28.4 ± 14.7	151
Cornea verticillata	46.1	173	28.4 ± 14.0	120
Tortuous vessels	26.4	99	31.9 ± 13.1	67
Posterior subcapsular cataract	7.2	27	31.4 ± 16.0	16
Dermatological	70.1	263	18.7 ± 14.7	147
Angiokeratoma	65.9	247	18.7 ± 13.9	139
Telangiectasia	22.1	83	26.1 ± 16.6	46

LV, left ventricular; TIA, transient ischaemic attack.

There is no evidence for an atypical variant of Fabry disease with manifestations limited to a single organ system, as has been reported previously involving the heart [3], kidney [4] and kidney plus heart [5]. In both genders, the number of organ systems involved rises progressively with age, although some signs and symptoms are more common in children than in adults.

Approximately 83% of males and 66% of females had neurological symptoms, the most prevalent of these being neuropathic pain. These symptoms began at an early age, being

Table 3. *Frequency and age at onset of specific signs and symptoms of Fabry disease in female patients (n = 396) enrolled in FOS – the Fabry Outcome Survey.*

	Frequency		Age at symptom onset (years)	
	Proportion of population (%)	Number of patients	Mean ± SD	Number of patients
Cerebrovascular	20.7	82	41.4 ± 15.9	55
Stroke	5.8	23	50.8 ± 14.6	20
TIA	7.3	29	46.8 ± 14.0	25
Neurological	65.9	261	21.2 ± 16.2	152
Pain attacks	50.0	198	18.2 ± 17.1	147
Chronic pain	30.6	121	23.0 ± 17.9	80
Cardiac	51.8	205	36.4 ± 18.6	133
Chest pain	20.5	81	44.2 ± 15.9	55
Palpitations	24.2	96	40.7 ± 16.5	68
LV hypertrophy	25.5	101	49.5 ± 11.0	62
Renal/urinary	36.9	146	36.8 ± 16.4	92
Proteinuria	32.8	130	36.9 ± 17.1	90
Haemodialysis	0.5	2	38.5 ± 2.0	2
Peritoneal dialysis	0	0	–	0
Transplantation	0.5	2	40.1 ± 1.2	2
Gastrointestinal	45.5	180	25.9 ± 18.5	127
Diarrhoea	21.0	83	23.9 ± 17.0	59
Abdominal pain	31.8	126	26.3 ± 20.3	94
Constipation	16.7	66	29.4 ± 20.7	47
Auditory	41.9	166	34.3 ± 18.7	111
Tinnitus	26.3	104	31.3 ± 17.5	72
Vertigo	27.5	109	33.6 ± 17.8	82
Sudden deafness	2.8	11	34.0 ± 18.4	10
Ophthalmological	49.7	197	32.0 ± 18.7	138
Cornea verticillata	38.9	154	32.0 ± 19.9	112
Tortuous vessels	10.1	40	41.8 ± 19.6	29
Posterior subcapsular cataract	3.5	14	54.7 ± 18.8	9
Dermatological	37.4	148	28.9 ± 17.1	91
Angiokeratoma	35.6	141	28.7 ± 16.9	86
Telangiectasia	9.3	37	39.0 ± 22.1	24

LV, left ventricular; TIA, transient ischaemic attack.

reported during childhood in males (mean age, 16.3 years) and during early adulthood in women (mean age, 21.2 years). Dermatological manifestations, which were more common in males than in females (70% versus 37%), began at an early age in males (mean age, 18.7 years) and somewhat later in females (mean age, 28.9 years). Other early manifestations of Fabry disease included those involving the gastrointestinal system, which began at a mean age of 23.3 years in males and 25.9 years in females. In total, some 56% of males and 45% of females with Fabry disease reported gastrointestinal problems.

Auditory signs and symptoms, including tinnitus, hearing difficulties or hearing loss, were found in 56% of males and 42% of females. Ocular manifestations were reported in 62.1% of males and nearly 50% of females.

Cardiac and renal manifestations of Fabry disease were reported to begin on average during the fourth decade of life in both men and women in FOS. Cardiac manifestations were reported in 61% of males and 52% of females, beginning at a mean age of 32.9 years in males and 36.4 years in females. Renal/urinary manifestations were reported in 57% of males and 37% of females, with onset at a mean age of 33.9 and 36.8 years, respectively (see Chapter 21). Cerebrovascular events (stroke, transient ischaemic attacks [TIAs] and prolonged reversible ischaemic neurological deficits) were less common, affecting approximately 20% of males and females; however, they may be observed in relatively young patients. The mean age for such events was 33.5 years in males and 41.4 years in females. The youngest patient to report a TIA was a boy aged 12 years. This is the first report of TIA in a child with Fabry disease.

These data confirm that female heterozygotes may exhibit the full range of disease manifestations and should no longer be considered as asymptomatic 'carriers'. However, these data and other clinical studies have shown that the signs and symptoms in females with Fabry disease are more variable than those in males, and that the disease appears to progress more slowly [6, 7]. The manifestations of Fabry disease in females are discussed in more detail in Chapter 30.

Children in FOS

As shown in Figure 1, there has been a steady increase in the number of patients younger than 18 years of age enrolled in FOS. In 2002, 10% of all patients included in FOS were children, but this proportion has increased to

17% in 2005 (see Table 4). Common clinical symptoms reported in children include acroparaesthesiae, decreased sweating and cardiac abnormalities [8] (see Chapter 31).

Mortality

Age and cause of death have been reported by those enrolled in FOS for 68 male and 39 female relatives who were presumed to have Fabry disease. The mean age at death (± SD) of affected male and female relatives was 44.9 ± 9.9 and 57.8 ± 14.3 years, respectively. This significant reduction in life expectancy is consistent with previous studies that have shown a reduced lifespan in males and females with Fabry disease [9, 10].

Enzyme replacement therapy

FOS data show, that the number of patients receiving agalsidase alfa has increased progressively over 3 years (Figure 2). In total, 483 patients are currently receiving ERT (60% males). Overall, 73% of all males and 46% of all females in FOS are receiving agalsidase alfa. Of these patients, 67 are children (29 girls and 38 boys). The proportion of women and children receiving ERT is

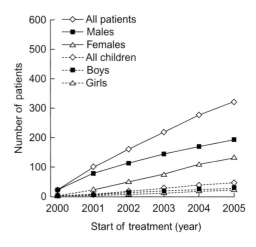

Figure 2. *Number of patients with Fabry disease enrolled in FOS – the Fabry Outcome Survey – starting enzyme replacement therapy each year. Data include patients for whom retrospective information was included in the database following enrolment.*

Table 4. *Proportion of men, women and children enrolled in FOS – the Fabry Outcome Survey – and receiving treatment with agalsidase alfa at the end of each year. Data for the proportions treated include patients for whom retrospective information was included in the database following enrolment.*

	Enrolled (%)			Treated (%)		
	Men	**Women**	**Children**	**Men**	**Women**	**Children**
2001	100	0	0	75	19	6
2002	49	40	10	64	27	10
2003	44	41	15	58	30	12
2004	41	42	17	53	33	13
2005	40	42	17	52	34	14

increasing (Table 4). Some 224 patients have now received treatment for more than 3 years. Analysis of data from the latest visit show that those patients who started treatment more recently are generally less severely affected than those who started ERT when it first became available (Figure 3). In 2001, the average age of females who started ERT was about 45 years; by 2005, younger heterozygotes with generally milder disease manifestations were receiving treatment (Figure 4).

Conclusions

The FOS database provides detailed information about the clinical manifestations of Fabry disease in a large cohort of patients. The size of this database will soon increase with the inclusion of patients currently enrolled in the US outcomes database for patients treated with agalsidase alfa (FIRE – Fabry International Research Exchange). Through FOS, significant clinical symptoms have

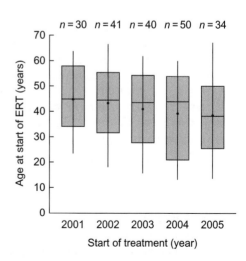

Figure 3. *Disease severity (as assessed by FOS – the Fabry Outcome Survey – adaptation of the Mainz Severity Score Index [FOS-MSSI]) at latest visit in males and females (combined) in FOS according to when they began enzyme replacement therapy. For an explanation of the FOS-MSSI, see Chapter 32.*

Figure 4. *Age of females in FOS – the Fabry Outcome Survey – when they started enzyme replacement therapy (ERT), according to year.*

been demonstrated in children and hetero-zygous females. Information gained from analyses of the FOS database may help to increase the awareness of Fabry disease in both genders and to avoid misdiagnoses and delays between the onset of symptoms and diagnosis.

References

1. Mehta A, Ricci R, Widmer U, Dehout F, Garcia de Lorenzo A, Kampmann C et al. Fabry disease defined: baseline clinical manifestations of 366 patients in the Fabry Outcome Survey. Eur J Clin Invest 2004;34:236–42

2. Galanos J, Nicholls K, Grigg L, Kiers L, Crawford A, Becker G. Clinical features of Fabry's disease in Australian patients. Intern Med J 2002;32:575–84

3. Sachdev B, Takenaka T, Teraguchi H, Tei C, Lee P, McKenna WJ et al. Prevalence of Anderson–Fabry disease in male patients with late onset hypertrophic cardiomyopathy. Circulation 2002;105:1407–11

4. Sawada K, Mizoguchi K, Hishida A, Kaneko E, Koide Y, Nishimura K et al. Point mutation in the α-galactosidase A gene of atypical Fabry disease with only nephropathy. Clin Nephrol 1996;45:289–94

5. Germain DP. A new phenotype of Fabry disease with intermediate severity between the classical form and the cardiac variant. Contrib Nephrol 2001;136: 234–40

6. Whybra C, Kampmann C, Willers I, Davies J, Winchester B, Kriegsmann J et al. Anderson–Fabry disease: clinical manifestations of disease in female heterozygotes. J Inherit Metab Dis 2001;24:715–24

7. Guffon N. Clinical presentation in female patients with Fabry disease. J Med Genet 2003;40:e38

8. Ries M, Gupta S, Moore DF, Sachdev V, Quirk JM, Murray GJ et al. Pediatric Fabry disease. Pediatrics 2005;115:e344–55

9. MacDermot KD, Holmes A, Miners AH. Anderson–Fabry disease: clinical manifestations and impact of disease in a cohort of 60 obligate carrier females. J Med Genet 2001;38:769–75

10. MacDermot KD, Holmes A, Miners AH. Anderson–Fabry disease: clinical manifestations and impact of disease in a cohort of 98 hemizygous males. J Med Genet 2001;38:750–60

17 Diagnosis of Fabry disease: the role of screening and case-finding studies

Gere Sunder-Plassmann[1] and Manuela Födinger[2]

[1]Division of Nephrology and Dialysis, Department of Medicine III, and [2]Clinical Institute of Medical and Chemical Laboratory Diagnostics, Medical University Vienna, Währinger Gürtel 18–20, A-1090 Vienna, Austria

In many patients, the diagnosis of Fabry disease is established rather late in the course of the disorder. Screening of newborns or case-finding studies among high-risk patient groups could, however, improve the clinical care of families with a hitherto unknown inherited trait. Hence, it is essential that awareness of this disease in the general population and among physicians is improved, so that early diagnosis and treatment can be achieved.

Introduction

The timely diagnosis of Fabry disease is difficult [1]. Early symptoms in childhood include acroparaesthesia and pain, which can be triggered by heat and fever, but these symptoms are often misinterpreted and only occasionally lead to the correct diagnosis [2]. The median age at diagnosis of Fabry disease was 28.6 years in a recent study from Australia [3]. Similarly, the median age at diagnosis was about 28 years among 688 patients recorded in FOS – the Fabry Outcome Survey – although the first symptoms occurred some 16 years earlier (Table 1).

Many patients with Fabry disease therefore have a long history of consultations with several different medical specialists and are often given the wrong diagnosis. Figure 1 shows the frequency of the most common erroneous diagnoses in patients included in the FOS database.

Who makes the diagnosis?

For patients enrolled in FOS, the medical specialists who most often establish the diagnosis of Fabry disease are nephrologists, followed by geneticists, although many other specialists may be involved (Figure 2). The potential for bias in these data, however, should be acknowledged. For example, the number of cases diagnosed by paediatricians may be high in those large centres that also diagnose and treat adult patients. Also, diagnoses by nephrologists may be indirect, with renal biopsies resulting in a correct diagnosis in patients where the disease was not initially suspected. Furthermore, geneticists may confirm the diagnosis of Fabry disease, although they are often not the first to suspect the disease.

Once an index patient has been identified, family members often play a major role in suspecting and diagnosing Fabry disease

Table 1. *Onset of symptoms and age at diagnosis of female and male patients with Fabry disease.*

	Females	Males
Number of patients	358	330
Median age at onset – years	13	9
(10–90th percentiles)	(6–44)	(5–25)
Median age at diagnosis – years	32	24
(10–90th percentiles)	(9–54)	(8–46)

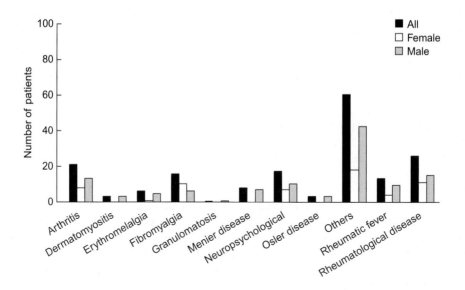

Figure 1. *Frequency of erroneous diagnoses in patients with Fabry disease enrolled in FOS – the Fabry Outcome Survey.*

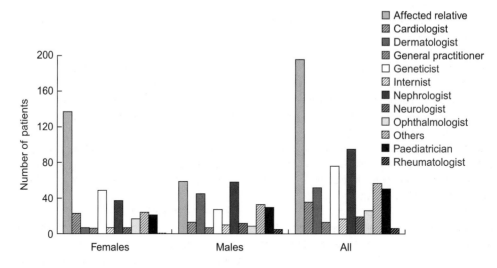

Figure 2. *Among patients enrolled in FOS – the Fabry Outcome Survey – relatives, nephrologists and geneticists suspect and diagnose Fabry disease most frequently.*

among relatives (Figure 2). The clinician has an important role in performing a pedigree analysis and in offering non-directive genetic counselling, proper diagnosis and adequate therapy for affected relatives (see Chapter 35).

Screening and case-finding

In general, screening involves conducting tests in apparently healthy populations to identify individuals at increased risk of a disease or disorder. Those identified may be offered a subsequent diagnostic test or procedure and/or, where available, a treatment or preventive medication.

Looking for additional illnesses in those with medical problems is termed case-finding [4].

Screening of newborns

Traditional newborn screening focuses on disorders for which early treatment prevents severe morbidity and mortality. In 1968, Wilson and Jungner delineated ten criteria that would justify population screening [5]. Many newborn screening task forces have reaffirmed these criteria as the standard for adding disorders to newborn screening programmes. A recent study showed that most paediatricians support diagnostic genetic testing of high-risk children, but are less supportive of expanding newborn screening [6]. In this study, willingness to expand newborn screening did not correlate with professional characteristics, such as subspecialty affiliation, but rather with personal interest in testing their own children.

Most recently, the American College of Medical Genetics (ACMG) has proposed newborn screening for 29 disorders that can be grouped into five categories: amino acid metabolism disorders, organic acid metabolism disorders, fatty acid oxidation disorders, haemoglobinopathies, and others [7]. In the months since their report was issued, many US states have expanded their newborn screening programmes. As of October 2005, ten states already mandate screening for all 29 conditions [8]. However, this policy has not been without criticism regarding the interests of the general population, as the evidence that such a screening policy is beneficial is uncertain [9].

Screening of newborns for Fabry disease has gained some interest in recent years because effective treatment is now available [10, 11]. Besides measuring enzyme activity in plasma or leukocytes (see Chapter 18), decreased α-galactosidase A activity

can be demonstrated in samples eluted from a dried blood spot collected on filter paper [12]. This assay was adapted for high-throughput screening [13, 14], but allows identification of only two-thirds of heterozygotes [15]. The α-galactosidase A protein eluted from blood spots can also be immuno-precipitated and the protein concentration and α-galactosidase activity measured [16]. Meikle and colleagues reported that newborn screening for Fabry disease by means of immune quantification assays and tandem mass spectrometry can show a sensitivity and specificity of 100% [17]. It is likely that electrospray tandem mass spectrometry will make screening for several different lysosomal diseases from dried blood spots feasible in the near future [18]. However, newborn screening for Fabry disease has not been recommended by the ACMG [7].

The reported incidence of Fabry disease of 1 in 117 000 [3] or 1 in 240 000 [19] live births may be an underestimation. In this context, recent screening of male newborns revealed an astonishingly high prevalence of Fabry disease in Italy, where 8 out of 22 058 children (1 in 2700) had a confirmed reduction in α-galactosidase A activity and mutations in the α-galactosidase A gene (M Spada, unpublished data). These data are provocative and need further confirmation.

Case-finding studies

Fabry disease can affect a wide range of organs. Medical specialists caring for patients suffering from renal disease, heart disease or stroke, for example, are likely to encounter individuals with undiagnosed Fabry disease. Making a correct diagnosis in these cases has the potential to improve medical care in the affected individual, as well as perhaps leading to identification of the disease in relatives.

Importantly, case-finding studies in dialysis patients have revealed a more than tenfold

Table 2. *Prevalence of Fabry disease among dialysis patients.*

Reference	All patients Number	%	Males Number	%	Females Number	%	Country	Assay
Utsumi *et al.* [22]	2/722	0.28	2/440	0.45	0/282	0	Japan	P
Desnick [23]	–	–	9/1903	0.47	–	–	USA	P/L
Spada & Pagliardini [14]	4/2991	0.13	4/1765	0.22	0/1226	0	Italy	BS
Linthorst *et al.* [24]	–	–	1/508	0.22	–	–	The Netherlands	WB
Nakao *et al.* [25]	–	–	6/514	1.17	–	–	Japan	P
Kotanko *et al.* [26]	4/2480	0.16	4/1516	0.26	0/964	0	Austria	BS
Ichinose *et al.* [27]	–	–	1/450	0.22	–	–	Japan	P
Bekri *et al.* [28]	1/106	0.94	–	–	–	–	France	L
Tanaka *et al.* [29]	5/696	0.7	4/401	1.00	1/295	0.33	Japan	P

P, α-galactosidase A activity in plasma; L, α-galactosidase A activity in leukocytes; BS, α-galactosidase A activity in dried blood spots; WB, α-galactosidase A activity in whole blood.

Table 3. *Prevalence of Fabry disease among patients with hypertrophic cardiomyopathy or left ventricular hypertrophy.*

Reference	Number	%	Country	Assay
Sachdev *et al.* [30]	6/153 males	3.92	UK	P
Chimenti *et al.* [31]	4/34 females	11.76	Italy	BX
Nakao *et al.* [32]	7/230 males	3.04	Japan	P

P, α-galactosidase A activity in plasma; BX, myocardial biopsy.

higher prevalence of Fabry disease among those with end-stage renal disease, compared with historical data obtained from large renal registries in the USA [20] and Europe [21]. The prevalence of Fabry disease among male or female patients suffering from end-stage renal disease is shown in Table 2.

Similarly, cardiologists have shown a high prevalence of Fabry disease among patients with left ventricular hypertrophy or hypertrophic cardiomyopathy (Table 3).

Among 721 young adults, aged 18–55 years, who presented with cryptogenic stroke, 21 out of 432 (4.9%) male patients, and 7 out of 289 (2.4%) female patients had Fabry disease, confirmed by mutational analysis of the α-galactosidase A gene [33]. By definition, this study excluded patients without typical risk factors for stroke, such as relevant nicotine abuse, significant carotid stenosis, severe obesity, cardiac emboli, patent foramen ovale, and coagulopathies, and also excluded those in whom there was no diagnosis made with regard to the aetiology of the stroke. Thus, based on an assumption that about 27% of juvenile strokes are of unknown aetiology, the authors estimated a prevalence of 1.2% for Fabry disease among all young patients with stroke.

Other patient populations that might harbour individuals with unknown Fabry disease include those who have multiple sclerosis or who present with chronic pain, rheumatic diseases or fever of unknown origin.

Conclusions

Diagnosis of Fabry disease is often delayed due to the rarity and variable nature of the disorder. This variability is reflected in the wide range of specialist physicians who diagnose the condition. Screening programmes and case-finding efforts may allow earlier diagnosis and hence earlier provision of effective enzyme replacement therapy.

References

1. Grunfeld JP. How to improve the early diagnosis of Fabry's disease? *Kidney Int* 2003;64:1136–7

2. Bodamer OA, Ratschmann R, Paschke E, Voigtländer T, Stöckler-Ipsiroglu S. Recurrent acroparaesthesia during febrile infections. *Lancet* 2004;363:1698

3. Meikle PJ, Hopwood JJ, Clague AE, Carey WF. Prevalence of lysosomal storage disorders. *JAMA* 1999;281:249–54

4. Grimes DA, Schulz KF. Uses and abuses of screening tests. *Lancet* 2002;359:881–4

5. Wilson J, Jungner F. Principles and practice of screening for disease. Public Health Papers, no. 34. Geneva: World Health Organization; 1968

6. Acharya K, Ackerman PD, Ross LF. Pediatricians' attitudes toward expanding newborn screening. *Pediatrics* 2005;116:e476–84

7. American College of Medical Genetics. Towards a uniform screening panel and system. Final report, 8 March 2005. http://mchb.hrsa.gov/screening

8. Newborn screening grows up. *Nat Med* 2005;11:1013

9. Mandavilli A. Screen savers. *Nat Med* 2005;11:1020–1

10. Eng CM, Guffon N, Wilcox WR, Germain DP, Lee P, Waldek S et al. Safety and efficacy of recombinant human α-galactosidase A replacement therapy in Fabry's disease. *N Engl J Med* 2001;345:9–16

11. Schiffmann R, Kopp JB, Austin HA, 3rd, Sabnis S, Moore DF, Weibel T et al. Enzyme replacement therapy in Fabry disease: a randomized controlled trial. *JAMA* 2001;285:2743–9

12. Chamoles NA, Blanco M, Gaggioli D. Fabry disease: enzymatic diagnosis in dried blood spots on filter paper. *Clin Chim Acta* 2001;308:195–6

13. Poeppl AG, Murray GJ, Medin JA. Enhanced filter paper enzyme assay for high-throughput population screening for Fabry disease. *Anal Biochem* 2005;337:161–3

14. Spada M, Pagliardini S. Screening for Fabry disease in end-stage nephropathies. *J Inherit Metab Dis* 2002;25 (Suppl. 1):113

15. Linthorst GE, Vedder AC, Aerts JM, Hollak CE. Screening for Fabry disease using whole blood spots fails to identify one-third of female carriers. *Clin Chim Acta* 2005;353:201–3

16. Fuller M, Lovejoy M, Brooks DA, Harkin ML, Hopwood JJ, Meikle PJ. Immunoquantification of α-galactosidase: evaluation for the diagnosis of Fabry disease. *Clin Chem* 2004;50:1979–85

17. Meikle PJ, Ranieri E, Simonsen H, Rozaklis T, Ramsay SL, Whitfield PD et al. Newborn screening for lysosomal storage disorders: clinical evaluation of a two-tier strategy. *Pediatrics* 2004;114:909–16

18. Li Y, Scott CR, Chamoles NA, Ghavami A, Pinto BM, Turecek F et al. Direct multiplex assay of lysosomal enzymes in dried blood spots for newborn screening. *Clin Chem* 2004;50:1785–96

19. Poorthuis BJ, Wevers RA, Kleijer WJ, Groener JE, de Jong JG, van Weely S et al. The frequency of lysosomal storage diseases in The Netherlands. *Hum Genet* 1999;105:151–6

20. Thadhani R, Wolf M, West ML, Tonelli M, Ruthazer R, Pastores GM et al. Patients with Fabry disease on dialysis in the United States. *Kidney Int* 2002;61:249–55

21. Tsakiris D, Simpson HK, Jones EH, Briggs JD, Elinder CG, Mendel S et al. Report on management of renal failure in Europe, XXVI, 1995. Rare diseases in renal replacement therapy in the ERA-EDTA Registry. *Nephrol Dial Transplant* 1996;11 (Suppl 7):4–20

22. Utsumi K, Kase R, Takata T, Sakuraba H, Matsui N, Saito H. Fabry disease in patients receiving maintenance dialysis. *Clin Exp Nephrol* 2000;4:49–51

23. Desnick R. Fabry disease: unrecognized ESRD patients and effectiveness of enzyme replacement on renal pathology and function. *J Inherit Metab Dis* 2002;25 (Suppl 1):116

24. Linthorst GE, Hollak CE, Korevaar JC, Van Manen JG, Aerts JM, Boeschoten EW. α-Galactosidase A deficiency in Dutch patients on dialysis: a critical appraisal of screening for Fabry disease. *Nephrol Dial Transplant* 2003;18:1581–4

25. Nakao S, Kodama C, Takenaka T, Tanaka A, Yasumoto Y, Yoshida A et al. Fabry disease: detection of undiagnosed hemodialysis patients and identification of a "renal variant" phenotype. *Kidney Int* 2003;64:801–7

26. Kotanko P, Kramar R, Devrnja D, Paschke E, Voigtländer T, Auinger M et al. Results of a nationwide screening for Anderson–Fabry disease among dialysis patients. *J Am Soc Nephrol* 2004;15:1323–9

27. Ichinose M, Nakayama M, Ohashi T, Utsunomiya Y, Kobayashi M, Eto Y. Significance of screening for Fabry disease among male dialysis patients. *Clin Exp Nephrol* 2005;9:228–32

28. Bekri S, Enica A, Ghafari T, Plaza G, Champenois I, Choukroun G et al. Fabry disease in patients with end-stage renal failure: the potential benefits of screening. *Nephron Clin Pract* 2005;101:c33–8

29. Tanaka M, Ohashi T, Kobayashi M, Eto Y, Miyamura N, Nishida K et al. Identification of Fabry's disease by the screening of α-galactosidase A activity in male and female hemodialysis patients. *Clin Nephrol* 2005;64:281–7

30. Sachdev B, Takenaka T, Teraguchi H, Tei C, Lee P, McKenna WJ et al. Prevalence of Anderson–Fabry disease in male patients with late onset hypertrophic cardiomyopathy. *Circulation* 2002;105:1407–11

31. Chimenti C, Pieroni M, Morgante E, Antuzzi D, Russo A, Russo MA et al. Prevalence of Fabry disease in female patients with late-onset hypertrophic cardiomyopathy. *Circulation* 2004;110:1047–53

32. Nakao S, Takenaka T, Maeda M, Kodama C, Tanaka A, Tahara M et al. An atypical variant of Fabry's disease in men with left ventricular hypertrophy. *N Engl J Med* 1995;333:288–93

33. Rolfs A, Böttcher T, Zschiesche M, Morris P, Winchester B, Bauer P et al. Prevalence of Fabry disease in patients with cryptogenic stroke: a prospective study. *Lancet* 2005;366:1794–6

18 Biochemical and genetic diagnosis of Fabry disease

Bryan Winchester and Elisabeth Young

Biochemistry, Endocrinology and Metabolism Unit, UCL Institute of Child Health,
Great Ormond Street Hospital, University College London, London, WC1N 1EH, UK

Fabry disease can be diagnosed in affected males by demonstrating a deficiency of α-galactosidase A in plasma and leukocytes. However, the enzymatic assay is unreliable for the detection of carriers, who can be detected reliably only by mutational analysis. All classic hemizygotes and over 90% of heterozygotes have an elevated level of urinary globotriaosylceramide (Gb_3). For male patients with lower than normal α-galactosidase activity or with an atypical clinical presentation, measurement of urinary Gb_3 and sequencing of the whole GLA gene must be carried out.

Biochemistry and structure of α-galactosidase A

A deficiency of α-galactosidase (ceramide-trihexosidase) was first shown to be the enzymatic defect in Fabry disease in 1967 by Brady and colleagues using radiolabelled globotriaosylceramide (Gb_3) as the substrate [1]. Subsequently, Kint [2] demonstrated that the α-galactosidase could act on the synthetic substrates p-nitrophenyl–α-D-galactoside and 4-methylumbelliferyl–α-D-galactoside and was specific for the α-anomeric galactosidic linkage. The introduction of synthetic substrates facilitated the assay of α-galactosidase activity for the diagnosis of Fabry disease [3] and the characterization and purification of the enzyme [4]. Investigation of α-galactosidase activity in normal individuals and residual activity in patients with Fabry disease revealed that there were two α-galactosidase isoenzymes, A and B, with activity towards the synthetic substrates [5]. α-Galactosidase A, which is thermolabile, accounts for most of the activity in normal tissues and is deficient in patients with Fabry disease. In contrast, α-galactosidase B, which is heat stable, accounts for the residual activity in patients

with Fabry disease, indicating that the two activities are genetically distinct. The purified enzymes have many similar physicochemical properties, but can be separated on the basis of charge. Antibodies raised against one do not cross-react with the other, supporting their genetic difference [4]. In fact, α-galactosidase B is an α-N-acetylgalactosaminidase that acts on natural substrates with terminal α-N-acetylgalactosaminyl residues [6, 7] and is defective in Schindler disease [8]. α-Galactosidase A does not catalyse the hydrolysis of the natural substrates of α-galactosidase B, whereas α-galactosidase B may act on some natural substrates with terminal α-galactosyl residues [9]. Therefore, as both enzymes act on synthetic α-galactoside substrates, a specific inhibitor of α-galactosidase B, α-N-acetylgalactosamine, is added to the assay mixture when measuring the α-galactosidase activity for diagnosing Fabry disease [10]. The genes encoding α-galactosidase A (*GLA*) and α-galactosidase B (*NAGA*) are localized on chromosomes Xq22.1 and 22q13, respectively, confirming that the two enzymes are genetically distinct. Cloning of the two genes suggested that they were evolutionarily related, with a predicted 46.9% identity of the amino acid sequence at the complementary DNA (cDNA) level and great similarity in the organization of a large section of the genes [11].

α-Galactosidase A is a glycoprotein and is synthesized as a precursor of 50 kDa, which is processed to a mature lysosomal form of 46 kDa following removal of a signal peptide during its transport to the lysosome via the mannose-6-phosphate (M6P) pathway [12]. The active enzyme is a homodimer that requires saposin B to act on its natural substrates in vivo [13]. As in Fabry disease, patients with a genetic deficiency of saposin B also accumulate the substrates for α-galactosidase A [14]. The predominant storage product in Fabry disease, and therefore the major natural substrate for α-galactosidase A, is Gb_3 [Gal($\alpha1\rightarrow4$)Gal($\beta1\rightarrow4$)Glc($\beta1\rightarrow1'$)Cer], also called CTH or GL-3. The hydrolysis of Gb_3 in vitro requires the addition of a detergent, usually sodium taurocholate. Another natural substrate is galabiosylceramide, [Gal($\alpha1\rightarrow4$) Gal($\beta1\rightarrow1'$)Cer] or Ga_2, which also accumulates in Fabry disease. Both of these neutral glycolipids consist of families of isoforms arising from heterogeneity in the fatty acid component of the ceramide [15]. Two other glycolipid substrates, which can accumulate in Fabry disease depending on the blood group and secretor status of the patient, are the blood group B and B1 glycosphingolipids, which have terminal α-galactosyl residues [9, 16]. α-Galactosidase A is a typical lysosomal acid hydrolase with an optimal activity towards natural and synthetic substrates at pH 3.8–4.6 [17]. The Michaelis constant (K_m) values for synthetic substrates are approximately one order of magnitude higher than for natural substrates.

Cloning of the GLA gene has permitted the production of recombinant human α-galactosidase A for enzyme replacement therapy (ERT) in Fabry disease [18, 19] and for structural analysis of the enzyme. Currently, two preparations are available, one of which (agalsidase alfa; Replagal®, TKT Europe AB) is produced in a continuous human cell line and the other (agalsidase beta; Fabrazyme®, Genzyme Corp.) in Chinese hamster ovary cells. Both proteins have the same amino acid sequence [20] but differ in their N-linked glycosylation because they are produced in different cell lines [21]. Three out of the four potential N-glycosylation sites are occupied in both preparations [22] but agalsidase beta has higher levels of sialic acid and M6P on its N-linked glycans than agalsidase alfa [21]. The rate of uptake of both preparations into fibroblasts via the M6P receptor is very similar and leads to the dispersal of accumulated Gb_3 [20]. The distribution of the two enzymes in knockout Fabry mice was comparable after intravenous administration. The enzymes have similar kinetics towards synthetic substrates [21] and show complete cross-reactivity [23].

The three-dimensional structure of recombinant human α-galactosidase A (agalsidase alfa) has been determined by X-ray crystallography at a resolution of 3.25 Å (Figure 1) [24]. It is a homodimeric molecule, with each monomer made up of two domains, one containing the active site and the other a β-sandwich of anti-parallel β-strands at the C-terminal. Co-crystallization with the product, galactose, revealed multiple interactions between the monosaccharide and parts of the first domain, confirming the location of the active site and suggesting that two aspartic acid residues could act as a nucleophile and acid/base in the catalytic mechanism. The distance between the two active sites is approximately 50 Å in both the free and liganded enzymes, suggesting that there is no cooperation between the sites. Comparison of the three-dimensional structures of α-galactosidase A and α-galactosidase B (α-N-acetylgalactosaminidase) confirms the structural similarity between the two enzymes [24, 25]. The absence of an 'N-acetyl recognition loop' in α-galactosidase A offers an explanation for the difference in substrate

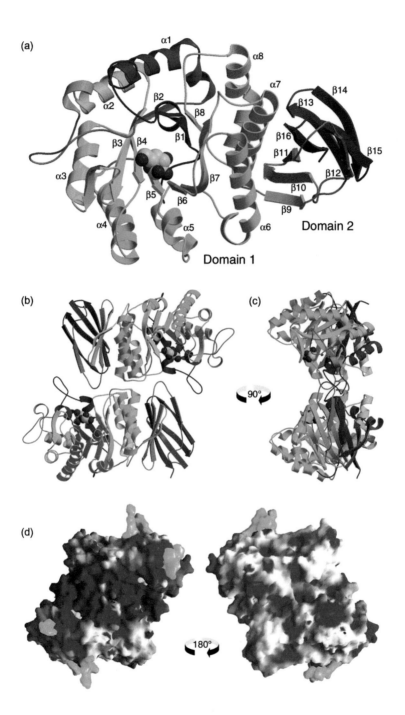

Figure 1. *The three-dimensional structure of recombinant human α-galactosidase. (a) Monomer showing two domains with an N-terminal (blue) and C-terminal (red). Galactose, with red and yellow atoms, is shown in the active site. β, beta strands; α, alpha helix. (b and c) Two views of the dimer. (d) Filled view of the model showing N-linked glycans in green. Degree of rotation of molecules is indicated. Reproduced with permission from [24].*

specificity. The X-ray crystal structures of free human α-galactosidase expressed in yeast and as a complex with an inhibitor, N-(N-benzyloxycarbonyl-6-aminohexyl)-α-D-galactopyranoside, have also been reported [26]. The three-dimensional structures have been used to understand the effects of mutations on the function of the enzyme (see Chapters 33 and 34).

Practical aspects of enzyme determination

α-Galactosidase A activity can easily be measured in plasma and leukocytes using the synthetic substrate 4-methylumbelliferyl-α-D-galactopyranoside [2, 3]. The effects of pH, temperature, inhibitors, anticoagulants and erythrocyte contamination on the activity of α-galactosidase A in plasma, serum, urine and

leukocytes have been investigated [3]. These findings were taken into account in the development of assays and establishment of reference ranges for α-galactosidase A in plasma and leukocytes, which have been used in our laboratory for over 30 years [27, 28] (Figures 2 and 3). Classically affected hemizygotes have very low or undetectable enzyme activity but some hemizygotes, for example those with the N215S mutation, may have higher residual activity in plasma and/or leukocytes. It is therefore important to confirm the mutation in these individuals. The α-galactosidase A activity in affected females can range from the low level found in affected males to well into the normal range, possibly due to skewed X-inactivation. Therefore, heterozygotes cannot be reliably defined by enzymatic analysis.

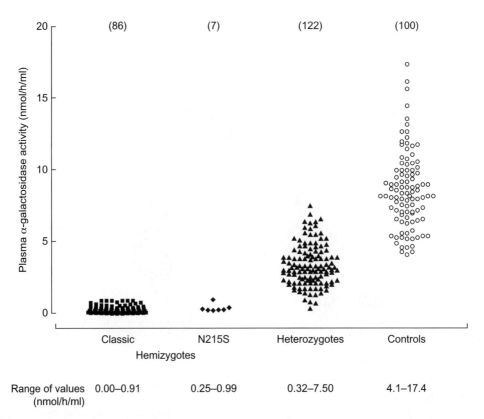

Figure 2. *Levels of plasma α-galactosidase in male hemizygotes with classic Fabry disease and with the N215S mutation, in female heterozygotes and in healthy control individuals. Numbers of subjects are given in parentheses.*

Pitfalls in plasma assays

As 100 μl of plasma/serum are used in the assay, a relatively strong acetate buffer is needed to maintain the incubation pH of 4.8. It is essential to add the inhibitor *N*-acetyl-galactosamine (final concentration, 100 mmol/l) to inhibit the α-*N*-acetylgalactosaminidase [10], which can account for up to 20% of the α-galactosidase activity in plasma. Pre-incubation of plasma at 37°C for 2 hours before the assay, decreased the α-galactosidase activity by approximately 80% [3]. In contrast, the activity was essentially unchanged when plasma was preheated at 25°C. To minimize the effect of denaturation and to ensure measurable hydrolysis of the substrate, assays are therefore performed at 30°C. Although there is no significant difference between the activity

in serum or plasma collected in tubes with ethylenediamine tetraacetic acid, heparin or acid-citrate-dextrose as anticoagulants, substances released from erythrocytes, for example haemoglobin, can significantly reduce fluorescence. This is corrected for by having a separate standard, standard blank and substrate blank for each sample assayed. The blank readings may vary considerably from sample to sample. The results from lipaemic plasma may be suspect because, depending on the severity of lipaemia, the solution may not clear after addition of the stopping reagent and this can affect the fluorescence. As with all diagnostic samples, another enzyme (e.g. β-hexosaminidase) should be assayed in the plasma/serum sample to ensure the viability of the sample.

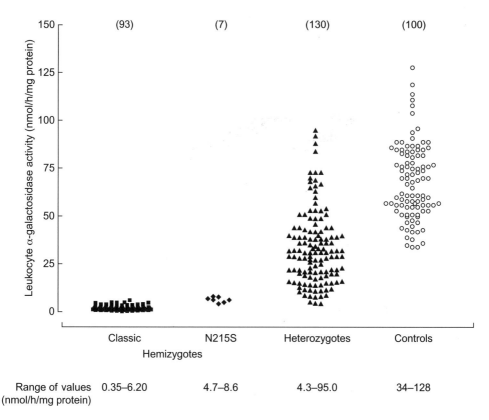

| Range of values (nmol/h/mg protein) | 0.35–6.20 | 4.7–8.6 | 4.3–95.0 | 34–128 |

Figure 3. *Levels of leukocyte α-galactosidase in male hemizygotes with classic Fabry disease and with the N215S mutation, in female heterozygotes and in healthy control individuals. Numbers of subjects are given in parentheses.*

Pitfalls in leukocyte assays

There are fewer pitfalls in the leukocyte assay than in the plasma assay. To solubilize the activity fully, leukocytes are homogenized in 0.5% sodium cholate [28], or frozen and thawed ten times [3], and the supernatant is used in the enzyme assays. The α-galactosaminidase activity accounts for only 5–10% of the total α-galactosidase activity in leukocytes, so the addition of N-acetylgalactosamine to the assay is not as important as in the plasma assay. However, it is recommended that it is included. As with plasma, haemoglobin contamination can quench the fluorescence but, again, this is usually not a problem, as contaminated erythrocytes can be removed by a haemolysis step in the leukocyte preparation. Another enzyme (e.g. β-galactosidase) should be assayed in the same extract to ensure the viability of the sample.

Male patients with residual α-galactosidase activity

There have been many reports of men with decreased but not absent α-galactosidase activity, who do not show the classic clinical phenotype of Fabry disease. Some of these patients have clinical variants, with the initial presenting symptoms restricted to a particular organ, for example the heart or kidneys, and such variants are often associated with particular mutations [5]. It is important to note that many of these mutations have also been found in patients with the classic phenotype, indicating that other factors affect the phenotype. The coding sequence variant, D313Y, which has approximately 60% of wild-type activity *in vitro* and decreased activity at neutral pH, leading to low plasma α-galactosidase activity, is not disease causing [29, 30]. It has an incidence of 0.45% in normal X chromosomes and has been found in combination with several disease causing missense mutations. The discovery of this pseudodeficiency allele emphasizes the need to sequence the GLA gene completely in the index case of newly diagnosed families with Fabry disease and to express novel missense mutations. Patients with an atypical clinical presentation and residual α-galactosidase activity should be investigated thoroughly before making a definitive diagnosis. This should include characterization of the residual α-galactosidase activity, measurement of urinary Gb_3 and sequencing of the whole GLA gene.

Prenatal diagnosis

Measurement of α-galactosidase A activity in cultured amniotic cells [31] and directly in chorionic villi [32] has been used for the prenatal diagnosis of Fabry disease. More recently, karyotype analysis followed by enzyme analysis and/or mutational analysis of a male fetus has become the usual procedure. With the advent of ERT, however, there are now very few requests for prenatal diagnosis of Fabry disease.

The availability of ERT has emphasized the importance of early diagnosis of Fabry disease after birth, even in newborns. Deficiency of α-galactosidase can be demonstrated in activity eluted from a dried blood spot collected on filter paper [33] (see Chapter 17).

Measurement of storage products

The accumulation of the major storage product, Gb_3, in various tissues is the hallmark of Fabry disease. Many methods have therefore been developed to detect and measure Gb_3, including thin-layer chromatography [34], gas-liquid chromatography [35], high-performance liquid chromatography [36] and an enzyme-linked immunosorbent assay using the verotoxin B subunit [37]. Glycosphingolipids can be detected and readily identified by various forms of mass spectrometry [38–41]. Initially, derivatization was necessary to prevent decomposition and is still used to achieve sensitivity. The advent of softer ionization methods and tandem mass spectrometry has permitted the analysis of small amounts of non-derivatized neutral and acidic glycosphingolipids, including detection of the isoforms due to heterogeneity in the sphingosine and fatty acid components. However, until recently, quantitative determination was handicapped by the lack of suitable internal standards. The synthesis of the novel internal standards C-17-Gb$_3$ [42], [d$_4$]C16- and [d$_{47}$]C24- isoforms of Gb$_3$ and Ga$_2$ [43] and [d$_{35}$]C18- Gb$_3$ [44] has overcome this problem. These standards and the development of simpler extraction and on-line purification procedures have permitted the rapid, automated and quantitative determination of non-derivatized Gb$_3$ in plasma and urine by liquid chromatography in conjunction with electrospray ionization tandem mass spectrometry [42, 44, 45]. Sonication of whole urine [46] or dilution of whole urine [45] was found to give reliable results without the need to separate the sediment and supernatant. The concentration of total Gb$_3$ is obtained by summating the concentrations of the individual isoforms of Gb$_3$ detected by using the mass spectrometer in the multiple-reaction monitoring mode [15, 42, 44–48]. This methodology has been used to establish reference ranges for total Gb$_3$ in plasma and urine from Fabry hemizygotes, heterozygotes and normal controls [15, 46, 47] (Table 1 and Figures 4 and 5).

Total Gb$_3$ was elevated in the plasma of 44 out of 48 classic hemizygotes studied, but not in some mildly affected male patients and those with the N215S mutation. Eight out of nine boys (ages ranging from 6 to 17 years) had elevated levels of Gb$_3$. Only 42% of female heterozygotes and only one of four N215S heterozygotes had elevated plasma levels of Gb$_3$. In contrast, all of the classic male hemizygotes and three of the seven patients with the N215S mutation had elevated urinary Gb$_3$ levels. The proportion of heterozygotes with elevated urinary Gb$_3$ was 95%, and all but one of the heterozygotes with a normal level of urinary Gb$_3$ were symptomatic. The urinary Gb$_3$ level was within the normal range for the N215S heterozygotes. Thus, urinary Gb$_3$ is a better marker of Fabry disease than plasma Gb$_3$, but does not detect some heterozygotes [47, 48]. Measurement of urinary and plasma Gb$_3$ by tandem mass spectrometry has been used to monitor ERT [45–50].

Attempts have been made to identify heterozygotes by obtaining a urinary lipid profile by tandem mass spectrometry [51] but this did not detect all female heterozygotes. Fingerprints of urinary sediment glycosphingolipids obtained using matrix-assisted laser desorption ionization time-of-flight mass spectrometry [52] indicated that there are significant differences in the composition of the glycosphingolipids amongst young, adult and atypical hemizygous and heterozygous patients. It is possible that these changes could be used to assess the severity, progress and pathophysiology of Fabry disease.

Table 1. *Proportion of hemizygous male and heterozygous female patients with Fabry disease (with or without the N215S mutation) with elevated levels of globotriaosylceramide (Gb$_3$) in plasma and urine.*

	Proportion of patients with raised Gb$_3$ levels			
	Hemizygotes	**N215S hemizygotes**	**Heterozygotes**	**N215S heterozygotes**
Plasma	44/48 (92%)	0/6 (0%)	27/64 (42%)	1/4 (25%)
Urine	41/41 (100%)	3/7 (43%)	78/82 (95%)	0/5 (0%)

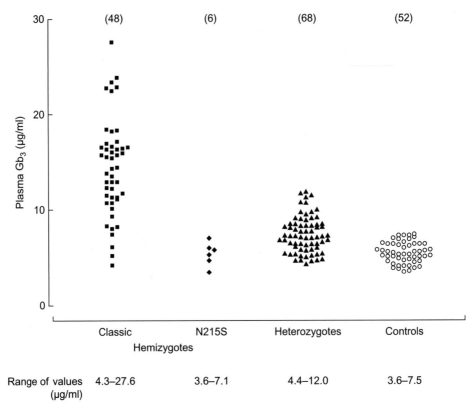

Figure 4. *Levels of plasma globotriaosylceramide (Gb₃) in male hemizygotes with classic Fabry disease and with the N215S mutation, in female heterozygotes and in healthy control individuals. Numbers of subjects are given in parentheses.*

Methods of genetic diagnosis

The *GLA* gene, which is located at Xq22.1, has been fully characterized [5, 53, 54]. It is 12 kilobases (kb) in length and contains seven exons, which have consensus intron/exon splicing sequences. There are several possible regulatory elements in the 5'-flanking region and an unmethylated CpG-rich island upstream of the initiation codon, which is characteristic of a housekeeping gene. The gene contains 12 Alu repetitive elements, about 20% of the gene. The mRNA (1.45 kb), which is unusual in lacking a 3'-untranslated sequence, encodes a protein of 429 amino acids, including the *N*-terminal signal peptide of 31 amino acids. Another unusual feature is the presence of three polymorphisms with a combined frequency of 10% in the 60 base pair

untranslated sequence before the initiation codon in the first exon [55]. One of these, -30G>A, which is found in 0.5% of normal individuals, gives rise to elevated plasma α-galactosidase activity [56]. In contrast, the pseudodeficiency allele (D313Y) lowers plasma α-galactosidase activity [29, 30].

Mutations in the *GLA* gene have been identified using a variety of strategies. Large gene rearrangements, which account for only 3–4% of the mutations, can be detected by Southern blot hybridization using full-length cDNA as the probe [57] or by multiplex polymerase chain reaction (PCR) of the gene in four fragments [58]. The sizes of the seven exons, 92–291 base pairs in length, lend themselves to amplification by PCR and detection of sequence changes by mutation

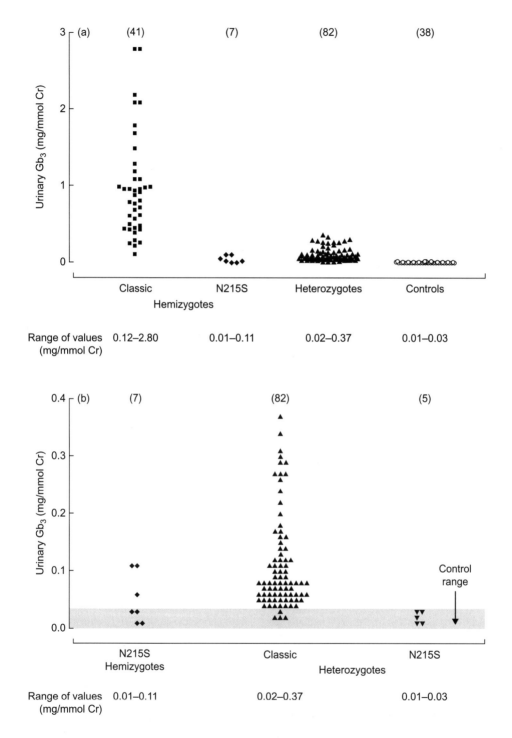

Figure 5. *Levels of urinary globotriaosylceramide (Gb₃) in (a) male hemizygotes with classic Fabry disease and with the N215S mutation, in female heterozygotes and in healthy control individuals, and (b) N215S hemizygotes, classic heterozygotes and N215S heterozygotes. The range of the control data is represented by the shaded bar. Numbers of subjects are given in parentheses. Cr, creatinine.*

screening methods. Single base changes and small deletions and insertions can be detected by single-strand conformation polymorphism analysis [55], chemical cleavage of mismatches with fluorescent detection [59] or denaturing high-performance liquid chromatography (DHPLC) [60], followed by sequencing of exons to identify the precise mutation. Direct sequencing of the entire coding sequence and flanking regions in both directions has also been used to identify mutations [61]. Mutations in the conserved 5'-splice donor sites and 3'-splice acceptor sites should be investigated further by northern blotting to define the effect on RNA processing.

Once the mutation in the index case has been identified, a specific test for the mutation is developed for investigation of family members. If the mutation alters an existing restriction enzyme site in the genomic DNA, the mutation can be detected by re-amplification of the DNA fragment and digestion with the enzyme. If the mutation does not alter a restriction site, a restriction site can be created using a primer containing an altered base (amplification-created restriction site) [62]. A specific mutation can also be rapidly detected by DHPLC analysis of the amplified fragment that contains the mutation and confirmed by sequencing [60]. Direct sequencing of the appropriate amplified fragment is a feasible strategy with the development of rapid and sensitive automated sequencers. Known single-point and small deletions can also be detected by a rapid, fluorophore probe-based technique that does not require gel electrophoresis [63]. Two probes with different fluorophores are designed to bind one base pair apart to a PCR product, with one probe covering the mutation. The proximity of the probes leads to fluorescence resonance energy transfer and emission of fluorescence of a specific wavelength. When such complexes are subjected to melting, the specific emission is lost and a melting curve can be recorded using a LightCycler

(Roche Diagnostics Corporation, USA). The mutant complex will hybridize less efficiently and melt at a lower temperature, enabling it to be detected even in heterozygotes.

Although the level of α-galactosidase activity in many female heterozygotes is lower than normal and the level of urinary Gb_3 is elevated, the only absolutely reliable method of carrier detection is identification of the family mutation in the GLA gene.

Types of mutations/ polymorphisms

To date, 363 different mutations have been reported in the GLA gene in the Human Gene Mutation Database (Cardiff, UK: http://www.hgmd.cf.ac.uk/ac/search/119272.html) that are believed to cause Fabry disease. Many have been shown by expression in vitro to abolish or markedly decrease α-galactosidase activity. Others are deduced to be disease causing because they are the only sequence change found in the patient's GLA gene and have not been found in normal controls. The Human Gene Mutation Database contains 245 missense and nonsense mutations, 18 RNA-processing defects, 22 small insertions 58 deletions, 4 indels (a deletion followed by an insertion), 10 gross deletions, 1 gross duplication and 5 complex mutations in which more than one mutational event appears to have occurred. Most are private mutations but some are recurrent, a few of which have been shown by haplotyping to occur in distantly related members of the same family. The majority of the recurrent mutations occur in CpG dinucleotides.

Conclusions

All males who are hemizygous for Fabry disease can be diagnosed by demonstrating a deficiency of α-galactosidase A activity in plasma and/or leukocytes. The mutation in the GLA gene should be determined. Female heterozygotes cannot be diagnosed reliably by enzymatic assay because of skewed inactivation of the X chromosome. Mutation analysis is necessary for the detection of female heterozygotes, and the affected families should be offered genetic counselling. Some individuals have α-galactosidase A activity below the normal reference range due to the presence of a pseudodeficiency allele. This can be confirmed by mutational analysis.

All classic hemizygotes have elevated levels of urinary Gb_3, whereas not all hemizygotes with variant forms of Fabry disease have elevated levels. Approximately 95% of female hetero-zygotes with classic disease have elevated levels of urinary Gb_3, whereas the proportion of heterozygotes with variant forms who have elevated Gb_3 levels is much lower. The pseudodeficiency allele does not cause elevation of urinary Gb_3. The levels of Gb_3 in plasma are not so informative, as only 92% and 42% of classic hemizygotes and hetero-zygotes, respectively, have elevated levels. Prenatal diagnosis of Fabry disease is possible by a combination of enzymatic assay and/or mutation analysis.

Acknowledgements

We acknowledge the collaboration of our colleagues in the Enzyme Diagnostic Laboratory at Great Ormond Street Hospital, London, and in the research laboratories of the Institute of Child Health, London, with whom we have worked for many years and without whom this chapter could not have been written.

References

1. Brady RO, Gal AE, Bradley RM, Martensson E, Warshaw AL, Laster L. Enzymatic defect in Fabry's disease. Ceramidetrihexosidase deficiency. *N Engl J Med* 1967;276:1163–7

2. Kint JA. Fabry's disease: α-galactosidase deficiency. *Science* 1970;167:1268–9

3. Desnick RJ, Allen KY, Desnick SJ, Raman MK, Bernlohr RW, Krivit W. Fabry's disease: enzymatic diagnosis of hemizygotes and heterozygotes. α-Galactosidase activities in plasma, serum, urine, and leukocytes. *J Lab Clin Med* 1973;81:157–71

4. Beutler E, Kuhl W. Purification and properties of human α-galactosidases. *J Biol Chem* 1972;247:7195–200

5. Desnick RJ, Ioannou YA, Eng CM. α-Galactosidase A deficiency: Fabry disease. In: Scriver CR, Beaudet AL, Sly WS, Valle D, editors. The metabolic and molecular bases of inherited disease. 8th edn. New York: McGraw-Hill; 2001. p. 3733–74

6. Dean KJ, Sung SS, Sweeley CC. The identification of α-galactosidase B from human liver as an α-N-acetylgalactosaminidase. *Biochem Biophys Res Commun* 1977;77:1411–17

7. Schram AW, Hamers MN, Tager JM. The identity of α-galactosidase B from human liver. *Biochim Biophys Acta* 1977;482:138–44

8. Desnick RJ, Schindler D. α-N-Acetylgalactosamin-idase deficiency: Schindler disease. In: Scriver CR, Beaudet AL, Sly WS, Valle D, editors. The metabolic and molecular bases of inherited disease. 8th edn. New York: McGraw-Hill; 2001. p. 3483–505

9. Asfaw B, Ledvinova J, Dobrovolny R, Bakker HD, Desnick RJ, van Diggelen OP et al. Defects in degradation of blood group A and B glycosphingo-lipids in Schindler and Fabry diseases. *J Lipid Res* 2002;43:1096–104

10. Mayes JS, Scheerer JB, Sifers RN, Donaldson ML. Differential assay for lysosomal α-galactosidases in human tissues and its application to Fabry's disease. *Clin Chim Acta* 1981;112:247–51

11. Wang AM, Desnick RJ. Structural organization and complete sequence of the human α-N-acetylgalactosaminidase gene: homology with the α-galactosidase A gene provides evidence for evolution from a common ancestral gene. *Genomics* 1991;10:133–42

12. Lemansky P, Bishop DF, Desnick RJ, Hasilik A, von Figura K. Synthesis and processing of α-galactosidase A in human fibroblasts. Evidence for different mutations in Fabry disease. *J Biol Chem* 1987;262:2062–5

13. Kase R, Bierfreund U, Klein A, Kolter T, Itoh K, Suzuki M et al. Only sphingolipid activator protein B (SAP-B or saposin B) stimulates the degradation of globotriaosylceramide by recombinant human lysosomal α-galactosidase in a detergent-free liposomal system. *FEBS Lett* 1996;393:74–6

14. Li SC, Kihara H, Serizawa S, Li YT, Fluharty AL, Mayes JS et al. Activator protein required for the enzymatic hydrolysis of cerebroside sulfate. Deficiency in urine of patients affected with cerebroside sulfatase activator deficiency and identity with activators for the enzymatic hydrolysis of GM1 ganglioside and globo-triaosylceramide. *J Biol Chem* 1985;260:1867–71

15. Mills K, Morris P, Lee P, Vellodi A, Waldek S, Young E et al. Measurement of urinary CDH and CTH by tandem mass spectrometry in patients hemizygous and heterozygous for Fabry disease. *J Inherit Metab Dis* 2005;28:35–48

16. Wherrett JR, Hakomori SI. Characterization of a blood group B glycolipid, accumulating in the pancreas of a patient with Fabry's disease. *J Biol Chem* 1973;248:3046–51

17. Dean KJ, Sweeley CC. Studies on human liver α-galactosidases. I. Purification of α-galactosidase A and its enzymatic properties with glycolipid and oligosaccharide substrates. *J Biol Chem* 1979; 254:9994–10000

18. Eng CM, Guffon N, Wilcox WR, Germain DP, Lee P, Waldek S et al. Safety and efficacy of recombinant human α-galactosidase A replacement therapy in Fabry's disease. N Engl J Med 2001;345:9–16

19. Schiffmann R, Kopp JB, Austin HA, 3rd, Sabnis S, Moore DF, Weibel T et al. Enzyme replacement therapy in Fabry disease: a randomized controlled trial. JAMA 2001;285:2743–9

20. Blom D, Speijer D, Linthorst GE, Donker-Koopman WG, Strijland A, Aerts JM. Recombinant enzyme therapy for Fabry disease: absence of editing of human α-galactosidase A mRNA. Am J Hum Genet 2003;72:23–31

21. Lee K, Jin X, Zhang K, Copertino L, Andrews L, Baker-Malcolm J et al. A biochemical and pharmacological comparison of enzyme replacement therapies for the glycolipid storage disorder Fabry disease. Glycobiology 2003;13:305–13

22. Ioannou YA, Zeidner KM, Grace ME, Desnick RJ. Human α-galactosidase A: glycosylation site 3 is essential for enzyme solubility. Biochem J 1998; 332 (Pt 3):789–97

23. Linthorst GE, Hollak CE, Donker-Koopman WE, Strijland A, Aerts JM. Enzyme therapy for Fabry disease: neutralizing antibodies toward agalsidase alpha and beta. Kidney Int 2004;66:1589–95

24. Garman SC, Garboczi DN. The molecular defect leading to Fabry disease: structure of human α-galactosidase. J Mol Biol 2004;337:319–35

25. Garman SC, Hannick L, Zhu A, Garboczi DN. The 1.9 Å structure of α-N-acetylgalactosaminidase: molecular basis of glycosidase deficiency diseases. Structure (Camb) 2002;10:425–34

26. Matsuzawa F, Aikawa SI, Doi H, Okumiya T, Sakuraba H. Fabry disease: correlation between structural changes in α-galactosidase, and clinical and biochemical phenotypes. Hum Genet 2005;117:317–28

27. Morgan SH, Rudge P, Smith SJ, Bronstein AM, Kendall BE, Holly E et al. The neurological complications of Anderson–Fabry disease (α-galactosidase A deficiency) – investigation of symptomatic and presymptomatic patients. Q J Med 1990;75:491–507

28. Donnai P, Donnai D, Harris R, Stephens R, Young E, Campbell S. Antenatal diagnosis of Niemann-Pick disease in a twin pregnancy. J Med Genet 1981; 18:359–61

29. Froissart R, Guffon N, Vanier MT, Desnick RJ, Maire I. Fabry disease: D313Y is an α-galactosidase A sequence variant that causes pseudodeficient activity in plasma. Mol Genet Metab 2003;80:307–14

30. Yasuda M, Shabbeer J, Benson SD, Maire I, Burnett RM, Desnick RJ. Fabry disease: characterization of α-galactosidase A double mutations and the D313Y plasma enzyme pseudodeficiency allele. Hum Mutat 2003;22:486–92

31. Brady RO, Uhlendorf BW, Jacobson CB. Fabry's disease: antenatal detection. Science 1971;172:174–5

32. Kleijer WJ, Hussaarts-Odijk LM, Sachs ES, Jahoda MG, Niermeijer MF. Prenatal diagnosis of Fabry's disease by direct analysis of chorionic villi. Prenat Diagn 1987;7:283–7

33. Chamoles NA, Blanco M, Gaggioli D. Fabry disease: enzymatic diagnosis in dried blood spots on filter paper. Clin Chim Acta 2001;308:195–6

34. Berna L, Asfaw B, Conzelmann E, Cerny B, Ledvinova J. Determination of urinary sulfatides and other lipids by combination of reversed-phase and thin-layer chromatographies. Anal Biochem 1999;269:304–11

35. Vance DE, Sweeley CC. Quantitative determination of the neutral glycosyl ceramides in human blood. J Lipid Res 1967;8:621–30

36. McCluer RH, Ullman MD, Jungalwala FB. High-performance liquid chromatography of membrane lipids: glycosphingolipids and phospholipids. Methods Enzymol 1989;172:538–75

37. Zeidner KM, Desnick RJ, Ioannou YA. Immuno-detection of glycolipid-bound recombinant verotoxin B subunit. Anal Biochem 1999;267:104–13

38. Sweeley CC, Dawson G. Determination of glyco-sphingolipid structures by mass spectrometry. Biochem Biophys Res Commun 1969;37:6–14

39. Hemling ME, Yu RK, Sedgwick RD, Rinehart KL, Jr. Fast atom bombardment mass spectrometry of glycosphingolipids. Glycosphingolipids containing neutral sugars. Biochemistry 1984;23:5706–13

40. Domon B, Costello CE. Structure elucidation of glycosphingolipids and gangliosides using high-performance tandem mass spectrometry. Biochemistry 1988;27:1534–43

41. Reinhold BB, Chan S-Y, Chan S, Reinhold VN. Profiling glycosphingolipid structural detail periodate-oxidation, electrospray, collision-induced dissociation and tandem mass-spectrometry. Organic Mass Spectrom 1994;29:736–46

42. Mills K, Johnson A, Winchester B. Synthesis of novel internal standards for the quantitative determination of plasma ceramide trihexoside in Fabry disease by tandem mass spectrometry. FEBS Lett 2002; 515:171–6

43. Mills K, Eaton S, Ledger V, Young E, Winchester B. The synthesis of internal standards for the quantitative determination of sphingolipids by tandem mass spectrometry. Rapid Commun Mass Spectrom 2005;19:1739–48

44. Fauler G, Rechberger GN, Devrnja D, Erwa W, Plecko B, Kotanko P et al. Rapid determination of urinary globotriaosylceramide isoform profiles by electrospray ionization mass spectrometry using stearoyl-d35-globotriaosylceramide as internal standard. Rapid Commun Mass Spectrom 2005; 19:1499–506

45. Boscaro F, Pieraccini G, la Marca G, Bartolucci G, Luceri C, Luceri F et al. Rapid quantitation of globotriaosylceramide in human plasma and urine: a potential application for monitoring enzyme replacement therapy in Anderson–Fabry disease. Rapid Commun Mass Spectrom 2002;16:1507–14

46. Mills K, Vellodi A, Morris P, Cooper D, Morris M, Young E et al. Monitoring the clinical and biochemical response to enzyme replacement therapy in three children with Fabry disease. Eur J Pediatr 2004;163:595–603

47. Young E, Mills K, Morris P, Vellodi A, Lee P, Waldek S et al. Is globotriaosylceramide a useful biomarker in Fabry disease? *Acta Paediatr Suppl* 2005;447:51–4

48. Kitagawa T, Ishige N, Suzuki K, Owada M, Ohashi T, Kobayashi M et al. Non-invasive screening method for Fabry disease by measuring globotriaosylceramide in whole urine samples using tandem mass spectrometry. *Mol Genet Metab* 2005;85: 196–202

49. Whitfield PD, Calvin J, Hogg S, O'Driscoll E, Halsall D, Burling K et al. Monitoring enzyme replacement therapy in Fabry disease – role of urine globotriaosylceramide. *J Inherit Metab Dis* 2005;28:21–33

50. Roddy TP, Nelson BC, Sung CC, Araghi S, Wilkens D, Zhang XK et al. Liquid chromatography-tandem mass spectrometry quantification of globotriaosylceramide in plasma for long-term monitoring of Fabry patients treated with enzyme replacement therapy. *Clin Chem* 2005;51:237–40

51. Fuller M, Sharp PC, Rozaklis T, Whitfield PD, Blacklock D, Hopwood JJ et al. Urinary lipid profiling for the identification of Fabry hemizygotes and heterozygotes. *Clin Chem* 2005;51:688–94

52. Touboul D, Roy S, Germain DP, Baillet A, Brion F, Prognon P et al. Fast fingerprinting by MALDI-TOF mass spectrometry of urinary sediment glycosphingolipids in Fabry disease. *Anal Bioanal Chem* 2005;382:1209–16

53. Bishop DF, Calhoun DH, Bernstein HS, Hantzopoulos P, Quinn M, Desnick RJ. Human α-galactosidase A: nucleotide sequence of a cDNA clone encoding the mature enzyme. *Proc Natl Acad Sci USA* 1986; 83:4859–63

54. Kornreich R, Desnick RJ, Bishop DF. Nucleotide sequence of the human α-galactosidase A gene. *Nucleic Acids Res* 1989;17:3301–2

55. Davies JP, Winchester BG, Malcolm S. Sequence variations in the first exon of α-galactosidase A. *J Med Genet* 1993;30:658–63

56. Fitzmaurice TF, Desnick RJ, Bishop DF. Human α-galactosidase A: high plasma activity expressed by the -30G>A allele. *J Inherit Metab Dis* 1997; 20:643–57

57. Bernstein HS, Bishop DF, Astrin KH, Kornreich R, Eng CM, Sakuraba H et al. Fabry disease: six gene rearrangements and an exonic point mutation in the α-galactosidase gene. *J Clin Invest* 1989;83:1390–9

58. Kornreich R, Desnick RJ. Fabry disease: detection of gene rearrangements in the human α-galactosidase A gene by multiplex PCR amplification. *Hum Mutat* 1993;2:108–11

59. Germain D, Biasotto M, Tosi M, Meo T, Kahn A, Poenaru L. Fluorescence-assisted mismatch analysis (FAMA) for exhaustive screening of the α-galactosidase A gene and detection of carriers in Fabry disease. *Hum Genet* 1996;98:719–26

60. Shabbeer J, Robinson M, Desnick RJ. Detection of α-galactosidase a mutations causing Fabry disease by denaturing high performance liquid chromatography. *Hum Mutat* 2005;25:299–305

61. Eng CM, Resnick-Silverman LA, Niehaus DJ, Astrin KH, Desnick RJ. Nature and frequency of mutations in the α-galactosidase A gene that cause Fabry disease. *Am J Hum Genet* 1993;53:1186–97

62. Blaydon D, Hill J, Winchester B. Fabry disease: 20 novel GLA mutations in 35 families. *Hum Mutat* 2001;18:459

63. Aoshima T, Sekido Y, Miyazaki T, Kajita M, Mimura S, Watanabe K et al. Rapid detection of deletion mutations in inherited metabolic diseases by melting curve analysis with LightCycler. *Clin Chem* 2000; 46:119–22

19 Natural history of Fabry disease

Atul Mehta[1] and Urs Widmer[2]

[1]Lysosomal Storage Disorders Unit, Department of Academic Haematology, Royal Free and University College Medical School, Rowland Hill Street, London NW3 2PF, UK; [2]Department of Internal Medicine, University Hospital Zurich, CH-8091 Zurich, Switzerland

Fabry disease is an X-linked condition that affects both men and women. The manifestations of this complex disease are progressive and multisystemic. The classic form is seen in both males and females, although the manifestations are often less severe in females and disease progression is generally delayed compared with males. This chapter describes the natural history of the classic form of the disease, as well as the different signs and symptoms in females, and atypical late-onset disease in males.

Classic Fabry disease

Although clinically heterogeneous, classic Fabry disease is usually a slowly progressive disease in which signs and symptoms change as the patient ages [1]. The clinical manifestations usually first become apparent in childhood or adolescence (Table 1). Lifespan is typically reduced in both males and females, and the main causes of death are renal failure, heart disease or stroke [2, 3].

Pain

Neuropathic pain typically appears during childhood [4, 5], and has been reported to affect 77% of men and 70% of women in adulthood [2, 3]. Data from FOS – the Fabry Outcome Survey – show that 64% of males and 83% of females experience neuropathic pain (defined as chronic pain, pain attacks, abdominal pain or joint pain). Pain may be chronic or experienced as episodic Fabry

Table 1. *Disease progression in patients with Fabry disease.*

Childhood and adolescence (≤ 16 years)	Early adulthood (17–30 years)
Acroparaesthesiae	More extensive angiokeratomas
Pain and Fabry disease crises	Proteinuria, lipiduria, haematuria
Angiokeratomas	Oedema
Raynaud phenomenon	Fever
Ophthalmological abnormalities, especially	Dyshidrosis (hypohidrosis, anhidrosis
cornea verticillata	and hyperhidrosis)
Hearing impairment	Lymphoedema
Dyshidrosis (hypohidrosis, anhidrosis	Heat sensitivity
and hyperhidrosis)	Diarrhoea, abdominal pain
History of non-specific bowel disturbances	**Later adulthood (> 30 years)**
History of lethargy and tiredness	Heart disease
	Impaired renal function
	Stroke or transient ischaemic attacks

Table 2. *Frequency and age at onset of specific signs and symptoms of Fabry disease in male (n = 318) and female (n = 337) patients enrolled in FOS – the Fabry Outcome Survey.*

	Frequency		Age at symptom onset (years)	
	Proportion of population (%)	Number of patients	Mean ± SD	Number of patients
Males				
Pain attacks	72	228	13 ± 12	165
Angiokeratomas	69	218	19 ± 14	130
Hypohidrosis	54	171	22 ± 16	105
Abdominal pain	40	128	23 ± 15	94
Diarrhoea	37	119	25 ± 17	79
Depression	24	76	32 ± 15	54
Proteinuria	48	154	33 ± 12	108
Hypertension	26	83	36 ± 13	53
Renal failure	20	64	36 ± 11	51
Left ventricular hypertrophy	43	136	39 ± 10	82
Stroke	9	28	39 ± 12	24
Angina	10	31	42 ± 5	22
Females				
Pain attacks	52	174	19 ± 17	123
Angiokeratomas	36	122	30 ± 17	73
Hypohidrosis	25	84	25 ± 21	56
Abdominal pain	30	102	24 ± 20	73
Diarrhoea	20	66	22 ± 17	46
Depression	21	72	37 ± 16	54
Proteinuria	34	113	39 ± 17	81
Hypertension	18	60	46 ± 15	32
Renal failure	3	9	44 ± 16	8
Left ventricular hypertrophy	26	86	50 ± 11	50
Stroke	6	21	52 ± 14	18
Angina	11	37	49 ± 13	19

'crises' or acroparaesthesiae. In FOS, pain attacks are reported by 72% of males and 52% of females (67% of boys; 45% of girls) (Table 2). Patients describe the pain as an excruciating burning sensation in the palms of the hands and soles of the feet, often radiating to the proximal extremities and occasionally to the abdomen. Pain may occur spontaneously but is exacerbated by temperature changes, fever, stress, physical exercise and alcohol [2].

Appearance

Hemizygous males often have a characteristic facial appearance – with prominent supra-orbital ridges, frontal bossing and thickening of the lips – which is recognizable from approximately 12–14 years of age [2] (Figure 1).

Angiokeratomas

Angiokeratomas are small, raised, dark red spots; they may be absent in patients with atypical Fabry disease [6]. Lesions typically

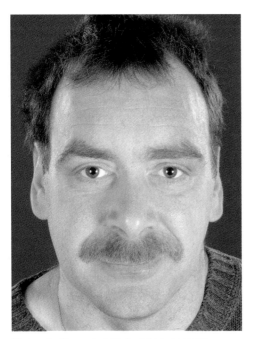

Figure 1. *Characteristic facial appearance.*

develop slowly and are predominantly found in the 'bathing trunk' area (genitalia, scrotum, buttocks and inner thighs), and on the back and around the mouth. Data from FOS show that approximately 70% of males and 35% of females have angiokeratomas (Table 2) and that these may first be observed during childhood. Angiokeratomas were reported in 39% of boys and 23% of girls in FOS (age at onset, 9.4 ± 3.3 years in boys and 13.7 ± 3.5 years in girls).

Dyshidrosis

Male patients commonly suffer from hypohidrosis or anhidrosis, which results in heat intolerance. Hypohidrosis may begin at a very early age [4]. In FOS, the mean age at onset of this symptom in children is before 10 years (9.3 ± 5.1 years in boys and 9.7 ± 6.3 years in girls). Patients do not tolerate exercise well and may suffer nausea, dyspnoea, lightheadedness and headache, or complete collapse with loss of consciousness [7]. There may also be reduced production of tears and saliva [8]. Rarely, cases of hyperhidrosis are reported.

Sensory organs

The eyes are affected in most patients with Fabry disease [9], and cornea verticillata (a whorl-shaped opacity) strongly suggests a diagnosis of Fabry disease, although it does not usually affect vision. Posterior subcapsular cataracts also occur, as do tortuous vascular lesions in the retina and conjunctiva, which sometimes cause severe visual loss.

FOS data suggest that tinnitus may also be an early sign of Fabry disease. This manifestation is reported in 27% of boys (age at onset, 12.3 ± 4.0 years) and 27% of girls (age at onset, 11.5 ± 4.1 years). Vertigo may also be reported. High-frequency sensorineural hearing loss is common [10].

Gastrointestinal symptoms

Gastrointestinal symptoms of Fabry disease tend to occur after meals and comprise recurrent bouts of abdominal pain in the mid and lower abdomen. Nausea, vomiting, abdominal distension, episodic diarrhoea and constipation may all occur. In many patients, gastrointestinal symptoms are similar to those associated with irritable bowel syndrome. Data from FOS suggest that gastrointestinal symptoms are one of the most common early manifestations of Fabry disease [5]. Diarrhoea was reported by 35% of boys and 24% of girls in FOS. Abdominal pain was experienced by 41% of boys and 38% of girls. This was the earliest symptom reported in girls (8.2 ± 4.8 years), and the second earliest in boys (7.0 ± 4.4 years) after diarrhoea (5.6 ± 4.3 years).

Renal function

Kidney involvement is common in classic Fabry disease and is an important cause of death. Abnormalities include proteinuria, haematuria, nephrotic syndrome and chronic renal failure requiring dialysis and/or renal transplantation [11, 12]. Proteinuria may be apparent during childhood. Data from FOS show that proteinuria occurs in 10% of boys and 17% of girls with Fabry disease. Onset of end-stage renal failure usually occurs in male patients when they are in their 30s and is not seen in childhood. Abnormalities of renal function are frequently seen in females, but end-stage renal failure is uncommon.

Cardiac function

Cardiac disease is one of the most frequent causes of death in patients with Fabry disease. Common cardiac defects include left and right ventricular hypertrophy, enlarged left atrium, heart valve abnormalities and conduction disturbances. Cardiac involvement may be the only symptom in some hemizygous males [6], and up to 5% of males with hypertrophic cardiomyopathy may have a 'cardiac' variant of Fabry disease [13] (see section below on 'Atypical variants of Fabry disease').

Nervous system

Cerebrovascular manifestations such as transient ischaemic attacks or stroke have been reported to affect 15–20% of patients with Fabry disease, and such attacks frequently recur and indicate a poor prognosis [14, 15]. Data from FOS show that some 6–9% of patients have experienced stroke; however, this value may be an underestimate of the true prevalence due to the high number of patients in the early stages of the disease who are included in this database. A recent study has indicated a prevalence of Fabry disease as high as 5% in males and 2.5% in females under the age of 55 years presenting with 'cryptogenic' stroke – that is, stroke occurring in the absence of other obvious risk factors [16]. Disturbed concentration, dizziness, dementia, headaches and learning difficulties also occur [2]. In addition, fatigue and depression have been reported in young patients.

The peripheral nervous system may also be affected, with disturbances of touch, pain and sensitivity to temperature.

Respiratory function

Significant airflow obstruction is common in patients with Fabry disease. Hence, smoking is particularly inadvisable as it seriously exacerbates pulmonary impairment [17]. Shortness of breath, tiredness and fatigue are common symptoms in early adulthood, and these symptoms arise as a result of cardiac, renal and pulmonary insufficiency. Asthma and reversible airways obstruction also occur [17].

Fabry disease in women and children

Although Fabry disease is an X-linked disorder, females are symptomatic in a high proportion of cases (see Chapter 30) (Table 2). Disease manifestations in females tend to occur at a later age than in males and are often less severe (see Chapter 32). Symptoms typically start in childhood, but the diagnosis is often difficult to establish in the index case and there is frequently a delay between the onset of signs and symptoms and diagnosis (see Chapter 16). FOS data on females [18] and children [5] with Fabry disease have recently been published.

Atypical variants of Fabry disease

There have been numerous reports in the literature regarding late-onset Fabry disease in males, generally presenting with features involving only a single organ system. It has been proposed that these so-called cardiac [6] and renal [19] variants arise as a result of missense mutations that are associated with sufficient residual enzyme activity to prevent symptoms in childhood and early adult life.

Within the FOS database, there are no clear data supporting the concept of single organ variants of Fabry disease. There are 18 individuals who currently report no signs and symptoms of Fabry disease, and there are three females (aged 19, 21 and 47 years) and one male (aged 19 years) who have reported only renal signs and/or symptoms to date. These data must be interpreted with care, as such reports of single organ involvement might be due to missing data in the

FOS database. Overall, FOS data suggest wide clinical heterogeneity.

Close scrutiny of the published literature on renal and cardiac variants shows that many of the patients do, in fact, have changes in other organ systems [17, 19]. Increasing numbers of patients with Fabry disease are being diagnosed following investigations of specific medical conditions such as hypertrophic cardiomyopathy, cerebrovascular disease and renal failure [16, 20, 21] (see Chapter 17). It may well be that many of these patients have mutations associated with residual enzyme activity (see Chapter 34), which could, in turn, be associated with a milder disease phenotype.

Cause of death in Fabry disease

Life expectancy is reduced for both males and females with Fabry disease. The surveys by MacDermott *et al.* [2, 3] indicate that life expectancy is decreased by approximately 20 years in males and 10–15 years in females.

To date, FOS has collected data on the cause and age of death for 107 affected relatives of patients (68 presumed hemizygous males and 39 presumed

Table 3. *Causes of death reported in male (n = 66) and female (n = 38) relatives of patients in FOS – the Fabry Outcome Survey – who are presumed to have had Fabry disease.*

Reported cause of death	Males	Females
Cardiac	11	8
Cardiac/renal	4	0
Cardiac/cerebrovascular	0	3
Renal	33	4
Renal/cerebrovascular	3	0
Cerebrovascular	5	5
Cancer	1	8
Vascular	2	2
Suicide	2	0
Lung	0	2
Gastric	0	1
Unknown	5	5

heterozygous females) (Figure 2). The peak decade of death among presumed hemizygous males is the fifth decade, and there are approximately equal numbers of males dying in their fourth and sixth decades. As shown in Table 3, the principal cause of death in these males was renal failure (*n* = 33), followed by cardiac (*n* = 11)

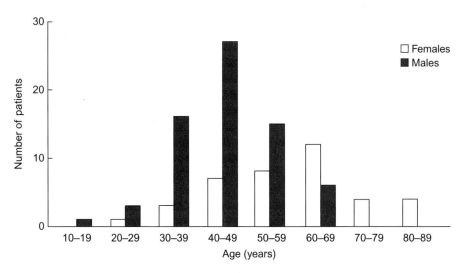

Figure 2. *Age at death in male (n = 68) and female (n = 39) relatives of patients in FOS – the Fabry Outcome Survey – who are presumed to have had Fabry disease.*

and cerebrovascular causes ($n = 5$); however, some deaths were also attributed to a combination of these causes (cardiac/renal, $n = 4$; renal/cerebrovascular, $n = 3$). The peak decade of death among presumed heterozygous females is the seventh decade, but there also appears to be an excess number of deaths in the fifth and sixth decades. The principal causes of death reported in females were cardiac in origin ($n = 8$) and cancer ($n = 8$). There also appears to be a significant number of premature deaths among females as a result of cerebrovascular disease ($n = 5$).

Conclusions

Fabry disease is a clinically heterogeneous, progressive X-linked disorder which results in a range of manifestations. Females tend to develop symptoms at a later age and of a lesser severity than males. Symptoms and signs typically begin in childhood and include pain, angiokeratomas, oedema, abnormalities of hearing, eye changes, dyshidrosis and gastrointestinal disturbances. Renal, cardiac and cerebrovascular complications cause premature death in both males and females.

It remains to be seen if enzyme replacement therapy can alter the natural history of Fabry disease. Data from FOS – the most comprehensive database on patients with Fabry disease – will help to answer this question.

References

1. Mehta A, Ricci R, Widmer U, Dehout F, Garcia de Lorenzo A, Kampmann C et al. Fabry disease defined: baseline clinical manifestations of 366 patients in the Fabry Outcome Survey. Eur J Clin Invest 2004;34:236–42

2. MacDermot KD, Holmes A, Miners AH. Anderson–Fabry disease: clinical manifestations and impact of disease in a cohort of 98 hemizygous males. J Med Genet 2001;38:750–60

3. MacDermot KD, Holmes A, Miners AH. Anderson–Fabry disease: clinical manifestations and impact of disease in a cohort of 60 obligate carrier females. J Med Genet 2001;38:769–75

4. Ries M, Ramaswami U, Parini R, Lindblad B, Whybra C, Willers I et al. The early clinical phenotype of Fabry disease: a study on 35 European children and adolescents. Eur J Pediatr 2003;162:767–72

5. Ramaswami U, Whybra C, Parini R, Pintos-Morell G, Mehta A, Sunder-Plassmann G et al. Clinical manifestations of Fabry disease in children: data from the Fabry Outcome Survey. Acta Paediatrica 2006;95:86–92

6. Nakao S, Takenaka T, Maeda M, Kodama C, Tanaka A, Tahara M et al. An atypical variant of Fabry's disease in men with left ventricular hypertrophy. N Engl J Med 1995;333:288–93

7. Shelley ED, Shelley WB, Kurczynski TW. Painful fingers, heat intolerance, and telangiectases of the ear: easily ignored childhood signs of Fabry disease. Pediatr Dermatol 1995;12:215–19

8. Cable WJ, Kolodny EH, Adams RD. Fabry disease: impaired autonomic function. Neurology 1982;32:498–502

9. Sher NA, Letson RD, Desnick RJ. The ocular manifestations in Fabry's disease. Arch Ophthalmol 1979;97:671–6

10. Hajioff D, Enever Y, Quiney R, Zuckerman J, Mackermot K, Mehta A. Hearing loss in Fabry disease: the effect of agalsidase alfa replacement therapy. J Inherit Metab Dis 2003;26:787–94

11. Tsakiris D, Simpson HK, Jones EH, Briggs JD, Elinder CG, Mendel S et al. Report on management of renal failure in Europe, XXVI, 1995. Rare diseases in renal replacement therapy in the ERA–EDTA Registry. Nephrol Dial Transplant 1996;11 (Suppl 7):4–20

12. Branton M, Schiffmann R, Kopp JB. Natural history and treatment of renal involvement in Fabry disease. J Am Soc Nephrol 2002;13 (Suppl 2):S139–43

13. Sachdev B, Takenaka T, Teraguchi H, Tei C, Lee P, McKenna WJ et al. Prevalence of Anderson–Fabry disease in male patients with late onset hypertrophic cardiomyopathy. Circulation 2002;105:1407–11

14. Mitsias P, Levine SR. Cerebrovascular complications of Fabry's disease. Ann Neurol 1996;40:8–17

15. Grewal RP, Barton NW. Fabry's disease presenting with stroke. Clin Neurol Neurosurg 1992;94:177–9

16. Rolfs A, Bottcher T, Zschiesche M, Morris P, Winchester B, Bauer P et al. Prevalence of Fabry disease in patients with cryptogenic stroke: a prospective study. Lancet 2005;366:1794–6

17. Rosenberg DM, Ferrans VJ, Fulmer JD, Line BR, Barranger JA, Brady RO et al. Chronic airflow obstruction in Fabry's disease. Am J Med 1980;68:898–905

18. Deegan P, Bähner AF, Barba-Romero MA, Hughes D, Kampmann C, Beck M. Natural history of Fabry disease in females in the Fabry Outcome Survey. J Med Genet 2006;43:347–52

19. Nakao S, Kodama C, Takenaka T, Tanaka A, Yasumoto Y, Yoshida A et al. Fabry disease: detection of undiagnosed hemodialysis patients and identification of a "renal variant" phenotype. Kidney Int 2003;64:801–7

20. Tanaka M, Ohashi T, Kobayashi M, Eto Y, Miyamura N, Nishida K et al. Identification of Fabry's disease by the screening of α-galactosidase A activity in male and female hemodialysis patients. Clin Nephrol 2005;64:281–7

21. Chimenti C, Pieroni M, Morgante E, Antuzzi D, Russo A, Russo MA et al. Prevalence of Fabry disease in female patients with late-onset hypertrophic cardiomyopathy. Circulation 2004;110:1047–53

20 The heart in Fabry disease

Aleš Linhart

2nd Department of Internal Medicine, 1st School of Medicine, Charles University, U Nemocnice 2, CZ-128 08 Prague 2, Czech Republic

Cardiac involvement is common in Fabry disease, both in hemizygous men and heterozygous women, and is one of the three major causes of morbidity and mortality. Storage of globotriaosylceramide occurs in various cells of the heart, including cardiomyocytes, conduction system cells, valvular fibroblasts, endothelial cells within all types of vessels, and vascular smooth muscle cells. Cardiac hypertrophy associated with depressed contractility and diastolic filling impairment is common. In addition, coronary insufficiency, atrioventricular conduction disturbances, arrhythmias and valvular involvement may be present. In patients with the atypical 'cardiac variant', the disease manifestations may be limited to the heart. Enzyme replacement therapy is now the treatment of choice for patients with Fabry disease, and preliminary results indicate promising effects not only on the renal and neurological manifestations of the disease but also on the cardiac manifestations.

Introduction

Cardiac involvement is one of the three major causes of morbidity and mortality in Fabry disease, together with end-stage renal disease and cerebrovascular events (Figure 1) [1, 2]. Lysosomal storage occurs within almost all cardiac tissues and leads to clinically important symptoms, including dyspnoea, chest pain, palpitations and syncope. These symptoms relate mainly to the development of progressive cardiac hypertrophy, conduction abnormalities and arrhythmias.

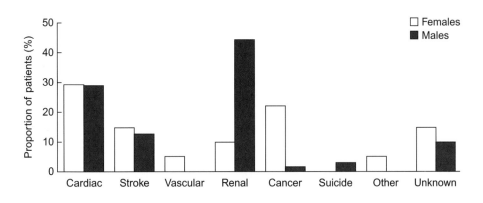

Figure 1. *The relative frequency of causes of death among 113 relatives of patients with Fabry disease in FOS – the Fabry Outcome Survey.*

Pathogenesis of the cardiac involvement

Storage of globotriaosylceramide (Gb₃) is found in various cells of the heart, including cardiomyocytes, conduction system cells, valvular fibroblasts, endothelial cells within all types of vessels, and vascular smooth muscle cells [3]. In women, a mosaic pattern caused by random X-chromosome inactivation is observed [4]. Gb₃ storage by itself, however, is unable to explain the observed level of cardiac hypertrophy, conduction abnormalities and other cardiac manifestations. Autopsy of an individual with Fabry disease who had an extremely hypertrophied heart revealed a relatively limited contribution (1–2%) of the stored material to the enormous increase in cardiac mass [5]. It appears that storage induces progressive lysosomal and cellular malfunctioning that, in turn, activates common signalling pathways leading to hypertrophy, apoptosis, necrosis and fibrosis (Figure 2). Energy depletion was recently proposed as the common denominator in multiple metabolic and even sarcomeric hypertrophic cardiomyopathies [6]. Energy depletion may also occur in Fabry disease, as suggested by the impairment in energy handling seen in skin fibroblasts [7]. This might be further supported by the observation of a decreased ratio of ATP to inorganic orthophosphate, as has been

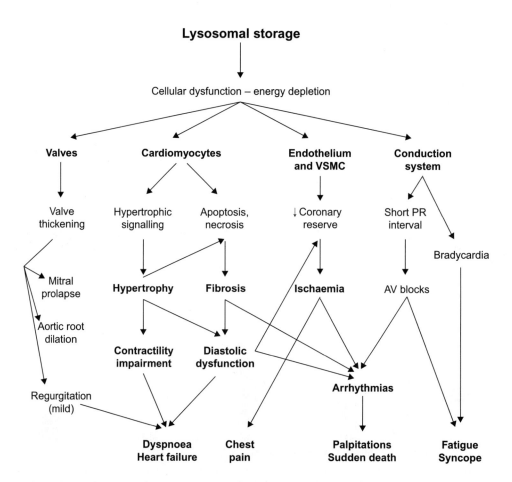

Figure 2. *Schematic showing the possible pathways between lysosomal storage and signs and symptoms of Fabry disease. VSMC, vascular smooth muscle cells; AV, atrioventricular.*

shown by magnetic resonance imaging (MRI) studies in patients with sarcomeric hypertrophic cardiomyopathies [8].

In summary, the natural history of Fabry disease is characterized by progressive hypertrophy of the cardiac muscle, with increasing interstitial and fibrotic changes. This is consistent with observations of relatively mild diastolic dysfunction in early stages of the disease and with the late appearance of signs and symptoms that might be observed in patients with restrictive cardiomyopathy [9]. The disease process is potentiated by absolute or relative ischaemia, occurring even in the absence of significant epicardial coronary artery disease. This might be mainly due to the increased oxygen demand of the hypertrophied muscle, decreased capillary density, increased diastolic filling pressures that impair blood flow throughout the subendocardial layers in diastole, and to the infiltration of small arterioles and

capillaries within endothelial cells and the smooth muscle layer [3, 10].

A similar pattern of progressive involvement is observed in the conduction system of the heart. Early stages of the disease are associated with accelerated conduction, and late stages are characterized by progressive bradycardia and atrioventricular conduction defects, frequently necessitating pacemaker implantation [11].

Cardiac hypertrophy

Left ventricular (LV) hypertrophy is the predominant finding, detected both by imaging techniques (echocardiography, MRI) (Figures 3 and 4) and by electrocardiography (ECG) (LV hypertrophy voltage criteria) (Figure 5) [9, 12, 13]. Histologically, hypertrophy is characterized by the absence of myofibrillar disarray, lysosomal inclusions within myofibrils and vascular structures, and a variable degree of fibrosis depending on the stage of the

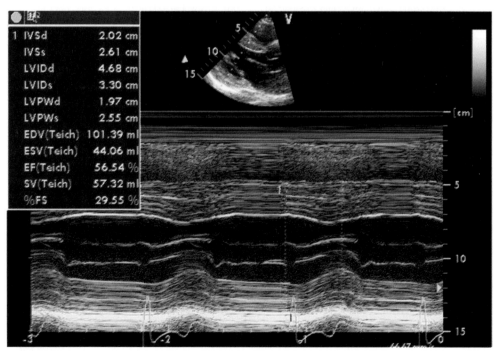

Figure 3. *Echocardiographic M-mode recording in a patient with Fabry disease, showing the concentric character of left ventricular hypertrophy with both diastolic interventricular septum (IVSd) and posterior wall (PWd) thickness exceeding 19 mm (normal values should not exceed 12 mm for either).*

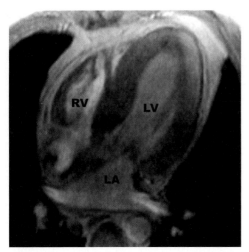

Figure 4. *Magnetic resonance imaging of a patient with Fabry disease, showing marked diffuse hypertrophy of the left ventricle (LV). LA, left atrium; RV, right ventricle.*

The hypertrophy is progressive and occurs earlier in men than in women. Early stages are characterized by concentric remodelling, progressing later to overt hypertrophy. In a large majority of patients, the hypertrophy is symmetrical; however, asymmetric septal hypertrophy, indistinguishable from that considered typical for sarcomeric cardio-myopathies, may be present in about 5% of all cases [9, 16]. Asymmetric hypertrophy may be associated with marked LV outflow obstruction. In these patients, treatment by alcohol ablation may bring substantial relief and stabilization, in spite of the progressive nature of the hypertrophy [17].

disease [5, 14]. Although the absolute amount of Gb_3 within cardiomyocytes is low, the heart contains the highest quantity of glycosphin-golipid compared with other organs (kidney, liver, skin) [5, 15].

Although early autopsy reports indicated important disease-related organ involvement in females heterozygous for Fabry disease, for a long time women were considered as carriers [18]. Due to random X-chromosome inactivation and the inability of cells express-ing the wild-type allele to cross-correct the metabolic defect, affected women may express symptoms that are similar to those of

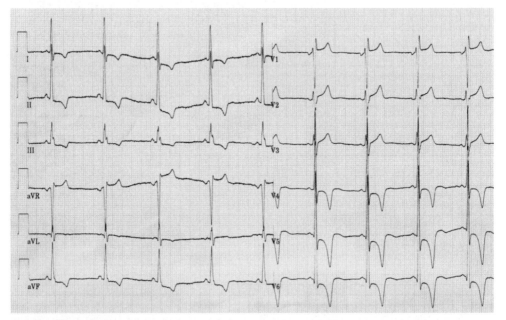

Figure 5. *Typical electrocardiogram tracing from a patient with Fabry disease, showing short PR intervals, marked electric left ventricular hypertrophy, and prominent ST depressions and T-wave inversions.*

hemizygous males [19, 20]. Cardiac involvement in women has recently been confirmed. However, symptoms are often milder, the onset delayed and disease progression slower than in men [21]. These observations have been confirmed by analysis of data from FOS – the Fabry Outcome Survey – in untreated patients (Figure 6), which shows the delayed onset of hypertrophy in females.

Magnetic resonance studies using gadolinium have provided new insights into the development of Fabry cardiomyopathy. In patients with LV hypertrophy, such studies have demonstrated late enhancement areas, corresponding to myocardial fibrosis, occurring frequently within the midwall of the posterolateral basal segments [22]. It appears that this finding characterizes late stages of LV involvement and is associated with decreased regional functioning, as assessed by strain and strain-rate imaging [23].

The right ventricle also appears to be affected by storage and hypertrophy. However,

the functional impact of right ventricular infiltration and hypertrophy is low, and right ventricular failure almost never complicates the course of the disease [24].

LV function

LV systolic function, measured by traditional parameters such as ejection fraction or fractional shortening, is seldom decreased [9, 25]. However, studies using tissue Doppler imaging and contractility assessment by strain-rate imaging documented a substantial decrease in contractile performance, occurring earlier in the longitudinal than in the radial dimension [23, 26]. FOS data show a progressive decline in midwall fractional shortening with age (Figure 7). This parameter reflects the contractility impairment that may be masked by the geometrical structural changes and may be undetectable by the measurement of ejection fraction or fractional shortening.

Diastolic dysfunction is a common feature of Fabry disease. In contrast to genuine restrictive cardiomyopathies, however, restrictive pathophysiology is found only rarely, mostly in extremely advanced stages of the disease that are associated with pronounced fibrosis. End-stage cardiac involvement may then present with restrictive pathophysiology [14, 27].

Ischaemia and coronary events

Traditional descriptions of Fabry disease report a high frequency of ischaemic events and myocardial infarctions. Data from the FOS database, however, suggest a low incidence of proven myocardial infarctions. By October 2005, the FOS database included 752 patients (393 heterozygous women and 359 hemizygous men). Only 13 myocardial infarctions were reported, representing a prevalence of less than 2%. On the other hand, angina and chest pain are frequent, being reported in FOS by almost 23% of females and 22% of males. This, together with frequently disturbed ECG patterns (Figure 5), including ST segment depressions and

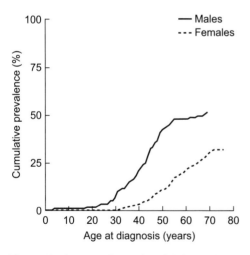

Figure 6. *Age at diagnosis of left ventricular hypertrophy among untreated men and women with Fabry disease in FOS – the Fabry Outcome Survey – showing a later onset and lower cumulative prevalence in women. Sixty-two out of 121 untreated males in FOS and 58 out of 183 untreated females have been diagnosed with left ventricular hypertrophy.*

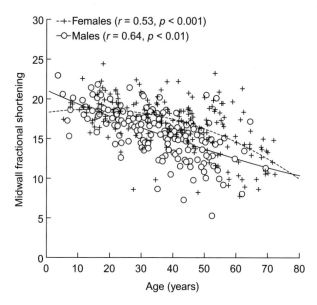

Figure 7. *Correlation of midwall fractional shortening with age in patients with Fabry disease in FOS – the Fabry Outcome Survey. Females n = 189, males n = 159.*

T-wave inversions, might be the cause of misdiagnosis of either acute or subacute myocardial infarction [28]. In addition, anginal pain and ECG changes are more frequent in patients with LV hypertrophy, in whom minor increases in markers of cardiac necrosis are possible. Epicardial coronary arteries, however, are only rarely occluded.

As shown by Kalliokoski and Elliott, patients with Fabry disease have a significantly reduced coronary flow reserve [29, 30]. This might be due to endothelial infiltration and dysfunction, potentiated by the increased oxygen demand of the hypertrophied ventricle and further aggravated by elevated diastolic filling pressures. In some cases, vasospasms may contribute to the anginal symptoms [31]. Most patients with Fabry disease who are investigated for chest pain have patent large coronary arteries. A history of revascularization due to the presence of stenotic lesions was reported in the FOS database in only five cases, representing a prevalence of less than 1%. However, as

underlined by the recent case report by Schiffmann and co-workers, the risk of death due to coronary artery disease should not be underestimated [32].

In addition to the infiltrative changes within the endothelial and muscular layers of arteries, patients with Fabry disease often accumulate a large number of risk factors for atherosclerosis, including high levels of blood lipids, hypertension and renal insufficiency. Another aggravating factor might be the prothrombotic state associated with the endothelial dysfunction caused by the disease [33]. However, it remains unclear to what extent these lesions are due to atherosclerosis or to infiltrative changes [3].

Electrophysiological abnormalities and arrhythmias
In most patients with Fabry disease, resting ECG patterns are perturbed. Besides high voltage and repolarization changes, a short PR interval is frequently found (Figure 5) [12]. The shortening is due to accelerated

atrioventricular (AV) conduction [34]. However, as in other lysosomal and glycogen storage diseases, pre-excitation with accessory pathways may also be present in patients with Fabry disease [35, 36]. With disease progression, conduction system dysfunction occurs, leading to bundle branch and AV blocks of varying degrees, requiring pacemaker implantation. In some patients, a pacemaker is needed due to symptomatic bradycardia, as progressive sinus node dysfunction is relatively frequent [11].

Palpitations and arrhythmias are common complaints in patients with Fabry disease. The most frequently encountered rhythm abnormalities include supraventricular tachycardias, atrial fibrillation and flutter. Non-sustained ventricular tachycardias (NSVT), however, were detected by 24-hour Holter monitoring, and cases of fatal malignant arrhythmias resistant to an implantable cardioverter defibrillator have been reported

[37, 38]. Ventricular arrhythmias were found mostly in very advanced stages of the disease. Studies showing the high incidence of NSVT on Holter monitoring support the regular use of this method to identify high-risk individuals who may benefit from cardioverter defibrillator implantation.

Valvular involvement

Valvular disease in patients with Fabry disease is due, in part, to infiltrative changes within valvular fibroblasts. Although pulmonary valvular involvement has been reported, valvular changes are found almost exclusively in the left heart valves, probably due to the higher haemodynamic stresses in the left side of the heart [39, 40]. This results in valvular thickening and deformation (Figure 8). In original reports, the prevalence of mitral valve prolapse was overestimated, probably due to the different diagnostic criteria used [41]. Subsequent reports confirmed the existence of mitral valve prolapse, but with a lower prevalence [9, 12].

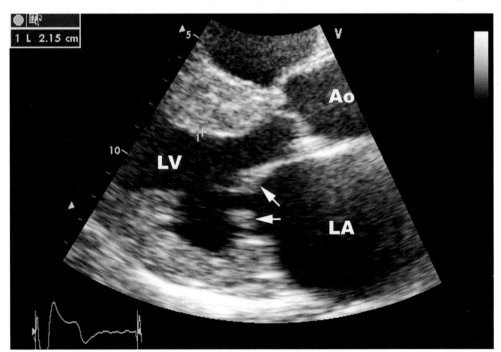

Figure 8. *Echocardiogram showing mild thickening of the mitral valve leaflets (arrows) in a patient with Fabry disease. Marked thickening of the interventricular septum is also present. Ao, Aorta; LA, left atrium; LV, left ventricle.*

Valvular regurgitant lesions are usually mild to moderate (Figure 9) and only rarely require surgical correction (3 cases out of 752 patients in FOS). At the level of the aortic valve, root dilation may contribute to valvular dysfunction and has been reported repeatedly, particularly in advanced stages of the disease [9, 25].

Cardiac variant

Early studies suggested that cardiac hypertrophy might be the sole or predominant manifestation of Fabry disease in a small number of male hemizygotes. Histopathological studies revealed Gb_3 storage located almost exclusively in the heart [5, 15, 42]. These cases, described as cardiac variants, were distinguished by relatively high residual α-galactosidase A activity. In addition, some mutations have been shown to be associated almost exclusively with this type of involvement [43].

Several studies have attempted to identify Fabry disease among patients with cardiac

hypertrophy [36, 44–47]. An early study by Nakao and co-workers identified seven unrelated patients with Fabry disease (3%) among 230 men with unexplained LV hypertrophy. A particularly important observation was made by Sachdev and co-workers, indicating that special attention should be paid to patients in whom unexplained LV hypertrophy is diagnosed after 40 years of age [44]. At this age, most male patients with Fabry disease have at least LV hypertrophy, which is not necessarily present in younger patients [9]. The negative findings of Ommen and co-workers is an understandable result of population selection [46]. As stated above, only about 5% of patients with Fabry disease have asymmetric septal hypertrophy, and even fewer have LV tract obstruction [16]. Therefore, the probability that patients with Fabry disease would be identified when investigating individuals referred for septal myectomy was *a priori* extremely low. The fact that diagnosing Fabry disease among individuals with LV

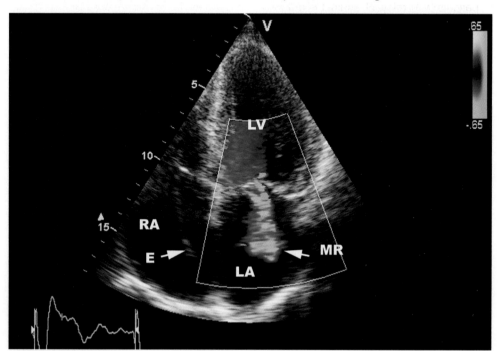

Figure 9. *Colour Doppler recording, illustrating mild to moderate mitral regurgitation (MR), in a patient with Fabry disease. In addition, bilateral atrial dilation can be seen and a pacemaker electrode (E) is visible. LA, left atrium; LV, left ventricle; RA, right atrium.*

hypertrophy may be subject to chance is documented by the strikingly high prevalence of Fabry disease among women with unexplained LV hypertrophy observed by Chimenti and colleagues, which contrasts with the negative result within the series explored by Arad and colleagues [36, 47].

Clinical symptoms

The predominant symptoms of cardiovascular involvement include dyspnoea and chest pain. In most patients, both symptoms are related to LV hypertrophy. The dyspnoea is mainly caused by diastolic dysfunction, although valvular regurgitation and/or systolic LV dysfunction may be the cause in some cases.

Anginal pain usually occurs even in the absence of stenotic coronary lesions, due to an increase in oxygen consumption and a decrease in coronary flow reserve. Coronary angiography should, however, be performed in patients with relevant anginal symptoms, as coronary stenosis may be encountered.

The third most frequent complaint includes palpitations and proven arrhythmias. The high frequency of life-threatening ventricular tachycardia, and the potential benefits of implantable cardioverter defibrillators should encourage the investigation of symptomatic patients by 24-hour Holter monitoring.

Finally, syncope may occur in patients with Fabry disease. Cardiac causes of syncope include high degrees of AV blockade or, more rarely, severe dynamic obstruction of the LV outflow tract.

Analysis of FOS data has confirmed the high prevalence of cardiovascular symptoms among women. However, the age of onset was delayed compared with that in hemizygous men (Figure 10).

Treatment issues

Although we have no formal proof of efficacy and prognostic improvement, all the usual measures for reducing cardiovascular risk are used in patients with Fabry disease,

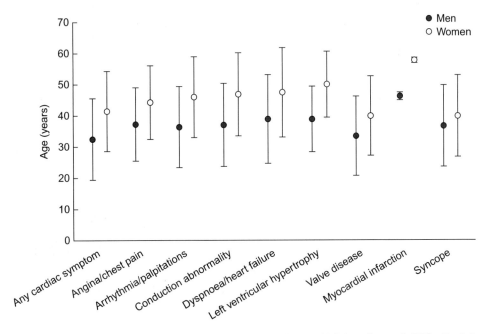

Figure 10. *The age of onset of symptoms among women and men with Fabry disease in FOS – the Fabry Outcome Survey – demonstrating the later onset of symptoms in women. Values are means ± SD.*

including statin therapy to lower lipid levels and antihypertensive treatment.

Patients should be treated according to the signs and symptoms they experience. Anti-anginal treatment should be given with care, as β-blockers may aggravate the tendency for symptomatic bradycardia and AV conduction impairment in some patients. Based on our experience, dihydropyridine calcium channel blockers are relatively effective and safe. Anti-aggregation therapy should be offered to all symptomatic patients.

Treatment for heart failure should be given to all symptomatic patients. Angiotensin-converting enzyme inhibitors or angiotensin receptor blockers should also be considered in asymptomatic individuals with LV hypertrophy. In addition, the potential nephroprotective effects of such treatment should be considered. Patients with advanced stages of heart disease, such as congestive heart failure, may be candidates for heart transplantation, as the intrinsic enzyme production within the graft should prevent its rapid deterioration [27].

Anticoagulant treatment should be initiated immediately in patients with supraventricular rhythm disturbances. In individuals with symptomatic bradycardia and/or AV conduction abnormalities, pacemaker implantation is frequently required. Patients with proven malignant arrhythmias may benefit from an implantable cardioverter defibrillator.

Septal alcohol ablation may be effective in patients with LV outflow tract obstruction. Other treatment modalities (surgical myectomy, mitral valve replacement) should be considered in individuals with unsuitable septal branch anatomy [17].

Enzyme replacement therapy (ERT) has recently been introduced in clinical practice. Agalsidase alfa, produced in human fibroblasts, is given at a dose of 0.2 mg/kg body weight every 2 weeks; agalsidase beta, produced in Chinese hamster ovary cells, is administered every 2 weeks at a dose of 1 mg/kg.

Several trials have been completed using both treatments, and have demonstrated the efficacy of ERT on neurological and renal manifestations of the disease and on quality of life [48–51]. None of these trials was designed specifically to demonstrate an improvement in cardiac structure and function. However, a phase III trial of agalsidase alfa has shown an improvement in the duration of the QRS complex, and bundle branch block was resolved in one patient [48]. In addition, results of cardiac biopsies performed during a phase III trial with agalsidase beta have shown that Gb_3 is cleared from endothelial cells within the myocardial capillaries [49]. Case reports and observational studies have also repeatedly suggested a significant improvement in LV structure and function with both treatments [52–55]. Furthermore, analysis of the FOS database has demonstrated long-term benefits of agalsidase alfa treatment on LV structure and function (see Chapter 37).

A case report has been published that describes an improvement in cardiac function after large doses of galactose – a competitive inhibitor of α-galactosidase A – in a patient with the cardiac variant of Fabry disease [56]. The clinical applicability of such therapy, however, remains unclear. The potential of other, more effective, small molecules, used as chaperones or as substrate deprivation mediators, is under investigation. Correction of the inherent genetic defect would represent the ultimate cure, and promising experimental studies are in progress. [57]

Conclusions

Cardiac involvement is a frequent finding in Fabry disease, both in hemizygous men and heterozygous women. Cardiac hypertrophy associated with depressed contractility and diastolic filling impairment is common, and coronary insufficiency, AV conduction disturbances, arrhythmias and valvular involvement may be present. Cardiac mortality appears to be a major problem in patients with Fabry disease. In those with the atypical 'cardiac variant', the disease manifestations may be limited to the heart. ERT is now the treatment of choice, and preliminary results indicate promising effects not only on the renal and neurological manifestations of the disease but also on the cardiac manifestations.

References

1. Mehta A, Ricci R, Widmer U, Dehout F, García de Lorenzo A, Kampmann C et al. Fabry disease defined: baseline clinical manifestations of 366 patients in the Fabry Outcome Survey. Eur J Clin Invest 2004;34:236–42

2. MacDermot KD, Holmes A, Miners AH. Anderson–Fabry disease: clinical manifestations and impact of disease in a cohort of 98 hemizygous males. J Med Genet 2001;38:750–60

3. Hulkova H, Ledvinova J, Poupetova H, Bultas J, Zeman J, Elleder M. Postmortem diagnosis of Fabry disease in a female heterozygote leading to the detection of undiagnosed manifest disease in the family. Cas Lek Cesk 1999;138:660–4

4. Uchino M, Uyama E, Kawano H, Hokamaki J, Kugiyama K, Murakami Y et al. A histochemical and electron microscopic study of skeletal and cardiac muscle from a Fabry disease patient and carrier. Acta Neuropathol (Berl) 1995;90:334–8

5. Elleder M, Bradova V, Smid F, Budesinsky M, Harzer K, Kustermann-Kuhn B et al. Cardiocyte storage and hypertrophy as a sole manifestation of Fabry's disease. Report on a case simulating hypertrophic non-obstructive cardiomyopathy. Virchows Arch A Pathol Anat Histopathol 1990;417:449–55

6. Ashrafian H, Redwood Ch, Blair E, Watkins H. Hypertrophic cardiomyopathy: a paradigm for myocardial energy depletion. Trends Genet 2003;19:263–8

7. Lücke T, Höppner W, Schmidt E, Illsinger S, Das AM. Fabry disease: reduced activities of respiratory chain enzymes with decreased levels of energy-rich phosphates in fibroblasts. Mol Genet Metab 2004; 82:93–7

8. Jung WI, Sieverding L, Breuer J, Hoess T, Widmaier S, Schmidt O et al. ^{31}P NMR spectroscopy detects metabolic abnormalities in asymptomatic patients with hypertrophic cardiomyopathy. Circulation 1998;97:2536–42

9. Linhart A, Palecek T, Bultas J, Ferguson JJ, Hrudova J, Karetova D et al. New insights in cardiac structural changes in patients with Fabry's disease. Am Heart J 2000;139:1101–8

10. Cecchi F, Olivotto I, Gistri R, Lorenzoni R, Chiriatti G, Camici P. Coronary microvascular dysfunction and prognosis in hypertrophic cardiomyopathy. N Engl J Med 2003;349:1027–35

11. Ikari Y, Kuwako K, Yamaguchi T. Fabry's disease with complete atrioventricular block: histological evidence of involvement of the conduction system. Br Heart J 1992;68:323–5

12. Kampmann C, Wiethoff CM, Martin C, Wenzel A, Kampmann R, Whybra C et al. Electrocardiographic signs of hypertrophy in Fabry disease-associated hypertrophic cardiomyopathy. Acta Paediatr Suppl 2002;439:21–7

13. Senechal M, Germain DP. Fabry disease: a functional and anatomical study of cardiac manifestations in 20 hemizygous male patients. Clin Genet 2003;63:46–52

14. Cantor WJ, Butany J, Iwanochko M, Liu P. Restrictive cardiomyopathy secondary to Fabry's disease. Circulation 1998;98:1457–9

15. von Scheidt W, Eng CM, Fitzmaurice TF, Erdmann E, Hubner G, Olsen EGJ et al. An atypical variant of Fabry's disease with manifestations confined to the myocardium. N Engl J Med 1991;324:395–9

16. Linhart A, Lubanda JC, Paleček T, Bultas J, Karetová D, Ledvinová J et al. Cardiac manifestations in Fabry disease. J Inherit Metab Dis 2001;24 (Suppl 2):75–83

17. Magage S, Linhart A, Bultas J, Vojacek J, Mates M, Palecek T et al. Fabry disease: percutaneous transluminal septal myocardial ablation markedly improved symptomatic left ventricular hypertrophy and outflow tract obstruction in a classically affected male. Echocardiography 2005;22:333–9

18. Burda CD, Winder PR. Angiokeratoma corporis diffusum universale (Fabry's disease) in female subjects. Am J Med 1967;42:293–301

19. Dobrovolny R, Dvorakova L, Ledvinova J, Magage S, Bultas J, Lubanda JC et al. Relationship between X-inactivation and clinical involvement in Fabry heterozygotes. Eleven novel mutations in the α-galactosidase A gene in the Czech and Slovak population. J Mol Med 2005;3:647–54

20. Morrone A, Cavicchi C, Bardelli T, Antuzzi D, Parini R, Di Rocco M et al. Fabry disease: molecular studies in Italian patients and X inactivation analysis in manifesting carriers. J Med Genet 2003;40:e103

21. Kampmann C, Baehner F, Whybra C, Martin C, Wiethoff CM, Ries M et al. Cardiac manifestations of Anderson–Fabry disease in heterozygous females. J Am Coll Cardiol 2002;40:1668–74

22. Moon JC, Sachdev B, Elkington AG, McKenna WJ, Mehta A, Pennell DJ et al. Gadolinium enhanced cardiovascular magnetic resonance in Anderson–Fabry disease. Evidence for a disease specific abnormality of the myocardial interstitium. Eur Heart J 2003;24:2151–5

23. Weidemann F, Breunig F, Beer M, Sandstede J, Stork S, Voelker W et al. The variation of morphological and functional cardiac manifestation in Fabry disease: potential implications for the time course of the disease. Eur Heart J 2005;26:1221–7

24. Kampmann C, Baehner FA, Whybra C, Bajbouj M, Baron K, Knuf M et al. The right ventricle in Fabry disease. Acta Paediatr Suppl 2005;447:15–18

25. Goldman ME, Cantor R, Schwartz MF, Baker M, Desnick RJ. Echocardiographic abnormalities and disease severity in Fabry's disease. J Am Coll Cardiol 1986;7:1157–61

26. Pieroni M, Chimenti C, Ricci R, Sale P, Russo MA, Frustaci A. Early detection of Fabry cardiomyopathy by tissue Doppler imaging. Circulation 2003; 107:1978–84

27. Cantor WJ, Daly P, Iwanochko M, Clarke JT, Cusimano RJ, Butany J. Cardiac transplantation for Fabry's disease. Can J Cardiol 1998;14:81–4

28. Becker AE, Schoorl R, Balk AG, van der Heide RM. Cardiac manifestations of Fabry's disease. Report of a case with mitral insufficiency and electrocardiographic evidence of myocardial infarction. Am J Cardiol 1975;36:829–35

29. Kalliokoski RJ, Kalliokoski KK, Sundell J, Engblom E, Penttinen M, Kantola I et al. Impaired myocardial perfusion reserve but preserved peripheral endothelial function in patients with Fabry disease. J Inherit Metab Dis 2005;28:563–73

30. Elliott PM, Kindler H, Shah JS, Sachdev B, Rimoldi O, Thaman R et al. Coronary microvascular dysfunction in male patients with Anderson–Fabry disease and the effect of treatment with α-galactosidase A. Heart 2006;92:357–60

31. Ogawa T, Kawai M, Matsui T, Seo A, Aizawa O, Hongo K et al. Vasospastic angina in a patient with Fabry's disease who showed normal coronary angiographic findings. Jpn Circ J 1996;60:315–18

32. Schiffmann R, Rapkiewicz A, Abu-Asab M, Ries M, Askari H, Tsokos M et al. Pathological findings in a patient with Fabry after 2.5 years of enzyme replacement. Virchows Arch 2006;448:337–43

33. DeGraba T, Azhar S, Dignat-George F, Brown E, Boutiere B, Altarescu G et al. Profile of endothelial and leukocyte activation in Fabry patients. Ann Neurol 2000;47:229–33

34. Pochis WT, Litzow JT, King BG, Kenny D. Electrophysiologic findings in Fabry's disease with a short PR interval. Am J Cardiol 1994;74:203–4

35. Murata R, Takatsu H, Noda T, Nishigaki K, Tsuchiya K, Takemura G et al. Fifteen-year follow-up of a heterozygous Fabry's disease patient associated with pre-excitation syndrome. Intern Med 1999; 38:476–81

36. Arad M, Maron BJ, Gorham JM, Johnson WH Jr, Saul JP, Perez-Atayde AR et al. Glycogen storage diseases presenting as hypertrophic cardiomyopathy. N Engl J Med 2005;352:362–72

37. Shah JS, Hughes DA, Sachdev B, Tome M, Ward D, Lee P et al. Prevalence and clinical significance of cardiac arrhythmia in Anderson–Fabry disease. Am J Cardiol 2005;96:842–6

38. Eckart RE, Kinney KG, Belnap CM, Le TD. Ventricular fibrillation refractory to automatic internal cardiac defibrillator in Fabry's disease. Review of cardiovascular manifestations. Cardiology 2000;94:208–12

39. Matsui S, Murakami E, Takekoshi N, Hiramaru Y, Kin T. Cardiac manifestations of Fabry's disease. Report of a case with pulmonary regurgitation diagnosed on the basis of endomyocardial biopsy findings. Jpn Circ J 1977;41:1023–36

40. Linhart A, Lubanda JC, Palecek T, Bultas J, Karetova D, Ledvinova J et al. Cardiac manifestations in Fabry disease. J Inherit Metab Dis 2001;24 (Suppl 2):75–83

41. Desnick RJ, Blieden LC, Sharp HL, Hofschire PJ, Moller JH. Cardiac valvular anomalies in Fabry disease. Clinical, morphologic, and biochemical studies. Circulation 1976;54:818–25.

42. Ogawa K, Sugamata K, Funamoto N, Abe T, Sato T, Nagashima K et al. Restricted accumulation of globotriaosylceramide in the hearts of atypical cases of Fabry's disease. Hum Pathol 1990;21:1067–73

43. Ishii S, Nakao S, Minamikawa-Tachino R, Desnick RJ, Fan JQ. Alternative splicing in the α-galactosidase A gene: increased exon inclusion results in the Fabry cardiac phenotype. Am J Hum Genet 2002; 70:994–1002

44. Nakao S, Takenaka T, Maeda M, Kodama C, Tanaka A, Tahara M et al. An atypical variant of Fabry's disease in men with left ventricular hypertrophy. N Engl J Med 1995;333:288–93

45. Sachdev B, Takenaka T, Teraguchi H, Tei C, Lee P, McKenna WJ et al. Prevalence of Anderson–Fabry disease in male patients with late onset hypertrophic cardiomyopathy. Circulation 2002;105:1407–11

46. Ommen SR, Nishimura RA, Edwards WD. Fabry disease: a mimic for obstructive hypertrophic cardiomyopathy? Heart 2003;89:929–30

47. Chimenti C, Pieroni M, Morgante E, Antuzzi D, Russo A, Russo MA et al. Prevalence of Fabry disease in female patients with late-onset hypertrophic cardiomyopathy. Circulation 2004;110:1047–53

48. Schiffmann R, Kopp JB, Austin HA 3rd, Sabnis S, Moore DF, Weibel T et al. Enzyme replacement therapy in Fabry disease: a randomized controlled trial. JAMA 2001;285:2743–9

49. Eng CM, Guffon N, Wilcox WR, Germain DP, Lee P, Waldek S et al. Safety and efficacy of recombinant human α-galactosidase A replacement therapy in Fabry's disease. N Engl J Med 2001;345:9–16

50. Schiffmann R, Floeter MK, Dambrosia JM, Gupta S, Moore DF, Sharabi Y et al. Enzyme replacement therapy improves peripheral nerve and sweat function in Fabry disease. Muscle Nerve 2003; 28:703–10

51. Moore DF, Altarescu G, Ling GS, Jeffries N, Frei KP, Weibel T et al. Elevated cerebral blood flow velocities in Fabry disease with reversal after enzyme replacement. Stroke 2002;33:525–31

52. Weidemann F, Breunig F, Beer M, Sandstede J, Turschner O, Voelker W et al. Improvement of cardiac function during enzyme replacement therapy in

patients with Fabry disease: a prospective strain rate imaging study. *Circulation* 2003;108:1299–301

53. Beck M, Ricci R, Widmer U, Dehout F, de Lorenzo AG, Kampmann C *et al*. Fabry disease: overall effects of agalsidase alfa treatment. *Eur J Clin Invest* 2004; 34:838–44

54. Spinelli L, Pisani A, Sabbatini M, Petretta M, Andreucci MV, Procaccini D *et al*. Enzyme replacement therapy with agalsidase beta improves cardiac involvement in Fabry's disease. *Clin Genet* 2004; 66:158–65

55. Komamura K, Higashi M, Yamada N. Improvement of cardiac hypertrophy and ventricular function in a man with Fabry disease by treatment with recombinant α-galactosidase A. *Heart* 2004;90:617

56. Frustaci A, Chimenti C, Ricci R, Natale L, Russo MA, Pieroni M *et al*. Improvement in cardiac function in the cardiac variant of Fabry's disease with galactose-infusion therapy. *N Engl J Med* 2001;345:25–32

57. Park J, Murray GJ, Limaye A, Quirk JM, Gelderman MP, Brady RO *et al*. Long-term correction of globotriaosylceramide storage in Fabry mice by recombinant adeno-associated virus-mediated gene transfer. *Proc Natl Acad Sci USA* 2003;100:3450–4

21 Renal manifestations of Fabry disease

Gere Sunder-Plassmann

Division of Nephrology and Dialysis, Department of Medicine III, Medical University Vienna, Währinger Gürtel 18–20, A-1090 Vienna, Austria

Cross-sectional and cohort studies clearly show that renal manifestations occur early in life in a significant proportion of children, in many women, and in almost all men with Fabry disease. These manifestations ultimately progress to end-stage renal disease in nearly all males and some female patients. The prevalence of cortical and parapelvic renal cysts is also increased in patients with Fabry disease. A total of 132 of the 507 adult patients in FOS – the Fabry Outcome Survey – (26%; 54 females, 78 males) presented with an estimated glomerular filtration rate of less than 60 ml/min/1.73 m² (chronic kidney disease stages 3–5). In FOS, 22 patients are on dialysis and 26 have a kidney graft. It is anticipated that enzyme replacement therapy will alter the natural history of kidney disease in patients with Fabry disease.

Introduction

Fabry disease affects the kidney in almost all male and in many female patients, resulting in end-stage renal disease (ESRD) and early death. This chapter gives an overview of the clinical course, histopathology and radiological findings in the kidney of patients with Fabry disease. Finally, renal replacement therapy will be discussed in the context of a hereditary nephropathy.

The progressive nature of renal involvement in patients with Fabry disease

Cross-sectional and cohort studies clearly show that renal manifestations (e.g. proteinuria or a decreased glomerular filtration rate [GFR]) occur early in life in a significant proportion of children, in many females and in almost all male patients with Fabry disease. These manifestations progress over time, leading to ESRD in nearly all males and some female patients.

Children

The clinical manifestations of classic Fabry disease between 4 and 16 years of age include mild proteinuria and urinary sediment containing globotriaosylceramide (Gb_3). In some cases, this may progress to ESRD during late adolescence [1]. A study of 35 children and adolescents (20 females, 15 males; age range, 1–21 years) from 25 European families demonstrated that all males, and the majority of females, show signs and symptoms of Fabry disease before adulthood. Six of these children (3 males, 3 females, all over 14 years of age) showed renal involvement with proteinuria (13% of males, 14% of females), and one boy had a decreased creatinine clearance of 62 ml/min [2]. More recently, Ries and colleagues reported a mean 24-hour protein excretion of 92 ± 45 mg (range, 33–213 mg) among 25 boys (age, 12.3 ± 3.5 years) who were referred to the National Institutes of Health [3]. The mean estimated GFR (eGFR) in these children was 144 ± 22 ml/min/1.73 m^2, and none presented with an eGFR of less than 110 ml/min/1.73 m^2. Among 82 children (40 males, 42 females) in FOS, three were reported to have haematuria, eight to have microalbuminuria and 12 to have proteinuria.

Women

Among 20 females from 13 European families (mean age, 38 years; range, 12–65 years), every individual showed clinical manifestations of Fabry disease. A reduced GFR was observed in 11 patients (55%), and one patient also presented with crescentic glomerulonephritis [4]. Another study of 60 obligate carriers from the UK (mean age, 44 years) found clinically relevant disease manifestations in 33% [5]. Two of these patients (3.3%) presented with ESRD at a mean age of 36 years; however, renal function or proteinuria was assessed only in 31.5% of these 60 patients during the last years of follow-up. In Australia, 21% of 38 females with Fabry disease were reported to have renal involvement [6]. Interestingly, in this study anhidrosis was reported to be predictive of renal manifestations in females. In FOS, 86 (35%) of 303 females were reported to have proteinuria, one patient was on dialysis, and two had received a renal transplant.

Men

A large cohort study from the UK, conducted between 1985 and 2000, showed a high prevalence of ESRD of 30.8% among 84 adult hemizygous males [7]. The mean age of patients at initiation of renal replacement therapy was 36.7 years, and the youngest patient was 18 years of age at the start of therapy. Proteinuria (> 0.15 g/24 hours or > 1+ on dipstick testing) was documented in 37 out of 44 patients, and abnormal renal function (serum creatinine > 120 µmol/l, creatinine clearance < 85 ml/min, or GFR ≤ 120 or > 160 ml/min/m^2) was reported in 28 out of 60 patients.

Branton and colleagues carefully examined the records of 105 male patients with Fabry disease from the USA who were seen between 1970 and 2000 at the National Institutes of Health [8, 9]. Seventy-eight of these patients developed proteinuria ($n = 66$, > 0.2 g/24 hours) and/or chronic renal insufficiency (sustained serum creatinine ≥ 1.5 mg/dl). The age at onset of non-nephrotic proteinuria was 34 ± 10 years (range, 14–55 years), and 50% of the patients developed proteinuria by the age of 35 years. All survivors developed proteinuria by 52 years of age. Nephrotic range proteinuria (> 3 g/24 hours) was seen in 19 out of 78 patients (18%) with renal disease. Thirty-nine patients presented with an increase of serum creatinine above 1.5 mg/dl. The median age at onset of chronic renal failure (creatinine > 1.5 mg/dl) was 42 years (range, 19–54 years) among 33 patients for whom the date of onset was available. During the observation period, 24 out of 105 patients (23%) developed ESRD at a median age of 47 years (range, 21–56 years), and all survivors developed ESRD by the age of 55 years. Arterial hypertension was observed in 30% of the 105 patients. Branton and colleagues also calculated the rate of decline of renal function in 14 patients in whom the onset of chronic renal failure (serum creatinine > 1.5 mg/dl) and the time of initiation of renal replacement therapy were available. The mean decrease in eGFR was −12 ± 8.1 ml/min/1.73 m^2 per year (range, −3.3 to −33.7 ml/min/1.73 m^2 per year). It is important to recognize that this somewhat rapid decrease in renal function was described in a very small population with a serum creatinine concentration far above 1.5 mg/dl in the majority of cases. It is therefore not appropriate to compare the time course of changes in serum creatinine in Fabry patients who have normal baseline creatinine concentrations with this cohort of patients who had mild to severe impairment of renal function at baseline.

Renal disease in FOS

The largest study of patients with Fabry disease published to date reported pro-

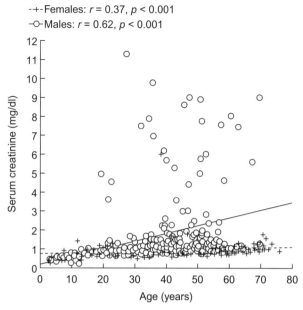

Figure 1. *Serum creatinine according to age in 590 patients (291 males, 299 females) with Fabry disease enrolled in FOS – the Fabry Outcome Survey.*

teinuria in 44% of males and 33% of females. In this huge group of 366 patients (201 males, 165 females) in FOS, ESRD was present in 17% of males (10% with renal transplants, 7% on dialysis) and in 1% of females (one patient on dialysis who subsequently received a renal transplant) [10].

At the time of the FOS analysis undertaken for this chapter, at least one serum creatinine level was available from 590 patients (83 children, 507 adults). The most recently reported creatinine concentrations for these patients, according to age and gender, are shown in Figure 1. Serum creatinine, however, is not an optimal tool for assessing kidney disease. It is generally accepted that a direct measurement of GFR is the best overall marker for renal function. Gold standard measurements of GFR (urinary clearance of inulin, iohexol, chromium ethylenediamine tetraacetate, etc.) are time consuming, expensive and not widely available. Serum creatinine-based eGFR values (using the

short Modification of Diet in Renal Disease [MDRD] formula [11]) are easy to calculate and it has been proposed that they should be used to provide rough estimates of overall kidney function. They also allow classification of patients into the different categories of chronic kidney diseases (CKD stages 1–5, [12]) (Table 1). The eGFR derived from the short MDRD formula [11], does not, however, show good agreement with measured GFR in patients with Fabry disease who have normal serum creatinine concentrations [13]. Furthermore, this formula underestimates measured GFR in individuals with high–normal (0.7–1.6 mg/dl) serum creatinine concentrations [14], and it has been recommended to report such GFR approximations only when estimated levels are less than 60 ml/min/1.73 m^2 (CKD stages 3–5).

Table 1 shows the number of male and female patients according to the different CKD categories, based on eGFR levels. As almost all hemizygotes develop symptomatic

Table 1. *Prevalence of chronic kidney disease (CKD) stages 1–5, as classified using the short form of the Modification of Diet in Renal Disease equation to estimate glomerular filtration rate (eGFR, based on the most recent serum creatinine concentration data), among adult patients with Fabry disease enrolled in FOS – the Fabry Outcome Survey.*

eGFR (ml/min/1.73 m^2)	CKD stage	Females (*n* = 256)	Males (*n* = 251)
> 90 and 60–89	1 and 2	202	173
30–59	3	51	44
15–29	4	0	11
< 15	5*	3	23

*Kidney transplant recipients and dialysis patients are not included.

renal disease and a significant proportion of heterozygotes with normal GFR will go on to develop signs of kidney damage, such as albuminuria, proteinuria, haematuria or specific findings on kidney biopsy, we have also included patients with an eGFR greater than 60 ml/min and no signs of kidney damage (combined CKD stages 1 and 2). A total of 132 of 507 patients (26%; 54 females, 78 males) presented with eGFR-based CKD stages 3–5. Data on albuminuria or proteinuria were available from 408

patients (adults and children; 192 females, 216 males). Figure 2 shows the most recent data on proteinuria according to age and sex in these 408 patients. Data on the presence or absence of haematuria were available from 391 patients. In total, 46 of the 196 females and 45 of the 195 males studied were reported to have haematuria.

Renal phenotype

There have been several reported cases of patients with signs and symptoms of Fabry

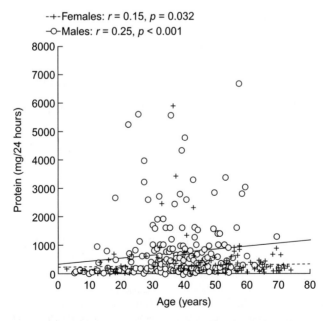

Figure 2. *Proteinuria according to age in 408 patients (216 males, 192 females) with Fabry disease enrolled in FOS – the Fabry Outcome Survey.*

disease confined to the kidneys. In some cases, however, other organ manifestations have not been excluded [15, 16]. Other reports have shown only mild renal involvement with proteinuria [17, 18], or described patients with renal variants that progressed to ESRD [19]. One report described a 20-year-old male with isolated proteinuria [20]. Family members, however, suffered from ESRD or presented with cardiac involvement. In FOS, to date, no patient has been described with disease confined to the kidneys.

Histopathology

The intracellular accumulation of glycosphingolipids is the histological hallmark of Fabry disease [21–23]. Deposition occurs primarily in the cells of blood vessel walls and, to a lesser degree, in renal glomerular and tubular epithelial cells, corneal epithelial cells, myocardial cells and ganglion cells of the autonomic nervous system, among others. The kidney is affected in all hemizygous males, as well as in many heterozygous females.

Light microscopy

In paraffin-embedded sections, glomerular visceral epithelial cells are enlarged and vacuolated, and tubules and blood vessels are also abnormal. In plastic-embedded sections of osmium-fixed tissues treated with toluidine or methylene blue, fine but darkly staining granular inclusions are present, corresponding to the vacuoles.

Immunofluorescence

Routine immunofluorescence microscopy is usually negative. In glomeruli with advanced lesions, however, immunoglobulin M and complement components (C3 and C1q) may be detectable in capillary walls and mesangial regions showing a segmental distribution and granular pattern.

Ultrastructure

Cellular inclusions within lysosomes have been described by various names, including zebra bodies, myelin figures, myelin-like figures or lamellated structures. They are surrounded by a single membrane and can be found in all cells, mainly podocytes and endothelial cells, regardless of the light microscopic features.

A recent study of 58 patients with a GFR of approximately 80 ml/min who were enrolled in a placebo-controlled trial of enzyme replacement therapy (ERT) [24] showed an extensive accumulation of Gb_3 in the kidneys before therapy [25]. The cellular inclusions varied considerably in quantity and morphology among the different cell types. Podocytes and distal tubular epithelial cells contained the highest concentrations of Gb_3, whereas proximal tubular epithelial cells were relatively unaffected. In some cell types, inclusions appeared as small, dark, dense-beaded granules; in others, they appeared as larger complex laminated bodies. There was also considerable Gb_3 accumulation in vascular endothelial cells, vascular smooth muscle cells, mesangial cells, interstitial fibroblasts and phagocytic cells of the renal cortex [25] (Figure 3).

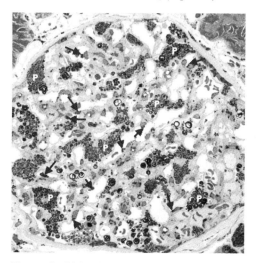

Figure 3. *Globotriaosylceramide accumulates in many cell types in the renal glomerulus as dark blue granules and scroll-like whorls, as shown here. Red arrows indicate endothelial accumulation; yellow arrows indicate mesangial cell accumulation; P, indicates podocyte accumulation (magnification, ×40 objective). Reproduced with permission from [25].*

With progression of the disease, fusion of podocyte foot processes can be observed. Focal glomerular and tubular epithelial necrosis, as well as thickening of glomerular and tubular basement membranes, were also reported [21, 26] and will finally result in segmental and global glomerulosclerosis, tubular atrophy and interstitial fibrosis [21]. In FOS, the results of biopsies of native kidneys of 19 patients (7 females, 12 males) were reported. All but two patients were reported to show lesions related to Fabry disease. The other cases were reported to present with focal segmental glomerulosclerosis (1 male aged 40 years, 1 female aged 43 years).

Renal imaging

Systematic examination of renal morphology in Fabry disease, using sonography, computed tomography or magnetic resonance imaging, was introduced recently [27, 28].

A large uncontrolled study of 122 patients showed a high prevalence of cortical and parapelvic cysts, as well as an increased echogenicity, decreased cortical thickness and decreased corticomedullary differentiation of the kidney [27]. Details of this study are given in Table 2. Another small case–control study also pointed to a high prevalence of parapelvic cysts in Fabry disease [28], as detected by computed tomography and magnetic resonance imaging (Table 3). Thus, the finding of renal cysts, especially parapelvic cysts, may suggest the presence of Fabry disease. Renal ultrasound data from 122 patients enrolled in FOS (Figure 4) confirmed these observations [29]. The analysis of FOS data did not, however, differentiate between cortical and parapelvic cysts. All three studies found an increase in the prevalence of renal cysts with age. The cause of cyst formation in Fabry disease, however, is currently unknown.

Table 2. *Prevalence of cortical and parapelvic renal cysts in patients with Fabry disease. Adapted with permission from [27].*

	Males (*n* = 76)			Females (*n* = 40)		
	US	**MRI**	**US and MRI**	**US**	**MRI**	**US and MRI**
Cortical cysts	17 (22.4%)	22 (29%)	11 (14.5%)	4 (10%)	8 (20%)	1 (2.5%)
Parapelvic cysts	11 (14.5%)	15 (19.7%)	7 (9.2%)	4 (10%)	7 (17.5%)	2 (5%)

US, ultrasound; MRI, magnetic resonance imaging.

Table 3. *Parapelvic renal cysts as detected by magnetic resonance imaging in patients with Fabry disease and matched controls. Adapted with permission from Macmillan Publishers Ltd [28].*

	Fabry disease (*n* = 24)		Matched controls (*n* = 19)	
	Cysts	**No cysts**	**Cysts**	**No cysts**
n (%)	12 (50%)	12 (50%)	1 (5.3%)	18 (94.7%)
Mean age (years)	36.3	35.8	61	33.1
Mean GFR$_{inulin}$ (ml/min)	80.3	95.9	–	–
Mean signal intensity ratio	1.47	1.18	1.14	1.10

GFR, glomerular filtration rate.

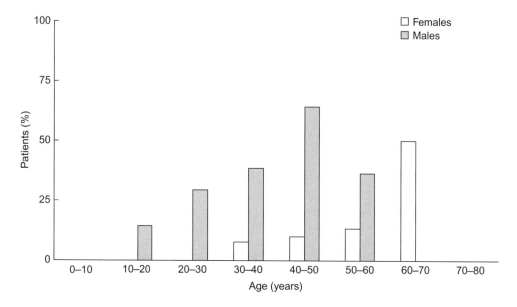

Figure 4. *Prevalence of renal cysts detected by ultrasound among 122 patients (65 males, 57 females) enrolled in FOS – the Fabry Outcome Survey – according to age and gender.*

The prevalence of simple renal cysts in the general population also increases with every decade of life (Table 4) [30]. In this context, it is worth mentioning that the occurrence of one or more simple cysts was associated with slightly reduced renal function in a population of hospitalized patients with cysts compared with patients without cysts [31]. Other causes of renal cyst formation include several inherited polycystic kidney diseases, including autosomal dominant polycystic kidney disease, autosomal recessive polycystic kidney disease, familial nephronophthisis and medullary cystic kidney disease [32], which can all lead to ESRD. In patients with ESRD, acquired cystic kidney disease (defined by the presence of three or more cysts per kidney in an individual on dialysis and the absence of an inherited polycystic kidney disease) may be present in about 10% of patients at the start of dialysis and affects a greater proportion of patients thereafter [33, 34]. The prevalence of acquired cystic kidney disease is directly related to the duration of dialysis (Figure 5), and the presence of acquired cystic kidney disease also increases the risk of renal cancer.

Table 4. *Prevalence of simple renal cysts in healthy individuals (n = 14 314). Adapted with permission from [30].*

Age range (years)	Males (n = 8703)	Females (n = 5611)
16–29	0%	0%
30–39	5.8%	3.4%
40–49	10.0%	5.7%
50–59	17.3%	9.1%
60–69	28.2%	13.4%
> 70	38.9%	28.2%
Total	**14.6%**	**7.6%**

Renal replacement therapy in patients with Fabry disease

A significant proportion of patients with Fabry disease is treated by dialysis or kidney transplantation [35]. In this context, small case series indicate that patients suffering from ESRD, either on dialysis [36, 37] or with a functioning renal graft [38], tolerate ERT very well and may even benefit from this treatment.

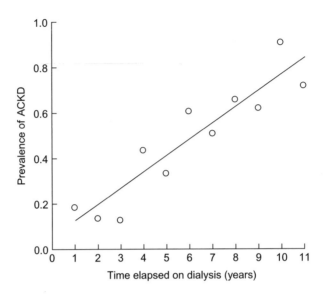

Figure 5. *Prevalence of acquired cystic kidney disease (ACKD) in patients on dialysis. Reproduced with permission from [34].*

Dialysis in Fabry disease

Before the widespread availability of dialysis, the mean age at death of hemizygous patients was 41 years [39]. Dialysis has increased life-expectancy in patients with Fabry disease [7]. However, a report on the prevalence of Fabry disease that identified 83 cases among 440 665 dialysis patients from Europe (0.0188%; 87% male) showed a less favourable 5-year survival rate of 41% in patients with Fabry disease, compared with 68% in patients with standard nephropathies [40]. Comparable data were reported by Thadhani *et al.*, who showed a similar prevalence, with 42 cases of Fabry disease among 250 352 dialysis patients enrolled in the United States Renal Data System (USRDS) (0.0167%; 88% male) [41]. In this study, the 3-year survival for patients with Fabry disease was 63%, compared with 74% for non-diabetic controls and 53% for diabetic controls.

Over the past few years, several case-finding studies have clearly shown that Fabry disease has been previously under-recognized in patients receiving dialysis. Systematic measurement of enzyme activity in whole blood, plasma, leukocytes or eluates of dried blood spots in large cohorts of dialysis patients disclosed a more than tenfold higher prevalence of Fabry disease among patients with ESRD than would be expected based on historical registry data [15, 42–48] (see also Chapter 17). It is worth mentioning that, to date, 22 patients on dialysis (4 of them after the start of ERT) are enrolled in FOS.

Kidney transplantation in Fabry disease

Some 40 years ago the first kidney transplantations in European patients with Fabry disease were performed in France in 1966 [49] and Switzerland in 1967 [50]. At this time, it was believed that renal transplantation may correct the metabolic defect in patients with Fabry disease [51–57]. This hypothesis was challenged by Clark *et al.* who suggested that the decrease in Gb_3 storage observed may reflect reduced production rather than enhanced clearance by the transplanted kidney [58]. A few years later, longitudinal studies showed that the activity of α-galactosidase A does not increase after successful kidney transplantion [59, 60].

Initially, it was thought that kidney transplantation was not justified in patients with Fabry disease [61]. One reason for this was reports of severe cardiac complications following successful kidney transplantation [62] and a high prevalence of life-threatening infectious episodes [63]; however, several case reports showed a favourable course following kidney transplantation [60, 64–70]. Recurrence of disease in the graft was rarely reported and occurred in most instances only many years after transplantation and was considered to be without major impact on patient or graft survival [71–75]. Interestingly, a study in a small series of transplanted patients with Fabry disease found an increased prevalence of activated protein C resistance associated with an increased risk of thrombosis and rejection [76].

In a study from the European Renal Association–European Dialysis and Transplant Association registry of 33 patients, graft survival at 3 years was no worse than in patients with other nephropathies (72% versus 69%), and patient survival after transplantation was comparable to that of patients under 55 years of age with standard nephropathies [40]. Excellent graft and patient survival was also reported from the USRDS registry [77, 78], Therefore, Fabry disease is currently not judged to be a contraindication for renal transplantation [35, 79, 80]. In FOS, 26 patients who had received kidney transplants (25 at entry into FOS, 1 after the start of ERT) were included at the time of this analysis.

Kidney donation from a living relative in patients with Fabry disease

Kidney donation from a living relative of a patient with Fabry disease is a very delicate issue, and clinical experience is documented in only a few case reports [49, 81–83].

Heterozygotes with normal kidney function and no outward signs and symptoms of Fabry disease, but who show evidence of extensive Gb_3 accumulation on kidney biopsy, have been recommended not to be used as donors [84]. This approach appears reasonable, because such kidneys may be prone to a rapid accumulation of glycolipids once transplanted in a hemizygous or heterozygous patient with ESRD. Furthermore, the donor may bear an increased risk of progression to ESRD. Hemizygous males should not be considered as kidney donors, even if there are no signs of kidney damage; however, they can receive a kidney from a living asymptomatic heterozygous relative (providing that kidney biopsy in the donor does not show extensive Gb_3 accumulation). However, the donation of a kidney by an asymptomatic heterozygous to a hemizygous patient may carry the risk of graft loss within a few years. Female patients with Fabry disease who have ESRD can receive a kidney from asymptomatic related heterozygotes. Receipt of a kidney from a living relative is not reported in FOS.

Conclusions

Data obtained from FOS and from other studies demonstrate that the kidney can be affected early in life, even during childhood, in males and females with Fabry disease. Progressive deterioration of renal function results in ESRD in the majority of hemizygotes at around the age of 50 years. ESRD may also be seen in some heterozygotes. Survival when on dialysis is impaired in patients with Fabry disease compared with patients with other kidney diseases; however, kidney transplantation offers comparable graft and patient survival to that observed in patients with other nephropathies. The ultimate goal of ERT and other therapies should be the prevention of disease manifestations.

References

1. Desnick RJ, Brady RO. Fabry disease in childhood. *J Pediatr* 2004;144:S20–6

2. Ries M, Ramaswami U, Parini R, Lindblad B, Whybra C, Willers I et al. The early clinical phenotype of Fabry disease: a study on 35 European children and adolescents. Eur J Pediatr 2003;162:767–72

3. Ries M, Gupta S, Moore DF, Sachdev V, Quirk JM, Murray GJ et al. Pediatric Fabry disease. Pediatrics 2005;115:e344–55

4. Whybra C, Kampmann C, Willers I, Davies J, Winchester B, Kriegsmann J et al. Anderson–Fabry disease: clinical manifestations of disease in female heterozygotes. J Inherit Metab Dis 2001;24:715–24

5. MacDermot KD, Holmes A, Miners AH. Anderson–Fabry disease: clinical manifestations and impact of disease in a cohort of 60 obligate carrier females. J Med Genet 2001;38:769–75

6. Galanos J, Nicholls K, Grigg L, Kiers L, Crawford A, Becker G. Clinical features of Fabry's disease in Australian patients. Intern Med J 2002;32:575–84

7. MacDermot KD, Holmes A, Miners AH. Anderson–Fabry disease: clinical manifestations and impact of disease in a cohort of 98 hemizygous males. J Med Genet 2001;38:750–60

8. Branton M, Schiffmann R, Kopp JB. Natural history and treatment of renal involvement in Fabry disease. J Am Soc Nephrol 2002;13 (Suppl 2):S139–43

9. Branton MH, Schiffmann R, Sabnis SG, Murray GJ, Quirk JM, Altarescu G et al. Natural history of Fabry renal disease: influence of α-galactosidase A activity and genetic mutations on clinical course. Medicine (Baltimore) 2002;81:122–38

10. Mehta A, Ricci R, Widmer U, Dehout F, Garcia de Lorenzo A, Kampmann C et al. Fabry disease defined: baseline clinical manifestations of 366 patients in the Fabry Outcome Survey. Eur J Clin Invest 2004;34:236–42

11. Levey AS. Clinical practice. Nondiabetic kidney disease. N Engl J Med 2002;347:1505–11

12. National Kidney Foundation (NKF) Kidney Disease Outcome Quality Initiative (K/DOQI) Advisory Board. K/DOQI clinical practice guidelines for chronic kidney disease: evaluation, classification, and stratification. Am J Kidney Dis 2002;39 (Suppl 2): S1–246

13. Kleinert J, Lorenz M, Hauser AC, Becherer A, Staudenherz A, Födinger M et al. Measurement of renal function in patients with Fabry disease. Acta Paediatr Suppl 2005;447:19–23

14. Rule AD, Gussak HM, Pond GR, Bergstralh EJ, Stegall MD, Cosio FG et al. Measured and estimated GFR in healthy potential kidney donors. Am J Kidney Dis 2004;43:112–19

15. Nakao S, Kodama C, Takenaka T, Tanaka A, Yasumoto Y, Yoshida A et al. Fabry disease: detection of undiagnosed hemodialysis patients and identification of a "renal variant" phenotype. Kidney Int 2003;64:801–7

16. Cybulla M, Schaefer E, Wendt S, Ling H, Krober SM, Hovelborn U et al. Chronic renal failure and proteinuria in adulthood: Fabry disease predominantly affecting the kidneys. Am J Kidney Dis 2005;45:e82–9

17. Sawada K, Mizoguchi K, Hishida A, Kaneko E, Koide Y, Nishimura K et al. Point mutation in the α-galactosidase A gene of atypical Fabry disease with only nephropathy. Clin Nephrol 1996;45:289–94

18. Germain DP, Shabbeer J, Cotigny S, Desnick RJ. Fabry disease: twenty novel α-galactosidase A mutations and genotype–phenotype correlations in classical and variant phenotypes. Mol Med 2002; 8:306–12

19. Rosenthal D, Lien YH, Lager D, Lai LW, Shang S, Leung N et al. A novel α-galactosidase a mutant (M42L) identified in a renal variant of Fabry disease. Am J Kidney Dis 2004;44:e85–9

20. Meroni M, Spisni C, Tazzari S, Di Vito R, Stingone A, Bovan I et al. Isolated glomerular proteinuria as the only clinical manifestation of Fabry's disease in an adult male. Nephrol Dial Transplant 1997;12:221–3

21. Alroy J, Sabnis S, Kopp JB. Renal pathology in Fabry disease. J Am Soc Nephrol 2002;13 (Suppl 2):S134–8

22. Cohen AH, Adler S. Fabry disease. In: Tisher CC, Brenner BM, editors. Renal pathology with clinical and functional correlations. 1st edn. Philadelphia: JB Lippincott Company; 1989. p. 1197–204

23. Bernstein J, Churg J. Heritable metabolic diseases. In: Jenette JC, Olson JL, Schwarts MM, Silva FG, editors. Heptinstall's pathology of the kidney. Philadelphia: Lippincott-Raven; 1999. p. 1289–92

24. Eng CM, Guffon N, Wilcox WR, Germain DP, Lee P, Waldek S et al. Safety and efficacy of recombinant human α-galactosidase A replacement therapy in Fabry's disease. N Engl J Med 2001;345:9–16

25. Thurberg BL, Rennke H, Colvin RB, Dikman S, Gordon RE, Collins AB et al. Globotriaosylceramide accumulation in the Fabry kidney is cleared from multiple cell types after enzyme replacement therapy. Kidney Int 2002;62:1933–46

26. Gubler MC, Lenoir G, Grunfeld JP, Ulmann A, Droz D, Habib R. Early renal changes in hemizygous and heterozygous patients with Fabry's disease. Kidney Int 1978;13:223–35

27. Glass RB, Astrin KH, Norton KI, Parsons R, Eng CM, Banikazemi M et al. Fabry disease: renal sonographic and magnetic resonance imaging findings in affected males and carrier females with the classic and cardiac variant phenotypes. J Comput Assist Tomogr 2004;28:158–68

28. Ries M, Bettis KE, Choyke P, Kopp JB, Austin HA, 3rd, Brady RO et al. Parapelvic kidney cysts: a distinguishing feature with high prevalence in Fabry disease. Kidney Int 2004;66:978–82

29. Kaiser E, Keune N, Whybra C, Kleinert J, Dehout F, Feriozzi S et al. Renal ultrasound analysis in Fabry disease: data from FOS – the Fabry Outcome Survey. Nephrol Dial Transplant 2005;20 (Suppl 5):v10

30. Terada N, Ichioka K, Matsuta Y, Okubo K, Yoshimura K, Arai Y. The natural history of simple renal cysts. J Urol 2002;167:21–3

31. Al-Said J, Brumback MA, Moghazi S, Baumgarten DA, O'Neill WC. Reduced renal function in patients with simple renal cysts. *Kidney Int* 2004;65:2303–8

32. Wilson PD. Polycystic kidney disease. *N Engl J Med* 2004;350:151–64

33. Dunnill MS, Millard PR, Oliver D. Acquired cystic disease of the kidneys: a hazard of long-term intermittent maintenance haemodialysis. *J Clin Pathol* 1977;30:868–77

34. Choyke PL. Acquired cystic kidney disease. *Eur Radiol* 2000;10:1716–21

35. Obrador GT, Ojo A, Thadhani R. End-stage renal disease in patients with Fabry disease. *J Am Soc Nephrol* 2002;13 (Suppl 2):S144–6

36. Kosch M, Koch HG, Oliveira JP, Soares C, Bianco F, Breuning F *et al.* Enzyme replacement therapy administered during hemodialysis in patients with Fabry disease. *Kidney Int* 2004;66:1279–82

37. Pisani A, Spinelli L, Sabbatini M, Andreucci MV, Procaccini D, Abbaterusso C *et al.* Enzyme replacement therapy in Fabry disease patients undergoing dialysis: effects on quality of life and organ involvement. *Am J Kidney Dis* 2005;46:120–7

38. Mignani R, Panichi V, Giudicissi A, Taccola D, Boscaro F, Feletti C *et al.* Enzyme replacement therapy with agalsidase β in kidney transplant patients with Fabry disease: a pilot study. *Kidney Int* 2004;65:1381–5

39. Colombi A, Kostyal A, Bracher R, Gloor F, Mazzi R, Tholen H. Angiokeratoma corporis diffusum - Fabry's disease. *Helv Med Acta* 1967;34:67–83

40. Tsakiris D, Simpson HK, Jones EH, Briggs JD, Elinder CG, Mendel S *et al.* Report on management of renal failure in Europe, XXVI, 1995. Rare diseases in renal replacement therapy in the ERA-EDTA Registry. *Nephrol Dial Transplant* 1996;11 (Suppl 7):4–20

41. Thadhani R, Wolf M, West ML, Tonelli M, Ruthazer R, Pastores GM *et al.* Patients with Fabry disease on dialysis in the United States. *Kidney Int* 2002;61:249–55

42. Utsumi K, Kase R, Takata T, Sakuraba H, Matsui N, Saito H *et al.* Fabry disease in patients receiving maintenance dialysis. *Clin Exp Nephrol* 2000;4:49–51

43. Linthorst GE, Hollak CE, Korevaar JC, Van Manen JG, Aerts JM, Boeschoten EW. α-Galactosidase A deficiency in Dutch patients on dialysis: a critical appraisal of screening for Fabry disease. *Nephrol Dial Transplant* 2003;18:1581–4

44. Kotanko P, Kramar R, Devrnja D, Paschke E, Voigtlander T, Auinger M *et al.* Results of a nation-wide screening for Anderson–Fabry disease among dialysis patients. *J Am Soc Nephrol* 2004;15:1323–9

45. Bekri S, Enica A, Ghafari T, Plaza G, Champenois I, Choukroun G *et al.* Fabry disease in patients with end-stage renal failure: the potential benefits of screening. *Nephron Clin Pract* 2005;101:c33–8

46. Desnick RJ. Fabry disease: unrecognized ESRD patients and effectiveness of enzyme replacement therapy on renal pathology and function. *J Inherit Metab Dis* 2002;25 (Suppl 1):116

47. Ichinose M, Nakayama M, Ohashi T, Utsunomiya Y, Kobayashi M, Eto Y. Significance of screening for Fabry disease among male dialysis patients. *Clin Exp Nephrol* 2005;9:228–32

48. Spada M, Pagliardini S. Screening for Fabry disease in end-stage nephropathies. *J Inherit Metab Dis* 2002;25 (Suppl 1):113

49. Grünfeld JP, Le Porrier M, Droz D, Bensaude I, Hinglais N, Crosnier J. [Renal transplantation in patients suffering from Fabry's disease. Kidney transplantation from an heterozygote subject to a subject without Fabry's disease]. *Nouv Presse Med* 1975;4:2081–5

50. Bühler FR, Thiel G, Dubach UC, Enderlin F, Gloor F, Tholen H. Kidney transplantation in Fabry's disease. *Br Med J* 1973;3:28–9

51. Philippart M, Franklin SS, Gordon A. Reversal of an inborn sphingolipidosis (Fabry's disease) by kidney transplantation. *Ann Intern Med* 1972;77:195–200

52. Krivit W, Desnick RJ, Bernlohr RW, Wold F, Najarian JS, Simmons RL. Enzyme transplantation in Fabry's disease. *N Engl J Med* 1972;287:1248–9

53. Desnick RJ, Raman M, Allen KY, Desnick SJ, Simmons RL, Anderson CF *et al.* Enzyme therapy in Fabry's disease by renal transplantation. *Proc Clin Dial Transplant Forum* 1972;2:27–35

54. Desnick RJ, Allen KY, Simmons RL, Woods JE, Anderson CF, Najarian JS *et al.* Fabry disease: correction of the enzymatic deficiency by renal transplantation. *Birth Defects Orig Artic Ser* 1973; 9:88–96

55. Philippart M. Fabry disease: kidney transplantation as an enzyme replacement technic. *Birth Defects Orig Artic Ser* 1973;9:81–7

56. Philippart M, Franklin SS, Leeber DA, Hull AR, Peters PC. Kidney transplantation in Fabry's disease. *N Engl J Med* 1973;289:270–1

57. Najarian JS, Desnick RJ, Simmons RL, Krivit W. Correction of enzymatic deficiencies by renal transplantation: Fabry's disease. *Bull Soc Int Chir* 1975;34:1–10

58. Clarke JT, Guttmann RD, Wolfe LS, Beaudoin JG, Morehouse DD. Enzyme replacement therapy by renal allotransplantation in Fabry's disease. *N Engl J Med* 1972;287:1215–18

59. Spence MW, MacKinnon KE, Burgess JK, d'Entremont DM, Belitsky P, Lannon SG *et al.* Failure to correct the metabolic defect by renal allo-transplantion in Fabry's disease. *Ann Intern Med* 1976;84:13–16

60. Donati D, Novario R, Gastaldi L. Natural history and treatment of uremia secondary to Fabry's disease: an European experience. *Nephron* 1987;46:353–9

61. Renal transplantation in congenital and metabolic diseases. A report from the ASC/NIH renal transplant registry. *JAMA* 1975;232:148–53

62. Kramer W, Thormann J, Mueller K, Frenzel H. Progressive cardiac involvement by Fabry's disease despite successful renal allotransplantation. *Int J Cardiol* 1985;7:72–5

63. Maizel SE, Simmons RL, Kjellstrand C, Fryd DS. Ten-year experience in renal transplantation for Fabry's disease. *Transplant Proc* 1981;13:57–9

64. Jacky E. [Fabry's disease (angiokeratoma corporis diffusum universale): benign course after kidney transplantation]. *Schweiz Med Wochenschr* 1976; 106:703–9

65. Sheth KJ, Roth DA, Adams MB. Early renal failure in Fabry's disease. *Am J Kidney Dis* 1983;2:651–4

66. Friedlaender MM, Kopolovic J, Rubinger D, Silver J, Drukker A, Ben-Gershon Z et al. Renal biopsy in Fabry's disease eight years after successful renal transplantation. *Clin Nephrol* 1987;27:206–11

67. Peces R, Aguado S, Fernandez F, Gago E, Gomez E, Marin R et al. Renal transplantation in Fabry's disease. *Nephron* 1989;51:294–5

68. Mazzarella V, Splendiani G, Tozzo C, Tisone G, Pisani F, Iaria G et al. Renal transplantation in patients with hereditary kidney disease: our experience. *Contrib Nephrol* 1997;122:203–6

69. Erten Y, Ozdemir FN, Demirhan B, Karakayali H, Demirag A, Akkoc H. A case of Fabry's disease with normal kidney function at 10 years after successful renal transplantation. *Transplant Proc* 1998;30:842–3

70. Mignani R, Gerra D, Maldini L, Bignardi L, Casanova S, Cambi V et al. Long-term survival of patients with renal transplantation in Fabry's disease. *Contrib Nephrol* 2001:229–33

71. Faraggiana T, Churg J, Grishman E, Strauss L, Prado A, Bishop DF et al. Light- and electron-microscopic histochemistry of Fabry's disease. *Am J Pathol* 1981;103:247–62

72. Mosnier JF, Degott C, Bedrossian J, Molas G, Degos F, Pruna A et al. Recurrence of Fabry's disease in a renal allograft eleven years after successful renal transplantation. *Transplantation* 1991;51:759–62

73. Sessa A, Meroni M, Battini G, Maglio A, Nebuloni M, Tosoni A et al. Renal transplantation in patients with Fabry disease. *Nephron* 2002;91:348–51

74. Gantenbein H, Bruder E, Burger HR, Briner J, Binswanger U. Recurrence of Fabry's disease in a renal allograft 14 years after transplantation. *Nephrol Dial Transplant* 1995;10:287–9

75. Van Loo A, Vanholder R, Madsen K, Praet M, Kint J, De Paepe A et al. Novel frameshift mutation in a heterozygous woman with Fabry disease and end-stage renal failure. *Am J Nephrol* 1996;16:352–7

76. Friedman GS, Wik D, Silva L, Abdou JC, Meier-Kriesche HU, Kaplan B et al. Allograft loss in renal transplant recipients with Fabry's disease and activated protein C resistance. *Transplantation* 2000;69:2099–102

77. Nissenson AR, Port FK. Outcome of end-stage renal disease in patients with rare causes of renal failure. I. Inherited and metabolic disorders. *Q J Med* 1989; 73:1055–62

78. Ojo A, Meier-Kriesche HU, Friedman G, Hanson J, Cibrik D, Leichtman A et al. Excellent outcome of renal transplantation in patients with Fabry's disease. *Transplantation* 2000;69:2337–9

79. Groth CG, Ringdén O. Transplantation in relation to the treatment of inherited disease. *Transplantation* 1984;38:319–27

80. Ramos EL, Tisher CC. Recurrent diseases in the kidney transplant. *Am J Kidney Dis* 1994;24:142–54

81. Puliyanda DP, Wilcox WR, Bunnapradist S, Nast CC, Jordan SC. Fabry disease in a renal allograft. *Am J Transplant* 2003;3:1030–2

82. Popli S, Molnar ZV, Leehey DJ, Daugirdas JT, Roth DA, Adams MB et al. Involvement of renal allograft by Fabry's disease. *Am J Nephrol* 1987;7:316–18

83. Schweitzer EJ, Drachenberg CB, Bartlett ST. Living kidney donor and recipient evaluation in Fabry's disease. *Transplantation* 1992;54:924–7

84. Wüthrich RP, Weinreich T, Binswanger U, Gloor HJ, Candinas D, Hailemariam S. Should living related kidney transplantation be considered for patients with renal failure due to Fabry's disease? *Nephrol Dial Transplant* 1998;13:2934–6

22 Neurological manifestations of Fabry disease

Raphael Schiffmann[1] and David F Moore[2]

[1]*Developmental and Metabolic Neurology Branch, National Institute of Neurological Disorders and Stroke, Building 10, Room 3D03, National Institutes of Health, Bethesda, Maryland 20892-1260, USA;* [2]*Section of Neurology, Department of Internal Medicine, University of Manitoba, Winnipeg, Canada*

The neurological manifestations of Fabry disease include both peripheral nervous system and CNS involvement, with globotriaosylceramide accumulation found in Schwann cells and dorsal root ganglia together with deposits in CNS neurones. The main involvement of the CNS is attributable to cerebrovasculopathy, with an increased incidence of stroke. The abnormal neuronal accumulation of glyco-sphingolipid appears to have little clinical effect on the natural history of Fabry disease, with the possible exception of some reported mild cognitive abnormalities. The pathogenesis of Fabry vasculopathy remains poorly understood, but probably relates, in part, to abnormal functional control of the vessels, secondary to endo-thelial dysfunction as a consequence of α-galactosidase A deficiency. Obstructive vasculopathy, either primarily due to accumulation of glycolipid or secondary to consequent inflammation and confounding vascular risk factors, may develop in response to abnormal endothelial and vessel wall function, similar in some respects to that observed with accumulation of cholesterol-laden lipids during atherosclerosis. Involvement of the peripheral nervous system affects mainly small Aδ and C fibres, and is probably causally related to the altered autonomic function and neuropathic pain found in Fabry disease. Other related neurological problems include hypohidrosis and other abnormalities associated with nervous system dysfunction.

Vasculopathy and stroke

The initial feature related to a blood vessel abnormality to be recognized in Fabry disease was angiokeratoma [1]. Although stroke was not mentioned in the original description of Fabry disease, this complication has been known for some time [2, 3]. In the CNS, vascular involvement has been well documented in the vertebrobasilar system and carotid circulation, but is thought to be more common in the vertebrobasilar or posterior circulation [4–7]. As a result, many neurological deficits may occur in a patient with Fabry disease. These include hemiparesis,

vertigo/dizziness, diplopia, dysarthria, nystagmus, nausea/vomiting, headaches, hemiataxia and dysmetria, cerebellar gait ataxia and, very rarely, cerebral haemorrhage [4]. Psychiatric behaviour and dementia have also been attributed to cerebral vasculopathy [8, 9]. Recent findings show that about 2–4% of patients with stroke in the general population aged 18–55 years have Fabry disease [10].

The cerebral vasculopathy of Fabry disease can be conveniently categorized into large- and small-vessel disease [4, 5]. Large-vessel

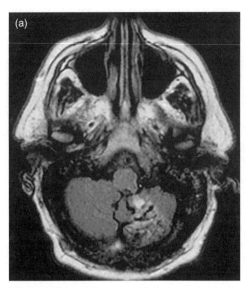 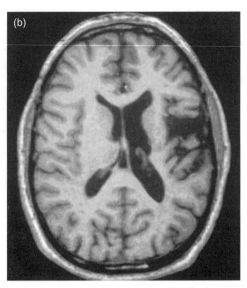

Figure 1. *Magnetic resonance image of a lesion caused by a large intracranial vessel occlusion in a patient with Fabry disease. (a) Left cerebellar hemisphere stroke caused by a vertebral artery occlusion (fluid-attenuated inversion recovery magnetic resonance image). (b) A left middle cerebral stroke in the area of the central sulcus (T1-weighted image).*

stroke is usually caused by occlusion or thrombosis of large intracranial vessels (Figure 1), although embolic strokes may also occur. As with typical vascular occlusions, stroke in Fabry disease is best seen by cranial magnetic resonance imaging (MRI) [11, 12]. Cerebral angiography is the 'gold standard' technique for demonstrating vessel obstruction. Magnetic resonance angiography, a non-invasive technique, has also been utilized (Figure 2) [13]. However, the false-positive rate for detection of intracranial stenosis is about 30% (M Chimowitz, personal communication). Another indicator of the susceptibility to large intracranial vessel disease is the frequently associated finding of dolichoectasia or the elongation and dilation of the affected vessel. This usually involves the basilar artery [4], although the carotid artery may also be affected (Figure 3).

Patients with Fabry disease present more commonly with small-vessel disease, either as a cause of symptomatic stroke or as clinically silent lesions found on neuroimaging, although radiological–pathological correlation studies remain to be carried out. These presumed small-vessel lesions are best seen on T2-weighted or fluid-attenuated inversion recovery (FLAIR) MRI (Figure 4). The lesions predominate in the white matter, mostly in the posterior periventricular and centrum semiovale region and are more prevalent with increasing age [5, 7, 14].

The mechanism by which α-galactosidase A deficiency and glycolipid accumulation causes this vasculopathy is not completely understood. We have hypothesized that Fabry vasculopathy is associated with abnormalities of blood components, blood flow and the vessel wall (Virchow's triad), leading to vascular dysfunction. The finding of increased soluble intercellular adhesion molecule-1, vascular cell adhesion molecule-1, P-selectin and plasminogen activator inhibitor and decreased thrombomodulin combined with increased monocyte CD11b expression confirms a prothrombotic state in Fabry disease [15]. Dysfunction of the cerebrovascular circulation has been shown in a number of studies using imaging end-

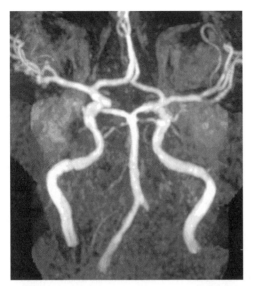

Figure 2. *Magnetic resonance angiogram, showing occlusion of the left vertebral artery in a patient with Fabry disease.*

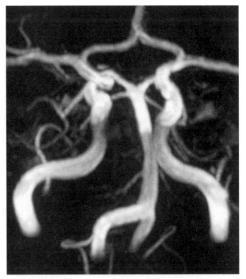

Figure 3. *Dolichoectasia: magnetic resonance angiogram, showing dilation of the carotid arteries and, to a lesser extent, the basilar artery.*

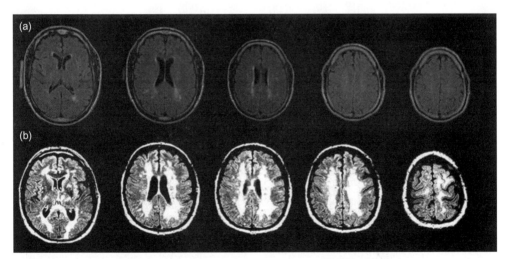

Figure 4. *(a) Serial axial fluid-attenuated inversion recovery (FLAIR) magnetic resonance image, demonstrating the posterior and periventricular predominance of Fabry leukoencephalopathy. (b) Serial axial FLAIR images of a patient with severe Fabry leukoencephalopathy, demonstrating grossly abnormal confluent white matter signal abnormality consistent with advanced disease. Both patients were clinically asymptomatic. Reproduced with permission from [5].*

points, such as cerebral perfusion (ml/100 g tissue/minute), cerebral blood flow velocity (cm/second) and cerebrovascular reactivity [5–7, 13, 16–20]. These studies found significant cerebral hyperperfusion in patients with Fabry disease compared with controls, predominantly in the posterior cerebral circulation. Hyperperfusion does not exist systemically, as indicated by normal cardiac output found in patients with Fabry disease compared with controls [16]. Interestingly, using post-ischaemic perfusion measurements, another group has shown a decreased hyperaemia in the forearm but an exaggerated hyperperfusion in the skin [21]. This finding suggests heterogeneity in the response to glycolipid storage of different vascular beds. We have subsequently demonstrated that cerebral hyperperfusion is a vascular phenomenon and not caused by neuronal overactivity [5].

Cerebral hyperperfusion is also associated with calcifications (end-organ damage) in the cerebral white matter and in the pulvinar or posterior thalamic regions (Figures 5 and 6) [6, 22]. There are also indications of abnormalities of cerebrovascular autoregulation and vasoreactivity [17, 23]. One can conclude from the above findings that Fabry disease has all

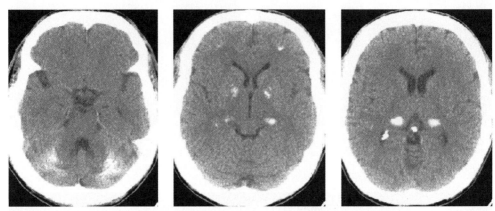

Figure 5. *Selected axial computed tomography scans, demonstrating dystrophic calcification of the subcortical arcuate fibres, globus pallidus, pulvinar and cerebellar corticomedullary junction in a severely affected patient with Fabry disease. Reproduced with permission from [6].*

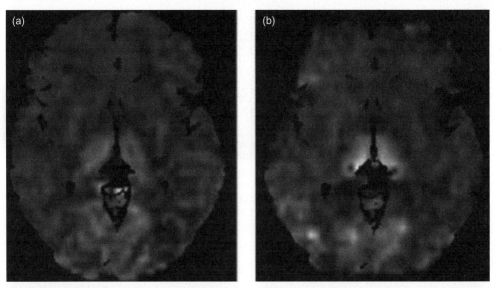

Figure 6. *Direct axial arterial spin tagging magnetic resonance images, demonstrating a relative increase in cerebral blood flow in the thalamus and posterior circulation at the anterior and posterior commissure plane in a patient (a) without and (b) with pulvinar calcifications (see right-hand panel of Figure 5). The dark thalamic regions in the pulvinar in (b) correspond to the damaged mineralized areas in the midst of the still hyperperfused pulvinar region. Reproduced with permission from [6].*

the features of a classic vasculopathy, in that there are abnormalities related to blood components, abnormalities related to blood flow and abnormalities related to the vessel wall, as shown by the disturbances in vasoreactivity and autoregulation.

We have also demonstrated an increased endothelium-dependent vascular reactivity to acetylcholine in the forearm vascular bed. This was still present after infusion of a competitive inhibitor of arginine, indicating an alteration in the function of non-nitric oxide pathways [20]. These findings, and the presence of dolichoectasia, led us to test the hypothesis that the vascular dysfunction in Fabry disease is due to increased release of reactive oxygen species, leading to increased oxidative stress and peroxynitrite formation, potentially resulting in persistent vasodilation [16]. Support for this hypothesis was indicated by the increased staining for 3-nitrotyrosine in dermal and cerebral blood vessels and in the increased nitrotyrosine and myeloperoxidase levels in the blood of patients with Fabry disease compared with controls [16, 19]. Using arterial spin tagging and MRI, we found an altered reactivity of the cerebral vasculature to ascorbate infusion, coupled with low blood levels of ascorbate, in patients with Fabry disease [19]. The decreased response to ascorbate may be caused by excessive release of reactive oxygen species. The reason for excessive production of reactive oxygen species in Fabry disease is unclear, but may be related to glycolipid accumulation altering endothelial caveolar function and mechano-transduction of arterial wall shear stress [24]. Excess $O_2 \cdot^-$ could react with nitric oxide (NO) to form peroxynitrite ($ONOO^-$) or dismutate to form H_2O_2, the putative endothelial-dependent hyperpolarizing factor. Both $O_2 \cdot^-$ and $ONOO^-$ cause dilation of the cerebral vasculature, suggesting that excess reactive oxygen species could not only lead to continued vasodilation but also to increased vulnerability to other vascular dysfunction, such as superimposed atherosclerosis [25].

Elevated levels of myeloperoxidase in the blood may also be related to the recent observation that atherosclerosis is accelerated in patients with Fabry disease. Indeed, we increasingly observe premature fixed coronary artery and cerebral artery disease in patients with Fabry disease [26]. Five of 26 patients (20%) who participated in our original pivotal trial developed complications of athero-sclerosis in their 40s [26]. Our findings in patients with Fabry disease (authors' un-published data) were recently confirmed by another group in an animal model, who found that α-galactosidase A deficiency accelerates atherosclerosis in mice deficient in apolipo-protein E [27]. These authors also found increased staining for 3-nitrotyrosine in aortic lesions and increased inducible NO synthase expression in vessel wall macrophages.

As not all patients with Fabry disease develop cerebral lesions, we were interested in identifying potential genetic modifiers of this process. In a prospective observational study, we evaluated 57 consecutive Fabry hemizygous male patients for brain FLAIR MRI lesions. We found that the -174G/C polymorphism of interleukin 6, the G894T polymorphism of endothelial NO synthase, the factor V G1691A mutation as well as the G79A and the A-13G polymorphisms of protein Z, but not the prothrombin G20210A variant or the methylenetetrahydrofolate reductase C677T, were significantly assoc-iated with cerebral lesions. These data suggest a relationship between a number of prothrombotic gene polymorphisms and the presumptive ischaemic small-vessel cerebral lesions in Fabry disease. This indicates that endogenous proteins may modulate cerebral vasculopathy in Fabry disease and will potentially allow the prospective identification of patients who are most at risk of developing these complications. Such complications are likely to be associated with a concomitant increase in oxidative stress and accelerated atherosclerosis, especially in genotypically susceptible individuals.

Peripheral neuropathy and hypohidrosis

The peripheral neuropathy in Fabry disease manifests as neuropathic pain, reduced cold and warm sensation and, possibly, gastro-intestinal disturbances. Patients with Fabry disease begin having pain towards the end of the first decade of life or during puberty [28, 29]. Children as young as 6 years of age have complained of pain, often associated with febrile illnesses, with reduced heat and exercise tolerance [30]. The patients describe the pain as burning, often associated with a deep aching sensation, or paraesthesiae. Some patients also have joint pain. Most of the 60–80% of patients with Fabry disease who develop neuropathic pain do so by the age of 20 years. Female heterozygotes may also develop neuropathic pain, with the same range of age at onset and clinical character-istics [31, 32]. In general, neuropathic pain in Fabry disease can be continuous or consist of episodic attacks brought about by changes in body or ambient temperature, as well as other stressful situations.

The neuropathy of Fabry disease is as-sociated with significantly increased cold and warm detection thresholds in the hands and feet [33, 34]. They are measured using a well-established biophysical quantitative sensory testing technique [35]. In addition, this neuropathy is associated with severe loss of intra-epidermal innervation at the ankle and, to a lesser extent, at the distal thigh [36]. Patients also have a reduced tolerance to exposure of their limbs to a cold challenge [37]. The findings described below indicate that Fabry disease is associated with a length-dependent peripheral neuropathy affecting predominantly the small myelinated (Aδ) fibres and unmyelinated (C) fibres. The mechanism of this neuropathy is unknown. In general, ischaemia of nerves caused by glycolipid accumulation in the vasa nervorum or an intrinsic nerve dysfunction have been suggested as potential causal mechanisms [33, 37, 38].

In patients with Fabry disease who have normal renal function, the only nerve conduction abnormality is an increased incidence of median nerve entrapment at the wrist (carpal tunnel syndrome). Although usually in the normal range, nerve conduc-tion parameters are significantly impaired compared with controls [34]. One group found nerve conduction of sympathetic skin responses to be generally preserved but of a lower amplitude [34]. The vibration threshold is usually normal in the feet, but some patients show an elevated threshold affecting the hands only, probably due to median nerve entrapment at the wrist [33]. However, another group found that vibration thresholds were significantly impaired in the distal forearm and hands [34]. Pathological examination of peripheral nerves (such as the sural nerve) typically shows a normal number of large myelinated fibres, but there is significant loss of unmyelinated fibres (Figure 7) [36, 39–42]. Groups of denervated Schwann cells can also be found. Glycolipid deposits are seen in the perineurium, as well as in the endothelial cells (Figure 7). The lipid deposits in sensory ganglia have been associated with the peripheral neuropathy itself as well as the neuropathic pain of Fabry disease [38, 40, 43, 44]. This abnormality is also seen in heterozygous females [44].

Most of the patients who suffer from neuropathic pain also have a deficiency in eccrine sweat gland function, but a one-to-one relationship between these symptoms has not been established [45]. As a result of eccrine sweat gland dysfunction, children and young adults often complain of poor exercise tolerance, resulting from lack of sweating and severe neuropathic pain [28, 29]. Patients with neuropathic pain also tend to have lower residual enzyme activity, and have mutations that lead to non-conservative amino acid substitution or to stop codons [46]. The sweating deficiency can be demon-strated using a global sweat test, the thermoregulatory sweat test [47–49], or by an

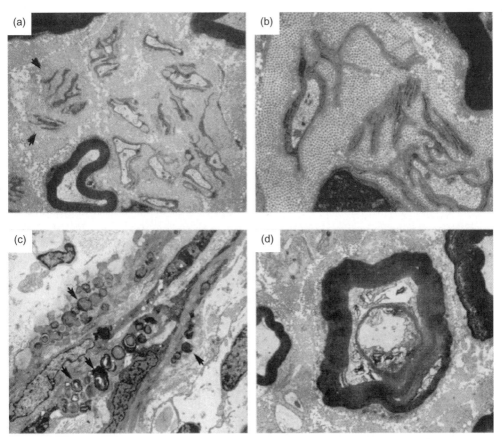

Figure 7. *Electron micrographs of sural nerve biopsy specimens from patients with Fabry disease. (a) Field of unmyelinated fibres with numerous denervated Schwann cells. A cluster of denervated Schwann cells appears at the left (arrows). (b) Several denervated Schwann cells at higher magnification, with two normal unmyelinated axons remaining. The perineurium of the nerves from the patients with Fabry disease typically has prominent lipid inclusions (c; arrows), but no lipid inclusions are present within the endoneurium (not shown). Although there is no detectable loss of large myelinated fibres in patients with Fabry disease who have preserved renal function, rare degenerating large fibres were seen (d). Reproduced with permission from [36].*

iontophoresis method using acetylcholine [45]. One recently developed form of the latter test is the quantitative sudomotor axon reflex test [50], which has shown a marked reduction in sweat output in adults and children with Fabry disease [28, 51].

Involvement of the dorsal root ganglions of the peripheral nervous system and sympathetic nervous system was previously thought to cause anhidrosis or hypohidrosis [38, 52]. Staining of dermal nerve endings for a pan-neuronal protein such as protein gene

product 9.5, however, demonstrated no decrease in the density of sweat gland innervation (Figure 8) [53]. Skin biopsies of patients with Fabry disease show the presence of sweat glands containing lipid inclusions, particularly in the myoepithelial cells [54–56]. The lack of nerve or sweat gland loss, normal neurophysiological testing [55], the non-neuropathic distribution of hypohidrosis [45] and the presence of storage material in sweat glands [54] indicate that a dysfunction of the glands, rather then a destructive process, plays a major role in

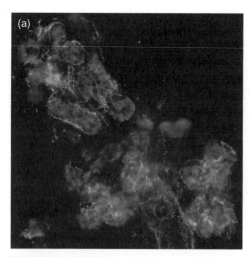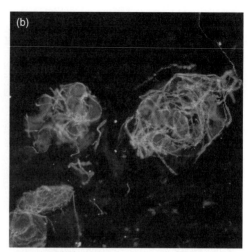

Figure 8. *Innervation of sweat glands. Representative staining of sweat glands in a punch skin biopsy at a site near the hip with protein gene product 9.5 (PGP 9.5) antibodies (a) in a control individual and (b) in an age-matched patient with Fabry disease. The staining density in the patient is at least as great as in the control, indicating no disturbance of innervation of the sweat glands in Fabry disease. Reproduced with permission from [53].*

the hypohidrosis of Fabry disease. Acute improvement in sweating 24–48 hours after intravenous administration of α-galactosidase A (agalsidase alfa) also supports the functional impairment of sweat glands in patients with Fabry disease [51]. Some authors have suggested that both the peripheral neuropathy and the hypohidrosis of Fabry disease are caused by an ischaemic process [57, 58]. Although the vascular elements supplying these systems contain storage material [54], the clinical, physiological and pathological characteristics of these disturbances do not support such a mechanism. Furthermore, blood flow to the skin was not found to be reduced in patients compared with controls [21].

Some of the manifestations of Fabry disease have been attributed to autonomic neuropathy [45]. There is no evidence of a global autonomic abnormality in Fabry disease, with normal plasma adrenaline and noradrenaline as well as preserved skin sympathetic responses [20, 33]. However, there are reports of significant orthostatic hypotension and syncope in patients with Fabry dis-

ease [59–61]. Some authors consider the abnormality of vasomotor control in Fabry disease to be an indication of a dysfunction of the autonomic nervous system [23, 62].

Despite these pathological abnormalities, the precise mechanism of neuropathic pain is unknown. It is likely that the increased levels of globotriaosylceramide in extra-lysosomal membranous compartments interfere with the function of critical proteins, such as ion channels. In general, neuropathic pain, whether of peripheral or central origin, is characterized by a neuronal hyperexcitability in damaged areas of the nervous system [63]. In peripheral neuropathic pain, damaged nerve endings exhibit abnormal spontaneous and increased evoked activity, partly due to an increased and novel expression of sodium channels [64]. The peripheral hyperexcitability may also be due to molecular changes at the level of the peripheral nociceptor, in dorsal root ganglia, in the dorsal horn of the spinal cord and in the brain [65]. These changes include abnormal expression and distribution of sodium channels [66], abnormal responses to endogenous pain-producing substances and cytokines (e.g. tumour necrosis factor), and an alteration of calcium influx into cells [65]. The neuronal hyperexcitability and corresponding molecular changes in neuropathic pain have many features in common with the cellular changes in certain forms of epilepsy [67]. This has led to the use of anticonvulsant drugs for the treatment of Fabry neuropathic pain, with some therapeutic efficacy [68, 69]. The mechanisms by which accumulated globotriaosylceramide causes nerve dysfunction, however, is not clear.

Conclusions

Recent years have brought a better understanding of the mechanism of the vasculopathy of Fabry disease. The data described above clearly show that the old dogma that ischaemic cerebral lesions in Fabry disease are due to bulging lipid-laden vascular endothelial cells encroaching upon the vessel lumen is incorrect. Although the exact mechanism is still poorly understood, it is likely to involve an interaction between the accumulating glycolipids and specific cellular proteins, leading to their dysfunction. The pathogenesis of the peripheral neuropathy and the pain that is associated with Fabry disease is even less well understood than that of the vasculopathy. Better awareness of the disease processes should lead to improved management of this disorder.

References

1. Anderson W. A case of "angeio-keratoma". *Br J Dermatol* 1898;10:113–17

2. Brown A, Mikne J. Diffuse angiokeratoma: report of two cases with diffuse skin changes, one with neurological symptoms and splenomegaly. *Glasgow J Med* 1952;33:361

3. Bethune J, Landrigan P, Chipman C. Angiokeratoma corporis diffusum (Fabry's disease in two brothers). *N Engl J Med* 1961;264:1280

4. Mitsias P, Levine SR. Cerebrovascular complications of Fabry's disease. *Ann Neurol* 1996;40:8–17

5. Moore DF, Altarescu G, Barker WC, Patronas NJ, Herscovitch P, Schiffmann R. White matter lesions in Fabry disease occur in 'prior' selectively hypometabolic and hyperperfused brain regions. *Brain Res Bull* 2003;62:231–40

6. Moore DF, Ye F, Schiffmann R, Butman JA. Increased signal intensity in the pulvinar on T1-weighted images: a pathognomonic MR imaging sign of Fabry disease. *Am J Neuroradiol* 2003;24:1096–101

7. Moore DF, Herscovitch P, Schiffmann R. Selective arterial distribution of cerebral hyperperfusion in Fabry disease. *J Neuroimaging* 2001;11:303–7

8. Mendez MF, Stanley TM, Medel NM, Li Z, Tedesco DT. The vascular dementia of Fabry's disease. *Dement Geriatr Cogn Disord* 1997;8:252–7

9. Liston EH, Levine MD, Philippart M. Psychosis in Fabry disease and treatment with phenoxybenzamine. *Arch Gen Psychiatry* 1973;29:402–3

10. Rolfs A, Bottcher T, Zschiesche M, Morris P, Winchester B, Bauer P et al. Prevalence of Fabry disease in patients with cryptogenic stroke: a prospective study. *Lancet* 2005;366:1794–6

11. Morgan SH, Rudge P, Smith SJ, Bronstein AM, Kendall BE, Holly E et al. The neurological complications of Anderson–Fabry disease (α-galactosidase A deficiency) – investigation of symptomatic and presymptomatic patients. *Q J Med* 1990;75:491–507

12. Grewal RP, McLatchey SK. Cerebrovascular manifestations in a female carrier of Fabry's disease. *Acta Neurol Belg* 1992;92:36–40

13. Moore DF, Altarescu G, Ling GS, Jeffries N, Frei KP, Weibel T et al. Elevated cerebral blood flow velocities in Fabry disease with reversal after enzyme replacement. *Stroke* 2002;33:525–31

14. Crutchfield KE, Patronas NJ, Dambrosia JM, Frei KP, Banerjee TK, Barton NW et al. Quantitative analysis of cerebral vasculopathy in patients with Fabry disease. *Neurology* 1998;50:1746–9

15. DeGraba T, Azhar S, Dignat-George F, Brown E, Boutiere B, Altarescu G et al. Profile of endothelial and leukocyte activation in Fabry patients. *Ann Neurol* 2000;47:229–33

16. Moore DF, Scott LT, Gladwin MT, Altarescu G, Kaneski C, Suzuki K et al. Regional cerebral hyperperfusion and nitric oxide pathway dysregulation in Fabry disease: reversal by enzyme replacement therapy. *Circulation* 2001;104:1506–12

17. Moore DF, Altarescu G, Herscovitch P, Schiffmann R. Enzyme replacement reverses abnormal cerebrovascular responses in Fabry disease. *BMC Neurol* 2002;2:4

18. Moore DF, Schiffmann R, Ulug AM. Elevated CNS average diffusion constant in Fabry disease. *Acta Paediatr Suppl* 2002;439:67–8

19. Moore DF, Ye F, Brennan ML, Gupta S, Barshop BA, Steiner RD et al. Ascorbate decreases Fabry cerebral hyperperfusion suggesting a reactive oxygen species abnormality: an arterial spin tagging study. *J Magn Reson Imaging* 2004;20:674–83

20. Altarescu G, Moore DF, Pursley R, Campia U, Goldstein S, Bryant M et al. Enhanced endothelium-dependent vasodilation in Fabry disease. *Stroke* 2001;32:1559–62

21. Stemper B, Hilz MJ. Postischemic cutaneous hyperperfusion in the presence of forearm hypoperfusion suggests sympathetic vasomotor dysfunction in Fabry disease. *J Neurol* 2003;250:970–6

22. Takanashi J, Barkovich AJ, Dillon WP, Sherr EH, Hart KA, Packman S. T1 hyperintensity in the pulvinar: key imaging feature for diagnosis of Fabry disease. *AJNR Am J Neuroradiol* 2003;24:916–21

23. Hilz MJ, Kolodny EH, Brys M, Stemper B, Haendl T, Marthol H. Reduced cerebral blood flow velocity and impaired cerebral autoregulation in patients with Fabry disease. *J Neurol* 2004;251:564–70

24. Laurindo FR, Pedro Mde A, Barbeiro HV, Pileggi F, Carvalho MH, Augusto O et al. Vascular free radical release. *Ex vivo* and *in vivo* evidence for a flow-dependent endothelial mechanism. *Circ Res* 1994;74:700–9

25. Wei EP, Kontos HA, Beckman JS. Mechanisms of cerebral vasodilation by superoxide, hydrogen peroxide, and peroxynitrite. *Am J Physiol* 1996; 271:H1262–6

26. Schiffmann R, Rapkiewicz A, Abu-Asab M, Ries M, Askari H, Tsokos M et al. Pathological findings in a patient with Fabry disease who died after 2.5 years of enzyme replacement. *Virchows Arch* 2005;448:1–7

27. Bodary PF, Shen Y, Vargas FB, Bi X, Ostenso KA, Gu S et al. α-galactosidase A deficiency accelerates atherosclerosis in mice with apolipoprotein E deficiency. *Circulation* 2005;111:629–32

28. Ries M, Gupta S, Moore DF, Sachdev V, Quirk JM, Murray GJ et al. Pediatric Fabry disease. *Pediatrics* 2005;115:e344–55

29. Ries M, Ramaswami U, Parini R, Lindblad B, Whybra C, Willers I et al. The early clinical phenotype of Fabry disease: a study on 35 European children and adolescents. *Eur J Pediatr* 2003;162:767–72

30. Mehta A, Ricci R, Widmer U, Dehout F, Garcia de Lorenzo A, Kampmann C et al. Fabry disease defined: baseline clinical manifestations of 366 patients in the Fabry Outcome Survey. *Eur J Clin Invest* 2004;34:236–42

31. MacDermot J, MacDermot KD. Neuropathic pain in Anderson–Fabry disease: pathology and therapeutic options. *Eur J Pharmacol* 2001;429:121–5

32. Whybra C, Wendrich K, Ries M, Gal A, Beck M. Clinical manifestation in female Fabry disease patients. *Contrib Nephrol* 2001;245–50

33. Luciano CA, Russell JW, Banerjee TK, Quirk JM, Scott LJ, Dambrosia JM et al. Physiological characterization of neuropathy in Fabry's disease. *Muscle Nerve* 2002;26:622–9

34. Dutsch M, Marthol H, Stemper B, Brys M, Haendl T, Hilz MJ. Small fiber dysfunction predominates in Fabry neuropathy. *J Clin Neurophysiol* 2002;19:575–86

35. Dyck PJ, O'Brien PC, Kosanke JL, Gillen DA, Karnes JL. A 4, 2, and 1 stepping algorithm for quick and accurate estimation of cutaneous sensation threshold. *Neurology* 1993;43:1508–12

36. Scott LJ, Griffin JW, Luciano C, Barton NW, Banerjee T, Crawford T et al. Quantitative analysis of epidermal innervation in Fabry disease. *Neurology* 1999; 52:1249–54

37. Hilz MJ, Stemper B, Kolodny EH. Lower limb cold exposure induces pain and prolonged small fiber dysfunction in Fabry patients. *Pain* 2000;84:361–5

38. Gadoth N, Sandbank U. Involvement of dorsal root ganglia in Fabry's disease. *J Med Genet* 1983; 20:309–12

39. Sima AA, Robertson DM. Involvement of peripheral nerve and muscle in Fabry's disease. Histologic, ultrastructural, and morphometric studies. *Arch Neurol* 1978;35:291–301

40. Gemignani F, Marbini A, Bragaglia MM, Govoni E. Pathological study of the sural nerve in Fabry's disease. *Eur Neurol* 1984;23:173–81

41. Bischoff A, Fierz U, Regli F, Ulrich J. [Peripheral neurological disorders in Fabry's disease (angiokeratoma corporis diffusum universale). Clinical and electron microscopic findings in a case]. *Klin Wochenschr* 1968;46:666–71

42. Kocen RS, Thomas PK. Peripheral nerve involvement in Fabry's disease. *Arch Neurol* 1970;22:81–8

43. Onishi A, Dyck PJ. Loss of small peripheral sensory neurons in Fabry disease. Histologic and morphometric evaluation of cutaneous nerves, spinal ganglia, and posterior columns. *Arch Neurol* 1974;31:120–7

44. Hozumi I, Nishizawa M, Ariga T, Inoue Y, Ohnishi Y, Yokoyama A et al. Accumulation of glycosphingolipids in spinal and sympathetic ganglia of a symptomatic heterozygote of Fabry's disease. *J Neurol Sci* 1989;90:273–80

45. Cable WJ, Kolodny EH, Adams RD. Fabry disease: impaired autonomic function. *Neurology* 1982;32:498–502

46. Altarescu GM, Goldfarb LG, Park KY, Kaneski C, Jeffries N, Litvak S et al. Identification of fifteen novel mutations and genotype–phenotype relationship in Fabry disease. *Clin Genet* 2001;60:46–51

47. Fealey R. Thermoregulatory sweat test. In: Low P, editor. Clinical autonomic disorders. Philadelphia: Lippincott-Raven; 1997. p. 245–57

48. Kang WH, Chun SI, Lee S. Generalized anhidrosis associated with Fabry's disease. *J Am Acad Dermatol* 1987;17:883–7

49. Kato H, Sato K, Hattori S, Ikemoto S, Shimizu M, Isogai Y. Fabry's disease. *Intern Med* 1992;31:682–5

50. Low P, Opfer-Gehrking T. The autonomic laboratory. *Am J Electroneurodiagn Technol* 1999;39:65–76

51. Schiffmann R, Floeter MK, Dambrosia JM, Gupta S, Moore DF, Sharabi Y et al. Enzyme replacement therapy improves peripheral nerve and sweat function in Fabry disease. *Muscle Nerve* 2003;28:703–10

52. Cable WJ, Dvorak AM, Osage JE, Kolodny EH. Fabry disease: significance of ultrastructural localization of lipid inclusions in dermal nerves. *Neurology* 1982; 32:347–53

53. Schiffmann R, Scott LJ. Pathophysiology and assessment of neuropathic pain in Fabry disease. *Acta Paediatr Suppl* 2002;439:48–52

54. Lao LM, Kumakiri M, Mima H, Kuwahara H, Ishida H, Ishiguro K et al. The ultrastructural characteristics of eccrine sweat glands in a Fabry disease patient with hypohidrosis. *J Dermatol Sci* 1998;18:109–17

55. Yamamoto K, Sobue G, Iwase S, Kumazawa K, Mitsuma T, Mano T. Possible mechanism of anhidrosis in a symptomatic female carrier of Fabry's disease: an assessment by skin sympathetic nerve activity and sympathetic skin response. *Clin Auton Res* 1996;6:107–10

56. Fukuhara N, Suzuki M, Fujita N, Tsubaki T. Fabry's disease on the mechanism of the peripheral nerve involvement. *Acta Neuropathol (Berl)* 1975;33:9–21

57. Inagaki M, Ohno K, Hisatome I, Tanaka Y, Takeshita K. Relative hypoxia of the extremities in Fabry disease. *Brain Dev* 1992;14:328–33

58. Thomas PK. The anatomical substratum of pain evidence derived from morphometric studies on peripheral nerve. *Can J Neurol Sci* 1974;1:92–7

59. Mutoh T, Senda Y, Sugimura K, Koike Y, Matsuoka Y, Sobue I et al. Severe orthostatic hypotension in a female carrier of Fabry's disease. *Arch Neurol* 1988;45:468–72

60. Menkes DL, O'Neil TJ, Saenz KK. Fabry's disease presenting as syncope, angiokeratomas, and spoke-like cataracts in a young man: discussion of the differential diagnosis. *Mil Med* 1997;162:773–6

61. Lien YH, Lai LW, Lui CY. Unexpected diagnosis of Fabry disease in an 80-year-old man with syncope. *Cardiology* 2001;96:115–16

62. Seino Y, Vyden JK, Philippart M, Rose HB, Nagasawa K. Peripheral hemodynamics in patients with Fabry's disease. *Am Heart J* 1983;105:783–7

63. Attal N, Bouhassira D. Mechanisms of pain in peripheral neuropathy. *Acta Neurol Scand Suppl* 1999;173:12–24; discussion 48–52

64. Jensen TS. Anticonvulsants in neuropathic pain: rationale and clinical evidence. *Eur J Pain* 2002; 6 (Suppl A):61–8

65. Zimmermann M. Pathobiology of neuropathic pain. *Eur J Pharmacol* 2001;429:23–37

66. Coward K, Plumpton C, Facer P, Birch R, Carlstedt T, Tate S et al. Immunolocalization of SNS/PN3 and NaN/SNS2 sodium channels in human pain states. *Pain* 2000;85:41–50

67. Backonja MM. Anticonvulsants (antineuropathics) for neuropathic pain syndromes. *Clin J Pain* 2000; 16:S67–72

68. Filling-Katz MR, Merrick HF, Fink JK, Miles RB, Sokol J, Barton NW. Carbamazepine in Fabry's disease: effective analgesia with dose-dependent exacerbation of autonomic dysfunction. *Neurology* 1989;39:598–600

69. Dougherty JA, Rhoney DH. Gabapentin: a unique anti-epileptic agent. *Neurol Res* 2001;23:821–9

23

Nervous system manifestations of Fabry disease: data from FOS – the Fabry Outcome Survey

Lionel Ginsberg[1]

Department of Neurology, Royal Free Hospital, Pond Street, London NW3 2QG, UK

FOS – the Fabry Outcome Survey – is the world's most comprehensive database of patients with Fabry disease (688 patients in total, as of March 2005; 330 males, 358 females). As would be predicted from smaller demographic studies, a high proportion of patients in FOS have developed neurological complications of Fabry disease. Thus, 13.2% (15.1% males, 11.5% females) have suffered an ischaemic stroke or transient ischaemic attack, usually at an early age. Patients in FOS who have experienced a cerebrovascular event are more likely to have advanced Fabry disease, with a significantly higher frequency of hypertension, renal insufficiency and cardiac disease than other patients in FOS.

Magnetic resonance imaging (MRI) has proved a useful tool for studying the cerebrovascular complications of Fabry disease. To date, the MRI scans of 84 patients in FOS have been reviewed by a central panel of neuroradiologists and neurologists – the world's largest series subjected to such analysis. The most common abnormal finding was the presence of non-specific white matter lesions. These lesions increased with patient age, and their frequency and severity were similar in males and females.

Regarding other neurological manifestations of Fabry disease, FOS has confirmed a very high frequency of neuropathic pain (76% males, 64% females), beginning in childhood or adolescence. A previously less well characterized association between epilepsy and Fabry disease has also been shown. In future, strategies will need to be developed to move from these demographic analyses to using FOS to study the pathogenesis of the neurological manifestations of Fabry disease, and the effects of treatment.

Introduction

The neurological features of Fabry disease span the entire nervous system – from small nerve fibres in the extremities to the cerebral cortex (Table 1) [1–3]. Neurological symptoms may be one of the first manifestations of Fabry disease in childhood [4]. In the form of ischaemic stroke, neurological disease is also one of the potentially life-threatening complications of the later stages of the condition, along with end-stage renal failure and cardiac dysfunction. Several published surveys have provided demographic information on the frequency of nervous system manifestations in Fabry disease [5–7]. The purpose of this chapter is to analyse the

[1]On behalf of the FOS CNS Working Group, comprising Lionel Ginsberg (Chair), Alessandro P Burlina (University Hospital of Padua, Padua, Italy), Renzo Manara (University Hospital of Padua, Padua, Italy), and Alan R Valentine, Brian Kendall and Atul Mehta (Royal Free Hospital, London, UK).

Table 1. *Neurological and sensory organ complications of Fabry disease.*

Central nervous system
- Ischaemic stroke
- Haemorrhagic stroke
- Epilepsy
- Cognitive impairment
- Behavioural problems

Peripheral nervous system
- Painful small fibre neuropathy
- Autonomic dysfunction

Sensory organs
- Ear – hearing loss, vertigo, tinnitus
- Eye – cornea verticillata, subcapsular cataract, retinal vascular tortuosity

natural history of the neurological complications of Fabry disease, using data from FOS – the Fabry Outcome Survey – which is now the world's most comprehensive database of patients with the disease. In FOS, the most frequently reported signs and symptoms of Fabry disease are neurological (84% males, 79% females) [8]. The discussion in this chapter will be restricted to the major CNS complications, in particular ischaemic stroke, and painful peripheral neuropathy. Disease of sensory organs; that is, the ear and eye, is described elsewhere (see Chapters 25 and 26, respectively), as are the gastrointestinal consequences of autonomic neuropathy (see Chapter 28). Technical and practical aspects of data collection in FOS are outlined in Chapter 15.

Ischaemic stroke

In keeping with previous studies [5–7, 9], the prevalence of ischaemic stroke and transient ischaemic attacks (TIAs) in the FOS cohort is high (Table 2). Thus, 91 (13.2%) of the 688 patients (330 males, 358 females) registered in

FOS by March 2005 had suffered a stroke or TIA. The prevalence was 15.1% in males (50 patients; 31 with ischaemic stroke, 19 with TIA) and 11.5% in females (41 patients; 21 with ischaemic stroke, 20 with TIA). These findings highlight the fact that female heterozygotes for this X-linked condition are not mere carriers, but are at risk of its life-threatening complications [6, 10]. The observed number of ischaemic strokes among males in FOS was 20.1 times that expected in a comparable general population, and among females was 7.8 times more than expected ($p < 0.001$)[2].

Also in line with previous reports, cerebrovascular events typically occur at an earlier age in FOS than in the general population. Fabry disease is increasingly being recognized as an important aetiological factor in young patients (aged 18–55 years) with 'cryptogenic' stroke [11]. Of the 50 male patients in FOS who had experienced an ischaemic stroke or TIA, 44 (88%) were under 55 years of age. Twenty-four (59%) of the 41 females were younger than 55 years. Similarly, 26 of the 31 strokes in male patients (84%) and 10 of the 21 in females (48%) occurred before the age of 55 years.

Vascular risk factors

The pathogenesis of ischaemic stroke in Fabry disease is likely to involve specific mechanisms related directly or indirectly to glycolipid deposition in vessel walls [12]. Indeed, it has been argued that patients with Fabry disease may be 'protected' from the usual degenerative vascular changes associated with age and other conventional risk factors, though recent clinical and laboratory studies suggest the opposite [12]. Either way, it would be valuable to know whether these factors might contribute to the risk of stroke in

[2]Reference data on prevalence of stroke and epilepsy in the general population were obtained from the Centre for Epidemiology at the National Board of Health and Welfare in Sweden. Prevalence by age and gender were available for diagnosed patients according to the ICD-10 classification. The code I63 (cerebral infarction) was used for 'stroke' and codes G40 and G41 (epilepsy and status epilepticus) were used for 'seizure disorders'. Mean prevalence data by age and gender from consecutive years 1998–2004 were used.

Table 2. *Prevalence of ischaemic stroke and transient ischaemic attacks in patients with Fabry disease.*

Study	Male	Female	Total
Morgan *et al.* [9]	3/7 (43%)	0/5 (0%)	3/12 (25%)
MacDermot *et al.* [5, 6]	22/98 (22%)	17/60 (28%)	39/158 (25%)
Galanos *et al.* [7]	9/29 (31%)	2/38 (5%)	11/67 (16%)
FOS (as of March 2005)	50/330 (15%)	41/358 (11%)	91/688 (13%)

FOS – the Fabry Outcome Survey.

Fabry disease. The FOS database at least permits a comparison of vascular risk factors between patients who have suffered a cerebrovascular event and those who have not. Data show that the proportion of smokers among patients with Fabry disease who had sustained an ischaemic stroke was no different from that among the other patients (approximately 25%). In contrast, the frequency of hypertension among patients who had had an ischaemic stroke was 42%, compared with 19% among the remaining patients in FOS ($p < 0.001$). This finding does not necessarily imply that hypertension acts as an independent risk factor for stroke in Fabry disease. Both hypertension and stroke may simply indicate advanced Fabry disease. This view is supported by the very high frequency of both co-existent end-stage renal disease among the stroke patients (21% compared with 6% in the other patients), and cardiac abnormalities (Table 3). A significantly higher proportion of patients in the stroke group had valvular heart disease, left ventricular hypertrophy or arrhythmia than the other FOS patients (Table 3). In some cases, these cardiac lesions presumably caused the stroke through thromboembolism [13]. Regarding other vascular risk factors such as serum lipid profiles, only limited data were available in FOS, but there were no obvious differences between the stroke group and the other patients.

Magnetic resonance imaging

Magnetic resonance imaging (MRI) has proved a useful tool for studying stroke and other CNS complications of Fabry disease. The documented MRI changes associated with Fabry disease include the effects of ischaemic stroke and haemorrhage, non-specific white and grey matter lesions [9, 13, 14], and vascular anomalies – particularly tortuosity and increased calibre of the larger vessels (dolichoectasia). These vascular findings have been attributed to weakening of the vessel wall as a result of glycolipid deposition [13]. Finally, a characteristic appearance of the posterior thalamus (pulvinar region) on T1-weighted scans has been de-

Table 3. *Prevalence of cardiac and renal complications of Fabry disease in patients in FOS – the Fabry Outcome Survey – who have or have not suffered an ischaemic stroke.*

	History of ischaemic stroke	No history of stroke
Hypertension	42%	19%*
End-stage renal failure	21%	6%*
Left ventricular hypertrophy	67%	29%*
Arrhythmia	29%	9%*
Valve disease	31%	13%*

*$p < 0.001$ versus patients with a history of ischaemic stroke.

scribed [15, 16]. This appearance is thought to be caused by microvascular calcification consequent on regional hyperperfusion [15]. All these features have been observed in patients in FOS.

To standardize MRI reporting in FOS, a working party of neuroradiologists and neurologists has been established with the aim of reviewing as many scans as possible. MRI scans from 84 patients have already been analysed by this central panel, who have identified abnormalities in 44 patients. By far the most common abnormal finding was the presence of non-specific white matter lesions (Table 4). In accordance with other studies [17], there was no gender difference in the severity of white matter involvement. The lesions did, however, tend to accumulate with age, again in agreement with previous publications [14]. The pathological significance of these white matter lesions remains uncertain, though their presence appears to correlate with stroke in Fabry disease [11]. The lesions rarely coincide with discrete clinical events and, although they are assumed to represent ischaemia, it has been argued that other processes contribute to their development, including demyelination [18].

Other CNS diseases

The FOS database is now large enough to be interrogated for the frequency of CNS disease other than stroke. Compared with the general population, there is no excess prevalence of common neurological conditions, such as Parkinson's disease and migraine, in FOS. Perhaps surprisingly – considering that dementia has been described in advanced Fabry disease [5] – there is also no increase in the prevalence of dementia. The cognitive impairment reported in some patients has been attributed either to the cumulative effects of cerebrovascular disease or to glycolipid deposition in neurones [19, 20]. The failure of FOS to demonstrate a higher proportion of patients with dementia than in the general population may be explicable in several ways. First, there is the issue of ascertainment, as only a minority of patients in FOS have undergone formal neuropsychological evaluation. Secondly, older patients with Fabry disease may currently be under-represented in FOS.

In contrast with Parkinson's disease and dementia, an excess prevalence of epilepsy has been observed in FOS. In males, the prevalence was 4%, which is 6.5 times that expected in a comparable general population; in females, the prevalence was 2%, or 4.5 times that expected ($p < 0.001$ for both)[2]. Like dementia, potential mechanisms for epilepsy in Fabry disease would include underlying cerebrovascular disease and glycolipid accumulation in neurones. However, these reports of epilepsy must be interpreted with caution. The comparator from the general population may not be ideally matched with the patients in FOS in terms of the 'activity' of the epilepsy – that is, whether the patient has had recent seizures. Furthermore, several of the patients with epilepsy in FOS came from just two families – one from the Czech Republic, the other from the UK. Such familial clustering may imply a second aetiology for epilepsy that is unrelated to Fabry disease.

Peripheral neuropathy

Some of the earliest and commonest symptoms encountered in Fabry disease are acroparaesthesiae and pain caused by

Table 4. Review of magnetic resonance imaging scans of 84 patients in FOS – the Fabry Outcome Survey – by a central panel of neuroradiologists and neurologists.

Abnormal	44 (52.4%)
● White matter lesions	38 (45.2%)
● Grey matter lesions	12 (14.3%)
● Cerebral haemorrhage	2 (2.4%)
● Dolichoectasia	18 (21.4%)
● Infarction	6 (7.1%)

a small fibre peripheral neuropathy. The pathogenesis of the peripheral neuropathy is thought to involve glycolipid deposition in dorsal root ganglia [21], with a predilection for those of small myelinated neurones [22]. This histological pattern is reflected in neurophysiological studies. Thus, quantitative sensory testing has shown preferential damage of cold sensation, which is conveyed by small myelinated fibres [9, 23].

In FOS as a whole, neuropathic pain was reported by 76% of males and 64% of females, beginning at a mean age of 9.4 and 16.9 years, respectively [8]. In a cohort of 82 paediatric patients in FOS, more than 60% reported neuropathic pain [4]. Less specific neuropsychiatric symptoms (including fatigue and depression) were seen in more than 40% of patients. Neuropathic pain has a major impact on quality of life in children and adults with Fabry disease. Not surprisingly, therefore, measures of health-related quality of life in patients in FOS were significantly lower than those reported for an age- and sex-matched normal population [24].

In addition to the painful sensory neuropathy, patients with Fabry disease also develop autonomic involvement. One of the most prominent autonomic symptoms is hypohidrosis, though this probably relates more to end-organ (sweat gland) glycolipid deposition than neural damage [25]. In FOS, 54% of males and 25% of females for whom a clinical evaluation was carried out had hypohidrosis.

Treatment

The effects of enzyme replacement therapy (ERT) on the neurological complications of Fabry disease are described in more detail elsewhere (see Chapter 39). For the purposes of the present discussion, it suffices to say that data from FOS have shown a beneficial effect of ERT on neuropathic pain and health-related quality of life [24], in line with previous controlled trials [26, 27]. Predictably, FOS has not yet been able to

demonstrate an effect of ERT on stroke. To do so, patients would need to be followed for much longer than the present duration of FOS. Large groups of patients would need to be compared for stroke incidence according to the age at which they started ERT and the duration of therapy. To date, ten patients have had ischaemic strokes while on ERT and two have had TIAs (see Chapter 41).

Other medications taken by patients with Fabry disease have been recorded in FOS. These records show that, despite the advent of ERT, many patients take regular analgesic medication and non-steroidal anti-inflammatory drugs (75% and 22%, respectively) [8]. Given recent evidence for the role of conventional risk factors in the pathogenesis of cerebrovascular events in Fabry disease [28], it is perhaps surprising that only 28.9% of patients in FOS were taking anticoagulant or antiplatelet therapy. Of patients who had suffered an ischaemic stroke or TIA, 69.7% were taking anticoagulant or antiplatelet medication. The proportion was only 18% in those who had not experienced an ischaemic cerebrovascular event.

Conclusions and future prospects

To date, FOS has proved a valuable resource for clarifying the epidemiology of ischaemic stroke, painful neuropathy and other neurological manifestations of Fabry disease. In future, the database will need to be used imaginatively to move from demographic information to insights into the pathogenesis, and the efficacy of treatment, of these neurological complications. One approach to studying pathogenesis would be to use the database to select groups of patients, for example those who have suffered an ischaemic stroke, and then to study these patients in greater detail in order to identify factors which distinguish them from other patients with Fabry disease, and from the remainder of the population. As for research into treatment, to demonstrate an effect of ERT on stroke incidence is inherently more difficult than showing its influence on painful neuropathy. As stated previously, the database would need to be large enough, and maintained for long enough, to follow groups of patients divided according to the age at which they started ERT and their duration of therapy.

References

1. Desnick RJ, Ioannou YA, Eng CM. α-Galactosidase A deficiency: Fabry disease. In: Scriver CR, Beaudet AL, Sly WS, Valle D, editors. The metabolic and molecular bases of inherited disease. 8th edn. New York: McGraw-Hill; 2001. p. 3733–74

2. Brady RO, Schiffmann R. Clinical features of and recent advances in therapy for Fabry disease. JAMA 2000;284:2771–5

3. Ginsberg L, Valentine A, Mehta A. Neurological rarity: Fabry disease. Pract Neurol 2005;5:110–13

4. Ramaswami U, Whybra C, Parini R, Pintos-Morell G, Mehta A, Sunder-Plassmann G et al. Clinical manifestations of Fabry disease in children: data from the Fabry Outcome Survey. Acta Paediatr 2006;95:86–92

5. MacDermot KD, Holmes A, Miners AH. Anderson–Fabry disease: clinical manifestations and impact of disease in a cohort of 98 hemizygous males. J Med Genet 2001;38:750–60

6. MacDermot KD, Holmes A, Miners AH. Anderson–Fabry disease: clinical manifestations and impact of disease in a cohort of 60 obligate carrier females. J Med Genet 2001;38:769–75

7. Galanos J, Nicholls K, Grigg L, Kiers L, Crawford A, Becker G. Clinical features of Fabry's disease in Australian patients. Intern Med J 2002;32:575–84

8. Mehta A, Ricci R, Widmer U, Dehout F, Garcia de Lorenzo A, Kampmann C et al. Fabry disease defined: baseline clinical manifestations of 366 patients in the Fabry Outcome Survey. Eur J Clin Invest 2004;34:236–42

9. Morgan SH, Rudge P, Smith SJ, Bronstein AM, Kendall BE, Holly E et al. The neurological complications of Anderson–Fabry disease (α-galactosidase A deficiency) – investigation of symptomatic and pre-symptomatic patients. Q J Med 1990;75:491–507

10. Deegan P, Baehner AF, Barba-Romero MA, Hughes D, Kampmann C, Beck M. Natural history of Fabry disease in females in the Fabry Outcome Survey. J Med Genet 2006;43:347–52

11. Rolfs A, Bottcher T, Zschiesche M, Morris P, Winchester B, Bauer P et al. Prevalence of Fabry disease in patients with cryptogenic stroke: a prospective study. Lancet 2005;366:1794–6

12. Schiffmann R, Ries M. Fabry's disease – an important risk factor for stroke. Lancet 2005;366:1754–6

13. Mitsias P, Levine SR. Cerebrovascular complications of Fabry's disease. Ann Neurol 1996;40:8–17

14. Crutchfield KE, Patronas NJ, Dambrosia JM, Frei KP, Banerjee TK, Barton NW et al. Quantitative analysis of cerebral vasculopathy in patients with Fabry disease. Neurology 1998;50:1746–9

15. Moore DF, Ye F, Schiffmann R, Butman JA. Increased signal intensity in the pulvinar on T1-weighted images: a pathognomonic MR imaging sign of Fabry disease. Am J Neuroradiol 2003;24:1096–101

16. Takanashi J, Barkovich AJ, Dillon WP, Sherr EH, Hart KA, Packman S. T1 hyperintensity in the pulvinar: key imaging feature for diagnosis of Fabry disease. Am J Neuroradiol 2003;24:916–21

17. Fellgiebel A, Müller MJ, Mazanek M, Baron K, Beck M, Stoeter P. White matter lesion severity in male and female patients with Fabry disease. Neurology 2005;65:600–2

18. Moore DF, Altarescu G, Barker WC, Patronas NJ, Herscovitch P, Schiffmann R. White matter lesions in Fabry disease occur in 'prior' selectively hypometabolic and hyperperfused brain regions. Brain Res Bull 2003;62:231–40

19. Mendez MF, Stanley TM, Medel NM, Li Z, Tedesco DT. The vascular dementia of Fabry's disease. Dement Geriatr Cogn Disord 1997;8:252–7

20. Tedeschi G, Bonavita S, Banerjee TK, Virta A, Schiffmann R. Diffuse central neuronal involvement in Fabry disease: a proton MRS imaging study. Neurology 1999;52:1663–7

21. Onishi A, Dyck PJ. Loss of small peripheral sensory neurons in Fabry disease. Histologic and morphometric evaluation of cutaneous nerves, spinal ganglia, and posterior columns. Arch Neurol 1974; 31:120–7

22. Kocen RS, Thomas PK. Peripheral nerve involvement in Fabry's disease. Arch Neurol 1970;22:81–8

23. Luciano CA, Russell JW, Banerjee TK, Quirk JM, Scott LJ, Dambrosia JM et al. Physiological characterization of neuropathy in Fabry's disease. Muscle Nerve 2002;26:622–9

24. Hoffmann B, Garcia de Lorenzo A, Mehta A, Beck M, Widmer U, Ricci R. Effects of enzyme replacement therapy on pain and health related quality of life in patients with Fabry disease: data from FOS (Fabry Outcome Survey). J Med Genet 2005;42:247–52

25. Cable WJ, Kolodny EH, Adams RD. Fabry disease: impaired autonomic function. Neurology 1982;32: 498–502

26. Schiffmann R, Kopp JB, Austin HA 3rd, Sabnis S, Moore DF, Weibel T et al. Enzyme replacement therapy in Fabry disease: a randomized controlled trial. JAMA 2001;285:2743–9

27. Schiffmann R, Floeter MK, Dambrosia JM, Gupta S, Moore DF, Sharabi Y et al. Enzyme replacement therapy improves peripheral nerve and sweat function in Fabry disease. Muscle Nerve 2003;28: 703–10

28. Altarescu G, Moore DF, Schiffmann R. Effect of genetic modifiers on cerebral lesions in Fabry disease. Neurology 2005;64:2148–50

24 Dermatological and soft-tissue manifestations of Fabry disease: characteristics and response to enzyme replacement therapy

Olivier Lidove[1], Roland Jaussaud[2] and Sélim Aractingi[3]

[1]Department of Internal Medicine, Bichat Hospital, Paris, France; [2]Department of Internal Medicine and Infectious Diseases, Robert Debré Hospital, Reims, France; [3]Department of Dermatology–Allergy, Hospital Tenon, Paris, France

Early manifestations of Fabry disease include dermatological and soft-tissue symptoms, such as angiokeratomas, acroparaesthesia, abnormal sweating (hypohidrosis and hyperhidrosis) and lymphoedema. Recognition of these symptoms is vital for the early diagnosis and treatment of Fabry disease. It is therefore important that dermatologists, as well as other specialists, are aware of the manifestations of Fabry disease. Clinical studies and data from FOS – the Fabry Outcome Survey – have suggested that enzyme replacement therapy with agalsidase alfa can improve sweating, heat intolerance and pain in patients with Fabry disease.

Introduction

Fabry disease, which was first described independently by a dermatologist (Johannes Fabry) and a surgeon (William Anderson) in 1898 [1, 2], is one of the genodermatoses and the second most prevalent lipid storage disorder in humans, after Gaucher disease. Some of the earliest manifestations of Fabry disease include corneal and lenticular opacities, skin lesions, acroparaesthesia, hypohidrosis and gastrointestinal symptoms [3, 4]. The onset of these symptoms typically occurs during childhood. Their recognition is therefore important for the diagnosis and early treatment of Fabry disease. Currently, however, there is often a delay of up to 15 years between the onset of symptoms and diagnosis, such that organ damage has already occurred by the time that Fabry disease is diagnosed.

This chapter reviews the dermatological and other soft-tissue manifestations of Fabry disease, and the effects of symptomatic treatment and enzyme replacement therapy (ERT) on these symptoms, with reference to clinical trials and data from FOS – the Fabry Outcome Survey.

Pathology of cutaneous lesions in Fabry disease

Glycosphingolipids are components of the plasma membrane that are degraded in the lysosome after internalization through an endocytic pathway. As a consequence of deficiency of α-galactosidase A in patients with Fabry disease, α-D-galactosyl glycosphingolipids, particularly globotriaosylceramide (Gb_3), accumulate in lysosomes and disrupt the function of affected cells.

The skin is a large and complex organ composed of the epidermis, dermis and hypodermis, which themselves have many cell types. Fabry disease affects mainly the endothelial vessels. Endothelial cells in the superficial dermis, just below the non-vascular epidermis, are therefore the main target of the disease. Vasa nervorum endothelial cells in the perineurium are also affected. In addition,

Gb$_3$ may accumulate in lysosomes of vascular pericytes, eccrine gland cells and dermal fibroblasts [5].

Angiokeratomas

Angiokeratomas are benign vascular skin lesions characterized by proliferation of dilated blood vessels in the upper dermis. They occur when accumulation of Gb$_3$ in dermal endothelial cells leads to vessel bulge and incompetence of the vessel wall, followed by secondary ectasia. They are the main cutaneous lesions found in patients with Fabry disease and may be the earliest physical sign of the disease, appearing in children between the ages of 5 and 15 years (mean age, 13.5 years) [6, 7]. They are found in 83% of males and 80% of females with Fabry disease [6]. Angiokeratomas spread with age to become visible on the lips, hands and toes. If the lesions occur on the genital mucosa, they may cause bleeding, especially during sexual intercourse. They may be isolated or clustered and appear as small red-to-black papules, with a smooth epidermal surface (Figure 1). As the disease progresses, the lesions grow, reaching a diameter of 10 mm, and become dark red to black, with a verrucous surface. Application of pressure empties – at least partially – the blood contained in the lesions. The distribution of angiokeratoma may be restricted to the 'swimsuit' area (the region between the umbilicus and the knees) or may be disseminated. Localized angiokeratomas

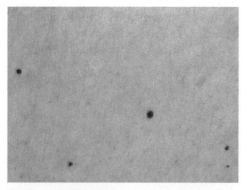

Figure 1. *Angiokeratoma in a patient with Fabry disease.*

on the soles, chin, ears and axillae may occur, and mucosal involvement has been reported [6–8].

Skin biopsies are not usually necessary to diagnose Fabry disease, as the diagnosis may be obtained by means of enzymatic/genetic analysis. Biopsies in patients with Fabry disease have revealed non-specific effects, with ectasia of subepidermal vessels that 'lift' the epidermis. Epidermal ridges are enlarged at the periphery of the angiokeratoma. In pressure areas, a variable degree of epidermal hyperplasia with orthokeratotic hyperkeratosis may occur. Accumulated glycosphingolipids are birefringent and, when viewed under polarized light, show a Maltese cross configuration.

Electron microscopy studies show electron-dense lysosomal inclusions in vascular endothelial cells, vascular pericytes, eccrine gland cells, dermal fibroblasts and the perineurium [9]. Immunolocalization can also be performed using sophisticated techniques such as immunoelectron microscopy. Such studies have confirmed that the intra-lysosomal deposits are composed of Galactose $\alpha \rightarrow$ Galactose $\beta \rightarrow$ Glucose [9].

It is important to note that angiokeratomas are not pathognomonic of Fabry disease, but are also found in patients with hereditary haemorrhagic telangiectasia, Fordyce disease, Schindler disease, fucosidosis and sialidosis. Angiokeratoma circumscriptum has been described in a patient in whom Fabry disease was excluded. The band-like distribution of angiokeratomas in this patient provided direct evidence that the condition reflected mosaicism of a hitherto unknown mutation [10]. In addition, it should be noted that during a pain crisis, the reddish-blue disseminated appearance of an angiokeratoma can lead to a misdiagnosis of meningitis.

Angiokeratomas are usually asymptomatic, although bleeding may occur in rare cases.

Cosmetic correction of the affected areas is possible using laser therapy. Argon laser therapy was one of the first techniques to be used clinically, although it is a continuous wave laser and leads to significant non-selective heating of surrounding tissues, which increases the risk of scarring. The variable pulse width neodymium:yttrium–aluminium–garnet (Nd:YAG) laser appears to be an alternative option in the treatment of angiokeratomas [11]. The use of combined treatment with erbium:YAG and 532 nm potassium titanyl phosphate (frequency-doubled Nd:YAG) lasers also leads to excellent cosmetic results without clinically visible scarring or recurrence (FG Bechara, personal communication). These procedures usually do not require anaesthesia. Other treatments include fine-needle electrocautery or surgical removal, both of which require local anaesthesia [12].

Sweating

Specific polyneuropathy and sweat gland infiltration often lead to sweating abnormalities in Fabry disease. The classic symptoms are hypohidrosis (reduced sweating) and anhidrosis (absence of sweating). These symptoms may have a significant effect on quality of life, causing fever, and heat and exercise intolerance [13].

Hypohidrosis

Hypohidrosis is a common and early manifestation of Fabry disease, with a higher prevalence in males than in females. In a study of the early clinical phenotypes of 35 European children and adolescents with Fabry disease, hypohidrosis was reported in 93% of males and 25% of females [3]. In a larger cohort of paediatric patients, enrolled in FOS, hypohidrosis or anhidrosis was reported in 25 out of 36 boys (70%) and hypohidrosis in 5 out of 29 girls (17%) [4]. In a quantitative analysis, Ries *et al*. [14] showed that sweat volume in a cohort of 25 boys with Fabry disease was 0.41 ± 0.46 $\mu l/mm^2$ compared with 0.65 ± 0.44 $\mu l/mm^2$ in age-matched controls. Hypohidrosis predisposes to acroparaesthesia by making sufferers intolerant of heat and exercise. Reduced tear production by the lacrimal glands and reduced saliva production may be associated with hypohidrosis in patients with Fabry disease. The resulting dry eyes and mouth may lead to a misdiagnosis of Gougerot–Sjögren syndrome [15].

Hyperhidrosis

Hyperhidrosis is much less common in patients with Fabry disease than hypohidrosis and appears to be more common in females than males. It has been reported in 14.5% of females (36 of 248 patients) and 4.1% of males (12 of 291 patients) in the FOS database. This compares with an estimated prevalence of 2.8% in the general population, according to a recent US study [16] and with a prevalence of primary palmar hyperhidrosis of 1% in the western population [17]. In the recently published study of the manifestations of Fabry disease in children in FOS, Ramaswami and colleagues reported hyperhidrosis in 1 of 36 boys (3%) and 5 of 29 girls (17%) [4]. It is likely that the hyperhidrosis is a manifestation of the peripheral neuropathy that occurs in Fabry disease.

When cutaneous and mucous glands are affected, it may be necessary for the patient to restrict the time they spend in a warm environment or undergoing physical activity. They may also require topical and systemic antiperspirant agents, and topical application of artificial lachrymal fluid and saliva [12].

Lymphoedema

Anderson cited lymphoedema as a clinical sign of Fabry disease in the original description of the disorder [1]. Lymphoedema also occurs in other lysosomal storage disorders, such as Kanzaki disease (α-N-acetylgalactosaminidase deficiency). In the absence of therapy, lymphoedema in Fabry disease can be complicated by erysipelas, with a risk of systemic infection.

Thus, lymphoedema may necessitate the use of compression stockings.

In patients with Fabry disease, lymphoedema appears to be related to the accumulation of glycolipids in the lymph vessels rather than to kidney or heart disease [18].

Severe lymphatic microangiopathy, leading to lymphoedema, has been described in Fabry disease [19]. This study showed that severe structural and functional changes in the initial lymphatics of the skin occur in both male and female patients with Fabry disease, regardless of whether lymphoedema is manifest.

In a further study of 14 patients (6 females, 8 males; mean age, 40 years; range, 15–55 years) with Fabry disease, the lymphatic microvessels of the skin were examined *in vivo* with fluorescence micro-lymphography, and intra-lymphatic pressure was measured [20]. Lymphoedema was present in seven patients. Twelve healthy controls were also studied. The assessments were repeated at a mean of 16 months (range, 12–24 months) after initiation of ERT. Fragmentation of the lymphatic network was found in all patients with Fabry disease but not in healthy controls. Severe structural and functional changes of the initial lymphatics of the skin were found, which might contribute to the formation of lymphoedema.

Acroparaesthesia

Acroparaesthesia is an early symptom of Fabry disease; it is common in male patients [8, 21] but has also been reported to occur in between 10 and 90% of female patients in various studies [6, 22, 23]. It is thought to result from ischaemia of the peripheral nerves secondary to abnormalities in endothelial perineurium cells and is characterized by tingling, chronic burning or nagging pain in the hands and feet. Acute episodes of incapacitating pain, lasting from a few minutes to several days, may develop [24]. These can occur spontaneously but may also be induced by heat, illness, stress or exercise. Fatigue, moderate fever and joint pain may be associated with these acute pain crises [25]. The presence of this symptom is likely to prompt a clinical examination of the hands, which often permits an associated diagnosis of Raynaud phenomenon, distal angiokeratoma or telangiectasia.

Facial dysmorphia

Males hemizygous for Fabry disease often have a characteristic facial appearance, with prominent supraorbital ridges, frontal bossing and thickening of the lips. This often leads to a misdiagnosis of acromegaly (excessive growth hormone) or Hurler disease. Richfield *et al.* have recently used photography to record the facial appearance of three patients before agalsidase alfa treatment and serially after 6–12 months of therapy. These photographs suggest that there is a gradual and subtle change in facial features with treatment [26].

Response to ERT
Data from clinical studies

There are few data available on the clinical effects of ERT in patients with Fabry disease. Moreover, no direct comparisons have been reported between agalsidase alfa and agalsidase beta.

Angiokeratoma

Thurberg and colleagues conducted a phase III, randomized, placebo-controlled 3-month trial, followed by a 30-month open-label extension study, to assess the effect of ERT with agalsidase beta on dermatological symptoms in 58 patients with Fabry disease [27]. A series of skin biopsies demonstrated a complete clearance of Gb_3 in deep vascular endothelial cells. The use of periodic dermal biopsies as a reliable monitor of sustained treatment efficacy is debatable, however, considering the ethical issues and alternatives, such as clinical monitoring.

Hypohidrosis

Schiffmann and colleagues conducted an open study to evaluate the effect of ERT on sweating [28]. Twenty-six male patients with Fabry disease were given agalsidase alfa for 36 months. The quantitative sudomotor axon reflex test (QSART) was used to measure the volume of sweat production triggered by transcutaneous ionophoresis.

The rate of sweating before infusion was 0.24 ± 0.33 µl/mm^2 in patients with Fabry disease ($n = 17$), compared with 1.05 ± 0.81 µl/mm^2 ($n = 38$; $p < 0.0001$) in controls. There was a significant improvement in the rate of sweating 24–72 hours after infusion of agalsidase alfa ($p = 0.04$, unilateral t-test) and sweating was normalized in four anhidrotic patients with Fabry disease. These data indicate that agalsidase alfa significantly improves the sweating related to small-fibre neuropathy.

It is important to note that QSART data were not available at baseline and were therefore analysed only at the end of the study. QSART may prove useful in future to optimize ERT, particularly as there was a decline in sweating a few days after infusion in many patients.

Hyperhidrosis

Limited data are available on the response of hyperhidrosis to ERT. Sympathetic skin responses to ERT have been investigated in seven male patients who received agalsidase alfa for 18 months ($n = 2$) or 24 months ($n = 5$) [29]. Before the start of therapy, the amplitudes of the sympathetic skin responses were small or absent, compared with a normal control group ($p < 0.0001$, t-test). In the second year of treatment with agalsidase alfa the sympathetic skin responses reached the range found in the control group, indicating a clinically relevant improvement in sympathetic function in these patients in response to ERT.

Neuropathy

Long-term ERT has been shown to have a positive effect on the neurological manifestations of Fabry disease (see Chapter 39), reducing pain and improving quality of life (see Chapter 40). Specifically, ERT for up to 3 years was associated with a significant improvement in the clinical manifestations of small-fibre neuropathy, increasing the threshold for peripheral detection of cold and warm stimuli and improving sweat function and vibratory perception [28, 30].

Vasculopathy

The vasculopathy associated with Fabry disease may be considered as a 'pseudovasculitis' of the small vessels. Nail-bed capillaroscopy is a simple method for examining tissue perfusion and has been used in the diagnosis of several vascular diseases. Nail-bed capillaroscopy was performed in eight patients with Fabry disease (5 females and 3 males from one family, 5 of whom were receiving ERT with agalsidase alfa) using a Nikin SMZ-10 stereomicroscope. The absence of some capillaries was noted in two patients, one of them receiving ERT. In three patients (one of whom was receiving ERT), capillaroscopy revealed fasciculated ramifications of some capillaries. Three patients, who were all receiving ERT, showed no abnormalities on capillaroscopy and also showed no symptoms of acroparaesthesia. Capillaroscopy may therefore be a promising method for evaluating small vessels in patients with Fabry disease [31].

Insights from FOS

The skin manifestations of Fabry disease have been analysed in 288 patients (94 female, 194 male) registered within FOS [C Orteu et al., unpublished data]. The diagnosis was first suspected by a dermatologist in 20.1% of affected men and 5.4% of woman. Forty-four per cent of woman were diagnosed as a result of an affected family member. The mean age at diagnosis for males was 25 ± 14 years (median, 23 years), and for females 35 ± 16 years (median, 38 years). Angiokeratoma and/or telangiectasia were reported in 73% of males and 38% of females, respectively. The median age at onset of angiokeratoma was 15 years in males (22 years for telangiectasia) and 26 years in females (43 years for telangiectasia). Heat intolerance was reported in 48% of males (median age at onset, 12 years) and 44% of females (median age at onset, 18 years). Most of these patients also had hypohidrosis, with a median age at onset of 13 and 29 years in males and females, respectively. Lymphoedema was reported in 22% of men (median age at onset, 39 years) and 14% of woman (median age at onset, 49 years).

The FOS database also attempts to characterize the extent of dermatological changes as mild, moderate or severe. Most patients report no change in their angiokeratoma whilst on ERT, but the tools for recording such clinical observations are relatively crude. The FOS database also has some quantitative subjective data on sweating, with individuals being asked to rate their sweating in comparison with other individuals before and after initiation of ERT. A complete absence of sweating was reported by 10 of 32 females and 23 of 46 males before the start of ERT. Three of these females and ten males reported an increase in sweating after the start of treatment. An additional 14 males claimed to be sweating less than others at the initiation of ERT; six of these reported improvements in sweating after ERT and four reported a deterioration.

Conclusions

It is particularly important to identify patients with Fabry disease because it has now been established that treatment can alter the course of the disease. However, diagnosis can sometimes be difficult, especially if the patient has relatively few symptoms. In such cases, the dermatologist can have a key role in achieving an early diagnosis. It is therefore important that dermatologists, as well as other specialists, are aware of the manifestations of Fabry disease. It will also be important to determine whether the beneficial dermatological effects of ERT reflect positive clinical changes in other major organs and organ systems affected by Fabry disease, such as the nervous, cerebrovascular and cardiovascular systems and the kidneys.

References

1. Anderson W. A case of "angeio-keratoma". *Br J Dermatol* 1898;10:113–17

2. Fabry J. Ein Beitrag zur Kenntnis der Purpura haemorrhagica nodularis (Purpura papulosa haemorrhagica Hebra). *Arch Dermatol Syphilol* (Berlin) 1898;43:187–201

3. Ries M, Ramaswami U, Parini R, Lindblad B, Whybra C, Willers I *et al.* The early clinical phenotype of Fabry disease: a study on 35 European children and adolescents. *Eur J Pediatr* 2003;162:767–72

4. Ramaswami U, Whybra C, Parini R, Pintos-Morell G, Mehta A, Sunder-Plassmann G *et al.* Clinical manifestations of Fabry disease in children: data from the Fabry Outcome Survey. *Acta Paediatr* 2006;95:86–92

5. Kanda A, Nakao S, Tsuyama S, Murata F, Kanzaki T. Fabry disease: ultrastructural lectin histochemical analyses of lysosomal deposits. *Virchows Arch* 2000;436:36–42

6. Larralde M, Boggio P, Amartino H, Chamoles N. Fabry disease: a study of 6 hemizygous men and 5 heterozygous women with emphasis on dermatologic manifestations. *Arch Dermatol* 2004;140:1440–6

7. Mohrenschlager M, Henkel V, Ring J. Fabry disease: more than angiokeratomas. *Arch Dermatol* 2004;140:1526–8

8. MacDermot KD, Holmes A, Miners AH. Anderson–Fabry disease: clinical manifestations and impact of disease in a cohort of 98 hemizygous males. *J Med Genet* 2001;38:750–60

9. Kanekura T, Fukushige T, Kanda A, Tsuyama S, Murata F, Sakuraba H *et al.* Immunoelectron-microscopic detection of globotriaosylceramide accumulated in the skin of patients with Fabry disease. *Br J Dermatol* 2005;153:544–8

10. Jansen T, Bechara FG, Happle R, Altmeyer P, Grabbe S. Angiokeratoma circumscriptum without metabolic disease. *Acta Paediatr Suppl* 2006; 451:121

11. Bechara FG, Huesmann M, Altmeyer P, Hoffmann K, Jansen T. Angiokeratoma of the glans penis: successful treatment with Nd:YAG laser. *Acta Paediatr Suppl* 2002;439:143

12. Mohrenschlager M, Braun-Falco M, Ring J, Abeck D. Fabry disease: recognition and management of cutaneous manifestations. *Am J Clin Dermatol* 2003; 4:189–96

13. Shelley ED, Shelley WB, Kurczynski TW. Painful fingers, heat intolerance, and telangiectases of the ear: easily ignored childhood signs of Fabry disease. *Pediatr Dermatol* 1995;12:215–9

14. Ries M, Gupta S, Moore DF, Sachdev V, Quirk JM, Murray GJ et al. Pediatric Fabry disease. *Pediatrics* 2005;115:e344–55

15. Cable WJ, Kolodny EH, Adams RD. Fabry disease: impaired autonomic function. *Neurology* 1982;32: 498–502

16. Strutton DR, Kowalski JW, Glaser DA, Stang PE. US prevalence of hyperhidrosis and impact on individuals with axillary hyperhidrosis: results from a national survey. *J Am Acad Dermatol* 2004;51:241–8

17. Ro KM, Cantor RM, Lange KL, Ahn SS. Palmar hyperhidrosis: evidence of genetic transmission. *J Vasc Surg* 2002;35:382–6

18. Jansen T, Bechara FG, Orteu CH, Altmeyer P, Mehta A, Beck M et al. The significance of lymph-oedema in Fabry disease. *Acta Paediatr Suppl* 2005;447:117

19. Amann-Vesti BR, Gitzelmann G, Widmer U, Bosshard NU, Steinmann B, Koppensteiner R. Severe lymphatic microangiopathy in Fabry disease. *Lymphat Res Biol* 2003;1:185–9

20. Gitzelmann G, Widmer U, Bosshard NU, Steinmann B, Koppensteiner R, Amann-Vesti BR. Lymphoedema in Fabry disease: pathology and therapeutic perspectives. *Acta Paediatr Suppl* 2006;451:122

21. Mehta A, Ricci R, Widmer U, Dehout F, Garcia de Lorenzo A, Kampmann C et al. Fabry disease defined: baseline clinical manifestations of 366 patients in the Fabry Outcome Survey. *Eur J Clin Invest* 2004;34:236–42

22. Whybra C, Kampmann C, Willers I, Davies J, Winchester B, Kriegsmann J et al. Anderson–Fabry disease: clinical manifestations of disease in female heterozygotes. *J Inherit Metab Dis* 2001;24:715–24

23. Deegan P, Bähner AF, Barba-Romero MA, Hughes D, Kampmann C, Beck M. Natural history of Fabry disease in females in the Fabry Outcome Survey. *J Med Genet* 2006;43:347–52

24. Birklein F. Mechanisms of neuropathic pain and their importance in Fabry disease. *Acta Paediatr Suppl* 2002;439:34–7

25. Morgan SH, Rudge P, Smith SJ, Bronstein AM, Kendall BE, Holly E et al. The neurological complications of Anderson–Fabry disease (α-galactosidase A deficiency) – investigation of symptomatic and presymptomatic patients. *Q J Med* 1990;75:491–507

26. Richfield R, Orteu CH, Fox N, Milligan A, Goodwin S, Hughes D et al. Fabry disease: changes in typical facial features in response to enzyme replacement therapy with agalsidase alfa. *Acta Paediatr Suppl* 2005;447:122

27. Thurberg BL, Randolph Byers H, Granter SR, Phelps RG, Gordon RE, O'Callaghan M. Monitoring the 3-year efficacy of enzyme replacement therapy in fabry disease by repeated skin biopsies. *J Invest Dermatol* 2004;122:900–8

28. Schiffmann R, Floeter MK, Dambrosia JM, Gupta S, Moore DF, Sharabi Y et al. Enzyme replacement therapy improves peripheral nerve and sweat function in Fabry disease. *Muscle Nerve* 2003; 28:703–10

29. Jardim LB, Becker J, Neto C, Nora D, Matte U, Pereira F et al. Improvement of sympathetic skin responses after enzyme replacement therapy in Fabry disease. *Acta Paediatr Suppl* 2006;451:133

30. Hilz MJ, Brys M, Marthol H, Stemper B, Dutsch M. Enzyme replacement therapy improves function of C-, Aδ-, and Aβ-nerve fibers in Fabry neuropathy. *Neurology* 2004;62:1066–72

31. López M, Barbado FJ, Torrijos A, Gómez-Cerezo J, Pagán B, Suárez I et al. Capillaroscopy in Fabry disease: study of a family. *Acta Paediatr Suppl* 2005; 447:106

25 Fabry disease and the ear

Annerose Keilmann[1], Stefan Hegemann[2], Guido Conti[3] and Daniel Hajioff[4]

[1]Department of Communication Disorders, University of Mainz, Langenbeckstrasse 1, D-55101 Mainz, Germany; [2]University Hospital Zurich, Department of ORL HNS, Zurich, Switzerland; [3]ENT Clinic, Catholic University of the Sacred Heart, Rome, Italy; [4]Royal National Throat, Nose & Ear Hospital, London, UK

Otological symptoms are common in patients with Fabry disease. Although they are not life threatening, they may severely affect quality of life. Data from FOS – the Fabry Outcome Survey – show that most patients experience hearing loss during their lifespan and that this hearing loss exceeds that of the normal population, as seen in ISO 7029 (International Institute of Standardization). The majority suffer from sensorineural hearing loss, with only a minority having mixed or conductive losses. Slowly progressive hearing loss predominates but the frequency of sudden hearing loss is elevated compared with the general population. About 85% of male patients over 50 years of age and 75% of female patients over 60 years of age suffer from hearing loss severe enough to justify the use of hearing aids. Preliminary data suggest that enzyme replacement therapy has a small beneficial effect in patients with mild or moderate hearing loss. Tinnitus is also much more frequent in patients with Fabry disease than in the normal population. About half of the male patients over 50 years of age and half of the female patients over 60 years of age suffer from tinnitus, as recorded in the FOS sign and symptom checklist. The FOS database provides little information on vertigo, however, as, until recently, it has not differentiated true vertigo from other forms of dizziness. Vestibular dysfunction does occur in Fabry disease but appears to be much less frequent than the 'vertigo' documented in the FOS sign and symptom checklist. The prevalence of non-specific dizziness appears to increase with age, with a smaller difference between genders than is the case for hearing loss.

Introduction

As patients with Fabry disease suffer from many life-threatening disorders, otological problems have been relatively neglected until recently. It is becoming increasingly apparent, however, that many patients experience hearing loss, for which hearing aids may not always provide adequate compensation, and tinnitus, which may adversely affect quality of life. It is possible that the beneficial effects of enzyme replacement therapy (ERT) might extend to these otological symptoms.

Initial results from FOS – the Fabry Outcome Survey – suggest that vertigo is very common, but these data have failed to distinguish true vertigo from non-specific dizziness. Patients with Fabry disease are particularly prone to orthostatic hypotension, which may result in dizziness and fainting, rather than true vestibular disease.

Histopathology

Although otological symptoms are quite common in patients with Fabry disease, there is only one report on temporal bone pathology in the world literature. Schachern *et al.* described the clinical histories, audiometric results and temporal bone findings in two patients with Fabry disease [1]. Both patients had a bilateral sloping sensorineural hearing loss at pure-tone audiometry, as seen in most affected patients. In the first patient, they found that the mucoperiosteum in the middle ear and mastoid was thickened by fibrosis, sparsely infiltrated with chronic inflammatory cells and covered by hyperplastic squamous epithelium. In the second patient, the mucosa of the middle ear was reported as thickened, hyperaemic and diffusely lined with hyperplastic epithelium. In both patients, focal areas of seropurulent effusion were observed throughout the middle ear. The ossicles appeared normal, with the exception of hyperostosis of the stapedial crura.

In the first patient, the organ of Corti was essentially normal. Mild cochlear hydrops was noted in the apical turn. Examination of the second patient revealed a moderate loss of outer hair cells in each turn and areas of tectorial membrane collapse. Endothelial cells lining the internal auditory artery, modiolar vessels and vas spirale appeared distorted because of their foamy vacuolized cytoplasm. In both patients, cells in the spiral ganglion were morphologically normal but were moderately decreased in number in the basal turn. The stria vascularis and the spiral ligament were atrophic in each turn.

The utricles and vestibules revealed no morphological abnormalities, but in the non-ampullated end of the superior semicircular canal, new bone filled the perilymphatic space in the first patient. In the second patient, a mild haemorrhage was found within the saccule of the left ear.

The investigators speculated that histopathological changes resulting in dysfunction in the ear were due both to direct effects on the ear from the accumulation of glycosphingolipids within the stria vascularis and ganglion cells, and to indirect effects resulting from vascular damage to other tissues.

Natural history of hearing loss in Fabry disease

Until recently, hearing loss in patients with Fabry disease has only been reported anecdotally and in small case series. MacDermot and colleagues described 98 male patients of whom 41% reported hearing loss, 78% had an abnormal audiogram and 38% suffered from tinnitus [2]. In a group of 22 consecutive hemizygous males (mean age, 39 years), Germain and colleagues found abnormal hearing in 12 patients and tinnitus in six patients [3]. Seven patients had experienced sudden hearing loss and five patients had progressive hearing loss. All cases of deafness were sensorineural and more than half of them were high frequency. In addition, seven out of the remaining ten patients demonstrated a high-frequency hearing loss without subjective impairment. In total, 86% of their patients had a measurable hearing loss. In this group, the incidence of hearing loss was significantly increased in patients with kidney failure or cerebrovascular lesions, but the investigators found no correlation with left ventricular hypertrophy.

Germain and co-workers, and Conti and Sergi did not detect evidence of retrocochlear pathology on auditory brainstem response in any of their patients [3, 4], which is consistent with the normal appearance of ganglion cells found by Schachern and colleagues [1].

According to Schuknecht's classification, the pattern in patients with Fabry disease most closely resembles a mixed strial and sensory type of presbyacusis [5–7]. Hegemann and colleagues postulated that the distorted vessels in the stria vascularis (presumably caused by globotriaosylceramide accumulation in the vascular epithelium) could be the major factor in Fabry-related hearing impairment (unpublished data). By contrast, the hydrops in the apical turn, as described by Schachern and colleagues [1], seems to be clinically insignificant. Hegemann and co-workers detected only one ear with a low-frequency hearing loss, and Ménière-like symptoms were not suspected from the medical questionnaires (unpublished data).

Limberger and colleagues found hearing loss in about 50% of their patients (unpublished data), and there was a positive correlation with the Mainz Severity Score Index [8].

The most complete survey of hearing impairment in Fabry disease was obtained from the FOS database and reported by Hegemann and colleagues (unpublished data). In this study of 566 patients, ear-related symptoms were found in 316 individuals. Pure-tone audiograms taken from 86 patients before ERT was initiated were analysed. Hearing loss was most commonly sensorineural: 45 ears in men (58%), 47 ears in women (50%). A purely conductive hearing loss was found unilaterally in only two patients (2%) and a mixed hearing loss was found in seven patients (8%; two females, five males).

Analysing the audiograms of each patient's worst ear according to the World Health Organization classification of impairments, disabilities and handicaps, which better reflects the functional impairment in an age-independent manner, produced a different picture. Eighty-four per cent of the patients were classified as normal, 12% as having a mild hearing impairment and only 2% as having a moderate or severe hearing impairment.

Comparison with age-matched values for a normal population (International Institute of Standardization; ISO 7029) demonstrated that hearing is almost invariably worse in patients with Fabry disease than in the general population. Hearing thresholds were consistently above the median value of the age-matched control group, even in patients whose audiograms could be classified as 'normal'. Male patients had earlier and more severe hearing loss than female patients.

Compared with the general population, hearing was affected to a slightly greater extent at the lower frequencies. Examining the configuration of the audiograms for every tested ear ($n = 172$), 55% were classified as normal, 24% were flat, including two deaf ears (1%), 12% showed a gently sloping high-frequency hearing loss and 7% a steeply sloping hearing loss. Low-frequency ascending and mid-frequency U-shaped audiograms accounted for only 1% each. A sloping audiogram configuration was found to be typical for age-related hearing impairment and was not necessarily associated with Fabry disease [9].

Figure 1 shows the mean values of all audiograms in FOS, including those from patients receiving ERT. It illustrates the typical shape of audiograms in patients with Fabry disease, with a gently sloping high-frequency hearing loss.

Progression with age

In general, the pattern of hearing loss in patients with Fabry disease resembles the age-related hearing loss in a normal population but starts earlier and progresses faster. MacDermot and colleagues reported on three patients without a family history of deafness who suffered from severe sensorineural and conductive hearing loss diagnosed under the age of 10 years, all of whom wore hearing aids [2]. Brief episodes of tinnitus were reported, starting between the ages of 12 and 15 years and continuing to adulthood, with varying degrees of severity. Germain and colleagues reported that normal hearing was most common in younger patients (their youngest was 19 years of age), while sensorineural hearing loss was more common in the older age groups [3]. Most of their patients over 40 years had a mild to

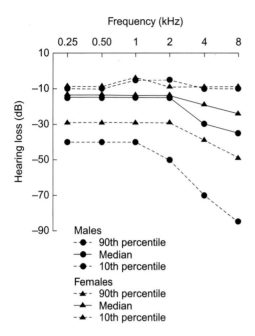

Figure 1. *Mean of all audiograms documented in FOS – the Fabry Outcome Survey – illustrating the typical audiogram configuration in male (n = 93) and female (n = 83) patients with Fabry disease.*

profound hearing loss. Keilmann examined four female and two male patients aged 7–17 years at baseline prior to ERT and 6 months after the initiation of therapy [10]. None of these patients complained about their hearing or had a measurable hearing loss. Hegemann and colleagues found that hearing loss in patients in the FOS database correlated strongly with age at all frequencies, as shown in Figure 2 (unpublished data).

Sudden hearing loss

Germain and colleagues, and Conti and Sergi found a high incidence of sudden onset or sudden progression of hearing loss [3, 4]. In neither study was there any evidence that retrocochlear pathology affected auditory brainstem response, which is consistent with the normal appearance of ganglion cells found by Schachern and co-workers [1]. The most likely explanation for sudden hearing loss is vascular pathology, such as repeated microvascular infarcts from stenosis or occlusion

of distorted small vessels caused by thickening of endothelial and smooth muscle cells. In addition, hypercoagulability in patients with Fabry disease might contribute to a reduced blood supply to the inner ear [11].

In contrast to the studies above, Hegemann and colleagues found a much lower incidence of sudden hearing loss among patients in the FOS database (unpublished data). Of the 566 patients with a complete symptom checklist, 32 (5.6%; 3.4% of the women, 7.7% of the men) reported at least one episode of sudden hearing loss (Table 1). Nevertheless, this is significantly more than would be expected from the estimated lifetime incidence of sudden hearing loss in the general population [12].

Audiograms were available from 15 of these patients with sudden hearing loss, and six of these audiograms were obtained before the start of ERT. However, data were not available around the time of the sudden hearing loss. Four of the audiograms showed an asymmetry between right and left ears. As bilateral symmetrical sudden hearing losses are rare, occurring in only 2% of individuals [13], Hegemann *et al.* speculated that in most patients with symmetrical audiograms, the reported episode of sudden hearing loss had

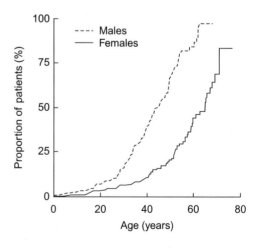

Figure 2. *Prevalence of subjective hearing loss in male and female patients with Fabry disease.*

Table 1. *Frequency of otological symptoms in the FOS – Fabry Outcome Survey – sign and symptom checklist and the age at first appearance.*

| Sign/symptom | Frequency of signs and symptoms | | | Age at onset (years) | | | |
	Total number assessed	Number with signs/ symptoms	%	Mean ± SD	Median	10th–90th percentile	n
Vertigo							
Female	299	89	29.8	34.8 ± 17.9	33.3	13.2–58.2	66
Male	311	100	32.2	29.3 ± 14.6	28.8	11.0–48.2	75
Tinnitus							
Female	299	90	30.1	30.6 ± 17.8	29.7	8.6–57.1	61
Male	311	104	33.4	28.7 ± 13.7	29.4	10.0–47.0	77
Sudden deafness							
Female	299	9	3.0	36.5 ± 20.0	35.5	6.8–65.2	8
Male	311	23	7.4	32.9 ± 12.6	37.3	16.7–44.9	14
Hearing impairment							
Female	299	70	23.4	40.7 ± 19.6	40.5	13.7–65.5	44
Male	311	142	45.7	33.0 ± 14.0	33.9	13.5–49.2	92

recovered completely or almost completely and the symmetrical hearing loss was the result of both ageing and slowly progressive Fabry disease. Based on this assumption, they estimated a rate of spontaneous recovery of 73%, which is similar to the recovery rate seen with sudden hearing loss in the general population.

Effects of ERT on hearing

As ERT has been available for only a few years, there is little information about the effects of ERT on hearing. Hajioff and colleagues described the response to ERT for the first time in a group of 15 hemizygous men (aged 25–49 years) randomized to placebo or agalsidase alfa replacement [14]. Four of these patients had bilateral and seven had unilateral high-frequency sensorineural hearing loss; two had a middle-ear effusion. The sensorineural hearing loss deteriorated both in the placebo and active treatment groups during the 6-month randomized controlled trial. Subsequently, over 18–30 months of open-label treatment, hearing improved to a small degree (5 dB) in 15 out of 20 ears at high frequencies.

Hajioff and colleagues have also described the effect of ERT with agalsidase alfa on hearing loss among patients in the FOS database (unpublished data). Twenty-six patients (8 women and 18 men) underwent audiometric follow-up at a median of 12 months (range 5–36 months) after starting ERT. The median hearing thresholds in this group appeared to improve at all frequencies by 3–5 dB, but these changes were only statistically significant at 4 kHz ($p = 0.03$). Hearing did not change significantly in ears with normal hearing or those with severe hearing loss. However, after correcting for the effects of non-specific age-related hearing loss by expressing hearing thresholds as deviations from the 50th centile of the normal population of that age (ISO 7029), ears with a mild or moderate hearing loss improved significantly by 4–7 dB at most frequencies over a median of 12 months. Hence, it was concluded that hearing is at the very least stabilized by ERT, and quite possibly improved in ears that are abnormal but not severely affected at baseline.

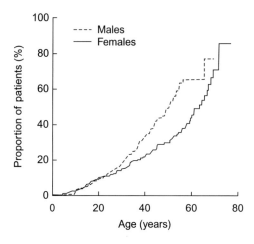

Figure 3. *Prevalence of tinnitus in male and female patients with Fabry disease.*

Tinnitus

Based on the data from the FOS sign and symptom checklist, tinnitus is more frequent than hearing loss in younger patients. The gender difference is less prominent than it is for hearing loss. The frequency of this symptom increases with age: about half of the male patients over 50 years of age and half of the female patients over 60 years of age complained of tinnitus (Figure 3, Table 1).

Unfortunately, the severity of tinnitus has not yet been documented in FOS. The severity of this symptom and its effect on quality of life may vary greatly. The updated FOS ear form will provide a more detailed description of the severity and effects of tinnitus.

Vertigo

De Groot described a patient with Fabry disease and Ménière syndrome (episodic vertigo). He also reviewed otological symptoms in 16 cases previously described by others; seven of these patients had dizziness and two had vertigo [15]. Bird and Lagunoff described two sisters and a brother with Fabry disease who experienced episodic vertigo and nystagmus [16]. Two of them also suffered from hearing loss and tinnitus.

Conti and Sergi found vestibular involvement in four of their 14 patients [4]. In three cases, caloric responses were bilaterally weak or abolished and in one case there was a unilateral weakness. Palla and colleagues investigated the vestibulo-ocular reflex during high-frequency head accelerations in 21 patients using the dual scleral search coil technique [17]. They found unilateral (nine patients) and bilateral (six patients) vestibular deficits in 71% of their patients. After 12 months of ERT, the average vestibular deficit tended to improve, but this change was not significant.

Based on data collected using the FOS sign and symptom checklist, vertigo seems to be as frequent as tinnitus and nearly as frequent as hearing loss in patients with Fabry disease (Figure 4, Table 1). The increasing incidence of vertigo with age is similar to that of tinnitus. However, on more detailed enquiry, most of those patients did not describe true vertigo suggestive of vestibular pathology; instead, they appeared to suffer from dizziness probably caused by orthostatic problems. For this reason, the FOS form for ear symptoms was updated in 2005. There are as yet insufficient data to determine the real prevalence of vestibular dysfunction.

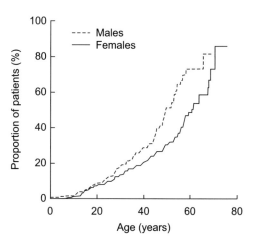

Figure 4. *Prevalence of non-specific 'vertigo' in male and female patients with Fabry disease.*

Conclusions

Otological problems, though not life-threatening, should be considered in all patients with Fabry disease as they may severely affect quality of life. Sensorineural hearing loss is very common and patients should undergo a careful audiological evaluation, as some of them could benefit from a hearing aid. Preliminary data suggest that ERT has a small beneficial effect on mild to moderate hearing loss. Hopefully, further data from FOS will allow a more detailed description of the tinnitus and vertigo that also appear to be common in Fabry disease.

References

1. Schachern PA, Shea DA, Paparella MM, Yoon TH. Otologic histopathology of Fabry's disease. *Ann Otol Rhinol Laryngol* 1989;98:359–63

2. MacDermot KD, Holmes A, Miners AH. Anderson–Fabry disease: clinical manifestations and impact of disease in a cohort of 98 hemizygous males. *J Med Genet* 2001;38:750–60

3. Germain DP. A new phenotype of Fabry disease with intermediate severity between the classical form and the cardiac variant. *Contrib Nephrol* 2001:234–40

4. Conti G, Sergi B. Auditory and vestibular findings in Fabry disease: a study of hemizygous males and heterozygous females. *Acta Paediatr Suppl* 2003; 443:33–7

5. Schuknecht HF. Presbycusis. *Laryngoscope* 1955; 65:402–19

6. Schuknecht HF. Further observations on the pathology of presbycusis. *Arch Otolaryngol* 1964; 80:369–82

7. Schuknecht HF, Gacek MR. Cochlear pathology in presbycusis. *Ann Otol Rhinol Laryngol* 1993;102:1–16

8. Whybra C, Kampmann C, Krummenauer F, Ries M, Mengel E, Miebach E *et al.* The Mainz Severity Score Index: a new instrument for quantifying the Anderson–Fabry disease phenotype, and the response of patients to enzyme replacement therapy. *Clin Genet* 2004;65:299–307

9. Mazzoli M, Van Camp G, Newton V, Giarbini N, Declau F, Parving A. Recommendations for the description of genetic and audiological data for families with nonsyndromic hereditary hearing impairment. *Audiological Med* 2003;1:148–50

10. Keilmann A. Inner ear function in children with Fabry disease. *Acta Paediatr Suppl* 2003;443:31–2

11. Friedman GS, Wik D, Silva L, Abdou JC, Meier-Kriesche HU, Kaplan B *et al.* Allograft loss in renal transplant recipients with Fabry's disease and activated protein C resistance. *Transplantation* 2000;69:2099–102

12. Hughes GB, Freedman MA, Haberkamp TJ, Guay ME. Sudden sensorineural hearing loss. *Otolaryngol Clin North Am* 1996;29:393–405

13. Nakashima T, Itoh A, Misawa H, Ohno Y. Clinico-epidemiologic features of sudden deafness diagnosed and treated at university hospitals in Japan. *Otolaryngol Head Neck Surg* 2000;123:593–7

14. Hajioff D, Enever Y, Quiney R, Zuckerman J, MacDermot K, Mehta A. Hearing loss in Fabry disease: the effect of agalsidase alfa replacement therapy. *J Inherit Metab Dis* 2003;26:787–94

15. De Groot WP. Angiokeratoma corporis diffusum Fabry. *Dermatologica* 1968;136:432–3

16. Bird TD, Lagunoff D. Neurological manifestations of Fabry disease in female carriers. *Ann Neurol* 1978;4:537–40

17. Palla A, Widmer U, Straumann D. Head-impulse testing in Fabry disease – vestibular function in male and female patients. *Acta Paediatr Suppl* 2003; 443:38–42

26 Ophthalmological manifestations of Fabry disease

Andrea Sodi[1], Alex Ioannidis[2] and Susanne Pitz[3]

[1]Department of Ophthalmology, University of Florence, Florence, Italy; [2]Department of Ophthalmology, Royal Free Hospital, London, UK; [3]Department of Ophthalmology, University of Mainz, Mainz, Germany

Ophthalmological manifestations are common in Fabry disease and result from the progressive deposition of glycosphingolipids in various ocular structures. The most specific ocular manifestations of Fabry disease are conjunctival vascular abnormalities, corneal opacities (cornea verticillata), lens opacities and retinal vascular abnormalities. These do not usually cause significant visual impairment or other ocular symptoms, but can nevertheless be important because they can act as markers of the disease, with diagnostic and prognostic implications. Being an external organ and easily investigated with minimally invasive technologies, the eye may be useful for monitoring the natural history of Fabry disease and the response to enzyme replacement therapy. FOS – the Fabry Outcome Survey – provides comprehensive data on the ocular manifestations of Fabry disease. As of March 2005, 173 of the 688 patients enrolled in FOS have undergone a detailed ophthalmological examination. Cornea verticillata was the most frequently reported ophthalmic abnormality in both hemizygous males and heterozygous females, and may represent a useful diagnostic marker. Tortuous vessels and Fabry cataracts were more frequent in males than in females. Vessel tortuosity was associated with a more rapid progression of the disease and may have some value in predicting systemic involvement.

Introduction

Ophthalmological manifestations are common in Fabry disease, affecting various ocular structures. They do not usually cause significant visual impairment or other ocular symptoms, but can nevertheless be important because some manifestations act as markers of the disease, with diagnostic and prognostic implications. Because the eye is an external organ, easily investigated with minimally invasive technologies, ocular abnormalities may also provide a useful means of monitoring the natural history of the disease and patients' response to enzyme replacement therapy (ERT).

Cornea verticillata, the most typical ocular sign in Fabry disease, was first described by Fleischer in 1910 [1], but it was only in 1925 that Weicksel recognized cornea verticillata as being related to Fabry disease [2]. In 1968, while studying a family with various cases of cornea verticillata, Franceschetti found that several members were affected by Fabry disease and reported an X-linked recessive model of inheritance for this metabolic disorder [3]. Subsequent investigators have reported that Fabry disease has significant clinical effects in female heterozygotes [4–6]. This is possibly due to the process of random X-inactivation.

Common ocular findings

Eye abnormalities in Fabry disease result from the deficient activity of the lysosomal hydrolase, α-galactosidase A. This deficiency leads to a progressive deposition of glycosphingolipids in some ocular structures [7–9]. The most specific ocular manifestations of Fabry disease are:

● conjunctival vascular abnormalities
● corneal opacities (cornea verticillata)
● lens opacities
● retinal vascular abnormalities.

Some other ophthalmological features have been described anecdotally in association with Fabry disease, but a possible correlation between these features and the metabolic impairment is unclear.

Conjunctival vessel abnormalities

The most characteristic ophthalmological manifestations are increased vessel tortuosity (Figure 1), venous vascular aneurysmal dilation and 'sludging' of the blood in the small blood vessels. These changes can be seen in any conjunctival area, but they are most commonly located in the inferior bulbar conjunctiva.

The histopathological abnormalities underlying the conjunctival vessel tortuosity are seen as electron-dense deposits, often with a lamellar structure, within the endothelial cells, pericytes and smooth muscle cells of the conjunctival vessel walls. This abnormal storage process induces degenerative changes that are responsible for the weak mechanical resistance of the vessel walls to blood pressure; after several years, this results in typical irregularities of the vessel course [10]. Similar deposits have been reported in all layers of the conjunctival epithelial cells and in the goblet cells [11–13].

Corneal opacities

Cornea verticillata consist of bilateral whorl-like opacities located in the superficial corneal layers, most commonly in the inferior corneal area. These opacities are typically cream coloured, ranging from whitish to golden-brown. They are termed cornea verticillata because the deposits are distributed in a vortex pattern. In the early stages, the opacities may form fine horizontal lines, but they later develop into curving lines, radiating from a point below the centre of the cornea and forming small whorls, before becoming almost straight at the periphery (Figure 2). They show some resemblance to the corneal opacities found after chronic administration of drugs, such as chloroquine or amiodarone, but the amiodarone-related opacities are slightly different as they consist of horizontal lines with some arborization at their extremities, giving a "cats' whiskers" appearance [14].

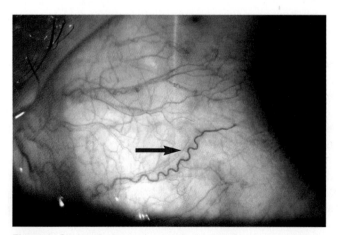

Figure 1. *Conjunctival vessel tortuosity (arrowed).*

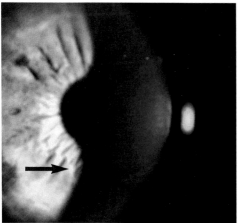
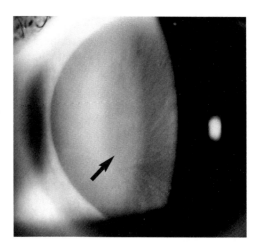
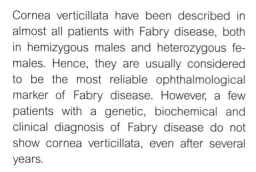

Figure 2. *Cornea verticillata (arrowed).*

Cornea verticillata have been described in almost all patients with Fabry disease, both in hemizygous males and heterozygous females. Hence, they are usually considered to be the most reliable ophthalmological marker of Fabry disease. However, a few patients with a genetic, biochemical and clinical diagnosis of Fabry disease do not show cornea verticillata, even after several years.

The cause of the vortex pattern of the corneal deposits is unknown. Various hypotheses cite the influence of ocular hydrodynamics, periodic blinking or ocular magnetic fields. Another possible cause is the centripetal movement of the renewing epithelial cells from the periphery towards the centre of the cornea [15–17].

There have been some reports of a subepithelial corneal haze, usually associated with the more typical whorl-like opacities. In most of these patients, the haze is diffuse and involves the whole cornea, but in some individuals it is limited to the central or limbal corneal area. It is generally brownish, or more rarely grey or whitish [18, 19]. The haze has been suggested to be an early manifestation of Fabry disease [20], although it has also been suggested to be a natural evolution of the vortex opacities [18].

Corneal pathology has been investigated both in hemizygous and heterozygous patients with Fabry disease [21–25]. The most relevant finding is the presence of intraepithelial deposits consisting of dense laminated cytoplasmic inclusions, both membrane-bound and lying freely in the cytoplasm. In a histopathological study of the cornea of a woman with Fabry disease, Weingeist and Blodi described subepithelial ridges composed of re-duplicated basement membrane and amorphous electron-dense material between the basement membrane and Bowman's layer. They suggested that the diffuse accumulation of sphingolipids in the corneal epithelium might be responsible for the diffuse corneal haze, while the whorl-like pattern might be determined by a series of subepithelial ridges [26]. However, these ridges have not been consistently reported in either heterozygous women or hemizygous men [11].

A more recent ultrastructural investigation revealed a disruption of the normal pattern of the basement membrane without any evident re-duplication of the basal lamina [27]. Possible corneal endothelium involvement in Fabry disease has been suggested by the finding of pigment and corneal guttae on the endothelium in two patients [28], but this has not been confirmed by other investigators.

Lens opacities

Two specific types of lens opacities have been reported in patients with Fabry disease: an anterior capsular or subcapsular cataract, and a radial posterior subcapsular cataract. Anterior capsular and subcapsular opacities are generally bilateral and wedge-shaped, with a radial distribution, and have their bases near the equator and their apices toward the centre of the anterior capsule. Posterior subcapsular cataracts are rare but very specific for the disease (and hence are called Fabry cataracts). They consist of linear whitish opacities located near the posterior capsule, and have a spoke-like appearance (Figure 3).

Fabry cataracts are not easily detected by direct observation using a slit lamp, and can often be missed on routine examination. They are best seen and imaged by retro-illumination, using the light reflected by the ocular fundus.

Laminated bodies have been described in the lens epithelium and stroma of patients with Fabry disease [11], but a histopathological study of a Fabry cataract has yet to be undertaken.

Retinal and choroidal vessel abnormalities

Retinal and choroidal vessel abnormalities are mainly represented by an increased tortuosity of the retinal vessels (sometimes with a 'corkscrew' appearance) associated with segmental venous dilation, arteriolar narrowing and arteriovenous nicking (localized constriction).

Retinal vessel tortuosity can be easily detected by simple ophthalmoscopy of the posterior segment of the eye. However, it is better appreciated using fluorescein angiography (Figure 4).

Electron microscopy reveals the presence of dense laminated cytoplasmic inclusions in the endothelial cells and pericytes of retinal vessels, closely resembling the lesions described in the conjunctiva [11, 16]. Similar lesions have been reported in all of the major vessels of the eye [11, 24, 25]. In choroidal arterioles and iris vessels, they are associated with similar accumulations in the smooth muscle cells of the vessel walls [11, 24]; inclusions were also found in both iris and retinal pigment epithelium [11, 24].

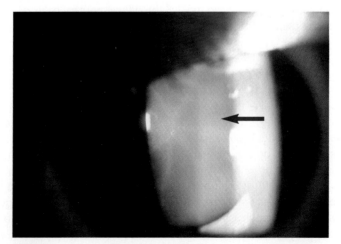

Figure 3. *Posterior subcapsular 'spoke-like' cataract (Fabry cataract; arrowed).*

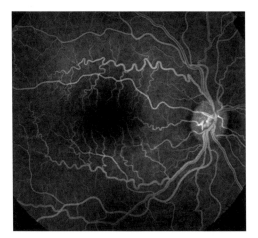

Figure 4. *Retinal vessel tortuosity (fluorescein angiography).*

Increased tortuosity of the retinal vessels is very common in patients with Fabry disease, but is not specific to this disease; the same abnormality can be observed in other retinal disorders, such as hypertensive retinopathy.

In addition to involvement of the larger retinal vessels, some authors have reported microvascular changes imaged using fluorescein angiography of the retina [29, 30]. These angiographic findings are not consistently observed in patients with Fabry disease and therefore cannot be considered typical of the disease.

Occasional ocular findings

Several other ocular manifestations have been described in association with Fabry disease, but have been reported only in isolated patients or in very small series. Sometimes the pathophysiological link with abnormal glycosphingolipid metabolism is unclear. The association of some of these vascular occlusive disorders with Fabry disease, although probably due to the compromised choroidal and retinal vasculature, is therefore hypothetical and requires further investigation.

Posterior segment of the eye

Most of the occasional ophthalmological findings involve the posterior segment of the

eye. There have been some cases of retinal artery and vein occlusions reported in association with Fabry disease [31–33], usually in patients under 30 years of age. An anterior ischaemic optic neuropathy has been observed in association with cilioretinal artery occlusion in a female carrier of Fabry disease [34]. A sudden decrease of visual acuity was reported in a young man with Fabry disease, together with pale areas in a lobular distribution on the eye fundus; this clinical picture is suggestive of choroidal ischaemia [35]. Fabry disease should therefore be considered in the differential diagnosis of ocular vascular occlusive disorders, especially in young patients.

Optic atrophy or papilloedema has been reported in several patients with Fabry disease, but the pathophysiology remains unclear [36]. Detection of papilloedema is facilitated by angiographic examination which, in the later phases, will show leakage of the dye from the borders of the disc. Myelinated nerve fibres have also been reported in association with Fabry disease [37].

Abnormalities of the peripheral retinal pigment epithelium have been described in an 18-year-old man with skin and kidney lesions typical of Fabry disease and a mutation of the *GLA* gene. Possible explanations for this uncommon finding are that there had been localized areas of vitreo-retinal traction, previous neuro-retinal detachment or choroidal ischaemia [38].

Anterior segment of the eye

Some rare ocular findings have also been reported that affect the anterior segment of the eye in patients with Fabry disease. Lid oedema has been described in several patients, usually in hemizygotes [19, 20], and angiokeratomas can occasionally be located on the skin of the lids. A dry eye syndrome has also been reported [39], sometimes in association with altered pupillary motility (reduced constriction with pilocarpine), suggesting that there is an impairment of autonomic function [40].

Visual field defects

The visual field was assessed in 27 patients with Fabry disease using Goldmann perimetry [18]. An enlargement of the blind spot was noted in 37% of the tested eyes. The enlargement was bilateral in most cases and was not associated with colour perception abnormalities. This defect might reflect subclinical involvement of the optic pathways, probably resulting from localized ischaemic events. Moreover, abnormalities of pattern-reversal visual-evoked responses have recently been reported in a child with Fabry disease [41].

Prevalence and clinical significance of ocular manifestations

The prevalence of the most significant eye abnormalities in Fabry disease are summarized in Table 1 [18, 20, 42–45]. Possible explanations for the differences in the reported prevalence of specific eye abnormalities in the various studies include underlying differences in demographic features (mainly age, sex and ethnic origin), genotype (determining different phenotypes) and technologies used to detect the eye signs, as well as the subjective evaluation of the investigators and, in a few cases, the influence of ERT.

An ophthalmological evaluation should be carried out in every patient in whom there is a clinical suspicion of Fabry disease. Some eye abnormalities are present in most individuals with Fabry disease and can be helpful in confirming the diagnosis in patients or in apparently healthy relatives, while other manifestations may be less specific. For example, conjunctival vessel abnormalities and cornea verticillata are both relatively common in Fabry disease. Cornea verticillata are highly sensitive for the diagnosis of Fabry disease (i.e. are present in almost all patients)

as well as being highly specific (i.e. rarely found in non-affected subjects). By contrast, conjunctival vessel tortuosity is encountered in a number of other diseases and its evaluation is subjective.

Furthermore, cornea verticillata can be easily detected on routine ophthalmological examination using a slit lamp. This is a non-invasive, inexpensive and simple procedure. Hence, cornea verticillata can be used as an ophthalmological marker for Fabry disease. The only drawbacks are that cornea verticillata (similar to other ophthalmological manifestatons of Fabry disease) do not result in visual symptoms and therefore do not cause patients to consult their doctor, and that general ophthalmologists are unfamiliar with this marker. For these reasons, ophthalmological screening programmes for Fabry disease have a low efficacy [46]. A campaign to inform general ophthalmologists about the recognition and clinical implications of cornea verticillata might increase the number of early diagnoses of Fabry disease.

It is difficult to follow-up ophthalmological features of Fabry disease with a standard examination. Assessing the degree of vessel tortuosity in the conjunctiva and fundus is highly subjective and non-specific. Lens opacities are either non-specific (e.g. anterior subcapsular cataracts) or very rare (e.g. 'spoke-like' Fabry cataracts). Cornea verticillata are useful for diagnosis, but changes over time are difficult to detect; clinical evaluation may be highly subjective, as corneal imaging is poorly reproducible and unreliable due to multiple technical photographic problems.

Based on a standard ophthalmological examination, changes in the ophthalmological features of Fabry disease can be detected reliably only when they become clinically obvious. They are therefore seldom useful in clinical practice for patient follow-up. Furthermore, ophthalmological abnormalities have not been observed in some patients.

Enzyme replacement therapy

One of the authors (AS) has seen a few instances of apparent regression of corneal opacities after ERT, detected using a slit lamp. However, quantification of the vortex opacities is highly subjective, and reliable methods of imaging cornea verticillata are still awaited. Hence, there are still questions about the use of cornea verticillata to monitor individual responses to therapy.

Future developments

Future developments may include an internationally agreed classification of the eye abnormalities that would allow 'scoring' of the severity of eye involvement. This, coupled with more sophisticated investigations (e.g. confocal corneal microscopy or colour Doppler imaging of orbital vessels), could enable the natural history of ocular manifestations to be elucidated as well as allowing the response to ERT to be monitored.

Ocular manifestations in FOS – the Fabry Outcome Survey

Assessment of eye abnormalities in patients with Fabry disease forms a significant part of FOS, an international database for all patients with Fabry disease who are receiving, or are candidates for, ERT with agalsidase alfa. As of March 2005, data have been collected from a total of 688 patients, of whom 173 (82 males, 91 females; about 25% of the FOS population) have undergone a detailed ophthalmological examination. This examination has paid particular attention to cornea and lens opacities (Fabry cataracts), and to the course of vessels in the conjunctiva and retina (grouped together as 'vessel tortuosity').

Data have been reported using a specific ophthalmological form (the eye examination form). The various signs have been classified simply as either present or absent, according to the subjective judgement of the examiner,

Table 1. *Prevalence of ocular manifestations of Fabry disease in published studies.*

		Ocular manifestation					
Study	Gender	Conjuctival vessel abnormalities	Cornea verticillata	Corneal haze	Anterior cataract	Posterior subcapsular cataract	Retinal vessel abnormalities
Spaeth and Frost [42]	6 males 3 females	41.6%	91.6%	NR	NR	50%	25%
Sher et al. [20]	37 males 25 females	78% 46%	94.5% 88%	NR NR	35% None	37% 14%	70% 25%
Orssaud et al. [18]	32 males	68.7%	43.7%	84.3%	15.6%	37.5%	56.2%
Nguyen et al. [43]	34 males 32 females	97.1% 78.1%	94.1% 71.9%	NR NR	41.2% 9.4%	11.8% None	76.5% 18.8%
Vaulthier et al. [44]	13 males 7 females	NR	65%	10%	NR	20%	55%
Fumex-Boizard et al. [45]	9 males 7 females	60%	90%	NR	NR	50%	90%

NR, not reported.

without any attempt to grade the severity of the abnormalities. Data analysis has focused particularly on prevalence (in the total FOS cohort and according to age and gender), concurrence of specific ocular manifestations in the same patient, and associations with systemic findings.

Overall prevalence

The presence of cornea verticillata has been reported in 76.9% of females and 73.1% of males; vessel tortuosity has been observed in 21.9% of females and 48.7% of males; and Fabry cataracts have been noted in 9.8% of females and 23.1% of males. Hence, in agreement with data from other studies [20, 42–45], cornea verticillata are the most common ophthalmic abnormality in Fabry disease in both hemizygous males and heterozygous females.

The prevalence of vessel tortuosity in FOS is lower than reported in previous smaller series [18, 20, 42–45]. This might be accounted for by the difficulties in evaluating the vessels objectively and by the lack of a clear distinction between tortuosity in the conjunctival and in the retinal vascular areas.

Tortuous vessels and Fabry cataracts (but not cornea verticillata) are more frequent in male than in female patients in the FOS database. This might be due to more severe clinical involvement in hemizygous males, or to some hormonal influence on ocular haemodynamics [47, 48] or lens structure.

Age- and gender-related prevalence

The prevalence of cornea verticillata was similar in males and females, as well as in different age groups. The prevalence of tortuous vessels and Fabry cataract, however, was lower in females than in males, and the prevalence of tortuous vessels increased significantly with age in males (Figure 5).

Ocular manifestations of Fabry disease can be detected in young children (to date, the youngest child in whom ocular manifestations have been found was 3 years old). This is consistent with previous reports of cornea verticillata in very young patients, including a 6-month-old child [20] and a fetus [22], and supports the case for ophthalmological examination of paediatric patients. At 20 years of age, approximately 30% of males and 25% of females had tortuous vessels, and approximately 20% of males and 10% of females had Fabry cataract. The frequency after 40 years of age was approximately 60% in males and 25% in females for tortuous vessels, and more than 30% in males and 15% in females for Fabry cataract.

Associations between eye abnormalities

Cornea verticillata may be the only eye abnormality observed in a patient with Fabry disease, and is not necessarily associated with vessel tortuosity. By contrast, vessel tortuosity rarely occurs as the only ocular sign in patients with Fabry disease.

Association between eye abnormalities and other signs and symptoms

Differences in disease progression were analysed using linear regression of disease severity, adjusting for age and sex. Disease severity was assessed by the Mainz Severity Score Index (MSSI) [49], as adapted for use in FOS. This is a scoring system developed to measure the severity of Fabry disease and to monitor its clinical course in response to ERT. There was no relationship between the presence of cornea verticillata and disease severity, as measured by the adapted MSSI. However, a significant relationship could be seen between the presence of vessel tortuosity and disease severity ($p = 0.01$): progression was more rapid in patients with tortuous vessels than in those without vessel tortuosity (Figure 6). Patients with vessel tortuosity also showed a more rapid deterioration in renal function, based on

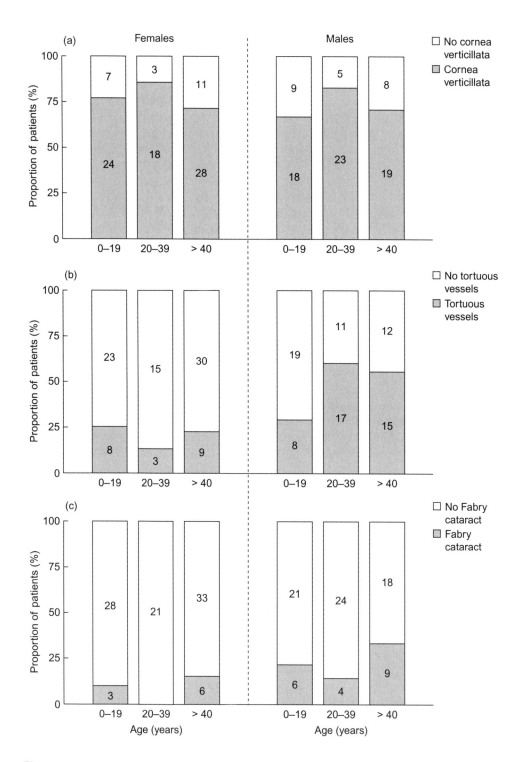

Figure 5. *Prevalence of (a) cornea verticillata, (b) tortuous vessels and (c) Fabry cataract according to age and gender in FOS – the Fabry Outcome Survey. Numbers in columns indicate numbers of patients.*

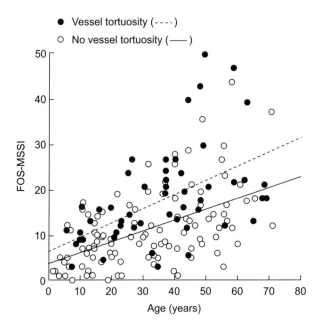

Figure 6. *Linear regression analysis showing the correlation between the Mainz Severity Score Index as adapted for use in FOS – the Fabry Outcome Survey (FOS-MSSI) and increasing age (i.e. disease severity) in patients in FOS with and without tortuous vessels.*

the estimated glomerular filtration rate ($p = 0.012$). Furthermore, the relationship between the increase in cardiac size (mean wall thickness) with age and vessel tortuosity was even more significant ($p < 0.0001$) (Figure 7). For Fabry cataracts, the numbers were too small to enable any valid conclusions to be drawn.

Conclusions

A review of published literature and analysis of the FOS database suggest the following conclusions regarding ocular manifestations of Fabry disease.

- The presence of cornea verticillata is highly sensitive and specific for Fabry disease in both male and female patients. Cornea verticillata can therefore be considered a useful ophthalmological marker for Fabry disease, although it should be

borne in mind that corneal opacities may also occur in patients taking certain drugs.

- In some cases, cornea verticillata can be an isolated occurrence, without the presence of other eye abnormalities.
- Tortuous vessels are common in Fabry disease, but are relatively non-specific for the disease.
- Posterior subcapsular cataracts with a spoke-like appearance are rare but, when present, may suggest a diagnosis of Fabry disease.
- The prevalence of cornea verticillata was similar in males and females as well as in different age groups; however, the frequency of tortuous vessels and Fabry cataracts was lower in females than in males.
- Eye abnormalities can also be detected in very young children.

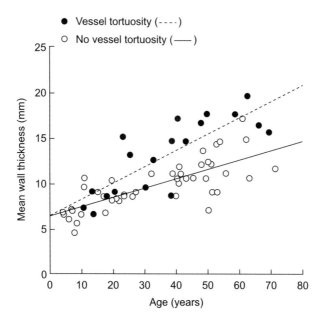

Figure 7. *Linear regression analysis showing the correlation between the heart mean wall thickness and increasing age (i.e. disease severity) in patients in FOS – the Fabry Outcome Survey – with and without tortuous vessels.*

- The presence of vessel tortuosity appears to be associated with a more rapid progression of Fabry disease.
- The study of eye abnormalities can aid diagnosis but does not significantly improve the accuracy of monitoring progression of the disease and its response to treatment. Technological developments are required before eye signs can be quantified and used successfully to monitor patients affected by Fabry disease.

References

1. Fleischer B. Uber eine eigenartige bisher nicht bekannte Hornhauttrubung [On an unusual thus far unknown type of corneal cloudiness]. *Graefes Arch Ophthalmol* 1910;77:136–40

2. Weicksel J. Angiomatosis bzw Angiokeratosis universalis (eine sehr seltene Haut-und Gefasserkrankung) [Angiomatosis or angiokeratosis universalis (a very rare disease of the skin and blood and lymphatic vessels)]. *Deutsch Med Wschr* 1925;51:898

3. Franceschetti AT. La cornea verticillata at ses relations avec la maladie de Fabry [Cornea verticillata (Gruber) and its relation to Fabry disease (angiokeratoma corporis diffusum)]. *Ophthalmologica* 1968;156:232–8

4. MacDermot KD, Holmes A, Miners AH. Anderson–Fabry disease: clinical manifestations and impact of disease in a cohort of 60 obligate carrier females. *J Med Genet* 2001;38:769–75

5. Whybra C, Kampmann C, Willers I, Davies J, Winchester B, Kriegsmann J et al. Anderson–Fabry disease: clinical manifestations of disease in female heterozygotes. *J Inherit Metab Dis* 2001;24:715–24

6. Mehta A, Ricci R, Widmer U, Dehout F, Garcia de Lorenzo A, Kampmann C et al. Fabry disease defined: baseline clinical manifestations of 366 patients in the Fabry Outcome Survey. *Eur J Clin Invest* 2004;34: 236–42

7. Germain DP. Maladie de Fabry (déficit en α-galactosidase A): physiopathologie, signes cliniques et aspects génétiques [Fabry's disease (α-galactosidase-A deficiency): physiopathology, clinical signs, and genetic aspects]. *J Soc Biol* 2002;196: 161–73

8. Hauser AC, Lorenz M, Sunder-Plassmann G. The expanding clinical spectrum of Anderson–Fabry

disease: a challenge to diagnosis in the novel era of enzyme replacement therapy. *J Intern Med* 2004;255: 629–36

9. Masson C, Cisse I, Simon V, Insalaco P, Audran M. Fabry disease: a review. *Joint Bone Spine* 2004;71: 381–3

10. Libert J, Toussaint D. Tortuosities of retinal and conjunctival vessels in lysosomal storage diseases. *Birth Defects Orig Artic Ser* 1982;18:347–58

11. Font RL, Fine BS. Ocular pathology in Fabry's disease. Histochemical and electron microscopic observations. *Am J Ophthalmol* 1972;73:419–30

12. Libert J, Tondeur M, Van Hoof F. The use of conjunctival biopsy and enzyme analysis in tears for the diagnosis of homozygotes and heterozygotes with Fabry disease. *Birth Defects Orig Artic Ser* 1976;12: 221–39

13. McCulloch C, Ghosh M. Ultrastructural changes in the cornea and conjunctiva of a heterozygous woman with Fabry's disease. *Can J Ophthalmol* 1984;19:192–8

14. Mantyjarvi M, Tuppurainen K, Ikaheimo K. Ocular side effects of amiodarone. *Surv Ophthalmol* 1998; 42:360–6

15. Dufier JL, Gubler MC, Dhermy P, Lenoir G, Paupe J, Haye C. La maladie de Fabry et ses manifestations ophtalmologique [Fabry's disease in ophthalmology]. *J Fr Ophtalmol* 1980;3:625–30

16. Roussel T, Grutzmacher R, Coster D. Patterns of superficial keratopathy. *Aust J Ophthalmol* 1984;12:301–16

17. Bron AJ. Vortex patterns of the corneal epithelium. *Trans Ophthalmol Soc UK* 1973;93:455–72

18. Orssaud C, Dufier J, Germain D. Ocular manifestations in Fabry disease: a survey of 32 hemizygous male patients. *Ophthalmic Genet* 2003;24:129–39

19. Rahman A. The ocular manifestations of hereditary dystopic lipidosis (angiokeratoma corporis diffusum universale). *Arch Ophthalmol* 1963;69:708–16

20. Sher NA, Letson RD, Desnick RJ. The ocular manifestations in Fabry's disease. *Arch Ophthalmol* 1979; 97:671–6

21. Tuppurainen K, Collan Y, Rantanen T, Hollmen A. Fabry's disease and cornea verticillata. A report of 3 cases. *Acta Ophthalmol (Copenh)* 1981;59:674–82

22. Tsutsumi A, Uchida Y, Kanai T, Tsutsumi O, Satoh K, Sakamoto S. Corneal findings in a foetus with Fabry's disease. *Acta Ophthalmol (Copenh)* 1984;62:923–31

23. Macrae WG, Ghosh M, McCulloch C. Corneal changes in Fabry's disease: a clinico-pathologic case report of a heterozygote. *Ophthalmic Paediatr Genet* 1985;5:185–90

24. Riegel EM, Pokorny KS, Friedman AH, Suhan J, Ritch RH, Desnick RJ. Ocular pathology of Fabry's disease in a hemizygous male following renal transplantation. *Surv Ophthalmol* 1982;26:247–52

25. Francois J, Hanssens M, Teuchy H. Corneal ultrastructural changes in Fabry's disease. *Ophthalmologica* 1978;176:313–30

26. Weingeist TA, Blodi FC. Fabry's disease: ocular findings in a female carrier. A light and electron microscopy study. *Arch Ophthalmol* 1971;85:169–76

27. Hirano K, Murata K, Miyagawa A, Terasaki H, Saigusa J, Nagasaka T et al. Histopathologic findings of cornea verticillata in a woman heterozygous for Fabry's disease. *Cornea* 2001;20:233–6

28. Grace EV. Diffuse angiokeratosis (Fabry's disease). *Am J Ophthalmol* 1966;62:139–45

29. Dantas MA, Fonseca RA, Kaga T, Yannuzzi LA, Spaide RF. Retinal and choroidal vascular changes in heterozygous Fabry disease. *Retina* 2001;21:87–9

30. Ohkubo H. Several functional and fluorescein fundus angiographic findings in Fabry's disease. *Ophthalmologica* 1988;196:132–6

31. Sher NA, Reiff W, Letson RD, Desnick RJ. Central retinal artery occlusion complicating Fabry's disease. *Arch Ophthalmol* 1978;96:815–7

32. Andersen MV, Dahl H, Fledelius H, Nielsen NV. Central retinal artery occlusion in a patient with Fabry's disease documented by scanning laser ophthalmoscopy. *Acta Ophthalmol (Copenh)* 1994;72:635–8

33. Oto S, Kart H, Kadayifcilar S, Ozdemir N, Aydin P. Retinal vein occlusion in a woman with heterozygous Fabry's disease. *Eur J Ophthalmol* 1998;8:265–7

34. Abe H, Sakai T, Sawaguchi S, Hasegawa S, Takagi M, Yoshizawa T et al. Ischemic optic neuropathy in a female carrier with Fabry's disease. *Ophthalmologica* 1992;205:83–8

35. Guenoun JM, Parc C, Monnet D, Brezin AP. [Loss of visual acuity due to choroidal ischemia in Fabry's disease]. *J Fr Ophtalmol* 2003;26:842–4

36. Velzeboer CM, de Groot WP. Ocular manifestations in angiokeratoma corporis diffusum (Fabry). *Br J Ophthalmol* 1971;55:683–92

37. Calmettes L, Deodati F, Suc JP, Bec P, Conte J, Pasternac A et al. Au sujet d'un noveau cas de maladie de Fabry [A new case of Fabry's disease]. *Bull Soc Ophtalmol Fr* 1967;67:1025–8

38. Jourdel D, Defoort-Dhellemmes S, Labalette P, Ryckewaert M, Hache JC. Anomalies pigmentaires rétiniennes associées à une maladie de Fabry [Retinal pigment anomalies associated with Fabry's disease]. *J Fr Ophtalmol* 1998;21:755–60

39. Klein P. Ocular manifestations of Fabry's disease. *J Am Optom Assoc* 1986;57:672–4

40. Cable WJ, Kolodny EH, Adams RD. Fabry disease: impaired autonomic function. *Neurology* 1982;32: 498–502

41. Liasis A, Ioannidis A, Thompson D, Davey C, Nischal K. Visual electrophysiology in patients with Anderson–Fabry disease. *Acta Paediatr Suppl* 2006;451:119

42. Spaeth GL, Frost P. Fabry's disease. Its ocular manifestations. *Arch Ophthalmol* 1965;74:760–9

43. Nguyen TT, Gin T, Nicholls K, Low M, Galanos J, Crawford A. Ophthalmological manifestations of Fabry disease: a survey of patients at the Royal Melbourne Fabry Disease Treatment Centre. *Clin Experiment Ophthalmol* 2005;33:164–8

44. Vauthier L, Cobut O, Depasse F, Dehout F, Van Maldergem L. Ophthalmological findings in a series of 20 patients with Fabry disease: preliminary results. *Acta Paediatr Suppl* 2006;451:118

45. Fumex-Boizard L, Cochat P, Fouilhoux A, Guffon N, Denis P. Relation entre les manifestations ophtalmologiques et les atteintes générales chez dix patients atteints de la maladie de Fabry [Relation between ocular manifestations and organ involvement in ten patients with Fabry disease]. *J Fr Ophtalmol* 2005;28:45–50

46. Hauser AC, Lorenz M, Voigtlander T, Fodinger M, Sunder-Plassmann G. Results of an ophthalmologic screening programme for identification of cases with Anderson–Fabry disease. *Ophthalmologica* 2004; 218:207–9

47. Harris-Yitzhak M, Harris A, Ben-Refael Z, Zarfati D, Garzozi HJ, Martin BJ. Estrogen-replacement therapy: effects on retrobulbar hemodynamics. *Am J Ophthalmol* 2000;129:623–8

48. Atalay E, Karaali K, Akar M, Ari ES, Simsek M, Atalay S *et al*. Early impact of hormone replacement therapy on vascular hemodynamics detected via ocular colour Doppler analysis. *Maturitas* 2005;50:282–8

49. Whybra C, Kampmann C, Krummenauer F, Ries M, Mengel E, Miebach E *et al*. The Mainz Severity Score Index: a new instrument for quantifying the Anderson–Fabry disease phenotype, and the response of patients to enzyme replacement therapy. *Clin Genet* 2004;65:299–307

27 Pulmonary involvement in Fabry disease

John D Aubert[1] and Frédéric Barbey[2]

[1]*Pneumology Division and* [2]*Nephrology Division, University Hospital (CHUV), 1011-Lausanne, Switzerland*

Pulmonary involvement in Fabry disease has received less attention than the effects of the disease on the kidneys, nervous system or heart. However, data from FOS – the Fabry Outcome Survey – are now helping to elucidate the pulmonary manifestations of Fabry disease. Twenty-three patients out of a cohort of 67 analysed in FOS have been identified with airway obstruction, as defined by a ratio of forced expiratory volume in 1 second to forced vital capacity of less than 0.7. This prevalence is much greater than would be expected in the general population, with the main risk factors appearing to be increasing age and male gender. Spirometric analysis has revealed that the airway obstruction is clinically much more similar to chronic obstructive pulmonary disease than to asthma. Although little is known about the anatomical changes responsible for airway obstruction in patients with Fabry disease, airway wall hyperplasia and/or fibrosis are potential causes. Treatment of patients with moderate or severe airway obstruction should include inhaled bronchodilators, and individuals who smoke should be encouraged to stop. Further studies and future analyses of FOS data should determine whether enzyme replacement therapy is able to help or prevent the pulmonary manifestations of Fabry disease.

Historical background

Although the original patient described by Fabry in 1898 had 'asthma', frequent respiratory tract infections, and died of lung disease at the age 43 years [1], reports of pulmonary involvement in Fabry disease are uncommon.

In 1972, Bartimmo and colleagues performed pulmonary function studies and pulmonary scintiphotography in three brothers aged 31, 34 and 38 years. In the absence of clinical or laboratory evidence of diffuse pulmonary parenchymal or vascular disease or dysfunction in these patients, the investigators concluded that pulmonary involvement had little clinical or functional impact on patients with Fabry disease, and that pulmonary symptoms were mainly associated with other conditions (i.e. cigarette smoking or cardiac disease) [2].

Before the findings of Bartimmo *et al.* were published, however, some interesting pathological data on lung involvement in Fabry disease had been reported. In 1947, Pompen and co-workers found that the bronchial mucosal cells in an autopsy case were much 'taller' than normal and the cytoplasm was vacuolated and pale [3]. Moreover, the bronchial and pulmonary vessels showed thickened walls due to hypertrophy and vacuolization of the smooth muscle fibres of the media. Abnormalities of the pulmonary vasculature had also been reported by others [4–6]. For example, in 1968, a histological and electron microscopic study of lung tissue carried out by Bagdade et al. revealed that the lipid inclusions in the lung were similar to those present in other tissues [4].

Hence, in contrast to kidney and heart involvement, it remained unclear for some time whether significant clinical or physiological pulmonary dysfunction occurs as a consequence of sphingolipid deposits. More recently, this has been clarified by several studies.

In 1978, Kariman and colleagues reported the case of a 32-year-old hemizygous man complaining of morning cough and exertional dyspnoea as a result of climbing two flights of stairs [7]. The patient was an active smoker, with a creatinine clearance rate of 110 ml/minute and a serum α_1-antitrypsin level within the normal range. Pulmonary function tests revealed severe obstruction, hyperinflation and a mild impairment of carbon monoxide diffusion, and the chest X-ray was compatible with severe bullous emphysema. The authors concluded that significant pulmonary involvement could occur even in the early stages of Fabry disease, before there was clinical evidence of multiple system involvement, and that cigarette smoking could be an aggravating factor.

In 1980, Rosenberg and colleagues carried out physiological studies and obtained ventilation and perfusion scans for seven patients with Fabry disease (6 males, 1 female) aged 29–64 years [8]. All were found to have significant airflow obstruction. Five of the patients were smokers, but the extent of obstruction in these individuals was disproportionate to that expected from cigarettes alone. In addition, cells obtained in the bronchoalveolar lavage fluid were found to have numerous sphingolipid deposits, suggesting that some of the functional abnormality might have resulted from intrinsic

airway disease. Moreover, as the majority of these patients also had a reduced diffusion capacity for carbon monoxide, the authors postulated that there was destruction of lung parenchyma, as suggested by the observation of hyperinflation and bullae on chest X-rays in three of the patients. Emphysema is a well-known mechanism for loss of elastic recoil in the lung.

In 1991, Smith and colleagues reported autopsy findings for a 52-year-old male with Fabry disease who had chronic airway disease and in whom numerous electron-dense inclusions were observed within pulmonary arteries, arterioles, veins and alveolar walls on electron microscopy [9]. There were also numerous deposits in the smooth muscle cells of the media of muscular pulmonary arteries and veins, and in the endothelial cells of all vessels and capillaries, as well as in the alveolar interstitial cells. However, Smith et al. did not conclude that accumulation of sphingolipids in the lung could have affected the respiratory function of their patient.

The most interesting and largest study on pulmonary involvement in Fabry disease was published recently by Brown et al. [10]. This study involved 25 affected men aged 16–54 years. Pulmonary complaints were common in these patients and included cough, wheeze or dyspnoea, but no haemoptysis. There were two cases of spontaneous pneumothorax, an incidence much greater than would be expected in the general population [11]. Nine patients (36%) had a reduced FEV_1:FVC ratio (ratio of forced expiratory volume in 1 second to forced vital capacity), consistent with airway obstruction, and six also had air trapping; four of the nine were non-smokers. The presence of obstructive impairment was strongly age dependent, as for heart and kidney involvement, with no patient younger than 26 years having a reduced FEV_1:FVC ratio. Interestingly, pulmonary symptoms were not associated with either cigarette smoking or cardiac disease, as previously suggested by Bartimmo et al. [2], and smokers with obstruction were not younger than non-smokers.

Eight of the nine patients underwent spirometry after receiving bronchodilator aerosol, and five (63%) of them exhibited a significant increase in FEV_1 [12]. There was no radiographic evidence of bullous emphysema, and single-breath diffusion capacity for carbon monoxide, which correlates with morphological emphysema, was normal in all patients [13]. A total of ten patients underwent methacholine challenge testing, and none of them exhibited a decline in FEV_1 of 20% or greater. This argues against airway inflammation, as disorders associated with extensive inflammatory changes (e.g. asthma, cystic fibrosis or chronic bronchitis) are frequently associated with positive challenge testing [14, 15]. The authors concluded that airway obstruction commonly occurs in patients with Fabry disease regardless of smoking history, and that it is strongly correlated with age, and most likely results from fixed narrowing of the airways by accumulated sphingolipids in bronchial epithelial and/or smooth muscle cells.

Recently, the Swiss Fabry group assessed pulmonary function in 44 patients with Fabry disease (27 men, 17 women). Twelve patients (9 men, 3 women) had an FEV_1:FVC ratio below 0.7, which is the cut-off point for defining chronic obstructive pulmonary disease (COPD); only one was an active smoker and one a previous smoker. FEV_1:FVC, expressed as a percentage of the predicted value, correlated with age ($p = 0.005$). The increase in FEV_1 after taking a β_2-agonist never exceeded 8% of the predicted value. These results confirm that there is a high prevalence of airway obstruction in Fabry disease, particularly in patients in the advanced stages of the disease [16].

Data from FOS

To date, spirometric data have been reported for 68 patients in FOS – the Fabry Outcome Survey. The data comprise FEV_1, FVC and the ratio of these two variables (available for 67 patients; Table 1), and are expressed as absolute values in litres or as a percentage of the predicted value according to the sex, age and height of each individual. This latter formulation is especially useful when comparing data from a cohort with heterogeneous anthropomorphic parameters.

There is no single worldwide accepted definition of airway obstruction. The simplest and most commonly used criterion has been established by the Global Initiative

Table 1. Summary of respiratory data from FOS – the Fabry Outcome Survey.

	With airflow obstruction*	Without airflow obstruction
Total number of patients	23	44
Males	14	17[†]
Females	9	26
Smokers	2	7
Past smokers	2	2
Non-smokers	4	13
Smoking status unknown	15	22
Age in years – mean (SD)	50 (9)	30 (15)

*Airflow obstruction is defined by an FEV_1:FVC ratio (ratio of forced expiratory volume in 1 second to forced vital capacity) below 0.7.
[†]One male smoker could not be classified as having airway obstruction, due to an absence of FEV_1 measurement.

on Obstructive Lung Disorders (GOLD) [www.goldcopd.com]. The cut-off FEV_1:FVC ratio is 0.7; if the ratio is below this value, patients are considered to have airway obstruction. Although straightforward, this definition may overestimate airway obstruction in older patients, as the FEV_1:FVC ratio declines with age. The definition put forward by the European Respiratory Society in 1995 takes this ageing effect into account, defining airway obstruction by an FEV_1:FVC ratio below 89% and 88% of the predicted value for females and males, respectively [17]. A consensus between the European Respiratory Society and GOLD criteria is expected in the near future.

The FEV_1:FVC ratios for patients in the FOS database are shown in Figure 1. Using the GOLD cut-off, 23 of 67 patients (34%; 9 females, 14 males) have airway obstruction (Figure 1a); according to the European Respiratory Society cut-off, 20 patients are considered to have airway obstruction (Figure 1b). Although these figures far exceed the prevalence of airway obstruction in the general adult population [18, 19], such cohorts are potentially biased by the two most frequent airway obstructive disorders, asthma and COPD, which occur in about 7% and 5%, respectively, of the general adult population.

Unfortunately, although the FOS database has information on 13 patients who are active or past smokers, and on 17 who have never smoked, the smoking status of 37 individuals is unknown. It is interesting to note that only two of the nine active smokers have significant obstruction based on the FEV_1:FVC ratio, suggesting that factors other than cigarette smoking are involved in this condition.

It is even more difficult to diagnose asthma in this population. In clinical practice, asthma is usually diagnosed when there is a compatible history of acute exacerbations with wheezing, cough and chest tightness, an atopic milieu (although this is not mandatory), and a significant response to bronchodilators on spirometry. As the precise mechanism of airway narrowing in Fabry disease is unknown, we cannot distinguish asthma from Fabry disease on the basis of spirometric reversibility. A thorough medical history must be obtained in order to identify with some confidence patients with Fabry disease who have clear bronchial asthma; this type of information is not available for the FOS cohort.

Despite these limitations, it is obvious that there are more patients with airway obstruction than expected within this cohort, especially in the male population aged 20–50 years. Moreover, five patients (1 female, 4 males), all aged 40–60 years, have severe obstruction according to the GOLD criterion (i.e. they have an FEV_1 < 50% of the predicted value; Figure 2). There is a significant correlation between FEV_1, expressed as a percentage of the predicted value, and age in the male population, even though the former parameter is already adjusted for age ($r = -0.64$, $p = 0.001$). This indicates that male patients with Fabry disease have an accelerated decline in FEV_1 of about 40 ml/year, compared with 25–30 ml in the general population [20]. There was no statistically significant correlation between age and FEV_1 expressed as a percentage of the predicted value, among female patients ($r = -0.24$).

Potential mechanisms of airflow limitation in Fabry disease

Several structural abnormalities of both the airways and the lung parenchyma can lead to airway obstruction. Although still the subject of some debate and active research, the structure–function relationship for both asthma and COPD have been well established [18, 21]. By contrast, almost nothing is known about the anatomical alterations that are responsible for airflow obstruction in patients with Fabry disease (Table 2). Some

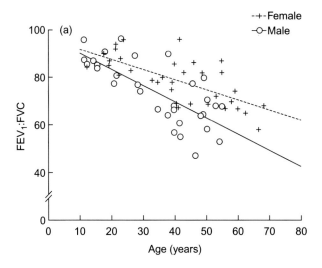

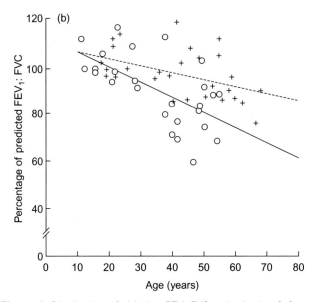

Figure 1 *Distribution of (a) the FEV$_1$:FVC ratio (ratio of forced expiratory volume in 1 second to forced vital capacity) according to age, and of (b) the FEV$_1$:FVC ratio expressed as a percentage of the predicted value for sex, age and height in patients with Fabry disease.*

mechanisms appear unlikely. Inflammatory cells have not been found in excess in the lungs of patients with Fabry disease. Acute and reversible bronchospasm, which is a classic feature of asthma, is not encountered in most patients. Moreover, acute reversibility testing with short-acting bronchodilators usually does not lead to an improvement in FEV$_1$ of the same magnitude as that seen in asthmatic patients [16]. Finally, airway hyper-responsiveness after a methacholine challenge test or administration of another

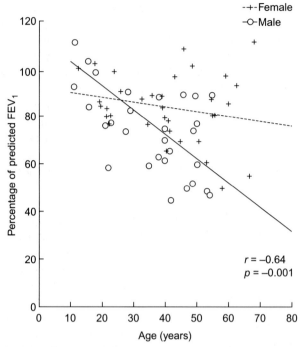

Figure 2. *Distribution of FEV$_1$ (forced expiratory volume in 1 second), expressed as a percentage of the predicted value for sex, age and height, in patients with Fabry disease. The percentage of predicted FEV$_1$ correlated significantly with age in men, but not in women.*

agonist has not been reported in patients with Fabry disease.

Based on clinical characteristics and pulmonary function tests, airflow obstruction in Fabry disease is similar to the fixed obstruction that characterizes COPD. Nevertheless, it is likely that the structure of airways and lung parenchyma in Fabry disease differs significantly from that in COPD. For example, recent published data show no evidence of emphysema in patients with Fabry disease

Table 2. *Potential mechanisms of airflow obstruction.*

Mechanism	Asthma	COPD	Fabry disease
Smooth muscle hyper-responsiveness	Yes	No	Probably no
Airway wall oedema	Yes	No	Probably no
Infiltration of inflammatory cells	Yes	Yes	?
Bronchial wall hypertrophy	Yes	Yes	?
Bronchial wall fibrosis	(Yes)	Yes	?
Smooth muscle hyperplasia/hypertrophy	Yes	(Yes)	?
Uncoupling of the smooth muscle from the adventitia	Yes	?	?
Loss of elastic recoil from the lung parenchyma	No	Yes	Probably no
Plugging of the airway lumen	Yes	(Yes)	Probably no

COPD, chronic obstructive pulmonary disease.

[10]. Airway wall thickening through hyperplasia and/or fibrosis is, among others, a potential alteration that could be responsible for airflow obstruction [19]. More studies on structure–function relationships are required to explain the pathophysiology of these clinical observations.

Treatment

There are no evidence-based recommendations for therapy in patients with Fabry disease who also have airflow obstruction; advice is therefore limited to the category of 'expert opinion'. All would agree that smokers with Fabry disease should be encouraged to stop smoking. It is likely that both active and passive smoking dramatically increase the risk of obstruction in these patients. Treatment of patients with moderate or severe obstruction, together with those who are symptomatic, should include the prescription of inhaled bronchodilators, such as long-acting β_2-agonists and atropine derivatives. There is no evidence, however, that steroids, either inhaled or systemic, are of any benefit in patients with Fabry disease, unless they have clinically apparent asthma. As with other chronic respiratory diseases, general measures, such as immunization against influenza and pneumococcal infection, are recommended.

The impact of enzyme replacement therapy on respiratory involvement in Fabry disease has not, to the best of our knowledge, been described. Long-term pulmonary function testing of patients receiving replacement therapy will be of utmost importance both for patients and for our understanding of the mechanisms involved.

Future areas of research

As respiratory involvement in Fabry disease has received little attention compared with other organ involvement, it will be important to gather more clinical data to characterize this manifestation of the disease. In particular, more extensive pulmonary function testing,

including plethysmography, assessment of carbon monoxide transfer factor, acute reversibility testing or bronchial hyper-responsiveness challenge, will provide a more complete picture of the respiratory disorder. Imaging, particularly with high-resolution computed tomography, is now powerful enough to analyse the structure of small airways in asthma, COPD and cystic fibrosis [22]. When lung tissue is available from patients with Fabry disease, either as surgical specimens or from post-mortem studies, thorough morphometric studies with adequate stereological tools would be extremely useful in correlating the airway remodelling at the microscopic level to functional alterations [23]. Biological in-vitro studies comparing airway smooth muscle cells and lung fibroblasts harvested from patients with Fabry disease with those from controls might enable alterations in the growth properties of these cells or abnormal resistance to apoptotic stimuli to be identified. The presence of circulating growth factors, which are abnormally expressed in Fabry disease, should also be sought in vitro using live target cells or tissue.

Conclusions

Much remains to be clarified regarding our understanding of pulmonary involvement in Fabry disease. An essential and yet unfulfilled objective remains the reliable and systematic description of affected individuals in a robust clinical database. It is hoped that the FOS database will soon be able to provide the necessary information to fulfil this objective.

References

1. Fabry J. Weiterer Beitrag zur Klinik des Angiokeratoma naeviforme. *Dermatol Wochenschr* 1930;90:339ff

2. Bartimmo EE Jr, Guisan M, Moser KM. Pulmonary involvement in Fabry's disease: a reappraisal follow-up of a San Diego kindred and review of literature. *Am J Med* 1972;53:755–64

3. Pompen A, Ruiter M, Wyers H. Angiokeratoma corporis diffusum (universale) Fabry as a sign of an unknown internal disease: two autopsy reports. *Acta Med Scand* 1947;128:235–46

4. Bagdade JD, Parker F, Ways PO, Morgan TE, Lagunoff D, Eidelman S. Fabry's disease. A correlative clinical, morphologic, and biochemical study. *Lab Invest* 1968;18:681–8

5. Ruiter M. Some further observations on angiokeratoma corporis diffusum. *Br J Dermatol* 1957;69:137–44

6. Wallace HJ. Angiokeratoma corporis diffusum. *Br J Dermatol* 1958;70:354–60

7. Kariman K, Singletary WV Jr, Sieker HO. Pulmonary involvement in Fabry's disease. *Am J Med* 1978; 64:911–12

8. Rosenberg DM, Ferrans VJ, Fulmer JD, Line BR, Barranger JA, Brady RO *et al*. Chronic airflow obstruction in Fabry's disease. *Am J Med* 1980;68:898–905

9. Smith P, Heath D, Rodgers B, Helliwell T. Pulmonary vasculature in Fabry's disease. *Histopathology* 1991;19:567–9

10. Brown LK, Miller A, Bhuptani A, Sloane MF, Zimmerman MI, Schilero G *et al*. Pulmonary involvement in Fabry disease. *Am J Respir Crit Care Med* 1997;155:1004–10

11. Melton LJ 3rd, Hepper NG, Offord KP. Incidence of spontaneous pneumothorax in Olmsted County, Minnesota: 1950 to 1974. *Am Rev Respir Dis* 1979;120:1379–82

12. Sourk R, Nugent K. Bronchodilator testing: confidence intervals derived from placebo inhalations. *Am Rev Respir Dis* 1983;128:153–7

13. Park SS, Janis M, Shim CS, Williams MH Jr. Relationship of bronchitis and emphysema to altered pulmonary function. *Am Rev Respir Dis* 1970;102:927–36

14. Mellis CM, Levison H. Bronchial reactivity in cystic fibrosis. *Pediatrics* 1978;61:446–50

15. Ramsdell JW, Nachtwey FJ, Moser KM. Bronchial hyperreactivity in chronic obstructive bronchitis. *Am Rev Respir Dis* 1982;126:829–32

16. Barbey F, Widmer U, Brack T, Vogt B, Aubert J. Spirometric abnormalities in patients with Fabry disease and effect of enzyme replacement therapy. *Acta Paediatr Suppl* 2005;447:105

17. Siafakas NM, Vermeire P, Pride NB, Paoletti P, Gibson J, Howard P *et al*. Optimal assessment and management of chronic obstructive pulmonary disease (COPD). The European Respiratory Society Task Force. *Eur Respir J* 1995;8:1398–420

18. Hogg JC, Wright JL, Wiggs BR, Coxson HO, Opazo Saez A, Pare PD. Lung structure and function in cigarette smokers. *Thorax* 1994;49:473–8

19. Riess A, Wiggs B, Verburgt L, Wright JL, Hogg JC, Pare PD. Morphologic determinants of airway responsiveness in chronic smokers. *Am J Respir Crit Care Med* 1996;154:1444–9

20. Brandli O, Schindler C, Kunzli N, Keller R, Perruchoud AP. Lung function in healthy never smoking adults: reference values and lower limits of normal of a Swiss population. *Thorax* 1996;51:277–83

21. James AL, Pare PD, Hogg JC. The mechanics of airway narrowing in asthma. *Am Rev Respir Dis* 1989;139:242–6

22. de Jong PA, Muller NL, Pare PD, Coxson HO. Computed tomographic imaging of the airways: relationship to structure and function. *Eur Respir J* 2005;26:140–52

23. Hogg JC, Chu F, Utokaparch S, Woods R, Elliott WM, Buzatu L *et al*. The nature of small-airway obstruction in chronic obstructive pulmonary disease. *N Engl J Med* 2004;350:2645–53

28 Gastrointestinal manifestations of Fabry disease

Satish Keshav

Department of Medicine, Royal Free and University College Medical School, Rowland Hill Street, London NW3 2PF, UK

The majority of individuals affected with Fabry disease report profound gastrointestinal symptoms, such as diarrhoea, abdominal pain and early satiety, which can have a profoundly negative effect on their quality of life. Without treatment, the disease is unremitting and progressive, with increasing amounts of lipid-rich materials being stored in a variety of cells, including intrinsic neurones of the intestinal tract. With the advent of enzyme replacement therapy, it is hoped that the pathological changes may be preventable, and even reversible, and recent data suggest that gastrointestinal symptoms are especially responsive to treatment. This supports the case for closer monitoring and evaluation of the gastrointestinal manifestations of Fabry disease, which could provide important insights that may help to optimize treatment strategies.

Introduction

Fabry disease is a rare, X-linked deficiency of α-galactosidase A, affecting approximately 2–5 individuals per 1 million live births. Typical presenting symptoms include acroparaesthesiae, hypohidrosis, cutaneous angiokeratomas and cornea verticillata. In hemizygous males, the condition manifests almost universally, while a proportion of heterozygous females are also affected [1, 2].

Clinical manifestations usually become apparent in childhood, and the diagnosis is frequently suspected on the basis of a positive family history. Approximately 60% of patients with manifest Fabry disease report gastrointestinal symptoms [3]. This compares with a prevalence of 77% for neuropathic pain, 78% for sensorineural deafness, 30% for renal failure and 24% for cerebrovascular disease. Although not usually life threatening, gastrointestinal symptoms can have a major negative impact on quality of life [2, 4–11]. Systematic studies of large numbers of patients, however, are lacking. Early indications are that enzyme replacement therapy (ERT) may have a positive effect on gastrointestinal symptoms and may potentially provide early evidence of overall treatment efficacy [5, 6, 11].

As yet, the pathophysiology of the altered gastrointestinal function in Fabry disease is poorly understood, with detailed investigation having been confined mainly to small patient groups and case studies. Clearly, therefore, further investigation and data collection could have an impact on our understanding of this important aspect of Fabry disease.

Gastrointestinal features of Fabry disease

The most commonly reported gastrointestinal symptom in affected patients is diarrhoea, with frequent loose bowel motions and cramping abdominal pain. Patients often complain of postprandial symptoms, including diarrhoea, urgency and flatulence. Stool frequency in patients with Fabry disease can be as high as 10–12 soft or semi-solid motions per day; however, in contrast to inflammatory bowel diseases, such as Crohn's disease and ulcerative colitis, patients do not typically report rectal passage of mucus or blood. In many patients, episodes of diarrhoea are interspersed with periods of normal, or even reduced, bowel activity, when they may complain of constipation; this alternating pattern is reminiscent of irritable bowel syndrome (IBS) [12].

Patients may also experience a sense of early satiety after meals, epigastric discomfort and abdominal bloating. These symptoms may lead them to avoid meals and to report a reduced appetite. Again, the symptoms of abdominal discomfort and bloating associated with meals are features of IBS. Altered gastric emptying, which is ameliorated by treatment with metoclopramide, has also been reported in Fabry disease [9]. Sharp or stabbing epigastric pain, dyspepsia and heartburn suggest alternative diagnoses, such as peptic ulcer disease or gastro-oesophageal reflux, and should prompt appropriate investigation and treatment.

MacDermot et al. described widespread gastrointestinal symptomatology in a cohort of adults with Fabry disease, and suggested that loss of weight and reduced body mass index (BMI) are associated with the disease [3]. Similarly, in a recent case report on the response to ERT, an improvement in gastrointestinal symptoms was accompanied by an increase in BMI [5]. Analysis of the current data in FOS – the Fabry Outcome Survey – on the other hand, does not suggest that reduced BMI is a feature of progressive Fabry disease, although the lack of reliable normative values makes this a difficult area to evaluate. Furthermore, serum protein, albumin, folate, vitamin B_{12}, calcium and phosphate levels are typically found to be normal, suggesting that malabsorption of

nutrients is not a major clinical feature; alternative diagnoses should be sought if these parameters are abnormal [1, 4]. Intestinal xylose absorption is unaffected, and endoscopic biopsies usually show normal villous architecture at the light microscopic level [4]. Interestingly, however, anaemia is a recently identified feature of Fabry disease, and may relate to renal and cardiac dysfunction and to systemic inflammation [13]. In clinical practice, physicians may encounter patients with severe gastrointestinal symptoms, a history of recent loss of weight and a reduced BMI. The effects of a reduced appetite, nausea, vomiting and diarrhoea may be implicated in such patients, although other factors, such as cardiac and renal disease, may also be important.

When evaluating a patient with α-galactosidase A deficiency and gastrointestinal symptoms, a careful history and examination provide good preliminary evidence for deciding on the likely aetiology. Care should be taken to document the severity of symptoms. For example, with diarrhoea, what is the average daily frequency of bowel movements, do they relate to meals, and is early satiety after meals a feature? Simple investigations, such as a full blood count, urea, electrolytes, serum albumin, liver enzymes, C-reactive protein and erythrocyte sedimentation rate, provide important information about the general nutritional state, extent of renal involvement and presence of a systemic inflammatory response. Serological testing for coeliac disease and estimation of haematological parameters, such as levels of iron, ferritin, saturation of transferrin, folic acid and vitamin B_{12}, should be performed routinely to exclude gastrointestinal disease causing malabsorption or occult blood loss [14]. Chronic pancreatitis is another important cause of diarrhoea, abdominal pain and weight loss, and should be excluded by careful clinical evaluation and appropriate imaging – for example, with abdominal radiography or ultrasound scanning, or with computed tomography or magnetic resonance imaging if the clinical suspicion is high.

In Fabry disease, endoscopic and colonoscopic appearances are typically normal, although microscopic examination of biopsies may demonstrate accumulation of lipid within the cytoplasm of enteric neurones [4]. In many cases, upper endoscopy and colonoscopy will be indicated to eliminate diagnostic uncertainty.

Functional testing of intestinal physiology may ultimately prove highly valuable in the evaluation of gastrointestinal manifestations of Fabry disease. For example, altered motility, secretion and bacterial overgrowth within portions of the small bowel may all contribute to the pathogenesis of diarrhoea; hence, tests to determine the rates of gastric emptying and colonic transit, and the presence of bacterial overgrowth in the small intestine, may yield important information. The appropriate tests, such as scintigraphic gastric emptying scans, and the relevant hydrogen breath tests, are not universally available; if possible, specialists with access to suitable facilities should evaluate patients with Fabry disease and gastrointestinal symptoms.

Pathophysiology

Deficiency of α-galactosidase A results in progressive intracellular accumulation of the cell membrane-derived glycolipid, globotriaosylceramide (Gb_3). Gb_3 accumulates within the cytoplasm and lysosomes of affected cells, and may be detected microscopically as a foamy deposit within the cell or ultrastructurally as electron-dense intralysosomal striped 'zebra-like' 0.5–0.75 μm bodies [4]. Gb_3 accumulates most prominently in endothelial, perithelial and perineural cells, cardiomyocytes, renal glomerular cells, and neurones. Small unmyelinated neurones, such as those responsible for peripheral pain perception and those in the enteric nervous system, are most affected [15, 16].

The pathogenesis of gastrointestinal symptoms remains unknown, although it is plausible that accumulation of Gb_3 in neurones of the submucosal and myenteric nerve plexuses causes enteric neuropathy. Gb_3 also accumulates in intestinal smooth muscle, and a direct myopathic effect, or combined myopathy and neuropathy, may be important [17, 18]. Enteropathy affecting the sympathetic and parasympathetic divisions of the autonomic nervous system is also possible, and autonomic nerve involvement has been reported in Fabry disease [19]. There is evidence of delayed gastric emptying, as assessed by radionuclide studies, which improves after metoclopramide therapy [9]. This abnormality may arise from dysfunction of the intrinsic enteric nervous system, as well as from parasympathetic dysfunction, and is seen, for example, in diabetes mellitus and following surgical vagotomy [20]. Other reported changes include formation of diverticula and saccules within the intestinal wall, which may also be related to disruption of muscle and nerve function [17, 18].

The lack of α-galactosidase A, which catalyses the breakdown of specific glycosylceramides, may also affect the accumulation of other lipids, such as isoglobotriaosylceramide (iGb_3), which was recently identified as an endogenous ligand for the CD1d molecule [21]. CD1d is homologous to major histocompatability complex class I molecules and is considered critical for the function of natural killer T lymphocytes (NKT cells), which bear a restricted subset of invariant T cell receptor molecules and recognize glycolipid antigens [22]. Until recently, the likely endogenous or exogenous ligand for NKT cells and CD1d had not been identified, and a synthetic form of a marine sponge-derived glycolipid, α-galactosylceramide, was the most widely used experimental ligand. Recent research, however, has identified endogenous iGb_3 and glycolipids derived from the cell walls of

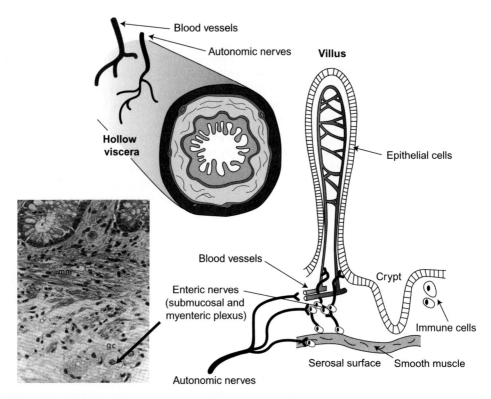

Figure 1. *Main features of the hollow gastrointestinal viscera that may be affected by Fabry disease, showing extrinsic nerve and blood vessel supply, and intrinsic structures including epithelial cells, immune cells, smooth muscle cells and the myenteric (Auerbach's) and submucosal (Meissner's) nerve plexuses. The inset, reproduced with permission from [4], illustrates globotriaosylceramide accumulation within ganglion cells of the submucosal nerve plexus, as seen by light microscopy; gc, ganglion cells; mm, muscularis mucosae.*

Gram-negative bacteria as the more likely physiological and pathophysiological ligands [21, 23]. The CD1d-dependent pathway of NKT cell activation is considered highly important in the maintenance of host defence in the intestine, and it is possible that some aspects of gastrointestinal symptomatology in Fabry disease may relate to as yet unidentified and subtle immunological alterations [24].

From the preceding discussion, it is apparent that almost all the cells and systems that contribute to intestinal structure and function may be affected by Fabry disease; the various targets are illustrated in Figure 1. The inset photomicrograph demonstrates the accumulation of glycolipid within enlarged

ganglion cells of the myenteric plexus. Less readily detected accumulation within epithelial cells, smooth muscle, myofibroblasts, vascular endothelial cells and immune cells may also have important effects that have yet to be defined.

Natural course

As with other manifestations of Fabry disease, gastrointestinal symptoms follow an unremitting progressive course. Data from FOS reveal that the occurrence of typical symptoms, such as diarrhoea and abdominal pain, increases progressively with time (Figure 2). Interestingly, heterozygous females are sometimes affected as severely as males, although there is a time lag in the development of symptoms in the majority of cases [1, 2, 8]. Thus, the curves charting the occurrence of symptoms for males and females diverge with time, although the final prevalence reached may be identical.

It is potentially difficult to determine whether common symptoms, such as diarrhoea and abdominal pain, which have a high prevalence in the general population and may arise from many causes, are attributable to Fabry disease. FOS data provide a potential diagnostic aid in this regard. Examination of the occurrence of diarrhoea and abdominal pain in patients enrolled in FOS, for example, shows that the proportion of patients affected increases with age and that the rate of accumulation of cases is greater for men than for women (Figure 2). This divergence of the occurrence curves would be predicted for symptoms associated with progressive Fabry disease. By contrast, for a clinical feature such as haemorrhoids, which, *a priori*, is unlikely to be related to progressive Fabry disease, no difference between the sexes is seen and the curves do not diverge appreciably (Figure 3). Interestingly, such

analysis suggests that constipation, which shows an equivalent prevalence in males and females, is also not related to progressive Fabry disease (Figure 3). More extensive and detailed collection of data is necessary to establish these relationships unequivocally, and to determine exactly which gastrointestinal symptoms and signs relate to Fabry disease, in order to use these more effectively to chart the progress of disease and the response to treatment.

Response to ERT

It is appropriate that most attention has focused on dermatological, neurological, renal and cardiac manifestations of Fabry disease, which are either most characteristic or have the most serious and life-threatening sequelae. However, it is now recognized that there is a large burden of gastrointestinal dysfunction among patients with Fabry disease, and a number of reports confirm that gastrointestinal symptoms are ameliorated by ERT [5, 6, 11]. Furthermore, debilitating gastrointestinal symptoms seem to respond rapidly to treatment, and the response

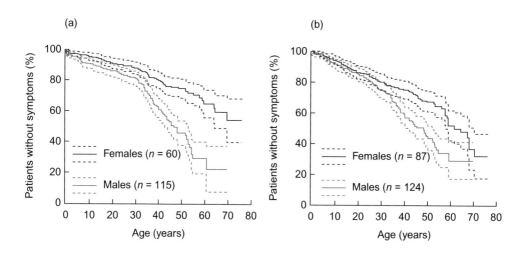

Figure 2. *Reported occurrence of (a) diarrhoea and (b) abdominal pain with age among patients entered in FOS – the Fabry Outcome Survey. The curves for males and females diverge as a result of the more rapid onset of symptoms in males. Nonetheless, it is evident for abdominal pain that the overall prevalence may be nearly equal in later life, and it is known that individual females may be as severely affected as males. Lines represent means ± 95% confidence intervals.*

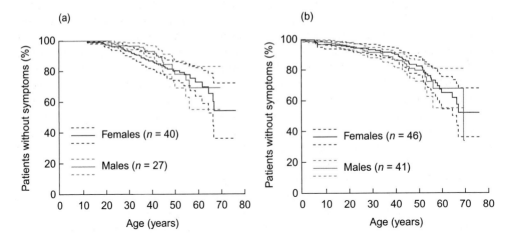

Figure 3. *Reported occurrence of (a) haemorrhoids and (b) constipation with age among subjects entered in FOS – the Fabry Outcome Survey. In contrast to Figure 2, there is a much lower overall occurrence of these symptoms and little divergence in the curves for males and females. By analysing symptoms in this way, it may be possible to distinguish symptoms that are likely to be due to progressive Fabry disease (where the occurrence increases markedly with time and presents earlier in males than in females) from symptoms that are likely to be incidental to the disease. Lines represent means ± 95% confidence intervals.*

may precede measurable changes in other parameters such as creatinine clearance and cardiac function, particularly for patients with severe established Fabry disease [25].

These preliminary data on the response of gastrointestinal manifestations to treatment are encouraging for the following reasons.
- Any demonstration that the established symptoms of Fabry disease can be reversed by therapy is highly welcome.
- If, as is surmised, the gastrointestinal manifestations are secondary to enteric neuronal damage, symptomatic improvement suggests that neuronal damage may be reversible.
- As the clinical response appears to be relatively rapid, it could be used in the evaluation and optimization of treatment for individual patients in a realistic timeframe, as well as to facilitate innovative treatment protocols (e.g. for heterozygous females or for paediatric patients) early in the course of the disease.

If gastrointestinal symptomatology can be ameliorated by treatment, this also presents a challenge to physicians to devise and evaluate specific, quantitative and reliable measures of Fabry-related gastrointestinal dysfunction that can be used in clinical studies. The FOS database, for example, already collects important relevant information, and the FOS Gastrointestinal Working Group is endeavouring to formulate a standardized, comprehensive and practical data collection tool that could be used as the basis of a 'Fabry gastrointestinal disease activity index', modelled, in part, on the successful and widely used Crohn's disease activity index [26].

Outstanding questions

Although Fabry disease is relatively rare, its study may yield insights that have broad relevance. Furthermore, with the recognition of clinical disease among heterozygotes, the true incidence of Fabry-related pathology may be higher than previously suspected. For example, in the context of cerebrovascular disease, heterozygosity for α-galactosidase A is now mooted as a potential risk factor for stroke at a young age [27]. In addition, diarrhoea and abdominal pain are two important symptoms in gastrointestinal practice that often, when they are not caused by identifiable organic pathology, indicate a form of IBS. This syndrome has an overall population prevalence of up to 15% in some communities [12]. The striking similarity in clinical findings between a typical case of Fabry-related gastrointestinal disease and diarrhoea-predominant IBS is summarized in Table 1. Is it possible that a proportion of patients with diarrhoea-predominant IBS are deficient in α-galactosidase A?

The pathophysiology of IBS is not understood, although there are indications that visceral nerve and smooth muscle function may be disrupted, possibly mainly via alterations in serotoninergic signalling. If it emerges that Fabry symptoms do relate to enteric neuronal dysfunction, might this reveal a general mechanism by which IBS arises in the general population, with enteric neuropathic changes caused by other distinct disease processes? Such questions can be addressed only by further clinical research.

Reversibility of pathological changes, particularly those affecting non-renewable cells, such as cardiomyocytes, renal glomerular cells and neurones, is a key determinant of the potential benefit of ERT and will, in part, guide the timing of therapy for at-risk groups. Because gastrointestinal symptoms may arise from damage to enteric neurones, the rapid response of such symptoms to therapy is intriguing. Enteric neurones can be studied in tissue sections from endoscopic biopsies, and the response to therapy can potentially be quantified at the pathological level. Although this involves invasive testing, serious consideration should be given to incorporating such measurements in clinical trials and surveys such as FOS. Antibodies to Gb_3 may allow quantitative or semi-quantitative evaluation of lipid loading, and the effect of ERT on this parameter in a tissue that, unlike the heart and kidney, can be accessed without undue risk to the patient, may prove a valuable adjunct.

While it is evident that heterozygous females may manifest clinical features of Fabry disease, the phenomenon is unexplained, as circulating levels of α-galactosidase A are usually adequate. One possible explanation is

Table 1. *Clinical features of the gastrointestinal manifestations of Fabry disease and diarrhoea-predominant irritable bowel syndrome.*

Fabry disease	Diarrhoea-predominant irritable bowel syndrome
Diarrhoea	Diarrhoea
Abdominal pain	Abdominal pain
Postprandial exacerbation of gastrointestinal symptoms	Postprandial bloating and abdominal pain
No rectal bleeding	No rectal bleeding
Normal 'routine' blood tests in early stages (i.e. blood count, urea and electrolytes, erythrocyte sedimentation, C-reactive protein)	Normal 'routine' blood tests (i.e. blood count, urea and electrolytes, erythrocyte sedimentation, C-reactive protein)
Normal upper endoscopy and colonoscopy (usually)	Normal upper endoscopy and colonoscopy
Symptoms associated with autonomic and enteric neuropathy	Syndrome associated with altered intestinal motility and nociception

that the abnormal enzyme exerts a dominant-negative effect. Alternatively, random inactivation of X chromosomes, which may be unbalanced, might provide an explanation, with markedly reduced tissue expression of α-galactosidase A in a proportion of critically important cells. This explanation would predict tissue mosaicism in the expression of α-galactosidase A and in the accumulation of Gb_3, which could potentially be investigated in intestinal tissue, where patches of epithelial cells in crypts and villi are derived from single stem cells [28]. Once more, an important pathophysiological question could be addressed by further research.

Finally, the intriguing possibility that α-galactosidase A deficiency results in the accumulation not only of glycolipids, such as Gb_3, but functionally critical species, such as iGb_3, which may have profound immunological effects, deserves further research. Alterations in CD1d-dependent antigen presentation and NKT cell function could have important effects in the gastrointestinal tract, and research in this area could provide important insights into gastrointestinal dysfunction, with implications beyond Fabry disease.

References

1. Mehta A, Ricci R, Widmer U, Dehout F, Garcia de Lorenzo A, Kampmann C et al. Fabry disease defined: baseline clinical manifestations of 366 patients in the Fabry Outcome Survey. Eur J Clin Invest 2004;34:236–42

2. Whybra C, Kampmann C, Willers I, Davies J, Winchester B, Kriegsmann J et al. Anderson–Fabry disease: clinical manifestations of disease in female heterozygotes. J Inherit Metab Dis 2001;24:715–24

3. MacDermot KD, Holmes A, Miners AH. Anderson–Fabry disease: clinical manifestations and impact of disease in a cohort of 98 hemizygous males. J Med Genet 2001;38:750–60

4. O'Brien BD, Shnitka TK, McDougall R, Walker K, Costopoulos L, Lentle B et al. Pathophysiologic and ultrastructural basis for intestinal symptoms in Fabry's disease. Gastroenterology 1982;82:957–62

5. Hoffmann B, Reinhardt D, Koletzko B. Effect of enzyme-replacement therapy on gastrointestinal symptoms in Fabry disease. Eur J Gastroenterol Hepatol 2004;16:1067–9

6. Dehout F, Roland D, Treille de Granseigne S, Guillaume B, Van Maldergem L. Relief of gastrointestinal symptoms under enzyme replacement therapy in patients with Fabry disease. J Inherit Metab Dis 2004;27:499–505

7. Ries M, Ramaswami U, Parini R, Lindblad B, Whybra C, Willers I et al. The early clinical phenotype of Fabry disease: a study on 35 European children and adolescents. Eur J Pediatr 2003;162:767–72. Epub 2003 Sep 20

8. MacDermot KD, Holmes A, Miners AH. Natural history of Fabry disease in affected males and obligate carrier females. J Inherit Metab Dis 2001;24:13–14; discussion 11–12

9. Argoff CE, Barton NW, Brady RO, Ziessman HA. Gastrointestinal symptoms and delayed gastric emptying in Fabry's disease: response to metoclopramide. Nucl Med Commun 1998;19:887–91

10. Nelis GF, Jacobs GJ. Anorexia, weight loss, and diarrhea as presenting symptoms of angiokeratoma corporis diffusum (Fabry–Anderson's disease). Dig Dis Sci 1989;34:1798–1800

11. Banikazemi M, Ullman T, Desnick RJ. Gastrointestinal manifestations of Fabry disease: clinical response to enzyme replacement therapy. Mol Genet Metab 2005;85:255–9

12. Cremonini F, Talley NJ. Irritable bowel syndrome: epidemiology, natural history, health care seeking and emerging risk factors. Gastroenterol Clin North Am 2005;34:189–204

13. Kleinert J, Dehout F, Schwarting A, de Lorenzo AG, Ricci R, Kampmann C et al. Anemia is a new complication in Fabry disease: data from the Fabry Outcome Survey. Kidney Int 2005;67:1955–60

14. Tumer L, Ezgu FS, Hasanoglu A, Dalgic B, Bakkaloglu SA, Memis L, Dursun A. The co-existence of Fabry and celiac diseases: a case report. Pediatr Nephrol 2004;19:679–81

15. Dutsch M, Marthol H, Stemper B, Brys M, Haendl T, Hilz MJ. Small fiber dysfunction predominates in Fabry neuropathy. J Clin Neurophysiol 2002;19:575–86

16. Schiffmann R, Floeter MK, Dambrosia JM, Gupta S, Moore DF, Sharabi Y et al. Enzyme replacement therapy improves peripheral nerve and sweat function in Fabry disease. Muscle Nerve 2003;28:703–10

17. Friedman LS, Kirkham SE, Thistlethwaite JR, Platika D, Kolodny EH, Schuffler MD. Jejunal diverticulosis with perforation as a complication of Fabry's disease. Gastroenterology 1984;86:558–63

18. Jack CI, Morris AI, Nasmyth DG, Carroll N. Colonic involvement in Fabry's disease. Postgrad Med J 1991;67:584–5

19. Sung JH. Autonomic neurons affected by lipid storage in the spinal cord in Fabry's disease: distribution of autonomic neurons in the sacral cord. J Neuropathol Exp Neurol 1979;38:87–98

20. Stacher G, Lenglinger J, Bergmann H, Schneider C, Brannath W, Festa A et al. Impaired gastric emptying

and altered intragastric meal distribution in diabetes mellitus related to autonomic neuropathy? *Dig Dis Sci* 2003;48:1027–34

21. Zhou D, Mattner J, Cantu C 3rd, Schrantz N, Yin N, Gao Y *et al.* Lysosomal glycosphingolipid recognition by NKT cells. *Science* 2004;306:1786–9

22. Kawano T, Cui J, Koezuka Y, Toura I, Kaneko Y, Motoki K *et al.* CD1d-restricted and TCR-mediated activation of Valpha14 NKT cells by glycosyl-ceramides. *Science* 1997;278:1626–9

23. Mattner J, Debord KL, Ismail N, Goff RD, Cantu C 3rd, Zhou D *et al.* Exogenous and endogenous glycolipid antigens activate NKT cells during microbial infections. *Nature* 2005;434:525–9

24. van de Wal Y, Corazza N, Allez M, Mayer LF, Iijima H, Ryan M *et al.* Delineation of a CD1d-restricted antigen presentation pathway associated with human and mouse intestinal epithelial cells. *Gastroenterology* 2003;124:1420–31

25. Tsambaos D, Chroni E, Manolis A, Monastirli A, Pasmatzi E, Sakkis T *et al.* Enzyme replacement therapy in severe Fabry disease with renal failure: a 1-year follow-up. *Acta Derm Venereol* 2004;84: 389–92

26. Best WR, Becktel JM, Singleton JW, Kern F Jr. Development of a Crohn's disease activity index. National Cooperative Crohn's Disease Study. *Gastroenterology* 1976;70:439–44

27. Giacomini PS, Shannon PT, Clarke JT, Jaigobin C. Fabry's disease presenting as stroke in a young female. *Can J Neurol Sci* 2004;31:112–14

28. Novelli MR, Williamson JA, Tomlinson IP, Elia G, Hodgson SV, Talbot IC *et al.* Polyclonal origin of colonic adenomas in an XO/XY patient with FAP. *Science* 1996;272:1187–90

29 Neuropsychiatric and psychosocial aspects of Fabry disease

Matthias J Müller

Department of Psychiatry, University of Mainz, D-55101 Mainz, Germany, and Clinic for Psychiatry and Psychotherapy Marburg-Sued, D-35039 Marburg, Germany

Fabry disease affects multiple organ systems, including the central nervous system. A high proportion of patients with Fabry disease are at increased risk of developing neuropsychiatric symptoms, such as depression and neuropsychological deficits. Due to both somatic and psychological impairment, health-related quality of life (QoL) is considerably reduced in patients with Fabry disease. Although the pathophysiological mechanisms of Fabry disease have not been fully elucidated, it is surmised that sphingolipid deposits in the endothelium of small cerebral vessels lead to regional cerebral ischaemia, which may be accompanied by neuropsychiatric symptoms. Furthermore, patients with Fabry disease are chronically distressed by pain attacks and additional somatic and psychosocial impairment. The available literature on psychiatric and neuropsychological findings, psychosocial adjustment and QoL during the natural course of Fabry disease in adults is reviewed in this chapter. Psychiatric symptoms, particularly depression, are highly prevalent in men and women with Fabry disease. Although more reliable data on neuropsychological deficits in the course of Fabry disease are needed, compelling evidence is available that almost all components of QoL are impaired in affected patients. As neuropsychiatric symptoms and poor psychosocial adjustment seem to contribute to the low QoL of patients with Fabry disease, early therapeutic intervention and prevention programmes, starting in childhood or adolescence, are strongly recommended.

Introduction

This chapter reviews the available literature on the psychiatric and neuropsychological signs and symptoms of Fabry disease that are closely related to the psychosocial and quality-of-life (QoL) aspects of the disease. The review will be confined to data on the natural course of the illness in adult patients. The clinical features of Fabry disease in children and adolescents, including psychosocial problems, are presented in Chapter 31, and the effects of enzyme replacement therapy (ERT) on psychosocial adjustment and QoL are reported in Chapter 40.

Patients with Fabry disease have a variety of signs and symptoms, including pain attacks and acroparaesthesia, angiokeratomas, corneal opacity, renal and cardiac impairment, hypohidrosis and anhidrosis, gastrointestinal symptoms, and cerebrovascular dysfunction with vertigo, headache and cerebral ischaemia. Although accurate data are lacking, clinical observations and a few published reports have shown that a high proportion of patients with Fabry disease are also at risk of developing neuropsychiatric symptoms, such as depression, suicidal tendencies and neuropsychological deficits. Due to both somatic and psychological impairment, health-related QoL is considerably reduced in patients with Fabry disease.

It has recently been shown that symptoms in female patients with Fabry disease, especially pain and neurological symptoms, are more frequent than was previously suspected [1]. Thus, the investigation of female patients with Fabry disease deserves particular clinical and scientific attention.

Methods
Literature review
The available literature (MedLine search, congress abstracts) on psychiatric symptoms, neuropsychological findings and QoL in men and women with Fabry disease has been qualitatively reviewed. Reports on data from FOS – the Fabry Outcome Survey – have been included in the review only if they relate to baseline data representing more or less the natural course of the disease. Furthermore, reports without explicit reference to neuropsychiatric findings or to a systematic assessment of QoL were excluded. The results are systematically summarized in tables. As the sample characteristics and the assessment methods vary considerably between the studies, no quantitative meta-analytical parameters will be reported.

Assessment instruments
The standardized assessment of neuropsychiatric signs and symptoms and psychosocial factors in Fabry disease is essential to obtain reliable and valid data that can be compared between research groups working on this and other diseases. Such standardized assessments are also important to determine the effects of ERT and other therapeutic options, for example analgesics and antidepressants, in patients with Fabry disease.

Table 1 summarizes the important psychosocial factors related to Fabry disease. Each of these psychosocial facets of the disease can be assessed by specifically developed techniques and instruments. Besides such detailed instruments to assess pain, psychosocial aspects, neuropsychiatric symptoms and QoL, global rating scales can be used to enable comparisons with other diseases. The most relevant psychiatric, psychological and social domains and assessment instruments that should be taken into account in studies on Fabry disease are pain (assessed using the Brief Pain Inventory), non-disease-specific health-related QoL (assessed using the EuroQol Group Instrument, EQ-5D) and generic QoL (assessed using the Medical Outcome Survey Short Form 36, SF-36) [2–8].

Results
Psychiatric signs and symptoms
There are few data regarding the occurrence of psychiatric disorders in patients with Fabry disease (Table 2) [9–12]. In a retrospective chart analysis study [10], 6 of 33 male patients with Fabry disease developed severe psychiatric conditions; all these patients also suffered from painful crises or painful neuropathy.

In a preliminary analysis of an ongoing study (MJ Müller and KM Müller, unpublished data), a high proportion of acutely depressed individuals (55%) was found in a sample of 36 patients with Fabry disease, corroborating earlier observations. Additionally, about one-third of male and more than two-thirds of female patients with Fabry disease had a lifetime diagnosis of major depression according to internationally established diagnostic criteria (Diagnostic and Statistical Manual of Mental Disorders – Fourth Edition, DSM-IV). In addition, a case series has been published on four female heterozygotes with Fabry disease who had severe depression [12]. In both our ongoing study and the published case series, a standardized assessment scale (Hamilton Depression Rating Scale, HAMD) was used to quantify the severity of depression.

In summary, psychiatric signs, symptoms and disorders appear to occur frequently in men

Table 1. *Psychosocial, psychological and neuropsychological factors in Fabry disease.*

Domain	Facet
Psychosocial and psychological characteristics	Sociodemographic data, biography and family history
	Family and social relationships
	Education and employment
	Friends and social support
	Socioeconomic status
	Personality traits and states
	Psychosocial stressors
	Somatic stressors (e.g. pain)
	Life events and daily hassles
	Coping strategies
Psychiatric signs, symptoms and disorders; psychosocial adjustment	Somatic and psychological complaints
	Depression and anxiety
	Psychotic symptoms and disorders
	Substance abuse and dependence
	Cognitive impairment and dementia
	Personality disorders
	Psychosomatic disorders
	Adjustment and stress disorders
Global adjustment, subjective well-being and quality of life	Social functioning
	Global psychosocial adjustment
	Subjective well-being
	Health-related quality of life
Neuropsychological status and cognitive function	General intellectual performance
	Learning and memory
	Attention
	Psychomotor performance
	Frontal executive function

and women with Fabry disease. Depressive disorders are apparently most prevalent, whereas psychotic syndromes have been reported only exceptionally.

Neuropsychological findings

Independently from, and in addition to, psychological and psychiatric symptoms, a substantial proportion of patients with Fabry disease will develop cerebral ischaemia with clinically evident cognitive impairment [13, 14], although systematic reports on neuropsychological deficits in patients with Fabry disease have, until now, been lacking. Table 3 lists the available literature on neuropsychological findings in patients with Fabry disease [9–11, 15].

Some of the case reports in Table 2 also appear in Table 3, demonstrating the overlap between neurocognitive and affective disorders in patients with Fabry disease. However, as only single case reports are currently available with regard to neuropsychological deficits (Table 3), the interpretation is limited. Moreover, different and only partially

Table 2. *Psychiatric signs and symptoms in patients with Fabry disease.*

Design	Sample characteristics	Age (years)	Gender	Assessment	Psychiatric findings	Reference
Case report (n = 1)	Neuropsychological deficits (see Table 3)	26	Male	Clinical description No standardized assessment	Paranoid thoughts, bizarre behaviour, hallucinations, episodic memory deficits	[9]
Case series (n = 33)	Not reported	Middle-aged	Male	Retrospective chart analysis No standardized assessment	6 patients with psychiatric disorders; 5 patients with depression, 2 committed suicide; 1 patient with a delirious state and cognitive impairment	[10]
Case report (n = 1)	Neurological and neuro-psychological disturbances (see Table 3)	52	Male	Clinical assessment No standardized assessment	Depression	[11]
Case reports (n = 4)	Single family Severe somatic symptoms	32, 48, 52, 67	Females	Semi-structured interview (HAMD) QoL (SF-36)	Reduced QoL, severe depression (HAMD > 25) with low mood, sleep disturbances, fatigue, reduced appetite, guilt feelings, hopelessness and suicidal ideations, one patient with a suicide attempt	[12]
Prospective control group study (preliminary results) (n = 36)	29 patients on ERT	36 ± 10	18 males, 18 females	Structured interview HAMD Self-reported depression Other standardized psychiatric rating scales	Significantly higher depression scores (HAMD) in male (8 ± 9) and female (14 ± 13) patients than in normal controls (2 ± 2) Life-time diagnosis of depression in 28% of male and 72% of female patients	(MJ Müller and KM Müller, unpublished data)

ERT, enzyme replacement therapy; HAMD, Hamilton Depression Rating Scale; QoL, quality of life; SF-36, Medical Outcome Survey, Short Form 36.

Table 3. *Neuropsychological deficits in patients with Fabry disease.*

Design	Sample characteristics	Age (years)	Gender	Assessment	Neuropsychological findings	Reference
Case report (*n* = 1)	Psychotic symptoms (see Table 2)	26	Male	Bender Gestalt test Wechsler Memory Scale Other tests	All results within normal values No individual results reported	[9]
Case report (*n* = 1)	Not reported	54	Male	Memory function; no specific information	High response latency Impaired memory function No neurological signs	[15]
Case report (*n* = 1)	Progressive cognitive decline (from 46 years) leading to unemployment	47	Male	Mini Mental Status Test (MMST) Digit span Memory tests Boston Naming Test Trail Making Test Stroop Test, Tapping etc.	MMST 16–20 points Reduced digit span Amnesic and aphasic symptoms, motor retardation, reduced verbal fluency, disturbed executive performance, personality changes (diagnosis: vascular dementia)	[14]
Case report (*n* = 1)	Speech disorder and memory complaints (from 50 years), depressed mood (see Table 2)	52	Male	Neuropsychological tests; no specific information	Impairment of general intelligence and memory	[11]
Case report (*n* = 1)	Unemployed (computer specialist)	23 Follow-up at 27 and 30 years	Male	Neuropsychological tests; no specific information	23 years: disorientation (time, location), attention and memory deficits 27 years: fully oriented, psychomotor retardation 30 years: no changes	[10]

standardized neuropsychological testing methods have been used. Patients with reported neuropsychological deficits also seem to have neurological abnormalities or substantial cerebral lesions documented by brain imaging techniques (not reported here).

Currently, the most comprehensive database on patients with Fabry disease is FOS, which includes baseline data prior to the start of ERT on more than 750 male and female patients, with a mean age of 35 years, from 11 countries [16, 17]. The frequency of cerebrovascular events (stroke or transient ischaemic attacks) and symptoms in the FOS database was about 18% for male (mean age, 36 years) and 13% for female patients (mean age, 50 years), indicating that CNS involvement is an important component in the natural history of the disease [17] (see Chapters 22 and 23). As of March 2005, 14% of females and 7% of males, for whom data were available in FOS, reported that they were taking antidepressant medication. In addition, 1% of males and 2% of females reported having made a suicide attempt.

The reports reviewed here do not provide any information on neuropsychological functions in patients with Fabry disease who have no discernible structural brain lesions. Subtle deficits in neuropsychological domains related to Fabry disease pathology, for example impaired attention or executive function, remain to be elucidated.

In a study of 36 moderately affected patients with Fabry disease (18 males, 18 females; one patient with a history of cerebral ischaemia) and 22 age- and gender-matched controls with comparable education (11.5 years on average), there was no significant difference in global intelligence quotient, as assessed by the German modification of the Wechsler Adult Intelligence Scale – the Hamburg Wechsler Intelligence Test for Adults (HAWIE) (Figure 1; Müller *et al.*, unpublished data).

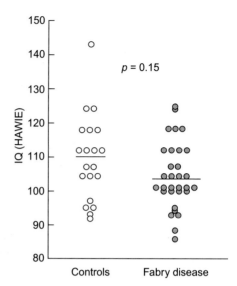

Figure 1. *Global intelligence quotient (IQ), as assessed by the German modification of the Wechsler Adult Intelligence Scale – the Hamburg Wechsler Intelligence Test for Adults (HAWIE) – in patients with Fabry disease and healthy controls. The horizontal line represents the mean value.*

Quality of life

Only a few studies have focused specifically on QoL in male and female patients with Fabry disease [18, 19]. From clinical practice, it is well known that many patients with Fabry disease have to cope with illness-related somatic and psychological impairments that can seriously diminish health-related QoL. Studies reporting QoL measures in adult patients with Fabry disease are summarized in Table 4 [16, 18–21].

These studies show that almost all areas of daily living are affected by the illness itself or by its psychosocial consequences. In the preliminary analysis of an ongoing study comparing 22 female and male patients with Fabry disease and 11 age- and gender-matched controls [21], 50% of patients with the disease had at least one diagnosis of affective disorder in their lifetime, and 45% had an additional somatic diagnosis. Patients with Fabry disease reported significantly more psychosocial stressors and showed

Table 4. *Studies including baseline quality-of-life assessment in patients with Fabry disease.*

Study design	Patients	Assessment and analysis	Outcome	Reference
Open longitudinal study of patients in FOS	73 males, 47 females	EQ-5D utility score (comparison with age- and gender-matched data from the normal UK population)	Significantly reduced EQ-5D utility score in males and females ($p < 0.05$); no difference between males and females	[16]
Open longitudinal study of patients in FOS	303 females	EQ-5D utility score (correlation with overall measure of disease severity using the FOS-MSSI)	Health-related QoL decreased with increasing age and increasing disease severity	[20]
Open longitudinal study	26 males, 7 females	EQ-5D (comparison with normative values from age- and gender-matched control groups)	Significantly reduced QoL in all 5 EQ-5D domains ($p < 0.05$) (mobility, self-care, usual activities, pain/discomfort, anxiety/depression)	[Bähner *et al.*, unpublished data]
Longitudinal control group study	11 males, 11 females	SF-36 (comparison between patients and healthy controls of similar age and gender distribution)	Significantly lower QoL values in all 8 SF-36 dimensions ($p < 0.05$) and in both composited scores (physical and mental health); no differences between male and female patients	[21]
Cross-sectional control group study	Males	SF-36 (comparison of male patients with Fabry disease with reference values from the US population and other chronic disease states (Gaucher disease, end-stage renal disease, stroke, AIDS)	Patients with Fabry disease had significantly ($p < 0.05$) lower QoL values in all 8 SF-36 domains compared with patients with Gaucher disease. Patients with Fabry disease had score profiles similar to patients with AIDS, with low values in all QoL domains. Cerebrovascular, cardiac and renal problems, as well as acroparaesthesiae and anhidrosis, were substantial predictors of low QoL	[18]
Open longitudinal study with baseline control group	38 males	SF-36, EQ-5D (comparison with an age-matched group of male patients with severe haemophilia and normative values)	Patients with Fabry disease had significantly lower QoL values in all 8 SF-36 domains compared with healthy controls ($p < 0.05$) and lower values in almost all SF-36 dimensions compared with patients with haemophilia	[19]

AIDS, acquired immunodeficiency syndrome; EQ-5D, EuroQol Group Instrument; FOS, Fabry Outcome Survey; FOS-MSSI, FOS adaptation of the Mainz Severity Score Index; QoL, quality of life; SF-36, Medical Outcome Survey, Short Form 36.

reduced QoL in all domains of the SF-36 questionnaire (Figure 2).

There was a significant correlation between the physical component of the SF-36 and the current pain level ($p < 0.001$), whereas depression ($p < 0.05$) and psychosocial distress ($p = 0.06$) were related to the mental component of QoL. The two QoL components were not significantly correlated to each other ($r = 0.30$).

Social support

In an additional analysis of 36 patients with Fabry disease and 22 controls (MJ Müller and KM Müller, unpublished data), the perceived social support, as assessed by questionnaire, was significantly lower ($p < 0.0005$) in the patients with Fabry disease. Moreover, both depression (HAMD) and pain levels (assessed by the Brief Pain Inventory) were

significantly inversely associated with the level of perceived social support (Figure 3) in patients with Fabry disease; that is, lower social support was associated with more intense pain (Figure 3a) and higher depression scores (Figure 3b).

Discussion

The present literature review on the neuropsychiatric and psychosocial aspects of Fabry disease reveals a paucity of reliable data. According to the available literature, depressive symptoms and disorders seem to occur frequently in males and females with Fabry disease. Depression is related to a high risk of suicide and elevated mortality, impaired psychosocial function and reduced QoL. This is consistent with other reports of depression occurring in the context of somatic illness, in wihch 20–50% of patients are found to suffer depressive episodes – for

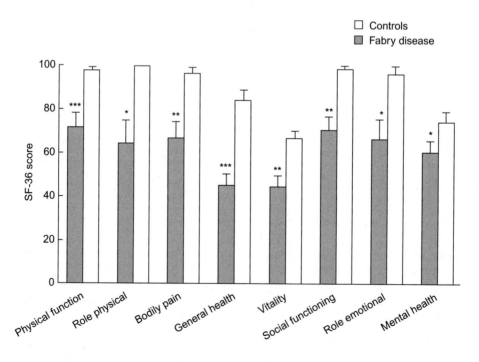

Figure 2. *Quality of life in patients with Fabry disease and controls [20], as assessed in all domains of the Short Form 36 (SF-36) questionnaire (good health = 100). *p < 0.05, **p < 0.01, ***p < 0.001 compared with controls (Mann–Whitney U-test).*

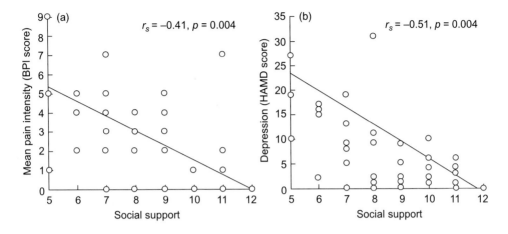

Figure 3. *Correlation between social support and (a) mean pain intensity experienced during the previous 24 hours, measured using the Brief Pain Inventory (BPI), and (b) depression, measured using the Hamilton Depression Rating Scale (HAMD), in patients with Fabry disease.*

example, after myocardial infarction, stroke, cancer and diabetes mellitus [22–26]. From these studies, we have learned that co-morbid untreated depression might reduce both the prognosis of the somatic illness and the patient's QoL [27, 28].

Depression is, in most cases, associated with feelings of hopelessness, passivity and pessimism, possibly leading to low treatment adherence and a high risk of substance abuse.

Some 10–25% of the general population suffer from at least one episode of major depression or anxiety disorder during their lives [29]. This makes it difficult to differentiate between depression related to Fabry disease and co-occurring psychiatric disorders. Nevertheless, it is important to diagnose psychiatric syndromes in patients with Fabry disease, as this will impact on therapeutic decisions.

In the light of these albeit limited prevalence figures and the available data from FOS, which show that approximately 10% of patients take antidepressant medication, depression and anxiety in patients with Fabry diseases would still appear to be under-recognized and under-treated.

The picture is less clear with regard to neuropsychological deficits. Whereas preliminary data did not reveal substantial differences in general intellectual functions between patients with Fabry disease and controls, clinical observations and case reports document that neuropsychological deficits do occur, often when neurological symptoms are clinically detectable. As structural brain abnormalities, particularly white matter lesions, are frequently found in relatively young male and female patients with Fabry disease [17, 30], future studies should focus on subtle neuropsychological findings at early stages of the disease and on the effects of ERT on cognitive and affective functions.

Almost all dimensions of QoL are substantially reduced in patients with Fabry disease [21], with the reduction comparable to that in very severe and life-threatening diseases [17–19].

Predictors of reduced QoL in Fabry disease are, in particular, cardiac, renal and cerebrovascular dysfunction, as well as pronounced pain and debilitating anhidrosis [18]. A close relationship between poor subjective physical health and pain, as well as between reduced mental health values (SF-36) and neuropsychiatric symptoms, especially depression, has been demonstrated in patients with Fabry disease [21]. These findings are in agreement with results in children and adolescents with Fabry disease [31]. In this latter study a different QoL assessment instrument was used (Child Health Questionnaire), and the results from nine boys less than 10 years of age with Fabry disease were compared with reference values for healthy control boys. Significantly worse QoL ratings were revealed for bodily pain and mental health scores in the children with Fabry disease, with pain scores being comparable to those of children with juvenile arthritis.

Fabry disease is often diagnosed 5–15 years after the onset of the first typical symptoms; that is, diagnosis often occurs only in adulthood [17]. This might contribute to the severe psychosocial impairment of patients with Fabry disease. Even after Fabry disease has been diagnosed, psychiatric symptoms often remain untreated [12].

Bio-psychosocial model of neuropsychiatric symptoms

The hypothetical development of depression, psychosocial impairment and reduced QoL in patients with Fabry disease is outlined below in a bio-psychosocial model.

Pathophysiological factors

Fabry disease is linked to a progressive accumulation of glycosphingolipids, particularly globotriaosylceramide, in visceral tissues and body fluids, especially vascular endothelial and smooth muscle cells [32]. Clinical manifestations include angiokeratomas, renal failure and neuropathy, as well as myocardial and cerebral ischaemia. Cerebrovascular

lesions are found in patients with Fabry disease, depending on age and the duration of disease manifestations. Particularly in the early stages of the diseases – in younger male and female patients – small vessels in the white matter of the brain seem to be primarily involved [30, 33]. In addition to increasing the risk of cerebral ischaemia and stroke (see Chapter 22), this vasculopathy is probably the pathophysiological basis of cognitive impairments in patients with Fabry disease. However, evidence for a relationship between neuropsychological findings and morphological alterations in the CNS of patients with Fabry disease, as assessed by brain imaging techniques such as magnetic resonance imaging, is currently lacking.

Psychological determinants

Fabry disease is a rare, hereditary chronic illness with frequent manifestations in childhood [17]. As mentioned above, diagnosis is often verified only 5–15 years after the onset of symptoms and, in many cases, more than one family member is affected [12]. Late diagnosis and many years in childhood and adolescence without appropriate treatment or even full acceptance that the reported symptoms are the result of an illness may severely hamper the development of social networks and active coping strategies.

The full impact of the chronic psychosocial distress associated with the highly individual course of Fabry disease is not established. However, it is well-known from other chronic, inherited or severe diseases, such as diabetes mellitus [34], heart failure [35] and cancer, that psychosocial aspects interact substantially with the somatic illness. Impaired psychosocial adjustment, involving lack of social support and isolation, unemployment and depression, has a strong negative influence on the disease process. Both the pathophysiological and psychosocial aspects of Fabry disease appear to determine subjective well-being and QoL.

Hypothetical model of neuropsychiatric symptoms

Thus, there are hypothetically two main factors in the development of possible neuro-psychiatric symptoms in patients with Fabry disease. On the one hand, cerebral isch-aemia might contribute to neuropsycho-logical deficits and psychiatric symptoms; on the other hand, chronic psychosocial distress seems to interact with individual coping resources. Both factors should not be regarded independently, as they have been shown to interact in other organic brain disorders with accompanying psychiatric symptoms (e.g. post-stroke depression [24]) Figure 4 shows a hypothetical model of neuropsychiatric symptoms in Fabry disease.

Stress and coping model

The psychological coping attempts and strategies during the course of a chronic illness can be interpreted within the frame-work of stress-coping models (Figure 5) [36, 37]. Such models are pragmatically helpful with regard to possible interventions, partic-ularly psychosocial therapies. Apart from 'objectively' distressing factors (e.g. somatic dysfunction, impairment and disability) sub-jective aspects of appraisal, and possibly inter-vening variables, such as the amount of perceived social support, have to be taken into account. In current stress models [37], psychosocial outcomes, including the ex-acerbation of psychiatric disorders (stress disorders, adjustment disorder, depression) are regarded as a consequence of an inter-action between individual coping resources and features of the illness.

According to Figure 5, not only the number and severity of objective or perceived stres-sors but also the availability and resilience of appropriate coping strategies and the per-ceived social support (i.e. to be accepted by others, to have others to talk to about problems, to receive help and support, etc.) are important in terms of long-term mental and physical outcomes. Social support is a

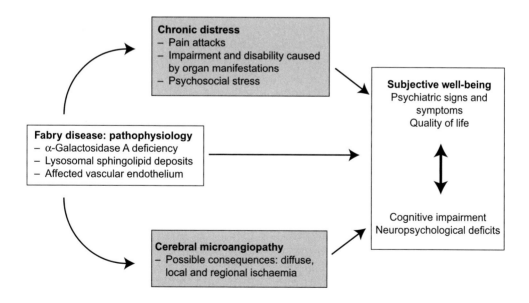

Figure 4. *Hypothetical model of neuropsychiatric symptoms in Fabry disease.*

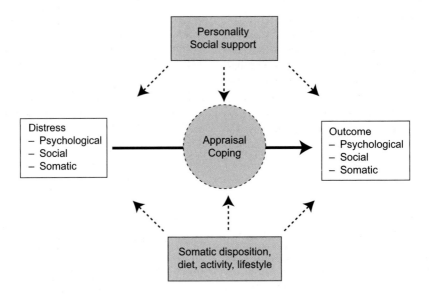

Figure 5. *Theoretical model of stress and coping in Fabry disease.*

well-known factor that moderates the influence of life-stress and illness on psychological well-being and psychiatric disorders [38, 39].

Social support seems to be of particular importance in disentangling the relationship between psychosocial factors, depression and QoL. In a preliminary analysis (MJ Müller and KM Müller, unpublished data), male and female patients with Fabry disease had a significantly lower level of perceived social support than controls. In the patients, depression and pain intensity were significantly inversely correlated with the level of perceived social support. This finding can be interpreted in two ways. First, patients with Fabry disease are more likely to develop depression and other psychiatric symptoms, leading to social isolation and reduced support. Alternatively, the difficulties associated with Fabry disease could lead to a tendency for patients to feel lonely, abandoned or isolated, even in adolescence or early adulthood. Low social support seems – particularly in females – to be related to a

higher risk of depression [40] and a higher level of pain [41]. Thus, in patients with Fabry disease, a vicious circle of mutually reinforcing negative factors (depression/pain and loss of social support) can develop (Figure 6).

Conclusions

The available literature and clinical observations provide evidence that psychiatric symptoms and neuropsychological deficits are not uncommon in the course of Fabry disease. In particular, the high rate of depression may contribute to the morbidity and mortality

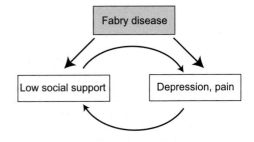

Figure 6. *Relationship between depression and social support in Fabry disease.*

of the disease in both females and males. The inclusion of psychiatric and psychosocial assessments in the routine examination of patients with Fabry disease could definitely benefit patients, as promising psychotherapeutic and psychopharmacological treatments are now available. The main areas of focus should be on awareness and early prevention of psychiatric disorders and suicidal tendencies, as well as on the long-term improvement of QoL in patients with Fabry disease.

References

1. Whybra C, Kampmann C, Willers I, Davies J, Winchester B, Kriegsmann J et al. Anderson–Fabry disease: clinical manifestations of disease in female heterozygotes. J Inherit Metab Dis 2001;24:715–24

2. Cleeland CS, Ryan KM. Pain assessment: global use of the Brief Pain Inventory. Ann Acad Med Singapore 1994;23:129–38

3. Cleeland CS, Nakamura Y, Mendoza TR, Edwards KR, Douglas J, Serlin RC. Dimensions of the impact of cancer pain in a four country sample: new information from multidimensional scaling. Pain 1996;67:267–73

4. Cleeland CS. Pain assessment: the advantages of using pain scales in lysosomal storage diseases. Acta Paediatr Suppl 2002;439:43–7

5. Brooks R, Rabin R, de Charro F. The measurement and valuation of health status using EQ-5D: a European perspective. New York: Kluwer Academic Publishers; 2003

6. Greiner W, Weijnen T, Nieuwenhuizen M, Oppe S, Badia X, Busschbach J et al. A single European currency for EQ-5D health states. Results from a six-country study. Eur J Health Econ 2003;4:222–31

7. Brazier JE, Harper R, Jones NM, O'Cathain A, Thomas KJ, Usherwood T et al. Validating the SF-36 health survey questionnaire: new outcome measure for primary care. BMJ 1992;305:160–4

8. Ware J, Kosinski M, Keller S. SF 36 physical and mental health summary scales: a user's manual. Massachusetts: The Health Institute, New England Medical Center; 1994

9. Liston EH, Levine MD, Philippart M. Psychosis in Fabry disease and treatment with phenoxybenzamine. Arch Gen Psychiatry 1973;29:402–3

10. Grewal RP. Psychiatric disorders in patients with Fabry's disease. Int J Psychiatry Med 1993;23:307–12

11. Mohanraj R, Leach JP, Broome JC, Smith DF. Neurological presentation of Fabry's disease in a 52 year old man. J Neurol Neurosurg Psychiatry 2002;73:340–2

12. Sadek J, Shellhaas R, Camfield CS, Camfield PR, Burley J. Psychiatric findings in four female carriers of Fabry disease. Psychiatr Genet 2004;14:199–201

13. Borsini W, Giuliacci G, Torricelli F, Pelo E, Martinelli F, Scordo MR. Anderson–Fabry disease with cerebrovascular complications in two Italian families. Neurol Sci 2002;23:49–53

14. Mendez MF, Stanley TM, Medel NM, Li Z, Tedesco DT. The vascular dementia of Fabry's disease. Dement Geriatr Cogn Disord 1997;8:252–7

15. Kaye EM, Kolodny EH, Logigian EL, Ullman MD. Nervous system involvement in Fabry's disease: clinicopathological and biochemical correlation. Ann Neurol 1988;23:505–9

16. Hoffmann B, Garcia de Lorenzo A, Mehta A, Beck M, Widmer U, Ricci R. Effects of enzyme replacement therapy on pain and health related quality of life in patients with Fabry disease: data from FOS (Fabry Outcome Survey). J Med Genet 2005;42:247–52

17. Mehta A, Ricci R, Widmer U, Dehout F, Garcia de Lorenzo A, Kampmann C et al. Fabry disease defined: baseline clinical manifestations of 366 patients in the Fabry Outcome Survey. Eur J Clin Invest 2004;34:236–42

18. Gold KF, Pastores GM, Botteman MF, Yeh JM, Sweeney S, Aliski W et al. Quality of life of patients with Fabry disease. Qual Life Res 2002;11:317–27

19. Miners AH, Holmes A, Sherr L, Jenkinson C, MacDermot KD. Assessment of health-related quality-of-life in males with Anderson–Fabry disease before therapeutic intervention. Qual Life Res 2002;11:127–33

20. Deegan P, Baehner AF, Barba-Romero MA, Hughes D, Kampmann C, Beck M. Natural history of Fabry disease in females in the Fabry Outcome Survey. J Med Genet 2006;43:347–52

21. Müller MJ, Müller KM, Dascalescu A, Fellgiebel A, Mann K, Scheurich A et al. Psychiatric symptoms and quality of life in patients with Fabry disease: preliminary results of a prospective study. Acta Paediatr Suppl 2005;447:114

22. Arolt V, Rothermundt M. Depressive disorders in patients with somatic illnesses. Nervenarzt 2003; 74:1033–52

23. Cheok F, Schrader G, Banham D, Marker J, Hordacre AL. Identification, course, and treatment of depression after admission for a cardiac condition: rationale and patient characteristics for the Identifying Depression As a Comorbid Condition (IDACC) project. Am Heart J 2003;146:978–84

24. Cassidy E, O'Connor R, O'Keane V. Prevalence of post-stroke depression in an Irish sample and its relationship with disability and outcome following inpatient rehabilitation. Disabil Rehabil 2004;26:71–7

25. Norton TR, Manne SL, Rubin S, Carlson J, Hernandez E, Edelson MI et al. Prevalence and predictors of psychological distress among women with ovarian cancer. J Clin Oncol 2004;22:919–26

26. Whittemore R, Melkus GD, Grey M. Self-report of depressed mood and depression in women with type 2 diabetes. Issues Ment Health Nurs 2004;25:243–60

27. Egede LE. Diabetes, major depression, and functional disability among US adults. Diabetes Care 2004; 27:421–8

28. Glassman AH. Does treating post-myocardial infarction depression reduce medical mortality? *Arch Gen Psychiatry* 2005;62:711–12

29. Andrade L, Caraveo-Anduaga JJ, Berglund P, Bijl RV, De Graaf R, Vollebergh W *et al*. The epidemiology of major depressive episodes: results from the International Consortium of Psychiatric Epidemiology (ICPE) Surveys. *Int J Methods Psychiatr Res* 2003; 12:3–21

30. Fellgiebel A, Müller MJ, Mazanek M, Baron K, Beck M, Stoeter P. White matter lesions severity in male and female patients with Fabry disease. *Neurology* 2005; 65:600–2

31. Ries M, Gupta S, Moore DF, Sachdev V, Quirk JM, Murray GJ *et al*. Pediatric Fabry disease. *Pediatrics* 2005;115:e344–55

32. Altarescu G, Moore DF, Pursley R, Campia U, Goldstein S, Bryant M *et al*. Enhanced endothelium-dependent vasodilation in Fabry disease. *Stroke* 2001;32:1559–62

33. Crutchfield KE, Patronas NJ, Dambrosia JM, Frei KP, Banerjee TK, Barton NW *et al*. Quantitative analysis of cerebral vasculopathy in patients with Fabry disease. *Neurology* 1998;50:1746–9

34. Lustman PJ, Clouse RE. Depression in diabetic patients: the relationship between mood and glycemic control. *J Diabetes Complications* 2005;19:113–22

35. Rodriguez-Artalejo F, Guallar-Castillon P, Pascual CR, Otero CM, Montes AO, Garcia AN *et al*. Health-related quality of life as a predictor of hospital readmission and death among patients with heart failure. *Arch Intern Med* 2005;165:1274–9

36. Lazarus R, Folkman S. Stress. Appraisal and coping. New York: Springer; 1984

37. Lazarus R. Stress and emotion. New York: Springer; 1999

38. Cobb S. Presidential Address – 1976. Social support as a moderator of life stress. *Psychosom Med* 1976;38:300–14

39. Cohen LH, McGowan J, Fooskas S, Rose S. Positive life events and social support and the relationship between life stress and psychological disorder. *Am J Community Psychol* 1984;12:567–87

40. Landman-Peeters KM, Hartman CA, van der Pompe G, den Boer JA, Minderaa RB, Ormel J. Gender differences in the relation between social support, problems in parent-offspring communication, and depression and anxiety. *Soc Sci Med* 2005;60: 2549–59

41. DePalma MT, Weisse CS. Psychological influences on pain perception and non-pharmacologic approaches to the treatment of pain. *J Hand Ther* 1997;10:183–91

30 Fabry disease in females: clinical characteristics and effects of enzyme replacement therapy

Patrick B Deegan[1], Frank Bähner[2], Miguel Barba[3], Derralynn A Hughes[4] and Michael Beck[2]

[1]Department of Medicine, University of Cambridge, Box 157, Addenbrooke's Hospital, Hills Road, Cambridge CB2 2QQ, UK; [2]University Children's Hospital, 55131 Mainz, Germany; [3]Internal Medicine Department, Albacete University Hospital, 37 Hermanos Falcó Street, 02006 Albacete, Spain; [4]Lysosomal Storage Disorders Unit, Department of Academic Haematology, Royal Free and University College Medical School, Rowland Hill Street, London NW3 2PF, UK

The availability of enzyme replacement therapy (ERT) and the possibility of improved organ function, quality of life and ultimately life expectancy has stimulated re-evaluation of the clinical expression of Fabry disease in females. Recent editions of general medical textbooks now recognize the burden of signs and symptoms found in heterozygotes. The use of the term carrier in this disorder has been questioned. FOS – the Fabry Outcome Survey – has reinforced the high prevalence of disease manifestations occurring in heterozygous females and now provides a mechanism for evaluating the natural history of disease and effects of ERT with agalsidase alfa in a large cohort of female patients.

Introduction

The realization that females heterozygous for mutations in the α-galactosidase A gene may experience significant manifestations of Fabry disease is relatively recent. Prior to the development of enzyme replacement therapy (ERT), medical literature relating to females with Fabry disease was confined to case reports, and small cohort studies and these were limited by preconceptions implicit in the notion of carrier status in an X-linked recessive condition. Disease-specific symptoms were said to be the exception [1, 2], often with a frequency of significant end-organ damage of no more than 1% in the female heterozygous population [3].

Until recently, general medical textbooks have emphasized that females are largely asymptomatic, citing the seminal article by Desnick *et al.* [3]. For example, it has been stated that: "Some heterozygous females… experience mild manifestations such as painful neuropathy, as well as other features of the disease" [4]. The following statements appear in another well-known general textbook: "heterozygous female subjects are usually asymptomatic or exhibit mild manifestations"; "corneal opacities and characteristic lenticular lesions are present in about 70 to 80 percent of asymptomatic heterozygotes"; "heterozygous female subjects may have corneal opacities, isolated skin lesions"; and "rare female heterozygotes may have manifestations as severe as those in affected male subjects" [5]. More recently published textbooks, however, reflect the changing view of the expression of Fabry disease in females. The most recent edition of the *Oxford Textbook of Medicine Reports*: "An unusual feature of Fabry's disease is the presence of clinical signs and symptoms in the majority of heterozygous female carriers of the condition, although these manifestations are usually less severe and of later onset than in affected hemizygous males" [6].

This changing view is reflected in an on-line updated version of *Harrison's Principles of Internal Medicine*, where in May 2005 it is written that: "Up to 70% of heterozygous females may exhibit clinical manifestations, including central nervous system and cardiac disease, but usually do not develop renal failure".

The peer-reviewed literature, recently stimulated by new prospects of therapy, has systematically documented disease expression in females. This chapter briefly reviews the current literature and describes the part played by FOS – the Fabry Outcome Survey – in defining the effects of Fabry disease in a large cohort of female patients, and its potential for assessing the effects of ERT.

Evidence for the effects of Fabry disease in female patients

Questionnaire studies of extensive cohorts of patients with Fabry disease have provided insight into the range of symptoms that female heterozygotes may experience [7, 8]. More recently, the introduction of ERT has demanded a thorough baseline assessment of all patients, including heterozygous females [9, 10]. It has now become clear that females may exhibit a range of severe disease manifestations, similar to that seen in male hemizygotes (Table 1). Heterozygous females should therefore be regarded as potential patients and not simply as carriers. Whybra and co-workers have gone so far as to postulate that this lysosomal storage disease should be considered as an X-linked dominant disease [9].

In a study of 60 obligate female carriers in a UK registry, MacDermot *et al.* found that 30% exhibited multiple and serious disease manifestations, including transient ischaemic

attacks, stroke and renal failure [7]. No patient investigated by Mehta *et al.* [10] or Whybra *et al.* [9] was entirely without clinical manifestations, and some symptoms were found in over 90% of patients.

Neuropathic pain

Neuropathic pain is reported to be a severe, disabling and common feature of Fabry disease in females. Most describe it as continuous, with exacerbations during illness and hot weather. Along with fatigue, neuropathic pain has a significant impact on quality of life (QoL). It has been reported in female patients as young as 4 years of age [9], with a median age of onset of 10 years, and may continue throughout life.

Quality of life

An evaluation conducted in Mainz showed that organ involvement in female patients with Fabry disease has a significant impact on QoL. Before initiating ERT, 15 female patients were asked to complete the short form 36 (SF-36) QoL questionnaire. The results were compared with those from a general German population and from patients with different chronic diseases. Female patients with Fabry disease had SF-36 scores that were substantially lower than those for the general female population. Female patients with Fabry disease also scored substantially lower than females with rheumatoid arthritis in 'general health', 'vitality', 'role emotional' and 'mental health' domains [11].

Cerebrovascular complications

Cerebrovascular complications of stroke and transient ischaemic attacks have been documented in 5–27% of heterozygous females [7, 8, 10], with one study finding them more frequently in female than in male patients (27% compared with 12%) [10]. Mitsias and Levine reported ten heterozygotes with cerebrovascular complications, such as memory loss, dizziness, ataxia, hemiparesis, loss of consciousness and hemisensory disturbance [12]. Corresponding

Table 1. *Literature review of the manifestations of Fabry disease in heterozygous female patients.*

	Whybra *et al.* [9]	Galanos *et al.* [8]	MacDermot *et al.* [7]	Mehta *et al.* [10]
n	20	38	60	165
Mean age (years)	NR	NR	44.9	41 ± 17
Angiokeratoma	55%	13%	35%	50%
Hypohidrosis	NR	11%	32%	NR
Acroparaesthesia	90%	53%	70%	64%
Left ventricular hypertrophy	55%	5% CM	19%	28%
Cardiac valve disease	NR	23%	48%	NR
Cardiac symptoms	NR	5–29%*	53%	65%
Proteinuria	NR	21%	NR	33%
Renal failure	55%	NR	3.3% ESRF	1% ESRF
			35% Abnormal RF	
Cerebrovascular disease	NR	5%	21%	27%
Vertigo/tinnitus/hearing loss	85%	NR	25%	47%
Ocular signs	70%	76%	NR	53%
Gastrointestinal symptoms	60%	11%	58%	50%
Lymphoedema	50%	3%	8%	NR

*Depending on definition.
CM, cardiomyopathy; ESRF, end-stage renal failure; NR, not reported; RF, renal function.

changes on magnetic resonance imaging (MRI), including diffuse white matter disease and infarction of the brainstem and thalamus, have been described [13–15]; however, Morgan *et al.* failed to find any changes on brain MRI in younger females [16]. Other neurovascular manifestations, including vertigo, tinnitus, hearing loss and hypohidrosis, are reported in approximately one-third of female patients, and Galanos *et al.* suggested that the presence of anhidrosis in females is predictive of later significant renal disease [8].

Renal involvement

Renal failure is a significant cause of premature death in male hemizygous patients with Fabry disease. In contrast, whilst proteinuria [17] and a reduction in renal function are well described in heterozygotes [18–20], progression to end-stage renal failure is infrequent, with only 1–2% of females requiring dialysis or transplantation [7, 10]. Histological evidence of renal changes has been found not only in those females with evidence of renal dysfunction but also in asymptomatic heterozygotes undergoing investigations as potential kidney donors [21]. Kriegsmann and co-workers published a case report of a 26-year-old female patient who was admitted to hospital because of fever of unknown origin and renal failure [22]. Extracapillary proliferative (crescentic) glomerulonephritis and granulomatous interstitial nephritis were identified by histological, immunohistochemical and electron microscopic analysis of a kidney biopsy, and Fabry disease was confirmed by further investigations [22].

Cardiac symptoms

Cardiac symptoms and evidence of structural cardiac disease, including septal hypertrophy, cardiomyopathy and mitral valve insufficiency, were reported by MacDermot *et al.* [7] and Whybra *et al.* [9]. Others have described palpitations in approximately one-third of females [8]. Arrhythmias and a requirement for pacemaker insertion have also been described [23], and Cantor and co-workers reported a 53-year-old female with restrictive cardiomyopathy requiring cardiac transplantation [24].

Gastrointestinal symptoms

Symptoms of diarrhoea, abdominal pain, constipation and vomiting, similar to those seen in irritable bowel syndrome, are described in 50–60% of females (Table 1). The aetiology of gastrointestinal disease is not known. However, the finding of electron-dense sphingolipids in neuronal and vascular tissue of the small bowel [25] suggests that it may be neurovascular in origin.

Mortality

The impact of Fabry disease on female survival remains unclear due to bias in ascertainment. Kaplan–Meier analysis of UK data provided by relatives and confirmed by examination of death certificates suggests a median cumulative survival of 70 years, some 15 years shorter than the reference UK population [7]. A study of deaths in 24 female relatives of patients with Fabry disease in FOS suggested a mean age of death of 55.4 ± 14.9 years, with cardiac disease being the most frequent cause [10].

FOS data
Patient demographics and clinical features

Data are currently available from 358 female patients recruited to the FOS database. The mean age at entry into FOS was 37.5 ± 18.3 years. Diagnosis was made at a mean age of 31.4 ± 17.1 years (n = 316), while the mean age at onset of symptoms was 19.1 ± 15.0 years (n = 214). Eighteen females did not have any symptoms reported (mean age at latest clinic visit, 26.1 ± 18.0 years). Patients have been recruited from 52 centres in 11 European countries.

The frequency and age at onset of disease-specific clinical features, as reported by the patient using a checklist of predefined clin-

ical features developed for FOS, are shown in Table 2. The most frequent features are neurological and cardiac, which are reported in 67% and 51% of patients, respectively. Neurological features are also the earliest to develop, beginning at an average age of 21.9 years, whereas cardiac features begin later, at an average age of 36.6 years. Self-reported indicators of renal involvement are recorded in 38% of patients and begin at an average age of 37.4 years. Other signs and symptoms involving the eye and gastro-intestinal system are also common, being observed in nearly 50% of the females for whom these data are available.

When the signs and symptoms are analysed in more detail, the predominant symptoms reported are acute attacks of pain (classed as neurological), affecting 52% of patients. The next most frequent features are angio-keratoma and cornea verticillata. A high proportion of patients (34%) are also reported to have proteinuria. Of the cardiac manifestations reported, left ventricular hypertrophy is found in 26% of the female population studied, and palpitations are reported by 21%.

Clinical investigations

Echocardiographic assessment of left ventricular mass (LVM) prior to starting ERT was available in 151 female patients in FOS. The mean LVM index (± SD) was 50.4 ± 25.7 g/m$^{2.7}$ at a mean age of 39.5 ± 17.6 years. Hypertrophic cardiomyopathy was considered to be present if the LVM index exceeded 50 g/m$^{2.7}$. Mean ventricular wall thickness was 10.9 ± 3.3 mm. The mean glomerular filtration rate (GFR) in 245 female patients enrolled in FOS prior to ERT was 77.1 ± 17.5 ml/min/1.73 m^2 at a mean age of 43.1 ± 14.6 years, excluding those below 18 years of age. Classification of renal function according to the Kidney Disease Outcomes Quality Initiative guidelines shows that, among females in FOS, 13% have stage III (moderate), 64% have

Table 2. *Frequency and age at onset of specific signs and symptoms of Fabry disease in heterozygous female patients enrolled in FOS – the Fabry Outcome Survey.*

Sign or symptom	Frequency		Age at onset (years)	
	% of population	*n*	Mean ± SD	*n*
Cerebrovascular	11.9	40	48.8 ± 14.6	33
Stroke	6.2	21	52.3 ± 14.4	18
TIA	7.1	24	45.2 ± 14.2	19
Neurological	67.4	227	21.9 ± 16.5	132
Pain attacks	51.6	174	18.7 ± 17.4	123
Chronic pain	30.6	103	22.8 ± 17.1	65
Cardiac	51.3	173	36.6 ± 18.2	106
Chest pain	19.3	65	44.8 ± 15.5	41
Palpitations	21.4	72	44.2 ± 16.0	51
LV hypertrophy	25.5	86	50.2 ±11.1	50
Renal/urinary	38.0	128	37.4 ± 16.7	85
Proteinuria	33.5	113	38.6 ± 17.3	81
Dialysis	0.6	2	38.5 ± 2.0	2
Transplantation	0.6	2	40.1 ± 1.2	2
Gastrointestinal	45.1	152	24.8 ± 18.4	102
Diarrhoea	19.6	66	22.1 ± 17.5	46
Abdominal pain	30.3	102	24.3 ± 19.7	73
Constipation	15.7	53	29.5 ± 18.8	36
Auditory	41.8	141	33.9 ± 19.0	87
Tinnitus	26.7	90	30.6 ± 17.8	61
Vertigo	26.4	89	34.8 ± 17.9	66
Sudden deafness	2.7	9	36.5 ± 20.0	8
Ophthalmological	46.6	157	32.7 ± 19.5	109
Cornea verticillata	36.5	123	32.7 ± 20.2	91
Tortuous vessels	6.8	23	45.1 ± 21.6	16
Posterior subcapsular cataract	3.6	12	53.5 ± 20.6	7
Dermatological	37.7	127	30.2 ± 17.4	75
Angiokeratoma	36.2	122	30.0 ±17.0	73
Telangiectasia	8.0	27	41.5 ± 20.8	18

LV, left ventricular; *n*, number of patients; TIA, transient ischaemic attack.

stage II (mild) and 22% have stage I (normal) renal function [26].

Proteinuria

A correlation between age and GFR was not seen in a subgroup of 41 female patients with proteinuria (protein > 300 mg/24 hours). The mean GFR was 70.1 ± 17.7 ml/min/1.73 m^2 at ages ranging from 17 to 71 years.

Disease severity and progression in untreated female patients

The LVM index (Figure 1) increases exponentially with age ($r = 0.78$, $p < 0.001$, $n = 151$), and the mean ventricular wall thickness increases in a more linear fashion with age ($r = 0.78$, $p < 0.001$, $n = 164$). Age is negatively correlated with estimated GFR (assessed using the Modification of Diet in Renal

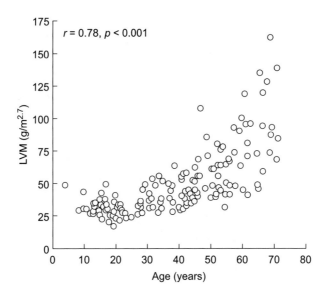

Figure 1. *Correlation between left ventricular mass (LVM) index and age in females with Fabry disease (n = 151) enrolled in FOS – the Fabry Outcome Survey.*

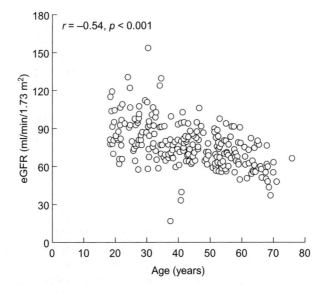

Figure 2. *Correlation between estimated glomerular filtration rate (eGFR, assessed using the Modification of Diet in Renal Disease [MDRD] equation) and age in females with Fabry disease (n = 245) enrolled in FOS – the Fabry Outcome Survey.*

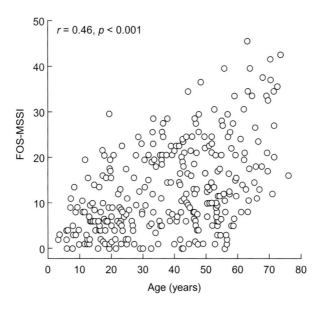

Figure 3. *Correlation between the modification of the Mainz Severity Score Index for the Fabry Outcome Survey (FOS-MSSI) and age in females with Fabry disease (n = 337) enrolled in FOS.*

Disease [MDRD] equation), with a decline in GFR of 0.62 ml/min/year (Figure 2; $r = -0.54$, $p < 0.001$, $n = 245$). In addition, age is negatively correlated with health-related QoL; however, there is no correlation after an adjustment has been made for the expected normal decline in QoL with age. 'Pain at its least' ($r = 0.26$, $p = 0.001$, $n = 195$) and 'pain right now' ($r = 0.23$, $p < 0.001$, $n = 195$), assessed using the Brief Pain Inventory, correlated positively with age. No significant correlation with age was found in relation to 'pain at its worst' ($r = 0.10$, $p = 0.15$, $n = 195$) or 'pain on average' ($r = 0.12$, $p = 0.10$, $n = 195$).

The modification of the Mainz Severity Score Index for FOS (FOS-MSSI) correlates positively with age (Figure 3; $r = 0.46$, $p < 0.001$, $n = 337$). It correlates inversely, however, with health-related QoL, as assessed using the European QoL (EQ-5D) utility score ($r = -0.41$, $p < 0.001$, $n = 134$),

a measure of the deviance of the EQ-5D scores from age- and gender-matched UK reference data [27–29] ($r = -0.34$, $p < 0.001$, $n = 134$), and with the visual analogue scale of the EQ-5D ($r = -0.42$, $p < 0.001$, $n = 111$).

Mortality

Mortality data, according to patient recall, are available for some relatives believed to have Fabry disease. The mean age at death in 39 female relatives was 57.8 ± 14.3 years (Figure 4).

Ascertainment bias

A potential limitation of the FOS database relates to ascertainment bias. The numbers of females and males within FOS are currently approximately equal. Theoretical considerations suggest that, assuming equal relative fecundity of males and females, heterozygotes should outnumber hemizygotes by two to one. We hypothesize that the shortfall is due to the relative under-representation of

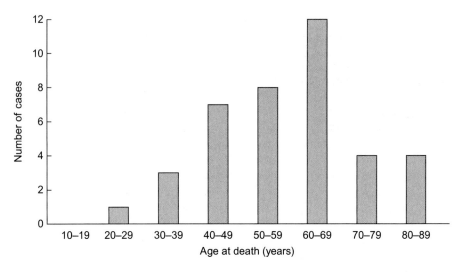

Figure 4. *Mortality data for female relatives of patients in FOS – the Fabry Outcome Survey – believed to have had Fabry disease (according to patient recall).*

unaffected females in FOS. A secular trend has become apparent over the first 5 years of FOS. Initially, when males outnumbered females, the severity of disease in females enrolled in FOS was higher than is now the case, as more young and asymptomatic women are recruited (see Chapter 16).

Relationship between X-inactivation, enzyme levels and disease severity

Current understanding of disease expression in females with X-linked disorders suggests that the severity of manifestations depends on the degree to which the normal X-chromosome is inactivated. Random skewing of X-inactivation may result in variation of expression of 25–75% of normal enzyme levels and, in cases of more severe or non-random skewing, expression levels of less than 25% may be seen. Preliminary studies by Morrone *et al.* have shown that there may be a correlation between skewing of X-inactivation in peripheral blood leukocytes and clinical expression of Fabry disease [30]. This finding requires confirmation. If this were the only factor, one might predict a straightforward relationship between blood enzyme activity and disease severity. Data on plasma or

leukocyte enzyme activity are available from 243 patients in FOS. Cross-tabulation with disease severity, as determined by the FOS-MSSI, demonstrated that among 96 patients with normal enzyme activity, 39% had a score above 20 (moderate disease severity), whereas 26 out of 147 patients (18%) with reduced enzyme activity had a score above 20. Thus, data from FOS do not support the use of enzyme activity in females as a marker of disease severity.

There are two X-linked disorders involving deficiency of lysosomal enzymes: Fabry disease and Hunter syndrome. In Hunter syndrome, clinical disease expression is exceptionally rare in females and, where observed, has been related to extreme Lyonization in almost all cases. This would suggest that the low levels of enzyme that are synthesized and secreted in all but extreme cases are sufficient to cross-correct deficient synthesis by abnormal cells. Cross-correction has been demonstrated in Hunter cells *in vitro*. This has not as yet been demonstrated in Fabry disease, and the fact that females with normal plasma enzyme activity may manifest moderately severe disease suggests that uptake of normal enzyme by abnormal cells may be defective. The clinical improvement achieved by ERT described below suggests, on the other hand, that cellular uptake of α-galactosidase A is possible *in vivo* in female patients.

ERT in females

The general effects of ERT are described later in this volume. ERT was initially evaluated in clinical trials of male patients. Bähner and co-workers evaluated the safety, efficacy and pharmacokinetics of agalsidase alfa (Replagal®; TKT Europe AB) administered intravenously to female patients with Fabry disease in an open-label, single-centre study [11]. Agalsidase alfa was shown to be well tolerated, and none of the female patients developed antibodies or experienced infusion reactions. The pharmacokinetic profile of agalsidase alfa in female patients is comparable to the pharmacokinetics in male patients. Mean levels of globotriaosylceramide – the lysosomal storage product in Fabry disease – in urinary sediment and plasma had decreased from baseline after 13, 27 and 41 weeks of ERT. A significant decrease in LVM from baseline was seen at weeks 27 ($p = 0.003$) and 41 ($p = 0.039$), and a significant reduction in the QRS duration was seen at week 27 ($p = 0.007$). Furthermore, there was a significant improvement in QoL. Renal function did not deteriorate in these 15 female patients over the 13–41 weeks of observation. It was concluded that ERT with agalsidase alfa was safe and effective in heterozygous females with Fabry disease [11].

Phenotypic heterogeneity and the lack of biomarkers have hindered the monitoring of responses to ERT. Whybra and co-workers therefore developed a scoring system – the MSSI – to measure the severity of Fabry disease and to monitor the clinical course of the disease in response to ERT [31]. Most male patients with Fabry disease were rated as severely or moderately affected on the MSSI, whereas most female patients were rated as moderately affected [31]. Although there was a trend towards a higher (worse) general score in males when compared with females ($p = 0.078$), this was no longer apparent after ERT. After 1 year of ERT, QoL had improved more in males than in females [32]. In those women with impaired health-related QoL (EQ-5D < 1), ERT was associated with an improvement in this important measure of outcome after 1 year of treatment (signed rank-sum test, $p < 0.05$, $n = 38$). This was equally the case when adjusted for age-related trends in QoL.

Analysis of organ-specific data from patients in FOS has demonstrated that cardiac structure and function improves and renal function is stabilized by ERT with agalsidase alfa (see Chapters 37 and 38). Analysis of the long-term effects of ERT in women is currently limited by the availability of follow-up data.

Conclusions

FOS has allowed investigators in many countries to pool their experience of patients with Fabry disease. In the case of disease expression in women, FOS has provided data to refute the long-held assumption that women with Fabry disease are rarely symptomatic. The data within FOS will be of immense value in addressing important issues relating to the pathogenesis of Fabry disease in women and their response to ERT.

References

1. Nakao S, Takenaka T, Maeda M, Kodama C, Tanaka A, Tahara M *et al*. An atypical variant of Fabry's disease in men with left ventricular hypertrophy. *N Engl J Med* 1995;333:288–93

2. Redonnet-Vernhet I, Ploos van Amstel JK, Jansen RP, Wevers RA, Salvayre R, Levade T. Uneven X inactivation in a female monozygotic twin pair with Fabry disease and discordant expression of a novel mutation in the α-galactosidase A gene. *J Med Genet* 1996;33:682–8

3. Desnick RJ, Ioannou YA, Eng CM. α-Galactosidase A deficiency: Fabry disease. In: Scriver CR, Beaudet AL, Sly WS, Valle D, editors. The metabolic and molecular basis of inherited disease. 8th edn. New York: McGraw-Hill; 2001. p. 3733–74

4. Jameson L, Kopp P. Principles of human genetics. In: Kasper DL, Braunwald E, Fauci A, Hauser S, Longo D, Jameson JL, editors. Harrison's priciples of internal medicine. 16th edn. New York: McGraw-Hill; 2004

5. McGovern M, Desnick R. Chapter 217. In: Goldman L, Ausiello D, editors. Cecil textbook of medicine. 22nd edn. Philadelphia: Elsevier; 2003. p. 1278–9

6. Cox TM. Metabolic disorders: lysosomal storage diseases. In: Warrell DA, Cox TM, Firth JD, Benz EJ, editors. Oxford textbook of medicine. 4th edn. Oxford: Oxford University Press; 2003. p. 119–120 and 416

7. MacDermot KD, Holmes A, Miners AH. Anderson–Fabry disease: clinical manifestations and impact of disease in a cohort of 60 obligate carrier females. *J Med Genet* 2001;38:769–75

8. Galanos J, Nicholls K, Grigg L, Kiers L, Crawford A, Becker G. Clinical features of Fabry's disease in Australian patients. *Intern Med J* 2002;32:575–84

9. Whybra C, Kampmann C, Willers I, Davies J, Winchester B, Kriegsmann J et al. Anderson–Fabry disease: clinical manifestations of disease in female heterozygotes. *J Inherit Metab Dis* 2001;24:715–24

10. Mehta A, Ricci R, Widmer U, Dehout F, Garcia de Lorenzo A, Kampmann C et al. Fabry disease defined: baseline clinical manifestations of 366 patients in the Fabry Outcome Survey. *Eur J Clin Invest* 2004;34:236–42

11. Bähner F, Kampmann C, Whybra C, Miebach E, Wiethoff CM, Beck M. Enzyme replacement therapy in heterozygous females with Fabry disease: results of a phase IIIB study. *J Inherit Metab Dis* 2003; 26:617–27

12. Mitsias P, Levine SR. Cerebrovascular complications of Fabry's disease. *Ann Neurol* 1996;40:8–17

13. Grewal RP, McLatchey SK. Cerebrovascular manifestations in a female carrier of Fabry's disease. *Acta Neurol Belg* 1992;92:36–40

14. Castro LH, Monteiro ML, Barbosa ER, Scaff M, Canelas HM. Fabry's disease in a female carrier with bilateral thalamic infarcts: a case report and a family study. *Rev Paul Med* 1994;112:649–53

15. Hasholt L, Sorensen SA, Wandall A, Andersen EB, Arlien-Soborg P. A Fabry's disease heterozygote with a new mutation: biochemical, ultrastructural, and clinical investigations. *J Med Genet* 1990;27:303–6

16. Morgan SH, Rudge P, Smith SJ, Bronstein AM, Kendall BE, Holly E et al. The neurological complications of Anderson–Fabry disease (α-galactosidase A deficiency) – investigation of symptomatic and presymptomatic patients. *Q J Med* 1990; 75:491–507

17. Yuen NW, Lam CW, Chow TC, Chiu MC. A characteristic dissection microscopy appearance of a renal biopsy of a Fabry heterozygote. *Nephron* 1997;77:354–6

18. Rodriguez FH Jr, Hoffmann EO, Ordinario AT Jr, Baliga M. Fabry's disease in a heterozygous woman. *Arch Pathol Lab Med* 1985;109:89–91

19. Van Loo A, Vanholder R, Madsen K, Praet M, Kint J, De Paepe A et al. Novel frameshift mutation in a heterozygous woman with Fabry disease and end-stage renal failure. *Am J Nephrol* 1996;16:352–7

20. el-Shahawy MA, Mesa C, Koss M, Campese VM. A 19-year-old female with fever, acroparesthesia, and progressive deterioration of renal function. *Am J Nephrol* 1996;16:417–24

21. Gubler MC, Lenoir G, Grunfeld JP, Ulmann A, Droz D, Habib R. Early renal changes in hemizygous and heterozygous patients with Fabry's disease. *Kidney Int* 1978;13:223–35

22. Kriegsmann J, Otto M, Wandel E, Schwarting A, Faust J, Hansen T et al. [Fabry's disease, glomerulonephritis with crescentic and granulomatous interstitial nephritis. Case of one family]. *Pathologe* 2003;24:439–44

23. Nakayama Y, Tsumura K, Yamashita N, Yoshimaru K. Dynamic left ventricular arterial pressure gradient and sick sinus syndrome with heterozygous Fabry's disease improved following implantation of a dual chamber pacemaker. *Pacing Clin Electrophysiol* 1999;22:1114–15

24. Cantor WJ, Daly P, Iwanochko M, Clarke JT, Cusimano RJ, Butany J. Cardiac transplantation for Fabry's disease. *Can J Cardiol* 1998;14:81–4

25. Sheth KJ, Werlin SL, Freeman ME, Hodach AE. Gastrointestinal structure and function in Fabry's disease. *Am J Gastroenterol* 1981;76:246–51

26. National Kidney Foundation (NKF) Kidney Disease Outcome Quality Initiative (K/DOQI) Advisory Board. K/DOQI clinical practice guidelines for chronic kidney disease: evaluation, classification, and stratification. *Am J Kidney Dis* 2002;39 (Suppl 2):S1–246

27. Kind P, Hardman G, Macran S. UK population norms for EQ-5D. York Centre for Health Economics discussion paper 1999;172

28. van Agt HM, Essink-Bot ML, Krabbe PF, Bonsel GJ. Test-retest reliability of health state valuations collected with the EuroQol questionnaire. *Soc Sci Med* 1994;39:1537–44

29. Brooks R. Quality of life measures. *Crit Care Med* 1996;24:1769

30. Morrone A, Cavicchi C, Bardelli T, Antuzzi D, Parini R, Di Rocco M et al. Fabry disease: molecular studies in Italian patients and X inactivation analysis in manifesting carriers. *J Med Genet* 2003;40:e103

31. Whybra C, Kampmann C, Krummenauer F, Ries M, Mengel E, Miebach E et al. The Mainz Severity Score Index: a new instrument for quantifying the Anderson–Fabry disease phenotype, and the response of patients to enzyme replacement therapy. *Clin Genet* 2004;65:299–307

32. Whybra C, Wendrich K, Ries M, Gal A, Beck M. Clinical manifestation in female Fabry disease patients. *Contrib Nephrol* 2001:245–50

31 Natural history and effects of enzyme replacement therapy in children and adolescents with Fabry disease

Uma Ramaswami[1], Rosella Parini[2] and Guillem Pintos-Morell[3]

[1]Department of Paediatric Endocrinology, Diabetes and Metabolism, Box 181, Addenbrooke's Hospital, Cambridge CB2 2QQ, UK; [2]Department of Paediatrics, S. Gerardo Hospital, Monza, Italy; [3]Department of Paediatrics, University Hospital 'Germans Trias i Pujol', Badalona, Spain

Many of the signs and symptoms of Fabry disease occur frequently in early childhood. These include acute and chronic neuropathic pain, acroparaesthesiae, hypohidrosis, angiokeratoma and gastrointestinal symptoms. Such manifestations occur in both boys and girls and may impair quality of life (QoL) and affect daily activities at home and school. Cornea verticillata is also commonly seen in affected children. In addition, although stroke, end-stage renal failure and heart failure are not found in children with Fabry disease, early signs of cerebrovascular, renal and cardiac involvement are encountered. Despite early manifestations of Fabry disease occurring in childhood, correct diagnosis is frequently delayed. Data from FOS – the Fabry Outcome Survey – and from clinical trials on the effects of enzyme replacement therapy (ERT) in children with Fabry disease have demonstrated that ERT with agalsidase alfa is well tolerated and has beneficial clinical effects on pain, QoL and gastrointestinal symptoms, at least in the short term. Early diagnosis is therefore important, because early initiation of ERT could potentially prevent or at least delay progression to end-stage organ failure.

Introduction

It has recently been recognized that the effects of Fabry disease are evident during childhood [1–3]. As in adults [4], manifestations of Fabry disease in children, including acute and chronic neuropathic pain, hypohidrosis, angiokeratoma and gastrointestinal symptoms, reduce quality of life (QoL) [1–3, 5]. Few data, however, are available on the efficacy of enzyme replacement therapy (ERT) in children with Fabry disease. This chapter discusses the natural course of Fabry disease in children and presents demographic data from FOS – the Fabry Outcome Survey. The efficacy and safety of ERT in preventing or delaying the onset of clinical manifestations of Fabry disease in children are also reviewed, with specific reference to FOS data.

Natural course of Fabry disease in children

Most patients with Fabry disease present with symptoms in early childhood, but these symptoms are not necessarily specific to the disease. As a result, there may be a significant delay in diagnosis. Fabry disease is progressive, and its characteristic life-threatening complications, including stroke, end-stage renal disease (ESRD) and cardiac failure, are not seen in childhood. The early clinical features of Fabry disease in children include poorly understood gastrointestinal manifestations, with alternating diarrhoea, constipation and abdominal bloating. In adults, a history of malabsorption, steatorrhoea and weight loss, with normal pancreatic enzymes, has been reported, but such symptoms are uncommon in children.

The burning and tingling sensation, and debilitating pain described in Fabry disease, known as acroparaesthesiae, is often the first presenting symptom in children. There has been anecdotal evidence of unexplained crying during infancy in children with Fabry disease, which is often diagnosed as colic. During childhood, they suffer from an acute onset of intense pain, predominantly in their hands and feet, and some children develop sudden abdominal pain, which may be mistaken for acute abdominal problems, such as appendicitis. These episodes are called Fabry crises and are usually precipitated by infections, fever, a change in temperature, or stress. Simple analgesics, opiates and gabapentin have been used with variable success. Fabry pain is debilitating, and often misdiagnosed in childhood. As in adults, it affects quality of life and normal childhood activities, such as participation in sport.

The characteristic skin rash with non-blanching small red lesions, known as angiokeratomas, seen in the groin, buttocks, abdomen and mucosal membrane of the mouth and lips, can appear in late childhood.

Cornea verticillata is common and can be seen by slit-lamp examination, performed by an experienced ophthalmologist, even in children under the age of 5 years. Tortuous retinal vessels and subcapsular cataracts are uncommon in children, but preliminary FOS data suggest that vessel tortuosity correlates with rates of progression of the systemic disease (see Chapter 26). The presence of subcapsular cataracts and retinal vessel tortuosity may also reflect disease severity, but there are currently too few data to be able to confirm this.

Hearing impairment, as a result of glue ear or due to sensorineural hearing loss at high and low frequencies, has been documented in children with Fabry disease. These symptoms, however, rarely occur in isolation and are usually accompanied by acroparaesthesiae and gastrointestinal manifestations.

Non-specific lethargy and myalgia are not uncommon in children with Fabry disease, but may be mistaken for rheumatological problems. In the author's experience, children with Fabry disease have difficulty in keeping up with their peers during sporting activities, because of excessive tiredness and decreased sweating.

Although cardiomyopathy and arrhythmias are uncommon in children with Fabry disease, mild valvular dysfunction is often revealed by echocardiography. Evidence of cardiomyopathy may be present in late childhood.

Proteinuria is documented mostly in late childhood, and ESRD has not been documented in patients below 18 years of age. Although most boys with classic Fabry disease who develop proteinuria will progress to ESRD, girls who present with proteinuria in their teenage years seldom progress to ESRD.

The burden of Fabry disease in young children is mainly due to debilitating pain, fever and pain crises, tiredness and lethargy, decreased sweating, impaired ability to participate in sports compared with peers, and gastrointestinal manifestations. It is therefore essential to have questionnaires that address these issues specifically, and which children themselves can complete. These questionnaires also aim to monitor functioning at school, relationships with peers and physical activity. Such a questionnaire is currently being evaluated in FOS.

FOS data

In March 2005, there were 119 patients in the FOS database who were under the age of 18 years (50 boys and 69 girls). The median age of these children at baseline evaluation was 12.7 years (range, 0.7–17.9 years), with a median age for boys of 11.1 years (0.7–17.8 years) and a median age for girls of 13.2 years (2.4–17.9 years) [5].

The children were reported to come from 86 families. In 44% of patients, the diagnosis was suspected from their family history. In the remaining patients, the diagnosis was suspected and confirmed by clinicians, including paediatricians, geneticists, dermatologists, general physicians, ophthalmologists, neurologists and nephrologists. Data for both the age at onset of symptoms and the age at diagnosis were available for 76 of the 119 patients (Table 1). For these 76 children, the mean age at diagnosis was approximately 10 years, and the delay between the onset of symptoms and diagnosis of Fabry disease was 2.8 ± 3.5 years (mean ± SD). The age at onset of symptoms was reported in only six of the remaining 43 patients. In many of the children detected by pedigree analysis, symptoms of Fabry disease had not yet developed.

The common signs and symptoms, including acroparaesthesiae, pain crises, angiokeratoma and gastrointestinal manifestations, were present in both male and female patients and were seen even in children below 10 years of age (Figure 1). Girls presented later than boys, with similar clinical manifestations [5].

Table 2 shows the frequency of different signs and symptoms of Fabry disease and age at onset in children in FOS, as of March 2005. The most frequently reported early clinical manifestations were gastrointestinal problems, pain attacks, hypohidrosis and cornea verticillata, all of which were reported in 30–50% of patients.

Other less frequent clinical features reported in children in FOS included claudication, Raynaud's syndrome, peripheral oedema, lymphoedema, headache, behavioural problems and anxiety, arrhythmias, chest pain, dyspnoea, left ventricular hypertrophy, palpitations, syncope and frequent infections.

Stroke, chronic kidney disease and heart failure, which together mainly account for the reduced lifespan of adults with Fabry disease, are not found in children. However, other cerebrovascular, renal and cardiac manifestations, as shown in Table 2, do occur in childhood, reflecting early onset of major organ involvement.

The symptoms of Fabry disease in children are likely to have an impact on QoL. Although detailed analyses of QoL data in children with Fabry disease are currently unavailable, limited data from Ries et al. [2] suggest that there is a decreased QoL.

Benefits of ERT

Data available in large outcomes databases such as FOS are important, not only for early diagnosis of Fabry disease in children but

Table 1. *Delay in diagnosis after onset of symptoms in patients below 18 years of age enrolled in FOS – the Fabry Outcome Survey. Values are means ± SD, with 95% confidence intervals and numbers of patients in parentheses.*

	Boys	Girls
Age at FOS entry (years)	11.0 ± 4.5	12.0 ± 4.6
	(9.7–12.3; $n = 50$)	(10.9–13.1; $n = 69$)
Age at onset of symptoms (years)	6.8 ± 3.3	8.2 ± 3.9
	(5.7–7.8; $n = 40$)	(7.0–9.4; $n = 42$)
Age at diagnosis (years)	9.1 ± 4.3	10.5 ± 4.5
	(7.8–10.4; $n = 45$)	(9.3–11.6; $n = 62$)
Delay in diagnosis (years)	2.4 ± 2.8	3.3 ± 4.1
	(1.4–3.3; $n = 37$)	(1.9–4.6; $n = 39$)

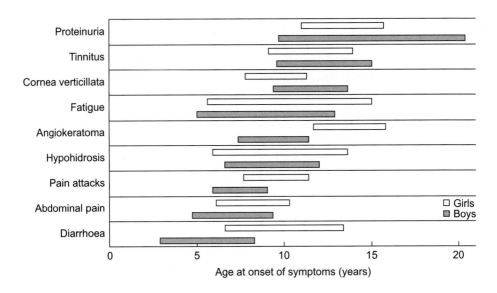

Figure 1. *Age at onset of symptoms in boys and girls with Fabry disease in FOS – the Fabry Outcome Survey. Bars represent the 95% confidence interval.*

also for understanding the natural history of the disease and predicting the rate of disease progression. This is particularly relevant in view of the recent introduction of ERT. The beneficial effects and safety of ERT have been demonstrated in adults with Fabry disease [6–10]. It is possible that ERT should be initiated early, as it offers the potential to change the natural course of this progressive disease.

In March 2005, there were 55 children (31 boys, 24 girls) from nine European countries receiving ERT in FOS (Table 3). Diagnosis of Fabry disease was confirmed in all patients by enzyme and/or DNA analysis.

At the start of therapy, 20 of the 55 children (13 boys, 7 girls) who were receiving ERT in FOS were younger than 12 years of age, and 35 (18 boys, 17 girls) were aged between 12 and 18 years. The median dose of agalsidase alfa was 0.2 mg (range, 0.17–0.23 mg), infused over 40 minutes every 2 weeks. It should be noted that all of the children and adolescents treated in two

European trials of paediatric patients have been entered into FOS and account for a third of this population (11 boys, 8 girls).

Data on the safety of ERT – as well as the effects of ERT on pain, QoL, hearing and gastrointestinal, cardiac and renal symptoms, have been analysed after 12 months of therapy.

Pain and QoL
The European QoL (EQ-5D) questionnaire was used to measure QoL (see Chapter 40). EQ-5D scores at the start of therapy (baseline) and after 12 months of therapy are shown in Figure 2 for the ten patients (6 boys, 4 girls) for whom paired QoL data were available in FOS. An improvement or no change in EQ-5D scores was observed in all ten patients (baseline scores were normal in those patients with no change in scores between baseline and 12 months).

The Brief Pain Inventory (BPI) (see Chapter 40 was completed by 11 patients (6 boys, 5 girls). The median age of these patients

Table 2. *Frequency and age at onset of specific signs and symptoms of Fabry disease in boys (n = 49) and girls (n = 66) enrolled in FOS – the Fabry Outcome Survey.*

	Frequency		Age at symptom onset (years)	
	Proportion of population (%)	Number of patients	Mean ± SD	Number of patients
Boys				
Diarrhoea	35	17	5.6 ± 4.3	12
Abdominal pain	41	20	7.0 ± 4.4	17
Pain attacks	67	33	7.4 ± 3.8	25
Hypohidrosis	49	24	9.3 ± 5.1	16
Angiokeratomas	39	19	9.4 ± 3.3	13
Anhidrosis	18	9	9.6 ± 6.7	6
Fatigue	16	8	10.3 ± 5.1	7
Telangiectasia	10	5	10.3 ± 5.4	5
Tortuous vessels	10	5	11.2 ± 4.5	4
Cornea verticillata	39	19	11.5 ± 4.0	16
Vertigo	16	8	11.9 ± 3.1	7
Tinnitus	27	13	12.3 ± 4.0	11
Proteinuria	10	5	15.0 ± 3.4	4
Depression	12	6	15.6 ± 3.9	3
Girls				
Diarrhoea	24	16	10.0 ± 6.4	16
Abdominal pain	38	25	8.2 ± 4.8	22
Pain attacks	45	30	9.5 ± 4.7	27
Hypohidrosis	21	14	9.7 ± 6.3	13
Angiokeratomas	23	15	13.7 ± 3.5	14
Anhidrosis	NR	NR	NR	NR
Fatigue	20	13	9.0 ± 5.5	10
Telangiectasia	8	5	13.8 ± 3.4	3
Tortuous vessels	5	3	10.4 ± 3.8	3
Cornea verticillata	45	30	9.6 ± 4.2	24
Vertigo	14	9	13.4 ± 3.3	9
Tinnitus	27	18	11.5 ± 4.1	14
Proteinuria	17	11	13.4 ± 3.2	10
Depression	9	6	12.7 ± 2.8	5

NR indicates that no girls enrolled in FOS reported this symptom.

was 14.7 years (range, 6.3–16.9 years). The median score at baseline for pain on average was 3 (range, 0–8) and the median change in score after 12 months of ERT was –1 (range, –6 to 4) (Figure 3). The median score at baseline for pain at its worse was 7 (range, 2–10) and the median change in score after 12 months of ERT was 0 (range, –7 to 7). Although only a small number of patients was studied, these results reveal an overall improvement in pain, with either improvement or no change from baseline in most patients.

Table 3. *Demographic data from 55 children receiving enzyme replacement therapy (ERT) in FOS – the Fabry Outcome Survey. Data are presented as means ± SD.*

	Boys (*n* = 31)	Girls (*n* = 24)
Age at entry into FOS (years)	12.3 ± 4.2	13.1 ± 4.6
Age at start of ERT (years)	12.3 ± 4.1	13.1 ± 4.5
Time on ERT (months)*	21.9 ± 12.3	16.4 ± 12.4

*Data correct as of March 2005.

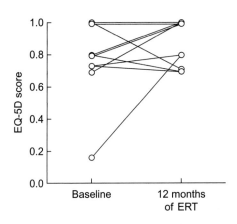

Figure 2. *Effect of 1 year of enzyme replacement therapy (ERT) on quality of life (QoL), as assessed using the European QoL (EQ-5D) questionnaire, in six boys and four girls in FOS – the Fabry Outcome Survey.*

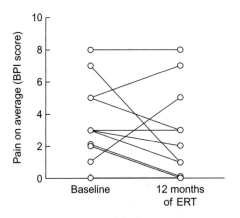

Figure 3. *Effect of 1 year of enzyme replacement therapy (ERT) on pain experienced on average, as assessed using the Brief Pain Inventory (BPI), in six boys and five girls in FOS – the Fabry Outcome Survey.*

Hearing

Hearing was assessed using pure-tone audiometry in patients older than 5 years. Audiometry data were available from ten patients at baseline and after 1 year of therapy. In nine of these patients, there was either no change or an improvement in hearing at high, medium and low frequencies.

Gastrointestinal symptoms

Eleven patients (4 boys, 7 girls) suffered from diarrhoea at baseline. After 12 months of therapy, there was a reduction in symptom frequency in ten of these patients from every day or more than once a week to once or twice or month or almost never. In one female, aged 18.3 years, the frequency of diarrhoea was documented as being the same after 9 months of ERT.

Renal features

Serial measurements of urine protein concentrations and glomerular filtration rate (GFR) were available at baseline and 1 year of therapy in only ten patients (4 boys, 6 girls). The mean age of these children at baseline was 14.5 years (range, 12.7–15.7 years in males; 9.1–17.3 years in females). Mean 24-hour urinary protein excretion was 229 mg/l (range, 77–615 mg/l) at baseline and 241 mg/l (range, 96–491 mg/l) after 1 year of therapy. Mean GFR, assessed using plasma ^{51}Cr-EDTA clearance, was 119 ml/min/1.73 m^2 (range, 72–221 ml/min/1.73 m^2) at baseline and 117 ml/min/1.73 m^2 (range, 84–143 ml/min/1.73 m^2) after 1 year of ERT. No patient showed deterioration in renal function after 1 year of therapy.

Cardiac features

Paired data for left ventricular (LV) mass at baseline and after 1 year of treatment were available in ten patients (4 boys, 6 girls). LV mass was within the normal range at baseline and after 1 year of ERT.

Safety of ERT

Eight patients (14.5%) reported 21 adverse events unrelated to treatment. Most of them ($n = 14$) were infections (ear, nose and throat infections, gastroenteritis); one case of recurrent tonsillitis was reported as serious. Six of these adverse events were exacerbations of abdominal pain or pain in the extremities related to Fabry disease. One patient had anaemia due to iron deficiency.

Thirty infusion-related reactions (1–8 per patient) were reported in ten patients (18.2%; 9 boys, 1 girl), giving an overall incidence of 1.3% (percentage of total number of infusions). Of these ten patients, five were below 12 years of age. By comparison, the percentage of adult patients experiencing infusion-related reactions has been calculated as approximately 13% (see Chapter 41). The most frequent symptoms of infusion reactions were rigors (6 patients), flushing (5 patients), pyrexia (5 patients), dyspnoea (3 patients), headache (3 patients) and nausea (3 patients). These reactions first occurred within the first 4 months of initiation of treatment (median, 2.8 months). One patient discontinued therapy due to severe infusion reactions and one due to multiple reactions of moderate severity; the majority of reactions were rated as mild (26; 86.7%).

In summary, infusion reactions in paediatric patients in FOS were generally mild and similar to those reported in adults.

Discussion

Fabry disease is a progressive disorder, with life-threatening complications by the time patients reach early adulthood. Early studies of ERT in Fabry disease focused on adult

males only. More recently, studies have clearly demonstrated that heterozygous women with Fabry disease should no longer be considered as asymptomatic carriers [11–16]. The burden of disease in children has also been documented [1, 17].

Clinical manifestations of Fabry disease are common in girls as well as boys, although they may be of later onset in girls. Healthcare workers therefore need to remain alert to signs and symptoms of Fabry disease in girls and boys. Given the non-specific nature of the clinical presentation of Fabry disease, the diagnosis in children should be suspected on the basis of a cluster of symptoms, including generalized pain, acroparaesthesiae, non-specific bowel disturbances, and hearing problems such as tinnitus and conductive or sensorineural hearing loss. When Fabry disease is a possible diagnosis, slit-lamp examination for cornea verticillata is useful, even in patients below 5 years of age, although its absence in early childhood does not exclude Fabry disease. In girls, it is essential to confirm the diagnosis by DNA analysis, as enzyme activity in heterozygous girls may be within the normal reference range. Family history, particularly concerning early deaths and renal, cardiac and neurological disease, is also important when Fabry disease is suspected.

Early treatment of Fabry disease, before irreversible organ damage occurs, is desirable. At the present time, however, there are no sensitive biomarkers to assess the efficacy of ERT when started before the onset of signs and symptoms. Until it is possible to show that the natural history of the disease is altered by starting therapy whilst the patient is asymptomatic, ERT will usually be indicated in children who are symptomatic. However, where there is a family history of severe disease, with very early onset of renal disease, cardiac disease or stroke, the clinician might consider treating asymptomatic children. As life-threatening complications of Fabry disease are very rare in children and not seen in individuals younger than 10 years of age, it is important that the indications for therapy in children are based on prevention of early complications of Fabry disease, such as pain crises, gastrointestinal and musculoskeletal problems and proteinuria, and on improving QoL.

The majority of boys in the FOS database were symptomatic at the start of ERT. However, the criteria for initiating ERT in females are less clear cut and, therefore, fewer girls within FOS are receiving treatment. The reasons for this inconsistency may be the cost implications in different countries and, more importantly, perhaps, the absence of specific guidelines for starting ERT in both males and females. In the UK, national guidelines have been developed for the management of all patients with Fabry disease (see Chapter 41). These will be reviewed annually but are an important milestone in the management of patients with Fabry disease.

In adult males who are not receiving ERT, the deterioration of renal function from early adulthood may reach 12 ml/min/year [18, 19]. Renal dysfunction is also common in females, although ESRD is infrequent. Beck *et al.* (2004) have shown that ERT with agalsidase alfa can stabilize or even improve renal function in patients in whom renal impairment is mild or moderate at baseline [10]. Significant improvements were not noted, however, in patients with ESRD. Early treatment therefore has the potential to reverse the underlying and otherwise inevitable renal failure in patients with Fabry disease.

Conclusions

The burden of Fabry disease in children is mainly due to neurological (e.g. pain crises) and gastrointestinal manifestations. Data from FOS are encouraging and indicate that ERT has beneficial effects on QoL, pain and gastrointestinal symptoms in children. Furthermore,

agalsidase alfa has a good safety profile and is well tolerated in children with Fabry disease.

It is very rare for children to present with life-threatening complications, such as cardiac failure, ESRD and stroke. Therefore, it is important to note that the outcome measures used in adults are not necessarily the most appropriate for assessing the efficacy of ERT in children.

References

1. Ries M, Ramaswami U, Parini R, Lindblad B, Whybra C, Willers I *et al*. The early clinical phenotype of Fabry disease: a study on 35 European children and adolescents. *Eur J Pediatr* 2003;162:767–72

2. Ries M, Gupta S, Moore DF, Sachdev V, Quirk JM, Murray GJ *et al*. Pediatric Fabry disease. *Pediatrics* 2005;115:e344–55

3. Ramaswami U, Whybra C, Parini R, Pintos-Morell G, Mehta A, Sunder-Plassmann G *et al*. Clinical manifestations of Fabry disease in children: data from the Fabry Outcome Survey. *Acta Paediatr* 2006;95:86–92

4. Hoffmann B, Garcia de Lorenzo A, Mehta A, Beck M, Widmer U, Ricci R. Effects of enzyme replacement therapy on pain and health related quality of life in patients with Fabry disease: data from FOS (Fabry Outcome Survey). *J Med Genet* 2005;42:247–52

5. Desnick RJ, Brady RO. Fabry disease in childhood. *J Pediatr* 2004;144:S20–6

6. Eng CM, Banikazemi M, Gordon RE, Goldman M, Phelps R, Kim L *et al*. A phase 1/2 clinical trial of enzyme replacement in Fabry disease: pharmacokinetic, substrate clearance, and safety studies. *Am J Hum Genet* 2001;68:711–22

7. Schiffmann R, Kopp JB, Austin HA 3rd, Sabnis S, Moore DF, Weibel T *et al*. Enzyme replacement therapy in Fabry disease: a randomized controlled trial. *JAMA* 2001;285:2743–9

8. Schiffmann R, Floeter MK, Dambrosia JM, Gupta S, Moore DF, Sharabi Y *et al*. Enzyme replacement therapy improves peripheral nerve and sweat function in Fabry disease. *Muscle Nerve* 2003; 28:703–10

9. Mehta A. Agalsidase alfa: specific treatment for Fabry disease. *Hosp Med* 2002;63:347–50

10. Beck M, Ricci R, Widmer U, Dehout F, de Lorenzo AG, Kampmann C *et al*. Fabry disease: overall effects of agalsidase alfa treatment. *Eur J Clin Invest* 2004; 34:838–44

11. Mehta A, Ricci R, Widmer U, Dehout F, Garcia de Lorenzo A, Kampmann C *et al*. Fabry disease defined: baseline clinical manifestations of 366 patients in the Fabry Outcome Survey. *Eur J Clin Invest* 2004;34:236–42

12. MacDermot KD, Holmes A, Miners AH. Natural history of Fabry disease in affected males and obligate carrier females. *J Inherit Metab Dis* 2001;24 (Suppl 2):13–4

13. MacDermot KD, Holmes A, Miners AH. Anderson–Fabry disease: clinical manifestations and impact of disease in a cohort of 60 obligate carrier females. *J Med Genet* 2001;38:769–75

14. Whybra C, Kampmann C, Willers I, Davies J, Winchester B, Kriegsmann J *et al*. Anderson–Fabry disease: clinical manifestations of disease in female heterozygotes. *J Inherit Metab Dis* 2001;24: 715–24

15. Kampmann C, Baehner F, Whybra C, Martin C, Wiethoff CM, Ries M *et al*. Cardiac manifestations of Anderson–Fabry disease in heterozygous females. *J Am Coll Cardiol* 2002;40:1668–74

16. Galanos J, Nicholls K, Grigg L, Kiers L, Crawford A, Becker G. Clinical features of Fabry's disease in Australian patients. *Intern Med J* 2002;32:575–84

17. Beck M, Whybra C, Wendrich K, Gal A, Ries M. Anderson–Fabry disease in children and adolescents. *Contrib Nephrol* 2001:251–5

18. Branton MH, Schiffmann R, Sabnis SG, Murray GJ, Quirk JM, Altarescu G *et al*. Natural history of Fabry renal disease: influence of α-galactosidase A activity and genetic mutations on clinical course. *Medicine (Baltimore)* 2002;81:122–38

19. Branton M, Schiffmann R, Kopp JB. Natural history and treatment of renal involvement in Fabry disease. *J Am Soc Nephrol* 2002;13 (Suppl 2):S139–43

32 Measurement of disease severity and progression in Fabry disease

Catharina Whybra, Frank Bähner and Karin Baron
Universitäts-Kinderklinik, Langenbeckstrasse 1, D-55101 Mainz, Germany

In the absence of a good biological marker, there is a need for a disease-specific scoring system to evaluate the severity and progression of Fabry disease and the response of the disease to treatment. This chapter describes the Mainz Severity Score Index (MSSI) and a recent derivative of this scoring system, the Fabry Outcome Survey Mainz Severity Score Index (FOS-MSSI), which has been adapted for use with the data collected in the FOS database. It has been shown that the FOS-MSSI is a useful tool for clinicians in evaluating the severity and progression of Fabry disease in adult patients.

Introduction

The availability of enzyme replacement therapy (ERT) for Fabry disease has led to the need for a convenient and sensitive means of monitoring disease progression and response to therapy. As no suitable biological marker has been discovered, a disease-specific scoring system is needed in order to describe the severity of disease (accurately representing the multisystemic nature of Fabry disease) and to allow monitoring of disease progression in individual patients. Ideally, this system should also be sensitive to changes induced by treatment.

Disease severity scores have already been successfully established for measuring the severity and clinical course of a number of diseases. One such example is the successful use of scoring systems in the field of haemato-oncology [1]. A scoring system has also already been developed for one of the lysosomal storage diseases, Gaucher disease. This system, the Zimran Severity Score Index, was initially developed in 1989 [2] and later modified in 1992 [3]. Until recently, however, there was no scoring system available for assessing the manifestations of Fabry disease.

Mainz Severity Score Index

The Mainz Severity Score Index (MSSI) was published in 2004 for use in patients with Fabry disease [4]. The development of this instrument was guided by the Zimran Severity Score Index and the general principles described by Rauchfuss [5]. The MSSI is composed of four sections that cover the general, neurological, cardiovascular and renal signs and symptoms of Fabry disease (Table 1). Each section includes a group of signs and symptoms that are associated with Fabry disease, and these are weighted according to their contribution to the morbidity of the disease.

The MSSI was developed using a relatively large patient group for such a rare orphan disorder, which affects an estimated 1 in 40 000 to 1 in 117 000 male live births [6, 7]. Thorough clinical evaluations were performed in 39 patients (24 males, 15 females) with Fabry disease both before and after 1 year of ERT with agalsidase alfa [4]. To assess the specificity of the MSSI, controls were also evaluated using the MSSI. The control group comprised 23 patients (9 males, 14 females) who presented with complaints similar to Fabry disease, but in whom the disease was subsequently excluded.

Table 1. The Mainz Severity Score Index (MSSI) and the Fabry Outcome Survey adaptation of the Mainz Severity Score Index (FOS-MSSI).

General score

Sign/symptom	Rating	MSSI score	FOS-MSSI score	Adaptation to signs and symptoms
Characteristic facial appearance	No	0	–	
	Yes	1	–	
Angiokeratoma	None	0	0	Any
	Some	1	1.5	
	Extensive	2	–	
Oedema	No	0	0	
	Yes	1	1	
Musculoskeletal	No	0	0	
	Yes	1	1	
Cornea verticillata	No	0	0	
	Yes	1	1	
Diaphoresis	Normal	0	0	
	Hypo/hyper	1	1	
	Anhidrosis	2	2	
Abdominal pain	No	0	0	
	Yes	2	2	
Diarrhoea/constipation	No	0	0	
	Yes	1	1	
Haemorrhoids	No	0	0	
	Yes	1	1	
Pulmonary	No	0	0	Breathing difficulties
	Yes	2	2	
New York Heart Association (NYHA) classification*	No	0	0	Angina
	Class I	1	–	
	Class II	2	2	
	Class III	3	–	
	Class IV	4	–	
Maximum score		**18**	**13.5**	

Neurological score

Sign/symptom	Rating	MSSI score	FOS-MSSI score	Adaptation to signs and symptoms
Tinnitus	No	0	0	Any
	Mild	1	1	
	Severe	2	–	
Vertigo	No	0	0	Any
	Mild	1	1	
	Severe	2	–	
Acroparaesthesia	No	0	0	Pain attacks
	Occasional	3	4	
	Chronic	6	6	Chronic pain
Fever pain crisis	No	0	–	
	Yes	2	–	
Cerebrovascular	No	0	0	
	Ischaemic lesions (in MRI/CT)	1	3	
	TIA/migraine etc.	3	6	TIA, PRIND
	Stroke	5	–	
Psychiatric/psychosocial				
Depression	No	0	0	
	Yes	1	1	
Fatigue	No	0	–	
	Yes	1	–	
Reduced activity level	No	0	–	
	Yes	1	–	
Maximum score		**20**	**15**	

continued

Table 1. The Mainz Severity Score Index (MSSI) and the Fabry Outcome Survey adaptation of the Mainz Severity Score Index (FOS-MSSI) (continued).

Cardiovascular score

Sign/symptom	Rating	MSSI score	FOS-MSSI score	Adaptation to signs and symptoms
Changes in cardiac muscle thickness	No	0	0	
	Thickening of wall/septum	1	–	
	LVH seen on ECG	6	6	
	Cardiomyopathy (< 15 mm)	8	10	Heart failure
	Severe cardiomyopathy (> 15 mm)	12	–	
Valve insufficiency	No	0	0	
	Yes	1	1	Valve disease
ECG abnormalities	No	0	0	
	Yes	2	2	Conduction abnormalities and arrhythmia
Pacemaker	No	0	0	
	Yes	4	4	Surgery
Hypertension	No	0	0	
	Yes	1	1	
Maximum score		**20**	**18**	

Renal score

Sign/symptom	Rating	MSSI score	FOS-MSSI score	Adaptation to signs and symptoms
Evidence of renal dysfunction	No proteinuria	0	0	
	Proteinuria	4	4	Haematuria/proteinuria
	Tubular dysfunction/low GFR or creatinine clearance	8	8	Renal failure
	End-stage renal failure (serum creatinine levels > 3.5 mg/dl)	12	–	
	Dialysis	18	18	Dialysis/transplantation
Maximum score		**18**	**18**	

*Limitation on physical activity according to NYHA classification is as follows. Class I: none; ordinary physical activity does not cause undue fatigue, palpitation, dyspnoea or anginal pain, but echocardiography reveals heart involvement. Class II: slight; comfortable at rest, but ordinary physical activity results in fatigue, etc. Class III: marked; comfortable at rest, but less than ordinary physical activity causes fatigue, etc. Class IV: unable to carry out any physical activity without discomfort; symptoms of cardiac insufficiency or of anginal syndrome may be present even at rest and physical activity increases discomfort.

CT, computed tomography; ECG, electrocardiography; GFR, glomerular filtration rate; LVH, left ventricular hypertrophy; MRI, magnetic resonance imaging; PRIND, prolonged reversible ischaemic neurological deficit; TIA, transient ischaemic attack.

Results showed that the MSSI of patients with Fabry disease was significantly higher than that of control patients with other severe debilitating diseases. The MSSI obtained for patients with Fabry disease indicated that, although more men than women had symptoms classified as severe (MSSI > 40), overall median total severity scores were not significantly different between male and female patients. After 1 year of ERT with agalsidase alfa, there was a significant ($p < 0.001$) reduction in the MSSI of patients with Fabry disease (by a median of 9 points). This study indicated that the MSSI may be a useful disease-specific measure for objectively assessing the severity of Fabry disease and for monitoring changes associated with ERT.

Development of a scoring system for use in FOS – the Fabry Outcome Survey

FOS is the world's most comprehensive database of patients with Fabry disease, which, at the time of the present analysis, contained data on 330 males and 358 females, including 69 girls and 50 boys younger than 18 years of age at entry into FOS. There is a need to evaluate disease severity, progression and response to treatment in this population. Therefore, a modified version of the MSSI, the FOS Mainz Severity Score Index (FOS-MSSI), has been developed for use with data collected in the FOS database (Table 1). This system is very similar to the original MSSI, but signs and symptoms are weighted in accordance with the data collected in FOS. As with the MSSI, there are sections relating to general, neurological, cardiovascular and renal disease manifestations. To assess the severity of disease, the total score obtained may be categorized as mild (≤ 18), moderate (19–38) or severe (> 38). As the FOS-MSSI is based only on dichotomous variables in the FOS signs and symptoms checklist, unlike the MSSI, it can only be used to give a description of the accumulated disease burden. At present, the FOS-MSSI has been assessed only using

data collected from patients with Fabry disease prior to ERT.

Patients from FOS

In total, 655 patients with Fabry disease for whom there were reports on clinical signs and symptoms were included in this study. This included 273 men (median age, 38 years; range, 18–81 years), 277 proven heterozygous women (median age, 44 years; range, 18–76 years), 45 boys (median age, 11 years; range, 1–17 years) and 60 girls (median age, 13 years; range, 3–18 years).

Changes in the FOS-MSSI score with age

There was a significant positive correlation between the overall accumulated FOS-MSSI score and age at the latest clinic visit in patients with Fabry disease of both genders (both $p < 0.001$) (Figure 1). Each subscore of the FOS-MSSI was also significantly correlated with age in male and female patients (all $p < 0.001$) (Figures 2 and 3). A recent study by Schaefer *et al.* [8] also found a significant relationship between age and overall FOS-MSSI score in male patients with missense mutations and in those carrying non-missense mutations. These data suggest that there could be a correlation between genotype and clinical severity.

In the subgroup of patients younger than 18 years of age at the latest visit, in both sexes there were significant correlations between the overall FOS-MSSI and age at that visit (girls, $p = 0.042$; boys, $p = 0.012$) (Figure 4). Significant correlations were observed between the neurological subscore and age for girls ($p = 0.004$) and boys ($p = 0.011$), but there were no significant correlations between the general, cardiac or renal subscores and age.

Disease severity

Comparing the severity classification of hemizygotes and heterozygotes using the FOS-MSSI (Figure 5), it was found that more

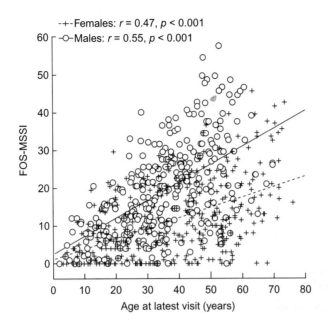

Figure 1. *Correlation between age at the latest clinic visit and disease severity as assessed by the Fabry Outcome Survey adaptation of the Mainz Severity Score Index (FOS-MSSI) in patients with Fabry disease (318 males, 337 females).*

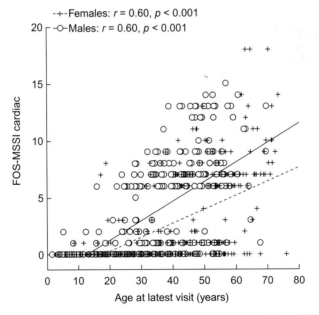

Figure 2. *Correlation between age at the latest clinic visit and the severity of cardiovascular manifestations of Fabry disease as assessed by the Fabry Outcome Survey adaptation of the Mainz Severity Score Index (FOS-MSSI) (318 males, 337 females).*

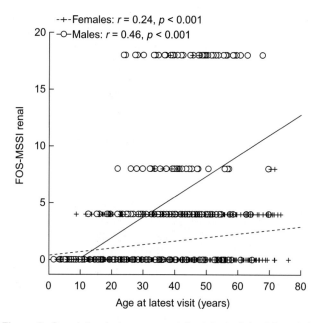

Figure 3. *Correlation between age at the latest clinic visit and the severity of renal manifestations of Fabry disease as assessed by the Fabry Outcome Survey adaptation of the Mainz Severity Score Index (FOS-MSSI) (318 males, 337 females).*

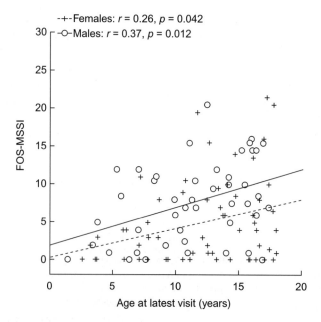

Figure 4. *Correlation between age at latest visit and disease severity as assessed by the Fabry Outcome Survey adaptation of the Mainz Severity Score Index (FOS-MSSI) in children (45 boys, 60 girls; aged < 18 years) with Fabry disease.*

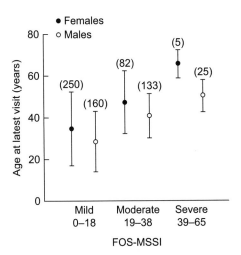

Figure 5. *Mean age (± SD) of male and female patients with Fabry disease according to the severity classification (mild, moderate or severe) on the Fabry Outcome Survey adaptation of the Mainz Severity Score Index (FOS-MSSI). Numbers of patients are shown in parentheses.*

males were classified as severely affected than females. The mean age of females in each classification group (mild, moderate and severe) was 6 or more years greater than for males with disease of the same severity. The average FOS-MSSI varies according to age and gender (Figure 1); the disease severity has a more rapid progression in males than in females, but the pattern is the same for females, with a delay of 10–20 years.

Discussion

The MSSI is a clinical scoring system, which was developed to assess the severity of signs and symptoms of Fabry disease and to monitor the progress of individual patients during ERT. Recently, an adaptation of this scoring system for use in FOS, the FOS-MSSI, has been used successfully to assess the severity of multisystemic disease in adults with Fabry disease.

Analyses have revealed a positive correlation between the FOS-MSSI and age in adults, indicating that, like the MSSI, this score reflects the progressive nature of Fabry disease with increasing disease severity over time. This is particularly true for those subscores that are most important for the morbidity of the disease, namely the cardiac and renal components. To improve sensitivity, the general, neurological and renal scores of the FOS-MSSI may need to be adjusted to better reflect the data available in FOS. Further modification of the FOS-MSSI is also necessary to make it more suitable for use in children.

Data from the FOS-MSSI demonstrate that women are usually at least 6 years older than men who have disease of the same severity. This compares with the approximate 10-year difference between development of comparable signs and symptoms in males and females in a similar cohort reported previously [9]. As already shown in a smaller population with the original MSSI [4], the overall FOS-MSSI was similar in male and female patients, highlighting the need for clinical evaluation and treatment of heterozygotes.

Conclusions

It has been shown that the FOS-MSSI is a useful and valid tool that can be used to evaluate disease severity and progression in adult patients with Fabry disease; however, there is room for further refinement of this index. In the absence of a good biochemical marker for monitoring clinical response to ERT, the FOS-MSSI may be used to monitor the progress of individual patients, although it probably does not always reflect the true morbidity of Fabry disease. It is conceivable that the combination of a biochemical marker and a clinical severity score may have better prognostic value for this multisystemic disease in the future.

References

1. Hughes D. The use of scoring systems in patients with haematological malignancy. *Acta Paediatrica Suppl* 2006;451:47–51

2. Zimran A, Sorge J, Gross E, Kubitz M, West C, Beutler E. Prediction of severity of Gaucher's disease by

identification of mutations at DNA level. *Lancet* 1989;ii:349–52

3. Zimran A, Kay A, Gelbart T, Garver P, Thurston D, Saven A *et al.* Gaucher disease. Clinical, laboratory, radiologic, and genetic features of 53 patients. *Medicine (Baltimore)* 1992;71:337–53

4. Whybra C, Kampmann C, Krummenauer F, Ries M, Mengel E, Miebach E *et al.* The Mainz Severity Score Index: a new instrument for quantifying the Anderson–Fabry disease phenotype, and the response of patients to enzyme replacement therapy. *Clin Genet* 2004;65:299–307

5. Rauchfuss HU. Die bildung von scores zur prognose von komplikationen. Ulm: Universität Ulm; 1984

6. Desnick RJ, Ioannou YA, Eng CM. α-Galactosidase A deficiency: Fabry disease. In: Scriver CR, Beaudet AL, Sly WS, Valle D, editors. The metabolic and molecular bases of inherited disease. 8th edn. New York: McGraw-Hill; 2001. p. 3733–74

7. Meikle PJ, Hopwood JJ, Clague AE, Carey WF. Prevalence of lysosomal storage disorders. *JAMA* 1999;281:249–54

8. Schaefer E, Mehta A, Gal A. Genotype and phenotype in Fabry disease: analysis of the Fabry Outcome Survey. *Acta Paediatrica Suppl* 2005; 447:87–92

9. MacDermot KD, Holmes A, Miners AH. Natural history of Fabry disease in affected males and obligate carrier females. *J Inherit Metab Dis* 2001;24 (Suppl 2):13–14

33 The genetic basis of Fabry disease

Andreas Gal, Ellen Schäfer and Imke Rohard

Institut für Humangenetik, Universitätsklinikum Hamburg-Eppendorf, Butenfeld 42,
22529 Hamburg, Germany

The coding region of the α-galactosidase A gene (GLA) consists of 1290 base pairs, is divided into seven exons and defines a polypeptide of 429 amino acids. The great majority of disease-related GLA mutations are unique ('private'). We have compiled a list of 429 mutations of the GLA gene from the published literature, including 306 point mutations (missense, nonsense and those affecting splice sites), 115 'short-length' rearrangements (affecting fewer than 60 nucleotides) and eight gross rearrangements (affecting one or more exons). Based on the number of different changes at any nucleotide position, there is no obvious 'hot spot' for point mutations, although mutations of CpG dinucleotides account for the majority of recurrent point mutations seen in unrelated families with Fabry disease. Remarkably, about one-third of the short-length rearrangements occur in exon 7, which accounts for only 22% of the coding region, suggesting that this part of the gene is susceptible to rearrangement. The recent elaboration of a putative three-dimensional structure of α-galactosidase A by X-ray crystallography may provide a better insight into how the enzyme works at the molecular level. This knowledge has recently been used for computer modelling of the structure of α-galactosidase A mutants and may result in improved understanding of the molecular pathology of the mutated protein. It is hoped that an increased understanding of structure/function correlates will help to develop alternative therapies or adjuvant treatments for Fabry disease.

Introduction

This chapter gives a short overview of the α-galactosidase A gene (*GLA*), which is mutated in Fabry disease, and the mutations found in the gene in health and disease. The term mutation refers to a permanent alteration of the genetic material. In daily practice, however, the word mutation is frequently (but incorrectly) associated only with a disease-causing effect. Due to this negative connotation, the neutral terms sequence variant, sequence alteration or allelic variant are used frequently in current literature.

Classification and nomenclature of mutations

From the point of view of pathology, only mutations that affect the phenotype (in a broad sense) are of relevance. These mutations can be divided into those that cause disease and those that are non-pathogenic. Clearly, non-pathogenic mutations may either be expressed phenotypically or be silent. From the point of view of genetics, mutations can be: familial – that is, transmitted from generation to generation within a family; or *de novo*, with a change first being detected in the index case. In terms of the change in the genetic material, we usually distinguish between novel mutations that have not been previously reported, and those that have already been documented in the literature. The fact that the same mutation has been found in two different patients may indicate either that the two individuals are (distantly) related or that we are dealing with recurrent mutations due to *de novo* events – that is, the same mutation has occurred independently on two occasions.

The prospect of computer-based mutation databases requires a uniform and unequivocal assignment of sequence variants. Following the initiative of a small group of human geneticists, recommendations have been put forward during the past decade to establish a standard nomenclature for describing mutations. Today, the majority of those working in the field largely agree on the 'Nomenclature for the description of sequence variations' that is posted on the HGV (Human Genome Variation) Society web page (http://www.genomic.unimelb.edu.au/mdi/). In view of the fact that mutation nomenclature is a specialized domain of human genetics that most readers of this book may not be familiar with, we have compiled a brief description of the currently used nomenclature.

In general, the abbreviated names (acronyms) of human genes are written in italic capital letters. This way, one can distinguish between the gene and its product, which is written in a regular font. For DNA, the capital letters A, C, G and T are used, corresponding to the nucleotides adenine, cytosine, guanine and thymine, respectively, whereas the three-letter amino acid code is preferred when describing a change at the protein level. The convention is that designation of nucleotide (DNA) changes begins with a number, and designation of protein changes with a letter. Thus, 100C>T (cytosine is replaced by thymine at position 100) is a nucleotide change, whereas C100T (more correctly Cys100Thr) is a missense mutation (cysteine

is replaced by threonine). The recommended designation helps to avoid confusion about whether A, C, G or T represent nucleotides or amino acids, which may occur if a shorthand (one-letter amino acid code) abbreviation is used. The description of any sequence change is always preceded by a letter indicating the type of sequence referred to:

- 'g' for genomic DNA
- 'c' for cDNA (complementary DNA)
- 'p' for protein.

Positions of amino acids and nucleotides (cDNA) are numbered starting, respectively, with the initiation methionine and the nucleotide A of the ATG-translation initiation triplet as number 1. For numbering nucleotides in introns (the intervening sequences between exons), the last nucleotide of the preceding exon (exons are the coding portions of the gene) and a plus sign are used at the beginning of the intron, such as 639+1G>A. Likewise, the designation consisting of the first nucleotide of the following exon and a minus sign correspond to the end of the intron, for example 640–1G>T. In this chapter, DNA mutations are described according to the *GLA* cDNA sequence GenBank U78027.1 or to the genomic sequence GenBank X14448.1 (http://www.ncbi.nlm.nih.gov/Genbank/).

Polymorphisms and rare sequence variants of the *GLA* gene

The term polymorphism refers to the existence of more than one normal allele at a gene locus, with a frequency of the minor (rare) allele greater than 1% in the normal population. If the frequency of the minor allele is less than 1%, it is referred to as a rare variant. Table 1 shows a list of common *GLA* gene polymorphisms and the frequencies of the minor (rare) alleles. The differences seen between unaffected controls and patients/carriers for Fabry disease, as determined in our laboratory, are probably due to the small sample sizes. Remarkably, the only coding variant (c.937G>T, p.Asp313Tyr) was detected about

Table 1. *DNA polymorphisms of the α-galactosidase A (GLA) gene. The top two rows show the number of individuals with the second allele, with percentages in parentheses, in the cohort of unaffected controls and patients with Fabry disease in the authors' laboratory. The bottom two rows show the haplotypes composed of five GLA DNA polymorphisms for two male patients with Fabry disease and the p.Trp340X mutation.*

| | Number (males/females) | 5'-UTR (c.–) | | | Intron 4 (c.640)* | Exon 6 | Intron 6 |
		30G>A	12G>A	10C>T	–16A>G	c.937G>T (p.Asp313Tyr)	c.1000–22C>T
Controls	86 (19/67)	1 (0.6)	5 (3.3)	8 (5.2)	12 (7.8)	8 (5.2)	20 (13.1)
Patients	55 (36/19)	2 (2.7)	5 (6.7)	3 (4.0)	12 (16.2)	3 (4.0)	11 (14.9)
p.Trp340X	Male (F50)	G	G	C	A	ND	C
p.Trp340X	Male (F94)	G	G	C	G	ND	T

5'UTR, 5'-untranslated region; ND, not determined.
*Three polymorphisms in intron 4 (c.639+68A>G, c.640–201del6 and c.640–146T>C) have not been typed in this analysis.

ten times more frequently (approximately 5%) in our cohort than the frequency of 0.45% reported originally [1].

The *GLA* gene and its mutations in Fabry disease

The *GLA* gene was mapped to the region q22.1 of the X chromosome. The coding part of the gene consists of 1290 base pairs (bp), is divided into seven exons, ranging in size from 92 to 291 bp, and defines a polypeptide of 429 amino acids. As expected for an X-chromosomal trait with reduced reproductive fitness of patients and increased frequency of spontaneous (*de novo*) mutations, most of the patients/families have different mutations; that is, the great majority of *GLA* mutations are unique ('private'). There are only a few reports of male patients carrying two different, and most likely disease-causing, *GLA* mutations on the same allele, such as p.Glu66Gln and p.Arg112Cys, or p.Leu89Arg and a 1 bp deletion in codon 303 [2, 3]. In contrast, about 5% of the patients carry a pathogenic *GLA* mutation and the non-disease-associated variant p.Asp313Tyr.

We have compiled a list of 429 *GLA* mutations published in the literature by ourselves and others (as of 31 December

2005). Figures 1 and 2 show the distribution of mutations over the seven coding exons, grouped according to the nature of the mutation; that is, point mutations (missense, $n = 240$, 55.9%; nonsense, $n = 48$, 11.2%; and those affecting splice sites, $n = 18$, 4.2%) and 'short-length' rearrangements (affecting fewer than 60 nucleotides, $n = 115$, 26.8%), whereas Table 2 lists the large rearrangements ($n = 8$; 1.9%) described to date.

The relative frequencies of different classes of mutations identified in patients registered in FOS – the Fabry Outcome Survey [4] – agree very well with the above data collected from the literature.

Based on the number of different changes at any nucleotide position, there is no obvious mutation 'hot spot', when considering all 288 point mutations (missense and nonsense) scattered over the 1290 bp coding region. However, there are some differences in the gross distribution of the different mutations. The data show a clustering of point mutations in exon 5, in which a total of 51 point mutations have been reported to date. Given the size of exon 5 (162 bp, comprising 12.6% of the coding

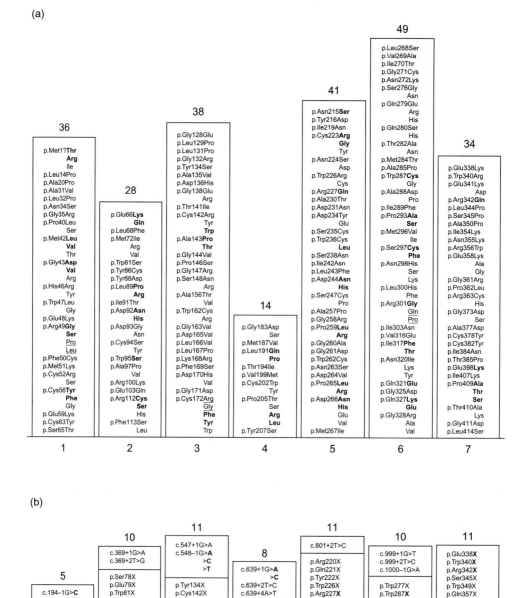

Figure 1. *(a) Missense point mutations of the GLA gene and (b) point mutations of the GLA gene that affect splice sites (top) or result in immediate termination of protein translation (nonsense mutation, bottom). Mutations are grouped according to their position in the seven exons and flanking intronic sequences. Numbers on top of the columns give the total number of mutations listed. Mutated variants are written in bold or underlined if they result from a change of the same nucleotide in the codon. If more than one mutated allele is known, the wild type is given only in the first line.*

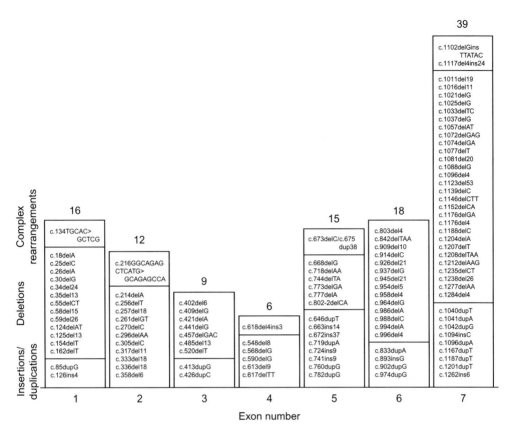

Figure 2. *Rearrangements affecting fewer than 60 base pairs of the GLA gene grouped according to their position in the seven exons and flanking intronic sequences, including complex rearrangements, deletions and insertions/duplications. Numbers on top of the columns give the total number of mutations listed.*

sequence) and the observation that it harbours 17.7% of all point mutations in the coding region shown in Figure 1, one can conclude that, of the seven *GLA* exons, exon 5 has the highest relative frequency of point mutations (3.15/10 bp), followed by exon 6 (198 bp and 56 point mutations; 2.83/10 bp) and exon 3 (178 bp and 45 point mutations; 2.53/10 bp). In total, exons 3, 5 and 6, which comprise 41.7% of the coding sequence, harbour 152 of the 288 point mutations (52.8%). CpG dinucleotides are known to be prone to point mutations due to methylation-induced deamination of 5-methyl cytosine. Of the 14 CpGs in the *GLA* coding sequence, point mutations have been described in ten (no point mutations of the CpG dinucleotides have yet been found in codons 39, 118,

Table 2. *Larger rearrangements of the α-galactosidase A gene affecting one or several exons. Mutations that are indented in the left-hand column have been characterized at the nucleotide level.*

Rearrangement	Location
Deletions	
402 bp	Exon 3
> 1.5 kb	Exons 5–7
1710 bp	Exons 5–7
3.2 kb	Exons 3–4
4519 bp	Exons 3–7
4651 bp	Exons 1–2
Duplications	
3.4 kb	Exon 2*
8112 bp	Intron 1–Exon 6

*E Schäfer and A Gal, unpublished data.

315/316 and 367/368). CpG-associated mutations account for the majority of recurrent
point mutations seen in families with Fabry
disease (Table 3).

About one-third (39 out of 115) of the small
rearrangements occur in exon 7, which
accounts for about 22% of the coding region.
This clustering of mutations suggests that this
part of the gene is susceptible to rearrangements. It has recently been recommended
that the term 'dup' (duplication) is used when
the mutation creates a run of two or more
bases. Compared with the earlier designation
'ins' or 'insertion' for this type of sequence
extension, 'dup' seems to be simpler, and
prevents confusion regarding the exact position introduced. For rearrangements in general, the most 3' (toward the end of the gene)
position possible should be arbitrarily assigned to have been changed. In Figure 2, we
have followed these most recent recommendations of the Nomenclature Committee
of the HGV Society.

Analysis of different mutation entries in
databases and in the literature shows that a
standard nomenclature is essential to compare data obtained in various laboratories;
for example, to determine whether a given
mutation has already been reported by
others. Figure 3 presents a typical example.
A 3 bp deletion (GAG) at position c.1072 has
been reported by Blanch *et al.* [5], whereas
Shabbeer *et al.* [6] reported a 3 bp deletion
(AGG) at position c.1070. As shown in
Figure 3, the two mutations seem to be
(structurally) identical.

If two mutations can be described by the
same formula, we might assume that we are
dealing with the same molecular change in
both cases. However, this is not necessarily
true, as it has been well documented that the
same mutation might occur several times
independently (recurrent mutation). Dis-
regarding this latter possibility may lead to
an underestimation of the natural variability

Table 3. *Recurrent point mutations in the
α-galactosidase A gene published in the literature.*

Very likely*	Putative†
p.Arg112His	p.Met296Ile
p.Arg112Cys	p.Trp204X
p.Ala143Pro	
p.Gln157X	
p.Asn215Ser	
p.Arg227Gln	
p.Arg227X	
p.Trp340X	
p.Arg342Gln	
p.Arg342X	
c.639 (IVS4)+919G>A	

*Independent occurrence of mutations was proven
(e.g. by family analysis and/or haplotyping).
†Detected in two or more apparently unrelated patients,
but no experimental proof was presented that the
mutations were independent.
Mutations due to changes in CpG dinucleotides are
underlined.

of the mutation spectrum and obscure the
fact that certain parts of the *GLA* gene are
prone to mutations. An independent origin of
recurrent mutations can be assumed if family
analysis suggests that the mutation occurred
de novo. In the cohort of patients in FOS, we
found two male cases with the p.Gln157X
mutation, both from Germany, in which the
patients' mothers did not carry the mutation;
that is, it appeared to arise *de novo*. Furthermore, a recurrent event can be assumed if
two patients with Fabry disease carry the
same *GLA* mutation on a different genetic
background. To examine this question, an
individual pattern of polymorphisms, which
consists of a number of different genetic
variants and is referred to as the haplotype,
is defined for each of the patients under
study. Table 1 shows the haplotypes of two
German male patients, both carrying the
c.1019G>A (p.Trp340X) mutation, for a total
of five *GLA* DNA polymorphisms. In view of
the fact that the two patients carry different
alleles for the intron 4 and intron 6 SNPs

```
                                        1070              1080
        GLA cDNA                CGGCAGGAGATTGGT

        c.1072delGAG            CGGCAG      ATTGGT

        c.1070delAGG            CGGC      AGATTGGT
```

Figure 3. *A 3 base pair deletion of the GLA gene has been described in two different ways by two groups of investigators. The top line shows the wild-type cDNA sequence and nucleotide positions, the middle line shows the assignment proposed by Blanche et al. [5] and the bottom line shows the designation given by Shabbeer et al. [6].*

(single nucleotide polymorphisms), it is likely that the two probands are unrelated and that this particular mutation has occurred independently on two occasions.

The frequency of *de novo* mutations in Fabry disease is unknown. Based on theoretical considerations, we have speculated that it might be approximately 3–10% of all cases [7]. Nine cases of molecularly proven *de novo* (novel) point mutations have been reported to date by ourselves and other investigators (Table 4) and an individual carrying a (recurrent) *de novo* p.Gln157X mutation has recently been detected in our laboratory (E Schäfer and A Gal, unpublished observation). The total number of different *GLA* point mutations compiled in this review is 306. Conservatively, we can assume that all but the ten *de novo* mutations were familial. In this case, the available data suggest that the minimum proportion of new mutations in the cohort studied here is 3.3% (10/306), which is similar to the figure (mentioned above) that has been derived from theoretical considerations.

The gene product

Recently, Garman and Garboczi [8] published the structure of human α-galactosidase A, determined by X-ray crystallography. α-Galactosidase A is a homodimeric glycoprotein. Each monomer contains five disulphide bonds (Cys52–Cys94, Cys56–Cys63, Cys142–Cys172, Cys202–Cys223 and Cys378–Cys382) and four possible *N*-glycosylation sites (Asn139, Asn192, Asn215 and Asn408).

Information on the putative three-dimensional structure of α-galactosidase A provides a better insight into how the enzyme works at the molecular level as well as a greater understanding of the molecular pathology of the mutated protein. This is especially the case for missense mutations, which represent the smallest possible structural change of the polypeptide – the replacement of one amino acid by another one. Based on their model, Garman and Garboczi [8] classified *GLA* missense mutations into three groups. First, mutations that perturb the active site of the enzyme by changing residues that either form the active centre itself or are essential for its correct three-dimensional structure; secondly, buried mutations that affect residues distant from the active site, although they adversely affect the folding and stability of the protein; thirdly, 'other' mutations that do not fall into either of the above categories,

Table 4. *De novo point mutations of the α-galactosidase A gene published in the literature.*

p.Leu32Pro
p.Met42Val
p.Cys56Tyr
p.Gln157X*
p.Ile219Asn
p.Asp231Asn
p.Trp287Gly
p.Gln330X
p.Cys382Tyr

*Identified in two (unrelated) patients (E Schäfer and A Gal, unpublished observation).

although their negative effect on the catabolic function of the molecule is evident, for example by disruption of an important disulphide bond or elimination of an *N*-carbohydrate attachment site.

By computer modelling of the structure of α-galactosidase A mutants, Matsuzawa and colleagues [9] have provided data suggesting that a number of *GLA* missense mutations associated with the classic disease phenotype should result in significant structural changes in functionally important regions of the polypeptide and thus in a dysfunctional and unstable enzyme. In contrast, other mutations located distant from the active site should result in small structural changes. Some of these latter enzyme variants, for example p.Met72Val, p.Gln279Glu and p.Met296Ile, which are known to be associated with a mild disease phenotype, had normal K_m and V_{max} values and showed residual catalytic activity. However, the mutant enzymes were posttranslationally inactivated and rapidly degraded. It has been shown that galactose may enhance the stability of the above-mentioned three 'mild' mutants expressed in lymphoblasts.

It is hoped that, eventually, knowledge of structure/function correlates for certain mutations may help to develop new therapies for Fabry disease, such as the use of chaperone molecules (see Chapter 43).

References

In recent years, several excellent reviews have been published on the *GLA* gene, its mutations and various aspects of Fabry disease. In order to avoid redundancy, the number of references has been kept to a minimum in this chapter. References to individual mutations are available on request from the authors.

1. Yasuda M, Shabbeer J, Benson SD, Maire I, Burnett RM, Desnick RJ. Fabry disease: characterization of α-galactosidase A double mutations and the D313Y plasma enzyme pseudodeficiency allele. *Hum Mutat* 2003;22:486–92

2. Ishii S, Sakuraba H, Suzuki Y. Point mutations in the upstream region of the α-galactosidase A gene exon 6 in an atypical variant of Fabry disease. *Hum Genet* 1992;89:29–32

3. Altarescu GM, Goldfarb LG, Park KY, Kaneski C, Jeffries N, Litvak S *et al*. Identification of fifteen novel mutations and genotype–phenotype relationship in Fabry disease. *Clin Genet* 2001;60:46–51

4. Schaefer E, Mehta A, Gal A. Genotype and phenotype in Fabry disease: analysis of the Fabry Outcome Survey. *Acta Paediatr Suppl* 2005;94:87–92; discussion 79

5. Blanch LC, Meaney C, Morris CP. A sensitive mutation screening strategy for Fabry disease: detection of nine mutations in the α-galactosidase A gene. *Hum Mutat* 1996;8:38–43

6. Shabbeer J, Yasuda M, Luca E, Desnick RJ. Fabry disease: 45 novel mutations in the α-galactosidase A gene causing the classical phenotype. *Mol Genet Metab* 2002;76:23–30

7. Schaefer E, Baron K, Widmer U, Deegan P, Neumann HP, Sunder-Plassmann G *et al*. Thirty-four novel mutations of the GLA gene in 121 patients with Fabry disease. *Hum Mutat* 2005;25:412

8. Garman SC, Garboczi DN. The molecular defect leading to Fabry disease: structure of human α-galactosidase. *J Mol Biol* 2004;337:319–35

9. Matsuzawa F, Aikawa SI, Doi H, Okumiya T, Sakuraba H. Fabry disease: correlation between structural changes in α-galactosidase, and clinical and biochemical phenotypes. *Hum Genet* 2005; 117:317–28

34 Genotype–phenotype correlation in Fabry disease

Markus Ries[1] and Andreas Gal[2]

[1]Developmental and Metabolic Neurology Branch, National Institute of Neurological Disorders and Stroke, National Institutes of Health, Bethesda, Maryland 20892-1260, USA; [2]Institut für Humangenetik, Universitätsklinikum Hamburg-Eppendorf, Butenfeld 42, 22529 Hamburg, Germany

A disease phenotype may be modulated by genetic and non-genetic modifiers. The correlation between genotype and phenotype is a statistical relationship that predicts a physical trait in a person or abnormality in a patient with a given mutation or a group of similar mutations. Analysis of genotype–phenotype correlations in Fabry disease is complicated by a number of factors, such as the high proportion of private mutations, the large phenotypic heterogeneity associated with the same mutation – both among patients from the same family and among those from unrelated families – and the fact that patients with Fabry disease may develop disease-related complications that are observed with high prevalence in the general population. Genotype-related information about the enzyme structure derived from crystallographic analysis, together with measurement of residual enzyme activity, can be of assistance in predicting the likelihood of a severe or attenuated phenotype. Individual genotypes may have pharmacogenomic implications; for example, the maximum possible clinical response to molecular chaperone therapy might be predicted from the correlation between the amount of residual enzyme activity and the associated clinical phenotype. Female heterozygotes exhibit significant phenotypic variability, which could be better understood given more comprehensive epidemiological data.

Introduction

The correlation between genotype (from the Greek *genos*, meaning race, offspring) and phenotype (from the Greek *phaino-*, from *phainein*, meaning to show) is defined as an above-chance probability of a distinct mutation being associated with a particular physical feature or abnormality. The genotype and phenotype share a statistical relationship. The more frequently a specific phenotype is observed in association with a certain genotype, the higher the likelihood that an unrelated person with the same genotype will show the traits or abnormalities observed in the population carrying the same allele(s). This relationship could be expressed as the positive predictive value (PPV) of a given genotype for a particular phenotype, as follows:

$$PPV = \frac{\text{Number of patients with mutation } M \text{ revealing trait } T}{\text{Number of patients with mutation } M \text{ revealing trait } T + \text{Number of patients with mutation } M \text{ not revealing trait } T}$$

Gaucher disease (OMIM 230800 type I; OMIM 231000 type III) provides a classic example of an established genotype–phenotype correlation in a lysosomal storage disorder. In this condition, homozygosity for the p.Leu483Pro

has been therapeutically elevated to 10%. Provided that the *in-vitro* results translate into clinical benefit, which must be confirmed in clinical trials, this kind of therapy may be useful for subsets of patients with Fabry disease associated with specific genotypes.

Female heterozygotes

In X-linked diseases, heterozygous females are commonly referred to as carriers. This term describes the genetic state of heterozygosity and, consequently, the likelihood of transmitting the given X-linked condition. However, the word 'carrier', by definition, does not provide any information on the female's disease phenotype in X-linked disorders. By reviewing published cases, Dobyns *et al.* estimated that, in Fabry disease, the penetrance in female heterozygotes is 70% (meaning that 70 out of 100 females have clinical manifestations). In the same study, the clinical severity of the disease in females was estimated as being, on average 4, on a scale from 0 (free from signs or symptoms) to 100 (full disease expression) [11]. However, it is difficult to define penetrance and expressivity reliably in females who are heterozygous for Fabry disease, because, at the time of writing, epidemiological data are incomplete.

Some authors have raised the question of whether Fabry disease is an X-chromosomal dominant or recessive condition. According to the principles summarized by Rimoin and colleagues, an X-chromosomal condition is dominant if the phenotype is similar in both genders and there is an excess of affected females compared with males. By contrast, in a recessive trait, males are affected almost exclusively [12]. In disease registries, females and males are represented at a ratio of approximately 1:1, whereas, statistically, there should be twice as many female heterozygotes as male hemizygotes. Investigators proposing that the condition is dominant will claim that females with Fabry disease are under-diagnosed, whereas those suggesting that the condition is recessive will contend that

cases of symptomatic females are over-reported. It is possible that the assessment of female heterozygotes with a mild phenotype is subject to ascertainment bias; that is, the signs and symptoms are not recognized as manifestations of Fabry disease and are consequently not referred to tertiary centres. Both groups agree that, in general, the onset of disease is later and the signs and symptoms tend to be milder in females than in males. Nevertheless, there is increasing evidence documenting high penetrance of Fabry disease in female carriers, with variable phenotypic expression, ranging from no clinical manifestations to the classic disease phenotype, including stroke and renal failure, as seen in hemizygous males [13–19].

In order to reflect the prevalence of symptomatic X-linked conditions in females more appropriately, Dobyns *et al.* proposed using only the term 'X-linked' trait, because the definitions 'X-linked recessive' or 'X-linked dominant' do not capture the wide spectrum of penetrance and expressivity [11]. The phenotype in heterozygotes may depend on a combination of factors, as is the case in their male relatives, such as the particular *GLA* mutation or autosomal and/or X-chromosomal modifier genes (see below). In addition, there are a number of issues specific to heterozygotes, such as the pattern of Lyonization in different organ systems, and sequence variants present on the wild-type *GLA* allele that may also modify the overall phenotype. For the clinical management and counselling of female heterozygotes, it is important to recognize that there is no surrogate marker available to predict the risk of complications, such as arrhythmias, stroke or renal failure.

Genetic modifiers

From the point of view of molecular pathology, Fabry disease may be considered as a metabolic vasculopathy beyond a single gene defect. Therefore, risk factors for cardiovascular and cerebrovascular disease, such as high blood pressure, elevated cholesterol levels and nicotine abuse, will adversely affect the phenotype in a given patient. Thus, the phenotype is probably also modified both by genetic factors unrelated to α-galactosidase A and by environmental factors. In a recent study, the presence of various DNA polymorphisms of genes encoding proteins of the inflammatory and coagulation system, such as interleukin 6 (c.-174G>C), p.Glu298Asp of endothelial nitric oxide synthase, the factor V p.Arg506Gln mutation, and the c.-13A>G and the IVS6 (intron F) +79G>A variants of the gene (*PROZ*) encoding the vitamin-K-dependent protein Z, were associated with an increased risk of cerebral lesions and stroke in patients with Fabry disease [20]. One might hypothesize that the relative influence of modifier genes may be greater in patients with residual enzyme activity than in those with no enzyme activity. In probands of the former group, *GLA*-unrelated factors may still have a significant effect on the extent of the *GLA*-mutation-defined residual enzyme activity and, consequently, on the overall phenotype, which would not be the case in the absence of residual enzyme activity.

Conclusions

Multivariate models based on large-scale systematic data collection are required to derive meaningful associations between genotype and phenotype in Fabry disease. In this context, FOS is likely to prove a valuable resource, providing important information for future efforts aimed at defining the different facets of the genotype–phenotype correlation.

Acknowledgements

This work was supported by the Intramural Research Program of the National Institute of Neurological Disorders and Stroke (National Institutes of Health, Bethesda, MD, USA).

References

1. Schäfer E, Baron K, Widmer U, Deegan P, Neumann HP, Sunder-Plassmann G et al. Thirty-four novel mutations of the *GLA* gene in 121 patients with Fabry disease. *Hum Mutat* 2005;25:412

2. Schiffmann R, Ries M. Fabry's disease – an important risk factor for stroke. *Lancet* 2005;366:1754–6

3. Goker-Alpan O, Schiffmann R, LaMarca ME, Nussbaum RL, McInerney-Leo A, Sidransky E. Parkinsonism among Gaucher disease carriers. *J Med Genet* 2004;41:937–40

4. Garman SC, Garboczi DN. The molecular defect leading to Fabry disease: structure of human α-galactosidase. *J Mol Biol* 2004;337:319–35

5. Branton MH, Schiffmann R, Sabnis SG, Murray GJ, Quirk JM, Altarescu G et al. Natural history of Fabry renal disease: influence of α-galactosidase A activity and genetic mutations on clinical course. *Medicine (Baltimore)* 2002;81:122–38

6. Altarescu GM, Goldfarb LG, Park KY, Kaneski C, Jeffries N, Litvak S et al. Identification of fifteen novel mutations and genotype–phenotype relationship in Fabry disease. *Clin Genet* 2001;60:46–51

7. Ries M. Quantitative analysis of the neuropathic and cerebrovascular correlates of hearing loss in Fabry disease. School of Medicine. Durham, NC: Duke University; 2005

8. Ries M, Moore DF, Robinson CJ, Tifft CJ, Rosenbaum KN, Brady RO et al. Quantitative dysmorphology assessment in Fabry disease. *Genet Med* 2006;8:96–101

9. Ries M, Gupta S, Moore DF, Sachdev V, Quirk JM, Murray GJ et al. Pediatric Fabry disease. *Pediatrics* 2005;115:e344–55

10. Fan JQ, Ishii S, Asano N, Suzuki Y. Accelerated transport and maturation of lysosomal α-galactosidase A in Fabry lymphoblasts by an enzyme inhibitor. *Nat Med* 1999;5:112–5

11. Dobyns WB, Filauro A, Tomson BN, Chan AS, Ho AW, Ting NT et al. Inheritance of most X-linked traits is not dominant or recessive, just X-linked. *Am J Med Genet A* 2004;129:136–43

12. Rimoin D, Connor J, Pyeritz RE. Emery and Rimoin's principles and practice of medical genetics. New York: Churchill Livingstone; 1997, p. 93–94

13. Guffon N. Clinical presentation in female patients with Fabry disease. *J Med Genet* 2003;40:e38

14. Gupta S, Ries M, Kotsopoulos S, Schiffmann R. The relationship of vascular glycolipid storage to clinical manifestations of Fabry disease: a cross-sectional study of a large cohort of clinically affected heterozygous women. *Medicine (Baltimore)* 2005;84:261–8

15. MacDermot KD, Holmes A, Miners AH. Anderson–Fabry disease: clinical manifestations and impact of disease in a cohort of 60 obligate carrier females. *J Med Genet* 2001;38:769–75

16. Mehta A, Ricci R, Widmer U, Dehout F, Garcia de Lorenzo A, Kampmann C et al. Fabry disease defined: baseline clinical manifestations of 366 patients in the Fabry Outcome Survey. *Eur J Clin Invest* 2004;34:236–42

17. Ries M, Ramaswami U, Parini R, Lindblad B, Whybra C, Willers I et al. The early clinical phenotype of Fabry disease: a study on 35 European children and adolescents. *Eur J Pediatr* 2003;162:767–72

18. Ries M, Schiffmann R. Fabry disease: angiokeratoma, biomarker, and the effect of enzyme replacement therapy on kidney function. *Arch Dermatol* 2005; 141:904–5; author reply 905–6

19. Whybra C, Kampmann C, Willers I, Davies J, Winchester B, Kriegsmann J *et al.* Anderson–Fabry disease: clinical manifestations of disease in female heterozygotes. *J Inherit Metab Dis* 2001;24:715–24

20. Altarescu G, Moore DF, Schiffmann R. Effect of genetic modifiers on cerebral lesions in Fabry disease. *Neurology* 2005;64:2148–50

Section 4:

Selected aspects of the clinical management of Fabry disease

35 A multidisciplinary approach to the care of patients with Fabry disease

Derralynn A Hughes, Sian Evans, Alan Milligan, Linda Richfield and Atul Mehta
Lysosomal Storage Disorders Unit, Department of Academic Haematology, Royal Free Hospital and University College Medical School, Rowland Hill Street, London NW3 2PF, UK

Although enzyme replacement therapy has had a considerable impact on the management of patients with Fabry disease, it is essential that attention is also given to general patient care. The varied clinical and psychological problems faced by patients with Fabry disease necessitate the involvement of doctors, nurses and allied professionals from a number of different specialties, as well as a wide range of concomitant treatments. It is therefore important that centres take a coordinated multidisciplinary approach to patient care, involving, for example, cardiologists, nephrologists, psychologists and specialist nurses. In addition, addressing the psychological needs of patients and their families, providing genetic counselling and family screening, and ensuring that treatment is made as convenient as possible (for instance, by making home therapy an option) are all likely to have a positive impact on the quality of life of those affected by Fabry disease.

Introduction

The availability of enzyme replacement therapy (ERT) has had a significant impact on the management of patients with Fabry disease. It remains essential, however, that attention is also given to general aspects of patient care. Consideration of the medical optimization of organ function and symptom control, the psychological impact of the condition and its inheritance, and issues relating to the delivery of ERT (e.g. in the home versus at specialist centres) are all relevant to any physician treating a patient with Fabry disease. This chapter will discuss the general provision of care for patients with Fabry disease, drawing particularly from experience gained in the UK.

The multidisciplinary team approach

The varied nature of the problems experienced by patients with Fabry disease necessitates the involvement of doctors, nurses and allied professionals from a number of different specialities. Coordination and regionalization of the services provided by these individuals allows development of significant clinical expertise, despite the relative rarity of this condition.

In the UK, a number of centres have now been designated by the Department of Health National Specialist Commissioning Advisory Group to offer treatment for Fabry disease and other lysosomal storage diseases (LSDs). The centres provide genetic counselling, diagnostic services, clinical assessment of patients and ongoing supportive care both for those requiring specific therapy, such as ERT, and for those in whom observation is currently appropriate. A lead physician with a particular interest and expertise in genetic and metabolic conditions should head the multidisciplinary team and coordinate appropriate assessment and investigation of patients. He or she will work alongside a team of specialist nurses with interest and expertise in the area of LSDs. After their initial assessment, patients may also be seen by other physicians appropriate for their individual case. Effective and high-quality care requires the involvement of a multispeciality and multidisciplinary team familiar with the range of clinical problems likely to be encountered (Table 1). The aim should be to provide a personal service which recognizes that each patient's experience of their condition will be very different.

All patients should have an initial baseline assessment of each organ system, including renal, cardiac and neurological function, and manifestations of the disease in the skin, eyes, ears and gastrointestinal tract should be recorded. The impact of the disease both on outward manifestations, such as pain and angiokeratoma, and on occult organ dysfunction should be assessed. Whilst most patients will experience some symptoms related to the disease, it is not unknown for patients to be subjectively asymptomatic but to exhibit significant proteinuria, renal dysfunction or left ventricular hypertrophy on

echocardiography. After the initial assessment, major organ system function should continue to be monitored in each patient on a regular basis, whereas other consultations, such as dermatological assessment, can be tailored to an individual patient's needs (see Chapter 42). Regular meetings of the multidisciplinary team should facilitate timely and appropriate decision-making with respect to therapy. It is especially important that any discussion of starting, modifying or ceasing ERT should involve the whole team, including those members involved in the home care of the patient.

Patients with Fabry disease often possess expert knowledge of the condition, after having suffered for many years with little information and lack of an accurate diagnosis. They not only become well versed in their own disease but are also often fully aware of new scientific and technical developments. Patients should be fully apprised of the investigations carried out, as progress and compliance are likely to be increased if the patient is part of any decision-making process. At the start of therapy, a patient contract may be drawn up between the patient and physician, outlining the rationale for therapy and the responsibilities of both

Table 1. *The core essential expertise and services that should be available at the treatment centre or in a neighbouring hospital. There should be clear policies and protocols for access to these services.*

- **Clinical services**
  - Lead consultant
  - Clinical nurse specialists
  - Paediatric specialists
  - Cardiology
  - Neurology
  - Dermatology
  - Ophthalmology
  - Audiology
  - Nephrology/haemodialysis
  - Gastroenterology
  - Palliative care
  - Physiotherapy/rehabilitation
  - Psychology and counselling

- **Diagnostic services**
  - Chemical pathology
  - Clinical genetics
  - Radiology
  - Haematology
  - Nuclear medicine
- **Support services**
  - Pharmacy facilities
  - Administrative support
  - Social services
  - Financial advice
  - Patient support
  - Primary care liaison

parties with respect to attendance at follow-up, compliance with ongoing care and issues related to recording data.

Role of the specialist nurse

In the UK, there are six designated regional specialist centres for the management of adults, adolescents and children with Fabry disease. Each of these centres includes clinical nurse specialists as part of the multidisciplinary team.

Specialist Fabry nurses may undertake a wide range of responsibilities that are complementary to those of clinicians and laboratory scientists. Specialist nurses often have a unique relationship with the patient and their wider family and can help them to cope with a chronic genetic disease. There is also the potential for nurses to explore issues that physicians may have less time to broach, such as the psychological/psychosocial effects of the disease, including emotional, relationship or sexual problems.

An important responsibility of the specialist nurse is the administration and monitoring of ERT. They may also ensure that patients who wish to self-administer at home are fully trained to do so, possibly with the assistance of family members.

The availability of ERT has significantly reduced the incidence of Fabry crises. Some patients, however, continue to experience neuronopathic pain and require advice on the adequate control and management of the occasional pain crisis. Most Fabry centres operate a telephone helpline manned by the nursing team, which provides advice and information on the disease for patients, relatives and other healthcare professionals.

Specialist nurses are also involved in explaining the FOS database to patients. In addition, they also administer and help patients to complete the various questionnaires, and provide patient data for the database.

Holistic care

Therapy in Fabry disease comprises both specific replacement of the deficient enzyme and supportive or adjunctive therapy for complications of the condition. Adjunctive therapies include treatment of pain, hypertension and angiokeratoma and should be available to all patients who are symptomatic (Table 2). There are no randomized controlled trials of these therapies in Fabry disease and the evidence for their effectiveness is largely derived from experience in other conditions. Aggressive control of other risk factors for cardiovascular disease, such as hypercholesterolaemia and smoking, is recommended. Hypertension should be vigorously controlled and, in the presence of proteinuria, an angiotensin-converting enzyme inhibitor would be recommended as first-line therapy, supplemented with a calcium-channel antagonist, if necessary. Sinus bradycardia is a common consequence of cardiac involvement in Fabry disease and β-blockers should therefore be avoided. Patients with cardiac arrhythmias should be treated with anti-arrhythmics and anticoagulants according to current guidelines. Special care should be exercised with the use of amiodarone, as this has been reported to result in cornea verticillata; that is, a phenocopy of Fabry disease.

Psychological care

The patient's journey to a diagnosis of Fabry disease is often long and tortuous, with many years of misdiagnosis and delay. The median age at diagnosis in men is 30 years, after up to 10 years of investigation and visits to as many as ten different specialists. The psychological impact of delayed diagnosis and of a lifetime of being dismissed as a hypochondriac, malingerer or somatizer may result in significant depression even when a diagnosis is finally reached. Anxiety concerning implications of the natural history of the disease and its treatment often replaces the initial relief of identifying the condition. Patients may express concerns

Table 2. *Symptomatic treatment of Fabry disease.*

- **Pain**
  - Chronic pain: anticonvulsants
    (e.g. carbamazepine, gabapentin, phenytoin)
  - Painful crises: non-steroidal anti-
    inflammatory drugs or opiates
- **Angiokeratoma**
  - Removal with argon laser therapy
- **Renal disease**
  - Proteinuria: angiotensin-converting enzyme
    (ACE) inhibitors and/or angiotensin receptor
    blockers
  - Renal failure: dialysis or transplantation
- **Cardiovascular disease**
  - Chest pain: anti-anginals (β-blockers,
    calcium antagonists, nitrates)
  - Heart failure: diuretics, ACE inhibitors,
    digoxin, angiotensin-receptor blockers,
  - Atrial ventricular tachyarrhythmia: anti-
    arrhythmics, anticoagulants, implantable
    cardioverter/defibrillator
  - Symptomatic bradycardia: pacemaker
- **Gastrointestinal symptoms**
  - Low-fat diet, motility agents, pancreatic
    enzyme supplementation
- **Hypertension**
  - Rigorous control, with, for example, ACE
    inhibitors; avoid β-blockers where there is
    sinus bradycardia
- **Hyperlipidaemia**
  - Statin therapy
- **Neurovascular disease**
  - Aspirin, clopidogrel

regarding the availability of therapy, the reversibility of their symptoms or organ dysfunction and the practicalities of receiving treatment. They will require support at each stage of diagnosis, assessment and treatment. This might be best provided by a specialist nurse who has developed a relationship with the patient; however, in some cases, psychological counselling or psychiatric assessment for depression may be necessary.

Written information concerning the disorder and advice as to the reliability of web sites should be made available to all newly diagnosed patients. They should also be provided with a named contact within the multidisciplinary team with whom they can discuss concerns between visits to the centre. Patients may also request social support and advice with respect to health benefits and life insurance, and should be placed in contact with a patient support group with access to patient advocacy.

Many patients will be most anxious for their children. Until recently, women have been labelled merely as carriers of this X-linked condition, who may therefore pass it on to their sons. Mothers therefore often experience significant feelings of guilt when they pass the disease on. The acknowledgement that women also manifest clinical problems due to Fabry disease has relieved some of this burden and allowed their own psychological engagement with the disease process.

Genetic counselling and family screening

Pedigree analysis should be undertaken for each patient presenting with Fabry disease. This should be done by physicians and nurses with specialized training and experience in genetic counselling. Pedigree analysis is aided by the FOS – Fabry Outcome Survey – pedigree tool and is used to identify potentially affected family members. In addition to genetic counselling, the Fabry nurse may be involved in any other counselling that is needed due to the multisystemic nature of the disease and its psychosocial effects on both affected and unaffected family members. Ethical issues (e.g. sharing information with family members, informing employers, antenatal diagnosis) are also important in the context of genetic diseases, not only for the individual patient but also for the patient's family. The Fabry nurse needs to be aware of these issues and to be able to discuss them with the patient and his/her family members as appropriate.

The provision of specialized genetic counselling is considered by the European Commission to be an essential requirement for highly predictive testing for serious disorders. Counselling must be non-directive. The main goal is to assist individuals or families to understand and cope with Fabry disease and not to reduce the incidence in the population or to uncover more cases. Whilst medically relevant genetic testing is considered an integral part of health service provision, genetic testing should never be imposed and must be a matter of free personal choice. A patient has the right to know, the right not to know and the right to change his or her mind at a later date. Appropriate explanations and adequate time should be allocated, and simple printed information that can be consulted after counselling has been shown to be extremely valuable. This might include information concerning the inheritance pattern of the condition, the likelihood of clinically significant disease, potential consequences and possibilities for therapy.

Written informed consent should be obtained prior to any genetic test, and confidentiality between family members must be maintained at all times. Access to genetic testing should be non-discriminatory according to age, sex or geographical location.

Family involvement

After the diagnosis of an index case of Fabry disease, other members of the family may self-present for screening for the condition. With appropriate consent, such individuals should undergo genetic counselling and later testing. Complete patient confidentiality should be maintained when assessing family members. Some families will opt for joint visits but, in these instances, individual consultations should be performed without reference to other family members. It may be that individual branches of a family have not disclosed their diagnosis and it is therefore advisable to avoid meetings of estranged relatives in the waiting room. It is, however,

important to include a patient's partner in any discussions, if desired by the patient. In many cases the partner of a patient with Fabry disease will also be the parent of an affected child and will also therefore require information and support both in their concern for their dependents and in their position as the unaffected person within the family.

Unaffected siblings may feel distanced from a family group going through the process of diagnosis and assessment for Fabry disease. Where possible, these children should be given the opportunity to learn about the condition and to attend patient and family group meetings.

Home therapy

The consequence of regional specialization of services is that most patients will travel some distance to their Fabry centre. Whilst hospital visits may reduce feelings of frustration and isolation, many patients find overly frequent visits stressful, time consuming and disruptive. The facility to administer ERT in the home will therefore limit the time spent at the hospital to that necessary for specialist investigation and consultation. In the UK and in certain other countries, enzyme infusions are initially given by specialist community nursing staff but, after sufficient training, may later be administered by the patient at home. Home-based therapy offers several advantages over hospital-based therapy; it removes the need to make frequent hospital visits, it restores independence and gives control of the disease to the patient, and it reduces utilization of hospital resources. Infusions may be integrated comfortably and conveniently into the patient's normal routine, reducing the impact of treatment on work and family life. The requirements for providing good quality home care are listed in Table 3.

Administering the first one or two infusions in the hospital allows careful monitoring for infusion reactions. In the unlikely event that

Table 3. *Basic requirements for the provision of good quality home care.*

- An effective system of close liaison between the hospital team, the patient and carer(s), and the home care services
- Convenient delivery of pharmaceuticals and clinical supplies to the patient's home and the availability of appropriate storage facilities
- Specialist nurses in the community to support home treatment, either administering the ERT or training the patient/carer to administer the infusions (training or treatment is individualized to each patient's specific needs)
- A clear policy for dealing with emergency home care nurse call-outs and management of potential adverse events, including drug-related reactions

---

an infusion reaction occurs, the acute event should be managed by slowing or stopping the infusion and administering hydrocortisone, chlorpheniramine, fluids and salbutamol, as appropriate. Prophylaxis with hydrocortisone and chlorpheniramine may then be given before further infusions. Once the patient is receiving uneventful infusions within the hospital, the treatment can be transferred to the home environment. Approximately 50% of patients will eventually learn self-cannulation and administration, and will depend on the home care service only for delivery of drug and infusion equipment and possibly for call-out assistance if problems are experienced with cannulation.

Conclusions

The phenotypic heterogeneity of Fabry disease requires that centres treating and assessing patients have access to a dedicated multidisciplinary team, including physicians and specialist nurses, with experience in a wide range of clinical specialities. Patients will differ, however, not only in the physical manifestations of the condition but also in their psychological response to it. Counselling and support should be provided throughout the process of diagnosis, investigation and therapy both for the index case and for affected and unaffected family members. Once a decision has been made to administer ERT, improvements in quality of life can be achieved by utilizing home-based therapy.

36 Development of enzyme replacement therapy for Fabry disease

Raphael Schiffmann and Roscoe O Brady

Developmental and Metabolic Neurology Branch, National Institute of Neurological Disorders and Stroke, Building 10, Room 3D03, National Institutes of Health, Bethesda, Maryland 20892-1260, USA

We describe the pathway to the development of enzyme replacement therapy (ERT) for Fabry disease with particular emphasis on the agalsidase alfa preparation. For both agalsidase alfa and beta enzyme preparations, initial studies were performed in a mouse model of Fabry disease. Subsequent placebo-controlled and open-label trials showed reduction in neuropathic pain and gastrointestinal symptoms and increased cold perception and sweating in patients with the disorder. Partial reversal of the vascular pathophysiology was also observed. Reports from uncontrolled studies suggest a cardiac benefit as well, and initial studies in women with Fabry disease suggest a decreased disease burden in those patients who are receiving ERT. Most encouraging are the data on safety and initial symptomatic efficacy of ERT in children as young as 7 years of age. We conclude that ERT in Fabry disease has a definite benefit. Long-term studies are necessary to assess to what extent it delays the occurrence of sentinel disease manifestations, such as cardiac events, end-stage renal disease, stroke and death.

Introduction

The concept of enzyme replacement for lysosomal storage disorders was suggested by de Duve in 1964 [1] and for sphingolipid storage disorders by Brady in 1966 [2]. The first step toward development of enzyme replacement therapy (ERT) for Fabry disease was the identification by Sweeley and Klionsky of ceramidetrihexoside, now called globotriaosylceramide (Gb$_3$, also known as GL-3), as the major accumulating glycosphingolipid in patients with this disorder [3]. Several years later, the enzymatic defect was established as insufficient activity of the enzyme ceramidetrihexosidase (α-galactosidase A), which catalyses the hydrolytic cleavage of the terminal molecule of galactose from Gb$_3$ [4, 5]. α-Galactosidase A was initially purified from small-intestinal tissue [4]. Later, it was isolated from human placental tissue [6].

An early investigation was carried out with α-galactosidase A isolated from human placental tissue [6], which was subsequently shown to contain two isozymes of α-galactosidase [7]. The first administration of lysosomal enzyme consisted of a single intravenous injection into two patients with Fabry disease that caused brief, but significant, reductions of Gb$_3$ in the blood [8]. α-Galactosidase A was rapidly cleared from the blood and was taken up by the liver to a major extent. The level of Gb$_3$ in the circulation fell rapidly from a threefold elevation to the normal range in both recipients. However, within 48–72 hours, it had returned to the pre-infusion value in both patients [8]. Similar results were obtained later by another group of investigators using α-galactosidase A isolated from human spleen and from human plasma [9]. Further investigations of ERT for

Fabry disease were delayed for many years until improved procedures were developed for the production and purification of larger quantities of α-galactosidase A. During the past 6 years, two preparations of α-galactosidase A have been tested: agalsidase alfa and agalsidase beta. Both have eventually been widely approved in Europe and in many other countries, but only agalsidase beta is currently approved in the USA.

ERT using agalsidase alfa
Preclinical studies

An α-galactosidase A knockout mouse was produced by disruption of exon three of the murine α-galactosidase A gene [10]. Although the phenotype of this mouse does not closely simulate that of humans with Fabry disease, the mice accumulate substantial amounts of Gb_3 in various organs and have proved useful for testing the biochemical responses to exogenous α-galactosidase A. Agalsidase alfa was produced and purified from a genetically engineered human cell line by Transkaryotic Therapies Inc. (Cambridge, MA, USA).

We first examined the reduction of accumulated Gb_3 in the organs of the α-galactosidase A knockout mouse. Mice were injected intravenously with agalsidase alfa at doses of 0.2 and 1.0 mg/kg (corresponding to 10 and 50 IU/kg, respectively) [11]. The influence of frequency of administration, as well as the dose, on the response to enzyme therapy was investigated. An acute course of treatment, consisting of three doses per week for 2.5 weeks (arm A), and a longer-term course, consisting of administration of enzyme once per week for 8 weeks (arm B), were given for each of the doses. Tissues were harvested 1 week after the final injection of enzyme in order to maximize the probability of observing a significant reduction in tissue Gb_3 levels. Gb_3 and α-galactosidase A activity levels in normal control mice and in untreated Fabry mice were compared with the levels in Fabry mice that received agalsidase alfa. Enzyme levels in liver and spleen in the Fabry mice

receiving ERT were between 200 and 300 nmol/hour/mg protein, which was three- to fourfold higher than in normal control animals, and were accompanied by normalization of Gb_3 levels in these organs [11]. The level of augmented enzyme activity exhibited a relatively long half-life in the tissues of these animals. In both 'acute' and 'chronic' injection protocols, however, no significant enzyme activity remained in the kidney at 7 days post-infusion when the lower dose (10 IU/kg) was administered. Higher doses resulted in a more than twofold increase from a mean of 1.5 nmol/hour/mg to 3.4 nmol/hour/mg. This value is considerably lower than the 53 nmol/hour/mg observed in normal control kidneys. It should also be noted that even though high levels of enzyme were not found in the kidney at the time of harvest, tissue Gb_3 concentrations were significantly reduced in both arms of the study by 40–60% (Figure 1).

α-Galactosidase A activity in the heart approached normal levels: 1.3 and 3.9 nmol/hour/mg in arm A for the low dose and high dose, respectively, and 0.5 and 2.4 nmol/hour/mg in arm B for the same doses (normal, 7 nmol/hour/mg protein). There was marked reduction of Gb_3 in the heart, ranging from 80% to 90% at all doses and at all dose frequencies [11].

In the liver and spleen, enzyme activity was clearly normalized by administration of exogenous enzyme. α-Galactosidase A activity was also significantly increased in the kidney and lung above that of untreated controls (Figure 1). Although we can estimate that, at the higher dose, near-normal enzyme activity was achieved in these tissues, at least transiently, the actual intra-organ cellular distribution was initially investigated only in the liver. Immunohistochemical studies showed the enzyme to be present in vascular endothelial cells, Kupffer cells and hepatocytes. We have recently completed a comprehensive immunohistochemical study in this mouse model. Agalsidase alfa, 0.5 mg/kg, or vehicle was

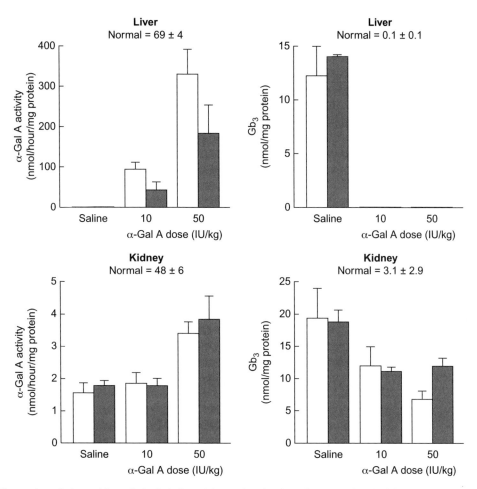

Figure 1. α-Galactosidase A (α-Gal A) activity and reduction of accumulated globotriaosylceramide (Gb₃) in the liver and kidneys of Fabry mice following administration of human α-galactosidase A (agalsidase alfa). Open bars, treatment arm A (three doses per week for 2.5 weeks); solid bars, treatment arm B (one dose per week for 8 weeks). Reproduced with permission from [11].

injected into the mice. Widespread staining was found in kidney glomerular and tubular cells, and in vascular endothelial cells only in the heart and aorta; staining was not seen in the brain (R Schiffmann *et al.*, unpublished data). The injected enzyme was visible in some other organs and tissues, such as bone marrow, spleen, adrenal gland and testes.

Clinical ERT studies in hemizygous males

A safety and dose-escalation trial was conducted in ten patients with Fabry disease. In this initial study, α-galactosidase A was purified from the conditioned medium of stably transfected human foreskin fibroblasts [12]. The doses given ranged from 0.3 to 4.7 IU/kg (0.007–0.1 mg/kg). Significant reductions in Gb₃ levels were found both in the liver and in shed renal tubular epithelial cells in the urine sediment, but there was no greater glycolipid reduction with the higher doses than with the lower doses. There was no significant reduction of plasma Gb₃ levels [12]. Immunohistochemical examination of percutaneous liver biopsy tissue showed

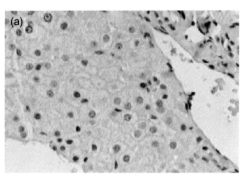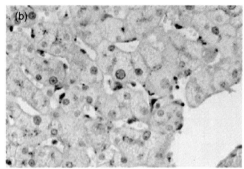

Figure 2. *Immunohistochemical localization of α-galactosidase A. A polyclonal rabbit anti-human α-galactosidase A antibody was used to stain liver biopsy sections from a patient in the study (a) just before treatment with α-galactosidase A and (b) 44 hours after treatment with α-galactosidase A. Reproduced with permission from [12].*

α-galactosidase A in sinusoidal endothelial cells, Kupffer cells and hepatocytes, suggesting diffuse uptake via the mannose 6-phosphate receptor (Figure 2).

The next step in the development of ERT in Fabry disease was a double-blind, placebo-controlled, 6-month trial with agalsidase alfa (0.2 mg/kg i.v. every 2 weeks) conducted in 26 hemizygous male patients [13]. The dose that was used was twice the highest dose used in the phase I study. In this study, as in all subsequent ones, α-galactosidase A was produced in a genetically engineered continuous human cell line (Transkaryotic Therapies Inc.). The main outcome measure was the effect of agalsidase alfa on the neuropathic pain experienced by all of the participants in this investigation [13]. Patients who received active enzyme had a significant ($p = 0.02$) reduction in pain compared with those in the placebo group (Figure 3) [13]. Pain-related quality of life scores declined more in patients receiving α-galactosidase A compared with placebo ($p = 0.05$). In the kidney, the proportion of glomeruli with mesangial widening decreased by a mean of 12.5% in patients receiving enzyme compared with a 16.5% increase for those on placebo ($p = 0.01$). A marked reduction in glycolipid deposits in renal vascular endothelial cells was observed in the enzyme group. This trial led to the approval of agalsidase alfa by

the European Agency for the Evaluation of Medicinal Products under special circumstances with post-marketing commitments.

In subsequent years, efforts were made to identify additional effects of agalsidase alfa, particularly on the neurological and renal aspects of the disease. Most of the studies described below were part of the original controlled trial described above and the open-label study with the same group of patients in the subsequent 4.5 years. Using $H_2^{15}O$ positron emission tomography in the initial trial [13], we found significant cerebral hyperperfusion in patients with Fabry disease compared with healthy controls [14].

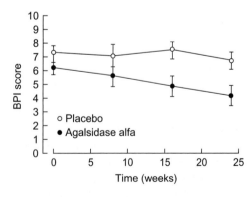

Figure 3. *Brief Pain Inventory (BPI) 'pain at its worst' scores for patients with Fabry disease given agalsidase alfa or placebo. Values are means ± SEM. Reproduced with permission from [13].*

Cerebrovascular hyper-reactivity to acetazol-amide infusion indicated poor vascular reconstriction and cerebrovascular dysregu-lation in Fabry disease [15]. These abnormal-ities were significantly improved in patients who received agalsidase alfa compared with those who received placebo [14, 15]. We also found increased staining for 3-nitro-tyrosine in dermal blood vessels in the same group of patients [14]. This staining was significantly reduced in the group given ERT and remained unchanged in the patients on placebo. More recently, we found a delayed reduction in cerebral blood flow following infusion of ascorbate, coupled with low blood ascorbate levels, in patients with Fabry disease [16]. The reactivity to ascorbate was partially reversed in patients on ERT compared with placebo. However, five out of the 25 patients in the original cohort devel-oped strokes and other vascular compli-cations while on ERT. Therefore, these func-tional vascular improvements cannot, at this point, serve as surrogate markers to predict the clinical response to agalsidase alfa infusions.

We also investigated the response to ERT of the small-fibre peripheral neuropathy of Fabry disease. Patients in the original place-bo group experienced a reduction in neuro-pathic pain, which was similar to that of the initial infused group, 6 months after crossing over to agalsidase alfa infusions [17]. Although there was a significant reduction in pain overall, pain scores for the whole group of 25 patients remained, on average, un-changed in the subsequent year of the open-label study (the 18-month time point). Using a well-established biophysical quantitative sensory testing procedure, we found a significant reduction in the threshold for cold and warm sensation in the foot over the first 3 years of ERT (Figure 4) [17]. We previously demonstrated that the small-fibre peripheral neuropathy of Fabry disease is associated with a marked reduction in epidermal inner-vation density [18]. The functional improve-ment in cold perception of about 10% was not associated with increased innervation density in the epidermis in this patient popu-lation [19]. At the 3-year time point, sweat function, as measured by a quantitative sudo-motor axon reflex test (QSART), improved 24–72 hours post-enzyme infusion compared with pre-infusion values [17]. The QSART res-ponse normalized in four anhidrotic patients. The thermoregulatory sweat test, a gold stan-dard sweat test involving exposure of sub-jects to environmental heat, confirmed the QSART results (Figure 5). These findings suggest that, at least in some patients, infus-ed α-galactosidase A acutely, but transiently, ameliorates the sweating function.

Renal function
We also studied the renal function of the 25 patients involved in our original placebo-controlled trial. One patient received a kidney transplant prior to starting ERT, and another patient left the study early for personal reasons. Effects on renal function were there-fore evaluated in only 23 patients [20]. The Modification of Diet in Renal Disease (MDRD) method, using serial measurements of serum creatinine, was used to follow renal function. Of the 23 patients, 11 had stage I renal dis-ease (MDRD glomerular filtration rate [GFR] $\geq$ 90 ml/min/1.73 m^2) at baseline, eight had stage II (MDRD GFR, 60 to < 90 ml/min/1.73 m^2) and four had stage III (GFR, 30 to < 60 ml/min/1.73 m^2) renal disease [20]. Mean MDRD GFR remained relatively stable for up to 36–54 months of ERT with agal-sidase alfa for the entire patient population. Mean baseline MDRD GFR was 88.3 ± 5.5 ml/min/1.73 m^2 ($n = 23$) and after 48 months of treatment it had declined only slightly to 75.1 ± 7.5 ml/min/1.73 m^2 ($p = 0.039$). This small decrease in mean MDRD GFR ap-peared to be driven primarily by the marked declines in GFR noted in the four patients with the worst renal function at baseline (Table 1) [20]. In these patients, mean MDRD GFR fell from 47.1 ± 4.7 ml/min/1.73 m^2 to 24.8 ± 7.2 ml/min/1.73 m^2 ($p = 0.098$) after

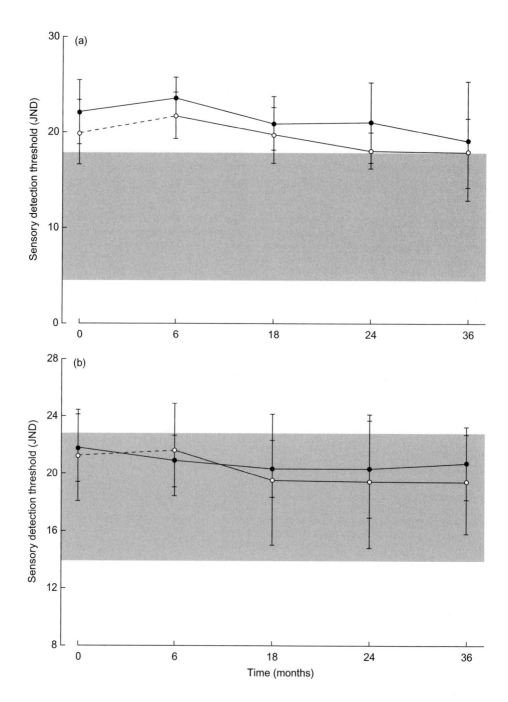

Figure 4. *Sensory detection thresholds, expressed as just noticeable difference (JND) units, over time (means ± SD). (a) Cooling detection thresholds in the foot (p < 0.001). (b) Warm detection thresholds in the foot (p = 0.006). Open circles, patients who started on placebo before crossing over to enzyme replacement therapy after 6 months; closed circles, patients who started on enzyme replacement therapy. The shaded area represents the tolerance interval for control subjects. Reproduced with permission from [17].*

Pre-infusion   7 days after infusion of agalsidase alfa

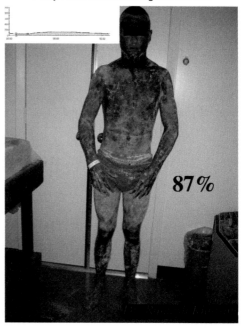

Figure 5. *Thermoregulatory sweat test in a patient before infusion of agalsidase alfa and 7 days after enzyme infusion in a patient who had been receiving enzyme replacement for 3 years. An iodine-starch combination was smeared on his body. Sweating transforms the colour of the starch powder from white to purple. In each panel, there is an insert depicting sweat testing using the quantitative sudomotor sweat test (QSART) performed on the same day. Sweating body surface area was 27% prior to enzyme infusion and 87% 7 days after infusion. In parallel, sweat output also increased, as measured by QSART. This figure demonstrates that agalsidase alfa acutely, but transiently, increases sweating of the anhidrotic patient with Fabry disease (courtesy of Dr R Khurana).*

48 months of therapy (representing an average rate of decline of approximately 5.2 ml/min/1.73 m^2 per year). It is noteworthy that during this 4- to 4.5-year period of observation, none of these patients with stage III renal disease progressed to end-stage renal failure while receiving ERT with agalsidase alfa. However, in the subsequent 2 years following the end of this 4- to 4.5-year extension study, despite continuing agalsidase alfa infusions at the same dose and frequency, two of these stage III patients were started on dialysis. Branton and co-workers identified 14 patients with chronic renal failure and documented a mean rate of decline of GFR of 12.2 ml/min/year over the next 4–4.5 years [21]. Their group was similar in age and baseline GFR to the four patients with stage III kidney disease in

the present study (Table 2). These observations suggest that ERT with agalsidase alfa slowed the decline in kidney function in this subgroup with severely reduced renal function. Proteinuria increased slightly from 1.08 ± 0.34 g/24 hours at baseline to 1.33 ± 0.45 g/24 hours ($p = 0.28$).

Mean plasma Gb$_3$ concentration at baseline was 11.4 ± 0.8 nmol/ml; this decreased to a mean of 5.8 ± 0.4 nmol/ml over the first 6 months of treatment with agalsidase alfa, and remained at this reduced level for the subsequent 48 months. ($p < 0.001$ for all time points compared with baseline) [19]. The urine sediment Gb$_3$ concentration at baseline was 2566 ± 299 nmol/g creatinine. A mean decrease of 58.8% was observed in 19 patients for whom urine sediment Gb$_3$ data

Table 1. *Glomerular filtration rate (GFR), as assessed by the Modification of Diet in Renal Disease method, in male patients with Fabry disease treated with agalsidase alfa for up to 54 months. Values are means ± SD for patients with stage I (GFR ≥ 90 ml/min/1.73 m²; n = 11), stage II (GFR 60–89 ml/min/ 1.73 m²; n = 8) and stage III (GFR 30–59 ml/min/1.73 m²; n = 4) renal disease at baseline.*

Duration of treatment (months)	Estimated GFR (ml/min/1.73 m²)		
	Stage I renal disease	Stage II renal disease	Stage III renal disease
0	110.4 ± 13.5	72.6 ± 10.4	47.1 ± 9.4
6	107.8 ± 17.5	78.6 ± 8.2	46.5 ± 12.1
12	107.9 ± 13.8	81.0 ± 12.8	39.8 ± 10.6
18	117.4 ± 10.1	77.9 ± 12.8	39.4 ± 13.0
24	112.6 ± 12.2	81.3 ± 19.9	40.5 ± 15.7
30	109.8 ± 14.6	83.0 ± 21.1	37.2 ± 17.3
36	114.6 ± 17.9	78.3 ± 22.9	32.9 ± 16.6
42	100.6 ± 12.2	74.5 ± 22.4	25.5 ± 10.6
48	101.1 ± 11.9	66.6 ± 16.6	24.8 ± 14.5
54	99.6 ± 8.7	69.7 ± 14.5	31.4 ± 24.3

Table 2. *Comparison of the rates of decline in glomerular filtration rate (GFR), as assessed by the Modification of Diet in Renal Disease method (ml/min/1.73 m²), in two populations of male patients with Fabry disease and chronic renal insufficiency.*

	Branton *et al.* [21]	Present study
Number of patients	14	4
Age (years)	39 ± 9	40.8 ± 3.8
Baseline GFR (ml/min/1.73 m²)	44 ± 10	47.1 ± 4.7
Rate of decline in GFR (ml/min/1.73 m² per year)	−12.2 ± 8.1	−5.2 ± 1.8
Range	(−3.3 to −33.7)	(−0.6 to −9.2)

were available after 48 months of agalsidase alfa treatment. It should be noted, however, that even though significantly reduced, glycolipid levels in urine remained markedly elevated compared with normal; therefore, the functional significance of such a reduction is unknown.

Effect of a higher frequency of ERT
Following the study described above, we identified 11 patients with a progressive decline in GFR of at least 5 ml/min/year despite 2.5–4.5 years of ERT. Serum creatinine was still in the normal range in half of the patients. The patients were entered in a prospective 2-year study of weekly infusion of agalsidase alfa at a dose of 0.2 mg/kg. Preliminary data showed that, after 18 months, the decline in GFR had stopped in seven of the 11 patients, while renal function continued to decline in the other four patients. These preliminary data suggest that at least some patients require a higher dose or a higher frequency of enzyme infusions for a therapeutic effect on renal function to be observed. It should be emphasized that stable renal function in patients on ERT with normal serum creatinine might not be due to a therapeutic

effect of enzyme infusions (Table 1). Renal glomerular function remains normal for years before the onset of decline [21].

Safety
The long-term follow-on study confirmed that agalsidase alfa infusions are safe overall. During the 4–4.5 years of ERT, all eligible subjects were able to transition to home therapy with no complications. Eight patients developed persistent IgG antibodies to agalsidase alfa, but IgE antibodies were not detected in any patient. There was no apparent relationship between the antibody status of the patient and the likelihood of a rapid decline in renal function. However, urinary Gb$_3$ concentrations declined less in patients with persistent IgG antibodies to agalsidase alfa [19].

Effect of ERT on the heart
Our studies were not designed to assess the effect of ERT on the cardiac manifestations of Fabry disease (see Chapter 37). Our original cohort, however, was followed over time with cardiac magnetic resonance imaging (for up to 18 months) and with echocardiography (for up to at least 3 years). Two blinded experienced individuals analysed our data. After 6 months of ERT, there was no difference between the enzyme and placebo groups (V Sachdev, unpublished data). Overall, we could not see much change. Echocardiograms showed that there was a trend towards increased cardiac mass, but there were large individual variations between patients. A few patients had marked increases in left ventricular mass (LVM) and some had decreases in LVM (V Sachdev, unpublished data). There was no consistent improvement in cardiac mass according to electrocardiograms. As there was no control group, it is not possible to say whether ERT modified the natural history of cardiac disease in our patients. The heart provides an example of the limits of a mouse model. Contrary to the marked reduction of Gb$_3$ concentrations in the heart of the mouse model of up to 80% [11, 22], substrate

reduction in human biopsies was no greater than 26% [23].

In summary, our studies indicate that ERT is safe, reduces neuropathic pain and improves cold perception, sweating and gastrointestinal symptoms. It probably has the potential to slow the progression of renal disease, but the frequency and dose at which agalsidase alfa should be used remain to be established. A therapeutic effect on the likelihood of stroke and on cardiomyopathy remains to be demonstrated.

Other reports on ERT
In the past 4 years, other groups have reported the results of ERT with agalsidase alfa, mostly from studies in Europe. Some of these studies were formal, whereas others were reports of data analyses from FOS – the Fabry Outcome Survey [24]. Most of the reports confirm the safety of ERT with agalsidase alfa and show a modest reduction in neuropathic pain, an improvement in quality of life and a possible reduction in LVM [24, 25]. Thus far, no randomized controlled study has shown a significant reduction in cardiac mass or other positive effect.

ERT in women
It is particularly difficult to evaluate a therapeutic effect in heterozygous females because they are clinically very heterogeneous. They manifest a wide range of severity of disease, from those who are essentially asymptomatic to women who have the same manifestations as a male with 'classic' Fabry disease [26]. Again, there are no controlled studies. There is one open-label report that used a clinical score to show progressive reduction in severity in male and female patients after 1 year of ERT [27].

ERT in children
We conducted a 6-month open-label prospective study as part of an investigation of 25 children initiated in Germany (Mainz), Canada (Toronto) and the US National Institutes of Health.

Twenty-three patients (95.8%) reported at least one adverse event; the majority of these were symptoms commonly seen in normal children and/or in untreated patients with Fabry disease. No patient was withdrawn from the study due to an adverse event and no patient died during the study. All serious adverse events were considered unrelated to agalsidase alfa (R Schiffmann et al., unpublished data). Adverse events related to infusion of agalsidase alfa were observed in seven patients (29.2%) and were managed for subsequent infusions with premedication and/or lengthening of the infusion duration. The most common infusion-related adverse events were rigors (16.7%), flushing, nausea, pyrexia (each 12.5%) and headache (8.3%). Only one patient had an infusion stopped prematurely due to an infusion-related reaction. One patient tested transiently positive for IgG antibodies to agalsidase alfa at week 9 but tested negative thereafter. No IgE antibodies were detected in any patient at any time point tested.

The pharmacokinetic profiles showed a biphasic serum elimination profile in all of these paediatric patients with Fabry disease following single and repeated doses of agalsidase alfa. Individual serum elimination half-lives were less than 5 hours, indicating that agalsidase alfa would not accumulate in serum following repeated infusions. There was no significant difference in pharmacokinetics between males and females. There was a significant increase in clearance in the younger (6.5- to 11-year-old) paediatric patients (M Ries et al., unpublished data). The cause of this difference is not known.

Renal function at baseline and at the end of the study was normal. Mean plasma Gb_3 levels decreased significantly (40%) in the males, while plasma levels in females, which were within the normal range at baseline, remained essentially unchanged. Urine sediment Gb_3 levels decreased by a median of 77.6% in male patients and by a median of 37.4% in female patients at week 26 (R Schiffmann et al. unpublished data). All patients had LVM indexed to height ($g/m^{2.7}$) within the normal range at baseline, as assessed by echocardiography. No clinically important changes from baseline in LVM for height were seen, except for decreases among a subgroup of three patients who had a high normal LVM for height (> 40 $g/m^{2.7}$) at baseline. There was a significant increase in the heart rate variability parameters, measured by 2-hour Holter monitoring, that were abnormal at baseline in males only. Diaries and quality of life questionnaires suggested a reduction in pain and gastrointestinal disturbances and an improvement in energy levels and quality of life (R Schiffmann et al., unpublished data). We have previously demonstrated hypohidrosis in children with Fabry disease by QSART. There was a trend towards improvement of sweat output in males when measured 14 days following infusion of agalsidase alfa (M Ries and R Schiffmann, unpublished data).

ERT using agalsidase beta

The development pathway for agalsidase beta was quite similar to that for agalsidase alfa. Agalsidase beta is produced in Chinese hamster ovary cells by the Genzyme Corporation (Cambridge, MA, USA). Using a similar α-galactosidase A knockout mouse model, a single dose or repeated doses (every 48 hours for eight doses) of α-galactosidase A at 0.3–10.0 mg/kg cleared hepatic Gb_3, whereas higher doses were required for depletion of Gb_3 in other tissues [22]. After a single dose of 3 mg/kg, hepatic Gb_3 was cleared for more than 4 weeks, whereas cardiac and splenic Gb_3 re-accumulated after 3 weeks [22]. These studies led to a phase I/II study where various combinations of five doses of 0.3–3 mg/kg were each shown to reduce plasma, renal and cardiac Gb_3 levels [23]. For the pivotal trial, the investigators settled on a dose of 1 mg/kg administered every 2 weeks in a double-blind placebo-controlled multicentre trial involving 58 patients [28]. Instead of looking for a clinical effect, the primary efficacy endpoint used by the investigators was the percentage of patients in whom renal microvascular endothelial deposits of Gb_3 were cleared (reduced to normal or near-normal levels) [28]. As expected, there was a significant reduction in deposits in vascular endothelial cells in the patients given ERT compared with those given placebo; the latter group experienced the same effect when crossed over to receive ERT. No significant clinical effects were observed in this study [29], but the results did allow accelerated approval of agalsidase beta, dependent on post-approval commitments to providing phase IV data, by the Food and Drug Administration in the USA and in Europe and other countries.

In open-label studies, a decreased LVM was later reported after ERT with agalsidase beta [30] and also an improvement in peripheral nerve function [31]. More recently, a phase IV double-blind placebo-controlled trial in patients with mild renal insufficiency was completed. The data are as yet unpublished but suggest a trend towards slowing the decline in renal function in patients on ERT compared with those on placebo. A larger study, with more statistical power, is likely to provide a greater degree of confidence in the effect of ERT on renal function.

Conclusions

Fabry disease is unique among the lyso-somal storage diseases in its complexity and its multiple clinical manifestations. The childhood clinical abnormalities, such as painful small-fibre neuropathy, hypohidrosis and gastrointestinal disturbances, mainly affect quality of life but are potentially reversible with ERT. On the other hand, the cardiac, cerebrovascular and renal compli-cations develop over decades and therapy needs to be aimed at preventing these disease manifestations. ERT seems to reverse at least some of the complications of Fabry disease but it remains to be demon-strated whether it is able to prevent or delay renal, cardiac and cerebrovascular events and prolong patient survival. In the absence of controlled trials, it will be difficult to tease out its specific effects in adults, as they may be confounded by better general medical care. However, there is still an opportunity to demonstrate a preventive effect of ERT by providing such treatment to children of all ages and prospectively studying the effect of age at treatment initiation on these clinical outcomes using appropriate statistical methods.

References

1. de Duve C. From cytases to lysosomes. *Fed Proc* 1964;23:1045–9

2. Brady RO. The sphingolipidoses. *N Engl J Med* 1966;275:312–18

3. Sweeley CC, Klionsky B. Fabry's disease: classification as a sphingolipidosis and partial characterization of a novel glycolipid. *J Biol Chem* 1963;238:3148–50

4. Brady RO, Gal AE, Bradley RM, Martensson E. The metabolism of ceramide trihexosides. I. Purification and properties of an enzyme that cleaves the terminal galactose molecule of galactosylgalacto-sylglucosylceramide. *J Biol Chem* 1967;242:1021–6

5. Brady RO, Gal AE, Bradley RM, Martensson E, Warshaw AL, Laster L. Enzymatic defect in Fabry's disease. Ceramidetrihexosidase deficiency. *N Eng J Med* 1967;276:1163–7

6. Johnson W, Brady R. Ceramidetrihexosidase from human placenta. *Methods Enzymol* 1972;XXVIII: 849–56

7. Kusiak JW, Quirk JM, Brady RO. Purification and properties of the two major isozymes of α-galactosidase from human placenta. *J Biol Chem* 1978;253:184–90

8. Brady RO, Tallman JF, Johnson WG, Gal AE, Leahy WR, Quirk JM et al. Replacement therapy for in-herited enzyme deficiency. Use of purified ceramide-trihexosidase in Fabry's disease. *N Engl J Med* 1973;289:9–14

9. Desnick RJ, Dean KJ, Grabowski G, Bishop DF, Sweeley CC. Enzyme therapy in Fabry disease: differential *in vivo* plasma clearance and metabolic effectiveness of plasma and splenic α-galactosidase A isozymes. *Proc Natl Acad Sci USA* 1979;76:5326–30

10. Ohshima T, Murray GJ, Swaim WD, Longenecker G, Quirk JM, Cardarelli CO et al. α-Galactosidase A deficient mice: a model of Fabry disease. *Proc Natl Acad Sci USA* 1997;94:2540–4

11. Brady RO, Murray GJ, Moore DF, Schiffmann R. Enzyme replacement therapy in Fabry disease. *J Inherit Metab Dis* 2001;24 (Suppl 2):18–24; dis-cussion 11–12

12. Schiffmann R, Murray GJ, Treco D, Daniel P, Sellos-Moura M, Myers M et al. Infusion of α-galactosidase A reduces tissue globotriaosylceramide storage in patients with Fabry disease. *Proc Natl Acad Sci USA* 2000;97:365–70

13. Schiffmann R, Kopp JB, Austin HA 3rd, Sabnis S, Moore DF, Weibel T et al. Enzyme replacement therapy in Fabry disease: a randomized controlled trial. *JAMA* 2001;285:2743–9

14. Moore DF, Scott LT, Gladwin MT, Altarescu G, Kaneski C, Suzuki K et al. Regional cerebral hyperperfusion and nitric oxide pathway dysregulation in Fabry disease: reversal by enzyme replacement therapy. *Circulation* 2001;104:1506–12

15. Moore DF, Altarescu G, Herscovitch P, Schiffmann R. Enzyme replacement reverses abnormal cerebrovascular responses in Fabry disease. *BMC Neurol* 2002;2:4

16. Moore DF, Ye F, Brennan ML, Gupta S, Barshop BA, Steiner RD et al. Ascorbate decreases Fabry cerebral hyperperfusion suggesting a reactive oxygen species abnormality: an arterial spin tagging study. *J Magn Reson Imaging* 2004;20:674–83

17. Schiffmann R, Floeter MK, Dambrosia JM, Gupta S, Moore DF, Sharabi Y et al. Enzyme replacement therapy improves peripheral nerve and sweat function in Fabry disease. *Muscle Nerve* 2003;28:703–10

18. Scott LJ, Griffin JW, Luciano C, Barton NW, Banerjee T, Crawford T et al. Quantitative analysis of epidermal innervation in Fabry disease. *Neurology* 1999; 52:1249–54

19. Schiffmann R, Ries M, Timmons M, Flaherty J, Brady R. Long-term therapy with agalsidase alfa for Fabry disease: safety and effects on renal function in a home infusion setting. *Nephrol Dial Transplant* 2006;21:345–54

20. Schiffmann R, Hauer P, Freeman B, Ries M, Scott LJC, Polydefkis M et al. Enzyme replacement therapy and intra-epidermal innervation density in Fabry disease. *Muscle Nerve* 2006;Mar 31 [Epub ahead of print]

21. Branton MH, Schiffmann R, Sabnis SG, Murray GJ, Quirk JM. Altarescu G et al. Natural history of Fabry renal disease: influence of α-galactosidase A activity and genetic mutations on clinical course. *Medicine (Baltimore)* 2002;81:122–38

22. Ioannou YA, Zeidner KM, Gordon RE, Desnick RJ. Fabry disease: preclinical studies demonstrate the effectiveness of α-galactosidase A replacement in enzyme-deficient mice. *Am J Hum Genet* 2001;68:14–25

23. Eng CM, Banikazemi M, Gordon RE, Goldman M, Phelps R, Kim L et al. A phase 1/2 clinical trial of enzyme replacement in Fabry disease: pharmacokinetic, substrate clearance, and safety studies. *Am J Hum Genet* 2001;68:711–22

24. Beck M, Ricci R, Widmer U, Dehout F, de Lorenzo AG, Kampmann C et al. Fabry disease: overall effects of agalsidase alfa treatment. *Eur J Clin Invest* 2004; 34:838–44

25. Hoffmann B, Garcia de Lorenzo A, Mehta A, Beck M, Widmer U, Ricci R. Effects of enzyme replacement therapy on pain and health related quality of life in patients with Fabry disease: data from FOS (Fabry Outcome Survey). *J Med Genet* 2005;42:247–52

26. Gupta S, Ries M, Kotsopoulos S, Schiffmann R. The relationship of vascular glycolipid storage to clinical manifestations of Fabry disease: a cross-sectional study of a large cohort of clinically affected heterozygote women. *Medicine (Baltimore)* 2005;84:261–8

27. Whybra C, Kampmann C, Krummenauer F, Ries M, Mengel E, Miebach E et al. The Mainz Severity Score Index: a new instrument for quantifying the Anderson–Fabry disease phenotype, and the response of patients to enzyme replacement therapy. *Clin Genet* 2004;65:299–307

28. Eng CM, Guffon N, Wilcox WR, Germain DP, Lee P, Waldek S et al. Safety and efficacy of recombinant human α-galactosidase A replacement therapy in Fabry's disease. *N Engl J Med* 2001;345:9–16

29. Wilcox WR, Banikazemi M, Guffon N, Waldek S, Lee P, Linthorst GE et al. Long-term safety and efficacy of enzyme replacement therapy for Fabry disease. *Am J Hum Genet* 2004;75:65–74

30. Weidemann F, Breunig F, Beer M, Sandstede J, Turschner O, Voelker W et al. Improvement of cardiac function during enzyme replacement therapy in patients with Fabry disease: a prospective strain rate imaging study. *Circulation* 2003;108:1299–301

31. Hilz MJ, Brys M, Marthol H, Stemper B, Dutsch M. Enzyme replacement therapy improves function of C-, Aδ-, and Aβ-nerve fibers in Fabry neuropathy. *Neurology* 2004;62:1066–72

37 Enzyme replacement therapy and the heart

Christoph Kampmann

Universitäts-Kinderklinik, Langenbeckstrasse 1, D-55101 Mainz, Germany

The heart is one of the major organs affected in patients with Fabry disease. Globotriaosylceramide (Gb₃) deposits are found in nearly all cardiac structures, including the myocardium, endocardium, endothelium and conduction cells, and in the autonomic nervous system. Clinically, these alterations result in a broad spectrum of cardiac signs and symptoms: patients with Fabry disease may present with angina, dyspnoea, fatigue, palpitations, syncope and alterations in cardiac autonomic control. Almost all male patients with classic Fabry disease will develop hypertrophic cardiomyopathy during their 30s, while female patients typically do so in their late 40s. Continuous enzyme replacement therapy (ERT) with agalsidase alfa results in a dramatic improvement in clinical cardiac symptoms in a substantial number of patients. These findings are consistent over the duration of treatment. There is also a reduction in dyspnoea and fatigue, which seems to be related to a significant improvement in myocardial function, and regression of angina, which may be the result of the significant reduction in heart mass combined with the clearance or reduction of Gb₃ deposits from the endothelium of the coronary arteries. Preliminary results from ongoing studies show normalization of disturbed autonomic regulation. Whether ERT will lead to a reduction in rhythm disturbances is a matter of ongoing clinical studies.

Introduction

The heart is one of the major organs affected in patients with Fabry disease. Deposits of globotriaosylceramide (Gb₃) are found in almost all cardiac structures, including the myocardium, endocardium, endothelium and conduction cells, as well as in the autonomic nervous system, which partially regulates heart rate variability [1–4]. The involvement of each of the cardiac structures results in different alterations in the heart/cardiovascular system. Involvement of the myocardium leads to progressive hypertrophic cardiomyopathy of all cardiac chambers, with increasing wall thickness and progressive deterioration of systolic and diastolic function [1, 5]. If the endocardium is affected, there is progressive alteration of the mitral and aortic valves (mainly thickening of the leaflets), whereas when the endothelium of the coronary vessels is affected, progressive coronary syndrome occurs. Gb₃ deposition in the cells of the conduction system can result in complex arrhythmias [6, 7], and involvement of the autonomic nervous system can lead to progressive disturbances in the regulation of heart rate and its variability [8, 9]. Clinically, these alterations result in a broad spectrum of cardiac signs and symptoms: patients with Fabry disease may present with angina, dyspnoea, fatigue, palpitations and syncope. There is an extremely high concordance between the clinical course of the disease and the degree of cardiac involvement. Furthermore, severe cardiac alterations account for the majority of deaths and the

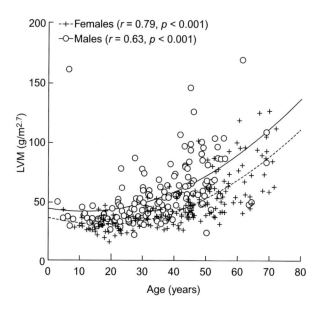

Figure 1. *Baseline cross-sectional data showing left ventricular mass (LVM) corrected for height in 182 female and 149 male patients with Fabry disease in FOS – the Fabry Outcome Survey.*

reduction in life expectancy and quality of life in patients with Fabry disease.

Although the inheritance of Fabry disease is X-chromosome linked, females are not just 'carriers' who transmit the disease, but are affected patients [10–12]. Observational studies, conducted in a large group of female patients with Fabry disease, showed that although heterozygous females usually develop signs and symptoms about 10–15 years later than males, these signs and symptoms ultimately develop to the same degree.

Almost all male patients with classic Fabry disease will develop hypertrophic cardiomyopathy during their 30s, while female patients typically do so in their late 40s. Data from FOS – the Fabry Outcome Survey – show that by approximately 36 years of age, 16–23% of patients suffer from angina, 22–28% from dyspnoea, 30–40% from fatigue, 13–16% from palpitations and 4–9% from syncope, regardless of gender.

Until 2001, when enzyme replacement therapy (ERT) was approved in Europe, only symptomatic treatment for Fabry disease was available, such as anti-congestive and anti-arrhythmic medication and, in the case of bradycardia, pacemaker implantation.

To understand the benefits of ERT on the heart, it is of utmost importance to recognize that cardiac involvement in Fabry disease progresses rapidly and is life threatening. The increase in left ventricular mass (LVM) (Figure 1) seen in untreated patients with Fabry disease results in a reduction in ventricular diastolic and systolic function. This can be demonstrated by measurement of midwall fractional shortening, which is a parameter of contractility and is decreased in hypertrophied hearts (Figure 2).

Potential of ERT in relation to cardiac involvement

In children and young adults, it is anticipated that ERT may be able to prevent development

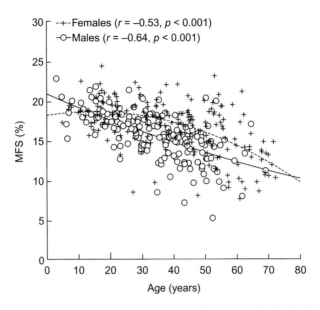

Figure 2. *Baseline cross-sectional data showing midwall fractional shortening (MFS) in 189 female and 159 male patients with Fabry disease in FOS – the Fabry Outcome Survey.*

of the serious cardiac alterations described above [13, 14]. However, it may not be possible to demonstrate the benefits of ERT until we have data from patients who have undergone continuous enzyme therapy over many years or even decades. In older patients, who already have extensive cardiac alterations, the situation is different because there is no way to reverse the damage caused by destruction of myocardial cells. Although the mechanisms of myocardial destruction in Fabry disease are not clearly understood, the myocardium loses its architecture and there is progressive fibrosis (or other causes of cell death) of contractile cells [10–12, 15–17].

Halting the progressive myocardial disease-related damage, slowing the speed of disease progression and reducing or normalizing heart mass and clinical symptoms are the aims of treatment. However, there are many factors that can affect the efficacy of treatment in individual patients. It has been shown for other lysosomal storage diseases,

such as Gaucher disease, that the general efficacy of ERT may be demonstrable within 2–3 years, whereas the appropriate individualization of dose may take much longer. Similarly, it can be speculated that dose individualization will take several more years of experience with ERT in Fabry disease because, to date, there is no surrogate marker that can be used to guide the enzyme replacement regimen.

Evidence of the benefits of ERT on cardiac manifestations

From the patients' perspective, the most important benefit of treatment is the reduction or elimination of clinical symptoms (e.g. a reduction or normalization of dyspnoea, angina, fatigue, palpitations and syncope). The first report of a biopsy-proven reduction of cardiac storage, regression of LVM and improvement of cardiac function in a patient with Fabry cardiomyopathy was described by Frustaci *et al.*, using infusions of high quantities of galactose, a competitive inhibitor of α-galactosidase A [5]. These changes were associated with enhanced residual enzyme activity. The major impact on LVM and function was believed to be related to a reduction in the size of auto-phagocytotic vacuoles within the myocardium.

The clinical improvement in systolic or diastolic function seen following ERT also seems to correlate with the reduction in myocardial mass [18]. It has been shown that ERT can remove Gb_3 deposits from endothelial cells in different organs [19, 20], but it remains questionable whether the removal of endothelial deposits from coronary arteries will improve coronary function [21].

Independently of age and gender, patients report a dramatic reduction in dyspnoea and angina within 6 months of starting ERT. Furthermore, observations over more than 4 years of continuous ERT revealed that, although Fabry disease is progressive in nature, no patient worsened clinically. It cannot be expected, however, that continuous ERT will eventually result in the total clearance of Gb_3 deposits from all cardiac tissues and structures, as Schiffmann et al. have shown that only the endothelial cells were cleared in a patient receiving recombinant α-galactosidase A over 2.5 years [22].

In phase III/IV double-blind placebo-controlled studies conducted in a small number of male patients at the Royal Free Hospital in London, UK, and at the Johannes Gutenberg University in Mainz, Germany, it was shown, using magnetic resonance imaging and echocardiography, that there was a reduction in LVM within 6 months of starting ERT with agalsidase alfa, compared with untreated patients [23, 24]. These findings were supported by open-label observations in female and male patients [25, 26].

Longitudinal multicentre echocardiographic follow-up examinations in a substantial number of patients showed that, within 1 year, there

was a substantial decrease in the thickness of the left ventricular walls (Figure 3a) and a reduction in LVM, which was combined with an increase in left ventricular midwall-related systolic function (Figure 4a). It was notable that there was normalization of mild cardiomyopathy in a number of patients. These findings have been consistent over the period of treatment.

Echocardiographic follow-up data from FOS over more than 3 years of ERT with agalsidase

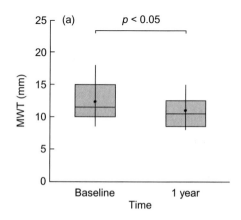

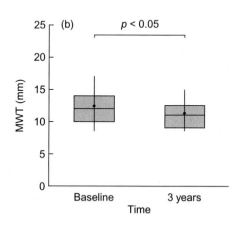

Figure 3. *Box plots of left ventricular mean wall thickness (MWT) at end-diastole in male and female patients with Fabry disease at baseline and after (a) 1 year (n = 83) and (b) 3 years (n = 75) of enzyme replacement therapy with agalsidase alfa. Means, dots; medians, horizontal lines; interquartile ranges, boxes; 10th–90th percentiles, vertical lines.*

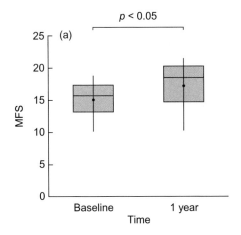

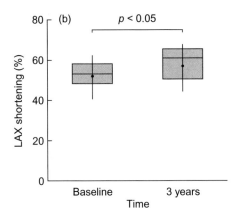

Figure 4. *Box plots of (a) left ventricular midwall fractional shortening (MFS) in male and female patients with Fabry disease at baseline and after 1 year of enzyme replacement therapy (ERT) with agalsidase alfa, and (b) left ventricular long-axis (LAX) (n = 79) shortening in male and female patients at baseline and after 3 years of ERT with agalsidase alfa (n = 52). Both midwall fractional shortening and long-axis shortening are parameters of left ventricular systolic function. Means, dots; medians, horizontal lines; interquartile ranges, boxes; 10th–90th percentiles, vertical lines.*

alfa showed that the left ventricular wall thickness decreased (Figure 3b) and systolic function improved (Figure 4b), underlining the consistency of treatment efficacy with agalsidase alfa over several years.

Follow-up of a small number of patients in whom ERT was interrupted revealed a rapid

increase in LVM combined with a new onset of dyspnoea, angina and palpitations, consecutively, followed by sudden death in one male patient. Thus, the benefits of ERT may be dependent on life-long enzyme substitution in order to avoid renewed deterioration.

Since ERT with agalsidase alfa has been available, many reports have been published documenting the different aspects of Fabry disease and the organ-specific effects of ERT. Nevertheless, there is much more to learn about the underlying pathophysiological mechanisms.

Conclusions

From the relatively limited experience of the effects of ERT on the heart, it can be concluded that continuous treatment with agalsidase alfa results in a dramatic improvement in cardiac symptoms in a substantial number of patients. The reduction and regression of dyspnoea and fatigue seem to be related to a significant improvement in myocardial function, and the regression of angina may be the result of the significant reduction in heart mass, combined with the clearance of Gb_3 deposits from the endothelium of the coronary arteries. Preliminary results from ongoing studies have shown normalization of disturbed autonomic regulation. Whether ERT will lead to a reduction in rhythm disturbances is currently being studied. To date, ERT does not serve as a substitute for other additive and supportive cardiac therapies, such as pacemaker implantation or anti-arrhythmic or anti-congestive medications, and specific cardiac treatment should not be withheld because a patient is receiving ERT.

References

1. Elleder M. New findings in pathology of storage. *Padiatr Padol* 1993;28:27–32

2. Kampmann C, Wiethoff CM, Perrot A, Beck M, Dietz R, Osterziel KJ. The heart in Anderson–Fabry disease. *Z Kardiol* 2002;91:786–95

3. Linhart A, Palecek T, Bultas J, Ferguson JJ, Hrudova J, Karetova D *et al.* New insights in cardiac structural

changes in patients with Fabry's disease. *Am Heart J* 2000;139:1101–8

4. Uchino M, Uyama E, Kawano H, Hokamaki J, Kugiyama K, Murakami Y *et al.* A histochemical and electron microscopic study of skeletal and cardiac muscle from a Fabry disease patient and carrier. *Acta Neuropathol (Berl)* 1995;90:334–8

5. Frustaci A, Chimenti C, Ricci R, Natale L, Russo MA, Pieroni M *et al.* Improvement in cardiac function in the cardiac variant of Fabry's disease with galactose-infusion therapy. *N Engl J Med* 2001;345:25–32

6. Igawa O, Miake J, Hisatome I. Ventricular tachy-cardias and dilated cardiomyopathy caused by Fabry disease. *Pacing Clin Electrophysiol* 2005;28:1142–3

7. Shah JS, Hughes DA, Sachdev B, Tome M, Ward D, Lee P *et al.* Prevalence and clinical significance of cardiac arrhythmia in Anderson–Fabry disease. *Am J Cardiol* 2005;96:842–6

8. Hilz MJ. Evaluation of peripheral and autonomic nerve function in Fabry disease. *Acta Paediatr Suppl* 2002;439:38–42

9. Hilz MJ, Brys M, Marthol H, Stemper B, Dutsch M. Enzyme replacement therapy improves function of C-, Aδ-, and Aβ-nerve fibers in Fabry neuropathy. *Neurology* 2004;62:1066–72

10. Kampmann C, Baehner F, Whybra C, Martin C, Wiethoff CM, Ries M *et al.* Cardiac manifestations of Anderson–Fabry disease in heterozygous females. *J Am Coll Cardiol* 2002;40:1668–74

11. Wendrich K, Whybra C, Ries M, Gal A, Beck M. Neurological manifestation of Fabry disease in females. *Contrib Nephrol* 2001;241–4

12. Whybra C, Kampmann C, Willers I, Davies J, Winchester B, Kriegsmann J *et al.* Anderson–Fabry disease: clinical manifestations of disease in female heterozygotes. *J Inherit Metab Dis* 2001;24:715–24

13. Ramaswami U, Whybra C, Parini R, Pintos-Morell G, Mehta A, Sunder-Plassmann G *et al.* Clinical mani-festations of Fabry disease in children: data from the Fabry Outcome Survey. *Acta Paediatr* 2006;95:86–92

14. Ries M, Ramaswami U, Parini R, Lindblad B, Whybra C, Willers I *et al.* The early clinical phenotype of Fabry disease: a study on 35 European children and adolescents. *Eur J Pediatr* 2003;162:767–72

15. Elleder M, Dorazilova V, Bradova V, Belohlavek M, Kral V, Choura M *et al.* [Fabry's disease with isolated disease of the cardiac muscle, manifesting as hypertrophic cardiomyopathy]. *Cas Lek Cesk* 1990; 129:369–72

16. Elleder M, Bradova V, Smid F, Budesinsky M, Harzer K, Kustermann-Kuhn B *et al.* Cardiocyte storage and

hypertrophy as a sole manifestation of Fabry's disease. Report on a case simulating hypertrophic non-obstructive cardiomyopathy. *Virchows Arch A Pathol Anat Histopathol* 1990;417:449–55

17. Koitabashi N, Utsugi T, Seki R, Okamoto E, Sando Y, Kaneko Y *et al.* Biopsy-proven cardiomyopathy in heterozygous Fabry's disease. *Jpn Circ J* 1999; 63:572–5

18. Weidemann F, Breunig F, Beer M, Sandstede J, Turschner O, Voelker W *et al.* Improvement of cardiac function during enzyme replacement therapy in patients with Fabry disease: a prospective strain rate imaging study. *Circulation* 2003;108:1299–301

19. Eng CM, Banikazemi M, Gordon RE, Goldman M, Phelps R, Kim L *et al.* A phase 1/2 clinical trial of enzyme replacement in Fabry disease: pharmaco-kinetic, substrate clearance, and safety studies. *Am J Hum Genet* 2001;68:711–22

20. Schiffmann R, Kopp JB, Austin HA 3rd, Sabnis S, Moore DF, Weibel T *et al.* Enzyme replacement therapy in Fabry disease: a randomized controlled trial. *JAMA* 2001;285:2743–9

21. Elliott PM, Kindler H, Shah JS, Sachdev B, Rimoldi OE, Thaman R *et al.* Coronary microvascular dysfunction in male patients with Anderson–Fabry disease and the effect of treatment with α-galac-tosidase A. *Heart* 2006;92:357–60

22. Schiffmann R, Rapkiewicz A, Abu-Asab M, Ries M, Askari H, Tsokos M *et al.* Pathological findings in a patient with Fabry disease who died after 2.5 years of enzyme replacement. *Virchows Arch* 2006;448: 337–43

23. Kampmann C, Ries M, Bähner F, Kim KS, Bajbouj M, Beck M. Influence of enzyme replacement therapy on Anderson–Fabry disease associated hypertrophic infiltrative cardio-myopathy. *Eur J Pediatr* 2002; 161:R5

24. MacDermot K, Brown A, Jones Y, Zuckerman J. Enzyme replacement therapy reverses the cardio-myopathy of Fabry disease; results of a randomized, double blind, placebo controlled trial. *Eur J Hum Gen* 2001;9:S92

25. Bähner F, Kampmann C, Whybra C, Miebach E, Wiethoff CM, Beck M. Enzyme replacement therapy in heterozygous females with Fabry disease: results of a phase IIIB study. *J Inherit Metab Dis* 2003; 26:617–27

26. Spinelli L, Pisani A, Sabbatini M, Petretta M, Andreucci MV, Procaccini D *et al.* Enzyme replace-ment therapy with agalsidase beta improves cardiac involvement in Fabry's disease. *Clin Genet* 2004; 66:158–65

38 Effect of enzyme replacement therapy with agalsidase alfa on renal function in patients with Fabry disease: data from FOS – the Fabry Outcome Survey

Andreas Schwarting[1], Gere Sunder-Plassmann[2], Atul Mehta[3] and Michael Beck[4]

[1]Department of Nephrology, University of Mainz, Langenbeckstrasse 1, 55101 Mainz, Germany; [2]Division of Nephrology and Dialysis, Department of Medicine III, Medical University Vienna, Währinger Gürtel 18–20, A-1090 Vienna, Austria; [3]Lysosomal Storage Disorders Unit, Department of Academic Haematology, Royal Free and University College Medical School, Rowland Hill Street, London NW3 2PF, UK; [4]Universitäts-Kinderklinik, Langenbeckstrasse 1, D-55101 Mainz, Germany

In the absence of large-scale placebo-controlled trials of enzyme replacement therapy (ERT) in patients with Fabry disease, FOS – the Fabry Outcome Survey – is providing valuable clinical data on the renal benefits of ERT with agalsidase alfa. Long-term longitudinal data in male and female patients with mild to moderate renal disease at baseline has clearly demonstrated a stabilization of renal function, compared with the decline seen in the period before treatment.

Introduction

Abnormalities of renal function are one of the most clinically significant features of Fabry disease and constitute an important cause of premature morbidity and mortality. Renal disease is often observed early in the course of Fabry disease [1] and is characterized by microalbuminuria, proteinuria, hypertension and a decreased glomerular filtration rate (GFR). It may ultimately progress to end-stage renal disease (ESRD) [2–6]. These abnormalities affect both males and females, although ESRD is uncommon in females. The renal manifestations of Fabry disease are discussed fully in Chapter 21.

Until recently, the clinical management of patients with Fabry disease was limited to symptomatic and supportive therapies only. Enzyme replacement therapy (ERT) with agalsidase alfa was licensed by the European Agency for the Evaluation of Medicinal Products in August 2001. The initial trials that led to the introduction of ERT focused on the effects of enzyme replacement on pain. However, patients in the early randomized double-blind trials of both agalsidase alfa [7] and agalsidase beta [8] underwent serial renal biopsies, which revealed that ERT had significant beneficial effects on renal histology. These included reduction in endothelial cell globotriaosylceramide content, reduction in mesangial widening and an increase in the number of histologically normal glomeruli. Most patients in the initial studies had normal renal function. There are no placebo-controlled studies assessing the impact of ERT on renal function in patients with Fabry disease. The effects of this intervention therefore have to be assessed using data from outcomes databases such as FOS – the Fabry Outcome Survey. There are, however, difficulties associated with such outcome studies (Chapter 14). The specific problems relating to assessing the impact of ERT on renal function in a patient database are described below.

Difficulties with registry studies
Measurement of outcome

The first issue is how should outcome be measured? One of the earliest signs of renal involvement in Fabry disease is the loss of the concentrating ability of the kidneys. However, isosthenuria is not easily detectable by routine methods. Proteinuria is another important feature of renal damage, although it is variable from day to day and depends on the GFR; a decline in the GFR, for example, is accompanied by reduced amounts of filtered protein. Thus, proteinuria should be adjusted for the amount of creatinine in the urine. In addition, females with Fabry disease frequently have proteinuria but only rarely develop ESRD, and proteinuria is often found in asymptomatic children. Overall, therefore, proteinuria does not appear to be a good index of the extent of renal damage, although the presence or absence of proteinuria (or the onset of microalbuminuria) may be a useful marker of the onset of damage and an indication to start ERT.

The GFR may be a better indicator of renal function, although there are issues concerning its measurement. It is convenient to estimate GFR from serum creatinine using the short MDRD (Modification of Diet in Renal Disease) formula, but this formula is not applicable to all categories of patients and has not been validated in children or in patients with normal or near-normal renal function. Creatinine clearance is not always an accurate measure of renal function and should be corrected for muscle mass, age, gender and race. In addition, it is essential that urine collections should be complete. Within an outcomes database, the patients who have been included will have undergone diverse measurements, and this variability may introduce further errors. A radioactive chromium-EDTA or DTPA clearance measurement is generally considered the 'gold standard', but has not been applied uniformly in FOS. Patients at an early stage of renal impairment may have a period of hyperfiltration; thus an elevated GFR (> 150 ml/min/1.73 m^2 in patients older than 18 years) may indicate early renal involvement.

Effect of concomitant medication

Another issue is that patients' concomitant medication is subject to variation. An improvement in pain may lead to a reduction in analgesic consumption that may, in turn, lead to an improvement in renal function. The successful treatment of blood pressure and, especially, the use of angiotensin-converting enzyme (ACE) inhibitors or angiotensin receptor blockers may result in a reduction in progression of renal failure, which is independent of the effect of concomitant ERT.

Database deficiencies

A third issue is that FOS is a multicentre outcomes survey. As such, the database lacks the consistency of a clinical trial, although there are basic similarities in the procedures used at each of the different participating centres. In addition, long-term follow-up data may be incomplete, and there is an ongoing need within such databases to maximize data recording.

Different organ systems

Finally, the effects of ERT are not necessarily consistent across different organ systems. Thus, a patient may demonstrate improvement in cardiac parameters (including reduction in left ventricular mass) and yet show deterioration in GFR, or may report substantial improvements in pain but little or no improvement in cardiac parameters.

Baseline characteristics of the patient cohort

The data reported here are from an analysis of the FOS database conducted in March 2005. At that time, there were 74 centres participating in FOS located in 11 European countries. These centres had enrolled a total of 688 patients, 401 of whom were receiving ERT with agalsidase alfa, with the remainder not receiving ERT. Of these 688 patients, 330 were male (including 50 boys < 18 years of age) and 358 were female (including 69 girls < 18 years of age). The age range of male patients was 0.75–80.9 years and for females was 2.5–78.5 years.

Of the 401 patients who were receiving ERT, 160 were female and 241 were male. These 401 patients included 55 children (31 boys, 24 girls). The age range of treated patients was 3.5–68.9 years for males and 3.5–76.1 years for females.

Duration of ERT and age at the start of treatment

The duration of agalsidase alfa therapy amongst the 401 treated patients is illustrated in Figure 1. In total, 219 patients (71 females, 148 males) had been receiving agalsidase alfa for 2 or more years, and 133 (31 females, 102 males) of these had been treated for 3 or more years. The age of patients at the start of agalsidase alfa therapy is shown in Figure 2, which illustrates the older age of female patients than male patients at the commencement of ERT. Although the mean and median ages at which patients with Fabry disease commenced agalsidase alfa therapy remained essentially unchanged between 2001 and 2004/2005, the range

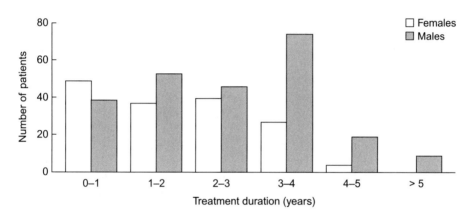

Figure 1. *Duration of treatment with agalsidase alfa in the 401 treated patients enrolled in FOS – the Fabry Outcome Survey – as of March 2005.*

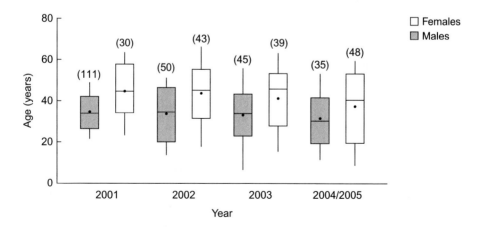

Figure 2. *Age at the start of treatment with agalsidase alfa in patients enrolled in FOS – the Fabry Outcome Survey – between 2001 and 2004/2005. Plots show means (dots), medians (horizontal lines) and 10th, 25th, 75th and 90th percentiles (box and whiskers) for the number of patients in parentheses.*

increased, demonstrating a progressively greater proportion of both younger and older patients starting treatment over time.

Symptom severity at the start of ERT

The Mainz Severity Score Index (MSSI) [9] is an overall measure of the clinical severity of Fabry disease. The scoring system has been adapted for use in FOS (FOS-MSSI), omitting the renal and cardiac laboratory assessments included in the original MSSI score (see Chapter 32). Figure 3 displays the severity of Fabry disease manifestations as assessed by the FOS-MSSI for patients commencing treatment between 2001 and 2004/05. The mean and median pretreatment FOS-MSSI scores declined over time between 2001 and 2004/05, indicating that physicians chose initially to commence agalsidase alfa therapy in the most severely symptomatic patients and later extended ERT to less severely affected patients, including a greater proportion of children and females.

Renal function before the start of ERT

Figure 4 shows renal function, presented as the estimated GFR (eGFR) calculated using the MDRD equation, prior to the start of ERT with agalsidase alfa and classified according to gender and year of commencement of ERT. The analysis includes all patients with eGFR data available at baseline who subsequently received agalsidase alfa (297 of the 401 treated patients). For males, the mean and median severity of renal dysfunction at the start of ERT with agalsidase alfa has decreased over time. Most patients commencing ERT have a baseline eGFR between 60 and 90 ml/min/1.73 m^2, which is defined as stage 2 chronic kidney disease (CKD) by the Kidney Disease Outcomes Quality Initiative classification.

Agalsidase alfa therapy and renal function

Figure 5 depicts the change in eGFR among adult patients with Fabry disease who have received agalsidase alfa therapy for 1, 2 or 3 years. All patients had renal involvement before treatment, with eGFR values in the range 30–89 ml/min/1.73 m^2. Data are excluded for those patients who were less than 18 years of age at the start of ERT, had normal renal function at baseline or had more than a 3-month interruption of ERT. An annual rate of decline

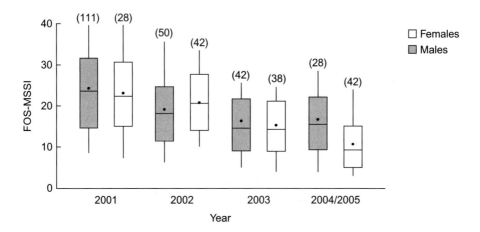

Figure 3. *Overall severity of Fabry disease in patients enrolled in FOS – the Fabry Outcome Survey – between 2001 and 2004/5. Disease severity is shown at the start of treatment with agalsidase alfa, and was assessed using the FOS adaptation of the Mainz Severity Score Index (FOS-MSSI), with higher scores indicating a greater disease severity. Plots show means (dots), medians (horizontal lines) and 10th, 25th, 75th and 90th percentiles (box and whiskers) for the number of patients in parentheses.*

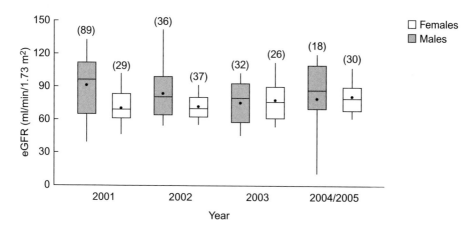

Figure 4. *Renal function in patients with Fabry disease enrolled in FOS – the Fabry Outcome Survey – between 2001 and 2004/5. Renal function is shown at the start of treatment with agalsidase alfa, and is presented as the estimated glomerular filtration rate (eGFR) derived from the Modification of Diet in Renal Disease equation. Plots show means (dots), medians (horizontal lines) and 10th, 25th, 75th and 90th percentiles (box and whiskers) for the number of patients in parentheses.*

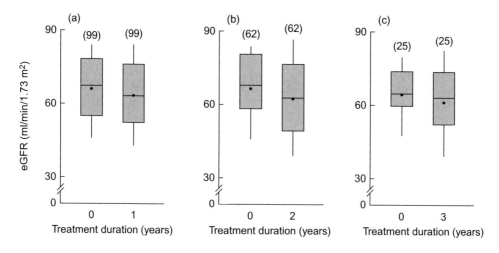

Figure 5. *The change in estimated glomerular filtration rate (eGFR) in all adult patients with Fabry disease in FOS – the Fabry Outcome Survey – after receiving agalsidase alfa therapy for (a) 1, (b) 2 or (c) 3 years. All patients had renal involvement before treatment, with eGFR values in the range 30–89 ml/min/1.73 m², as calculated using the Modification of Diet in Renal Disease equation. Plots show means (dots), medians (horizontal lines) and 10th, 25th, 75th and 90th percentiles (box and whiskers) for the number of patients in parentheses.*

in GFR of approximately 12 ml/minute in untreated patients with Fabry disease was demonstrated by Branton and colleagues [10]. In comparison with this benchmark, agalsidase alfa therapy appears to slow the decline in renal function in adult patients with Fabry disease with a baseline eGFR of 30–89 ml/min/1.73 m². Mean and median eGFR values at baseline and after 1, 2 and 3 years of agalsidase alfa therapy are summarized by gender in Table 1. The effect of agalsidase alfa in preserving renal function was approximately equal in males and females. After 2 years of treatment, only one out of 28 males experienced a fall in eGFR below 30 ml/min/1.73 m². Likewise, among the 34 female patients, only one experienced a fall in eGFR below 30 ml/min/1.73 m² (declining to 29.97 ml/min/1.73 m²) during 2 years of agalsidase alfa therapy.

Figure 6 and Table 2 show the serial changes in eGFR for patients with a baseline eGFR of 30–89 ml/min/1.73 m² after 2 and 3 years of ERT in a subgroup of patients for whom complete serial eGFR values were available. Again, these data clearly demonstrate a stabilization of renal function after long-term treatment with agalsidase alfa.

Detailed analysis of the FOS database reveals two further lines of evidence, that strongly support a beneficial effect of agalsidase alfa treatment on renal function.

The first of these analyses involved a subgroup of patients for whom GFR data were available from 1 year before treatment, at the start of treatment (baseline) and 1 year after the start of treatment (12 patients with CKD stage 2 and 8 patients with CKD stage 3 at baseline). Renal function in the 12 patients (10 females and 2 males; mean age, 40 years; range, 19–71 years) with baseline CKD stage 2 declined significantly ($p < 0.05$) in the year before the start of treatment. There was a similar decline in renal function in the eight patients (4 females and 4 males; mean age, 49 years; range, 29–69 years) with CKD stage 3 during the year before the start of treatment, although this did not reach significance.

Table 1. *Changes in estimated glomerular filtration rate (eGFR) in adult patients with Fabry disease in FOS – the Fabry Outcome Survey – after receiving agalsidase alfa therapy for 1, 2 or 3 years. All patients had renal involvement before treatment, with eGFR values in the range 30–89 ml/min/1.73 m², as calculated using the Modification of Diet in Renal Disease equation.*

Gender	n	Mean age (years)	Time point	eGFR (ml/min/1.73 m²)	
				Mean	Median (range)
Patients given 1 year of therapy with agalsidase alfa					
Female	52	48.3	Baseline	66.8	66.7 (32.0–89.5)
			Year 1	65.2	64.5 (29.3–87.4)
Male	47	41.9	Baseline	66.0	68.3 (38.4–89.5)
			Year 1	63.2	61.7 (26.1–113.0)
Patients given 2 years of therapy with agalsidase alfa					
Female	34	48.3	Baseline	65.6	64.3 (32.0–89.5)
			Year 2	63.1	63.5 (30.0–97.7)
Male	28	40.3	Baseline	69.4	73.1 (39.4–89.5)
			Year 2	63.3	63.0 (12.8–92.4)
Patients given 3 years of therapy with agalsidase alfa					
Female	13	45.5	Baseline	68.4	64.2 (47.6–89.5)
			Year 3	66.3	65.6 (48.9–88.2)
Male	12	40.7	Baseline	65.6	69.3 (38.4–84.5)
			Year 3	60.6	62.4 (23.9–91.2)

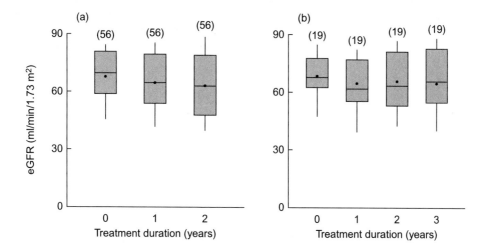

Figure 6. *Serial changes in estimated glomerular filtration rate (eGFR) after (a) 2 and (b) 3 years of agalsidase alfa therapy in all adult patients with Fabry disease in FOS – the Fabry Outcome Survey. All patients had a baseline eGFR of 30–89 ml/min/1.73 m², as calculated using the Modification of Diet in Renal Disease equation. Plots show means (dots), medians (horizontal lines) and 10th, 25th, 75th and 90th percentiles (box and whiskers) for the number of patients in parentheses.*

Table 2. *Changes in estimated glomerular filtration rate (eGFR) in adult patients with Fabry disease in FOS – the Fabry Outcome Survey – after receiving agalsidase alfa therapy. Data are given for subsets of patients with complete serial eGFR values over 2 or 3 years of treatment. The baseline eGFR was 30–89 ml/min/1.73 m², as calculated using the Modification of Diet in Renal Disease equation.*

				eGFR (ml/min/1.73 m²)	
Gender	**n**	**Mean age (years)**	**Time point**	**Mean**	**Median (range)**
Patients given 2 years of therapy with agalsidase alfa					
Female	30	47.4	Baseline	66.2	66.0 (32.0–89.5)
			Year 1	63.5	62.8 (29.3–86.4)
			Year 2	63.1	63.5 (30.0–93.4)
Male	25	40.0	Baseline	69.5	74.9 (39.4–89.5)
			Year 1	65.9	67.7 (26.1–103.9)
			Year 2	63.3	60.7 (12.9–92.4)
Patients given 3 years of therapy with agalsidase alfa					
Female	9	43.2	Baseline	66.4	64.2 (47.6–89.5)
			Year 1	62.6	61.4 (39.0–82.0)
			Year 2	64.5	63.1 (46.6–93.4)
			Year 3	63.6	64.3 (48.9–88.2)
Male	10	40.1	Baseline	70.1	73.4 (39.9–84.5)
			Year 1	66.0	65.1 (34.4–96.4)
			Year 2	66.6	63.0 (43.2–86.7)
			Year 3	66.2	72.3 (34.1–91.2)

After 1 year of treatment, however, the progressive loss of GFR had been stabilized in both groups of patients (Figure 7a [11]).

In 13 of these 20 patients, follow-up data for 2 years after the start of treatment were available (8 patients with CKD stage 2 and 5 patients with CKD stage 3 at baseline). Again, in contrast to the decline in GFR before the start of ERT, renal function remained stable in both groups over 2 years (Figure 7b [11]). There was no clear effect of concomitant therapy in these 20 patients; five used ACE inhibitors or angiotensin receptor blockers at the start of ERT, another five used these drugs at other times, and information on concomitant renal-protective medication was not available for the remaining ten patients.

The second analysis of FOS data involved a multivariate study of 1040 serum creatinine measurements from 201 patients with Fabry disease, aged 20–60 years. All patients had serum creatinine concentrations below 2 mg/dl and had received ERT with agalsidase alfa for up to 4.7 years. Both pretreatment and treatment data were used to examine independent predictors of changes in serum creatinine.

Independent positive associations were found between serum creatinine concentrations and age, gender and body mass index (BMI) (all $p < 0.01$) and an inverse association was noted between serum creatinine and time on agalsidase alfa therapy ($p < 0.05$, $R^2 = 23\%$) (Table 3), as defined by the following equation:

$$\text{Serum creatinine} = 0.662 + (0.003 \times \text{age}) + 0.007(\text{age} \times \text{gender}) + (0.005 \times \text{BMI}) - 0.017(\text{ERT} \times \text{treatment duration}).$$

Effect of agalsidase alfa on renal function in children

To assess renal function in paediatric patients with Fabry disease, the Counahan–Barratt equation [12] was used to determine

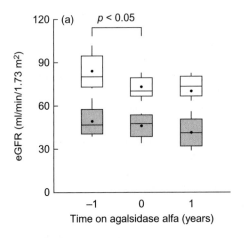
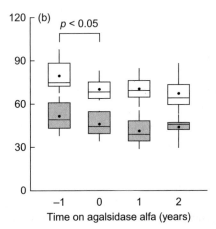

Figure 7. *Serial changes in estimated glomerular filtration rate (eGFR) in adult patients with Fabry disease enrolled in FOS – the Fabry Outcome Survey. Patients were followed from 1 year before the start of treatment with agalsidase alfa to (a) 1 year and (b) 2 years after the start of treatment. The eGFR was calculated using the Modification of Diet in Renal Disease equation. Plots show means (dots), medians (horizontal lines) and 10th, 25th, 75th and 90th percentiles (box and whiskers) for (a) twelve patients with stage 2 and eight patients with stage 3 renal disease at baseline, and (b) eight patients with stage 2 and five patients with stage 3 renal disease at baseline. Open boxes, stage 2 renal disease; shaded boxes, stage 3 renal disease. Reproduced with permission from [11].*

Table 3. *Independent associations of serum creatinine with time on agalsidase alfa enzyme replacement therapy (ERT) in 201 patients with Fabry disease in FOS – the Fabry Outcome Survey.*

	Independent variable	*p*
Age	0.0028	< 0.0001
Age × gender	0.0072	< 0.0001
Body mass index	0.0053	0.004
Time × ERT	−0.0171	0.04

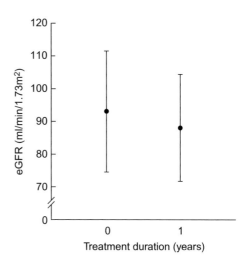

Figure 8. *Mean change in estimated glomerular filtration rate (eGFR) in patients with Fabry disease who were under 18 years of age at enrolment in FOS – the Fabry Outcome Survey – at baseline and after 1 year of treatment with agalsidase alfa. The eGFR was calculated using the Counahan–Barratt equation [12]. Values are means ± SD for 21 patients.*

the eGFR at baseline and after 1 year of agalsidase alfa therapy. Figure 8 gives the mean eGFR at baseline and after 1 year of agalsidase alfa therapy for 21 of 55 paediatric patients treated with agalsidase alfa for whom serum creatinine data were available. Mean and median values for eGFR at baseline and after 1 year of agalsidase alfa therapy are summarized by gender in Table 4.

At baseline, 12 of the 21 patients had eGFR values less than 90 ml/min/1.73 m^2 and seven patients had normal eGFR values in the range of 90–135 ml/min/1.73 m^2. The remaining two patients (boys aged 3.4 and 12.7 years) had baseline eGFR values above 135 ml/min/1.73 m^2. From the preliminary paediatric data presented in Figure 8 and Table 4, it can be concluded that renal function, on average, remained stable in this subgroup of patients receiving agalsidase alfa therapy for 1 year, as would be expected at this early stage of the disease. The small decrease in mean eGFR was driven by the two children with a high eGFR at baseline. Both of these boys showed apparent 'improvement' in their renal function after 1 year of agalsidase alfa therapy, as indicated by a large decrease in their eGFR from above 135 ml/min/1.73 m^2 to less than 99 ml/min/1.73 m^2. This preliminary conclusion, however, must be considered tentative in view of the small number of patients and the recognized unreliability of eGFR values above 90 ml/min/1.73 m^2.

Effect of agalsidase alfa on proteinuria

Figure 9 depicts the effects of agalsidase alfa treatment on proteinuria (measured as total protein in 24-hour urine collections). In 40 patients with longitudinal data on proteinuria at the start and after 1 and 2 years of treatment, no significant change could be detected (Figure 9a). Similarly, in a group of 12 patients with longitudinal data available over a 3-year treatment period, ERT with agalsidase did not affect the mean or median levels of proteinuria. It should be remembered, however, that there are limitations concerning the use of proteinuria as an accurate measure of renal damage.

Discussion and conclusions

ERT with agalsidase alfa leads to stabilization of renal function in patients with CKD stages 1 and 2. Among 17 male patients receiving ERT and with a baseline eGFR in

Table 4. *Mean and median changes in estimated glomerular filtration rate (eGFR) in patients with Fabry disease who were under 18 years of age at enrolment in FOS – the Fabry Outcome Survey – at baseline and after 1 year of treatment with agalsidase alfa. The eGFR was calculated using the Counahan–Barratt equation [12].*

Gender	n	Mean age at baseline (years)	Time point	eGFR (ml/min/1.73 m²) Mean	eGFR (ml/min/1.73 m²) Median (range)
Girls	9	14.1	Baseline	87.5	87.9 (70.7–101.4)
			Year 1	82.2	77.4 (71.5–100.0)
Boys	12	10.7	Baseline	97.3	87.1 (75.7–146.4)
			Year 1	93.8	90.7 (77.0–150.5)

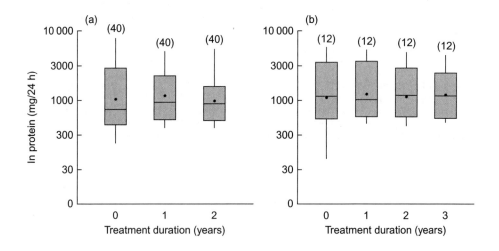

Figure 9. *Effect of agalsidase alfa on proteinuria in (a) 40 adult patients treated for 2 years and (b) 12 adult patients treated for 3 years in FOS – the Fabry Outcome Survey. The patients were followed longitudinally, and proteinuria was measured in 24-hour urine samples. Plots show means (dots), medians (horizontal lines) and 10th, 25th, 75th and 90th percentiles (box and whiskers) for the number of patients in parentheses. Note the natural log (ln) scale.*

the range 30–60 ml/min/1.73 m² (stage 3 CKD), mean eGFR declined by less than 4 ml/min/1.73 m² per year. The rate of decline in GFR of 12.2 ml/min/1.73 m² per year reported by Branton *et al.* [10] in a cohort of 39 comparable untreated male patients with Fabry disease is clearly much higher than the values observed in patients who were receiving ERT with agalsidase alfa in FOS. In fact, more than half (62.5%) of the

39 patients reported by Branton *et al.* progressed to ESRD within 4 years, whereas none of the patients in FOS progressed to ESRD during 30–54 months of treatment. Renal function in both men and women with a baseline eGFR of 60–90 ml/min/1.73 m² (stage 2 CKD) was stabilized after 1–2 years of ERT following a deterioration in the year before treatment. Further long-term analyses of renal data from the increasing numbers of

patients receiving agalsidase alfa in FOS should not only further demonstrate the beneficial effects on renal function in adults, but should also help to determine whether ERT prevents the development of renal disease in patients starting treatment in childhood.

References

1. Ramaswami U, Whybra C, Parini R, Pintos-Morell G, Mehta A, Sunder-Plassmann G et al. Clinical manifestations of Fabry disease in children: data from the Fabry Outcome Survey. Acta Paediatr 2006;95:86–92

2. MacDermot KD, Holmes A, Miners AH. Anderson–Fabry disease: clinical manifestations and impact of disease in a cohort of 60 obligate carrier females. J Med Genet 2001;38:769–75

3. MacDermot KD, Holmes A, Miners AH. Anderson–Fabry disease: clinical manifestations and impact of disease in a cohort of 98 hemizygous males. J Med Genet 2001;38:750–60

4. Whybra C, Kampmann C, Willers I, Davies J, Winchester B, Kriegsmann J et al. Anderson–Fabry disease: clinical manifestations of disease in female heterozygotes. J Inherit Metab Dis 2001;24:715–24

5. Mehta A, Ricci R, Widmer U, Dehout F, Garcia de Lorenzo A, Kampmann C et al. Fabry disease defined: baseline clinical manifestations of 366 patients in the Fabry Outcome Survey. Eur J Clin Invest 2004;34:236–42

6. Deegan P, Bähner AF, Barba-Romero MA, Hughes D, Kampmann C, Beck M. Natural history of Fabry disease in females in the Fabry Outcome Survey. J Med Genet 2006;43:347–52

7. Schiffmann R, Kopp JB, Austin HA III, Sabnis S, Moore DF, Weibel T et al. Enzyme replacement therapy in Fabry disease: a randomized controlled trial. JAMA 2001;285:2743–9

8. Eng CM, Guffon N, Wilcox WR, Germain DP, Lee P, Waldek S. Safety and efficacy of recombinant human α-galactosidase A replacement therapy in Fabry's disease. N Engl J Med 2001;345:9–16

9. Whybra C, Kampmann C, Krummenauer F, Ries M, Mengel E, Miebach E et al. The Mainz Severity Score Index: a new instrument for quantifying the Anderson–Fabry disease phenotype, and the response of patients to enzyme replacement therapy. Clin Genet 2004;65:299–307

10. Branton MH, Schiffmann R, Sabnis SG, Murray GJ, Quirk JM, Altarescu G et al. Natural history of Fabry renal disease: influence of α-galactosidase A activity and genetic mutations on clinical course. Medicine (Baltimore) 2002;81:122–38

11. Schwarting A, Dehout F, Feriozzi S, Beck M, Mehta A, Sunder-Plassmann G. Enzyme replacement therapy and renal function in 201 patients with Fabry disease. Clin Nephrol 2006 (In press)

12. Counahan R, Chantler C, Ghazali S, Kirkwood B, Rose F, Barratt TM. Estimation of glomerular filtration rate from plasma creatinine concentration in children. Arch Dis Child 1976;51:875–8

39 Neurological effects of enzyme replacement therapy in Fabry disease

Raphael Schiffmann[1] and David F Moore[2]

[1]Developmental and Metabolic Neurology Branch, National Institute of Neurological Disorders and Stroke, Building 10, Room 3D03, National Institutes of Health, Bethesda, Maryland 20892-1260, USA; [2]Section of Neurology, Department of Internal Medicine, University of Manitoba, Winnipeg, Canada

Enzyme replacement therapy (ERT) reverses the resting hyperperfusion and the abnormal regional vascular reactivity response induced by acetazolamide. ERT also normalizes the blunted cerebral perfusion response to ascorbate and reduces 3-nitro-tyrosine staining of dermal blood vessels. The function of the peripheral nervous system is also improved by ERT, with reduction in neuropathic pain and an improvement in the detection threshold for cold and warm sensation in the hands and feet. Improvement in sweating and heat tolerance has also been recorded following ERT. Despite these positive results, ERT does not completely normalize the function of the peripheral nervous system, and a reduction in the incidence of stroke remains to be demonstrated.

Introduction

Enzyme replacement therapy (ERT) is the first specific therapy for Fabry disease. It has been available only for the past 5–6 years, so it is a little early to reach any definitive conclusions about whether this therapy can reduce the morbidity associated with CNS disorders, such as stroke. In order to appreciate fully the difficulty in assessing the effect of ERT on the neurological aspects of Fabry disease, one needs to understand the nature of these abnormalities (see also Chapter 22). In general, neurological abnormalities (as well as non-neurological abnormalities) associated with Fabry disease can be divided into potentially reversible deficits/abnormalities, such as hypohidrosis, neuropathic pain or thermal sensation deficits, and non-reversible but preventable deficits, such as ischaemic stroke [1]. One might expect that it would be easier to assess the effect of ERT on potentially reversible aspects of Fabry disease than on, for example, reduction of stroke risk. The latter can be demonstrated prospectively only by observational studies on a relatively large cohort of patients over a prolonged period of time. The relatively low rate of stroke events makes the demonstration of the effect of a preventive therapy particularly difficult in a rare disease with few affected patients. Furthermore, general therapies, such as antiplatelet agents and statins, are highly effective in stroke prevention, making it very difficult to identify the specific effects of ERT [2, 3].

In this chapter, we concentrate on the effect of ERT on vascular dysfunction, small-fibre neuropathy (pain and thermal threshold), hypohidrosis and the incidence of stroke in patients with Fabry disease.

Effect of ERT on the vasculopathy of Fabry disease

Because of the expected difficulty in demonstrating an effect of ERT on stroke risk, we hypothesized that the vasculopathy of Fabry disease is associated with abnormalities in blood components, blood flow and vascular wall or endothelial function (Virchow's triad), resulting in vascular dysfunction and representing a vascular diathesis. If so, this vascular diathesis should improve with disease-specific therapy and potentially serve as a surrogate indicator of vascular risk reduction, including ischaemic stroke [4]. As described in Chapter 22, we found that a prothrombotic state exists in patients with Fabry disease, with cerebral hyperperfusion and an excessively prolonged vasodilatory response to acetazolamide (altered arterial wall reactivity) [5], increased nitrotyrosine staining in dermal blood vessels and a delayed decrease in cerebral perfusion in response to ascorbate [4].

The effect of ERT on cerebral vascular perfusion and function was examined as part of two 6-month randomized controlled trials of agalsidase alfa conducted at the National Institutes of Health (NIH; Bethesda, MD, USA). In our initial study, using $H_2{}^{15}O$ and positron emission tomography (PET), we found a significant decrease in resting cerebral blood flow in patients on ERT compared with the placebo group (Figure 1). This indicates at least a partial reversal of the cerebral hyperperfusion seen in this disorder [4]. The decrease in resting cerebral blood flow was confirmed using two other methods, one for measuring blood perfusion and the other for measuring cerebral blood flow velocity (transcranial Doppler) [6, 7].

In the initial study, we also examined the response of the cerebral vasculature to acetazolamide, a drug that maximally dilates the cerebral blood vessels by decreasing the pH of the extracellular space of the vessel wall [8]. Cerebral blood vessels of patients with Fabry disease remained maximally dilated significantly longer than controls [5]. We found that agalsidase alfa reverses the excessive reactivity to acetazolamide compared with placebo after 6 months of treatment (Figure 2). This finding suggested an altered cerebral

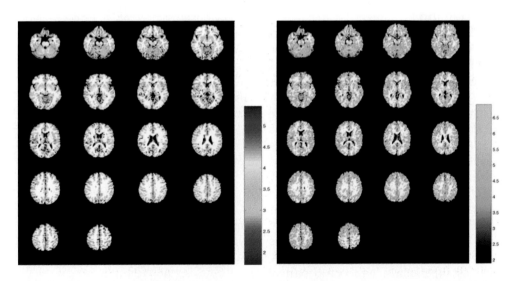

Figure 1. *(Left panel) Regional cerebral blood flow (rCBF) standard parametric t-mapping (SPM{t}) showing significantly increased blood flow in patients with Fabry disease (n = 26) compared with controls (n = 10) after template co-registration of individual positron emission tomography (PET) studies. (Right panel) Resting rCBF SPM{t} map showing significantly decreased rCBF in patients on enzyme replacement therapy (n = 14) compared with the placebo group (n = 12) after template co-registration of individual PET studies. No significant decrease in rCBF occurred in the placebo group compared with the treated group. Increasing SPM{t} voxel values above the threshold are shown by the coloured bars. Reproduced with permission from [4].*

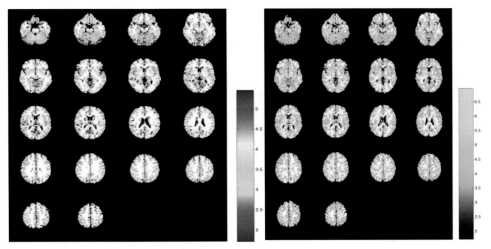

Figure 2. *Regional cerebral blood flow (rCBF) standard parametric t-mapping (SPM{t}) after an acetazolamide challenge, showing significantly increased blood flow in patients with Fabry disease (n = 26) compared with normal controls (n = 10). (Left panel) The rCBF 30 minutes after infusion of acetazolamide was significantly greater in patients with Fabry disease in many brain regions, with a posterior predominance. No significant rCBF elevation was found in the control group compared with Fabry patients (results not shown). (Right panel) SPM{t} map showing significantly lower rCBF 30 minutes after acetazolamide challenge in patients given enzyme replacement therapy (n = 13) compared with the placebo group (n = 9). Increasing SPM{t} voxel values above the threshold are shown by the coloured bars. Reproduced with permission from [5].*

vasomotor tone in the blood vessels of patients with α-galactosidase A deficiency, and may be related to the mechanism of the dilated cerebral vasculopathy or dolichoectasia noted in Fabry disease. As evidence of cellular access of intravenously infused α-galactosidase A beyond the vascular endothelial cells is lacking, the improved response to acetazolamide suggests a role for vascular endothelial cells in the CNS aspects of Fabry disease.

In another randomized placebo-controlled trial, we tested the hypothesis that reactive oxygen species (ROS) contribute to the cerebral hyperperfusion in Fabry disease by assessing the response of cerebral blood flow to the intravenous infusion of 1 g ascorbate over 4 minutes, a known scavenger of ROS [9]. This study, using quantitative arterial spin tagging and magnetic resonance imaging, confirmed the cerebral hyperperfusion seen with PET, and also demonstrated that healthy controls and patients on ERT responded similarly to ascorbate infusion by a decrease in cerebral blood flow [6]. The patients on placebo had a significant delay in the reduction of cerebral blood flow, again suggesting a defect in vessel reactivity, possibly due to an excess production of ROS in Fabry disease (Figure 3) [6]. This finding was supported by the observation of significantly increased staining for 3-nitrotyrosine in dermal and cerebral blood vessels of patients with Fabry disease [4] and in the increased 3-nitrotyrosine and myeloperoxidase in the blood of patients with the disease compared with controls [6]. In the initial NIH randomized controlled trial, we found a significant reduction in dermal 3-nitrotyrosine staining in patients receiving ERT, suggesting reduction in the potentially toxic effect of ROS secondary to peroxynitrite formation (Figure 4) [4].

Despite the significant improvement in the function of the cerebral vasculature, four of

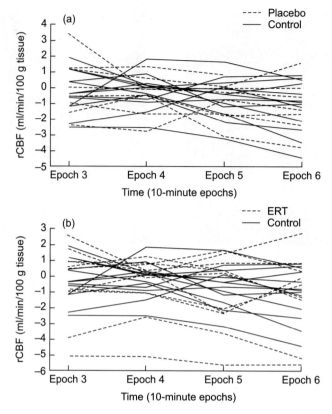

Figure 3. *Comparison between the change in regional cerebral blood flow (rCBF) after infusion of ascorbate between (a) patients with Fabry disease given placebo and normal control individuals, and (b) patients with Fabry disease given enzyme replacement therapy (ERT) and normal control individuals. The only significant difference in rCBF was between the normal controls and the patients with Fabry disease given placebo (analysis of variance of repeated measures), with the placebo group showing a decreased responsiveness to ascorbate. Reproduced with permission from [6].*

25 patients in our original study followed for 4.5 years on ERT developed non-debilitating strokes and one patient had a transient ischaemic attack. One stroke involved a large vessel (vertebral artery occlusion) and the others were small-vessel strokes. Based on our experience and that of others, strokes also continue to occur in patients on agalsidase beta [10], and there is no indication of a marked reduction in stroke risk in the first few years following initiation of ERT in adulthood. To our knowledge, however, no formal study has addressed this question. The lack of an observed clinical effect can be explained in a number of ways. First, there may be a small therapeutic effect that cannot be detected in the relatively small number of patients studied. It is also possible that the infused α-galactosidase A does not have access to the entire thickness of cerebral vessels and therefore leaves untreated a significant component of the vessel wall (Figure 5). In addition, the intermittent nature of ERT and the possibility

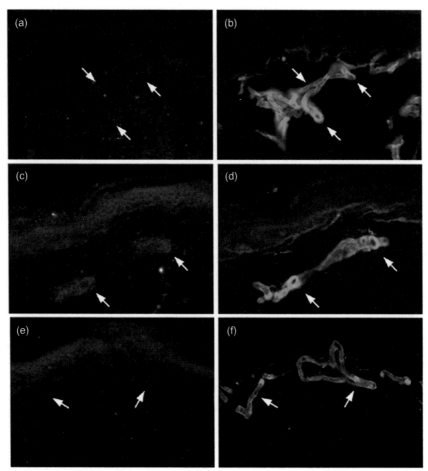

Figure 4. *Dermal nitrotyrosine (a, c, e) and laminin (b, d, f) immunohistochemical localization in control skin and in patients with Fabry disease before and after enzyme replacement therapy (ERT). (a) Control skin showing nitrotyrosine staining (rhodamine filter, ×10 magnification) and laminin staining. (b) Fluorescent filter, ×10 magnification of dermal vessels (arrows) and stratum basalis (same section). (c) and (d) Nitrotyrosine staining before ERT. Significant perivascular staining (arrows) after ERT dermal vascular staining is no longer apparent (e, f).*

of pre-existing irreversible structural changes in the vasculature may limit the effect of ERT when initiated in adulthood. It remains to be demonstrated whether better stroke prevention can be obtained when ERT is begun in childhood.

Effect of ERT on the peripheral nervous system

Our studies, and those of others, focused on neuropathic pain scores, sensory detection threshold for cold, warmth and vibration, sweat function and epidermal innervation density. There was also an attempt to study the effect of ERT on hearing in Fabry disease, which we shall briefly describe.

Neuropathic pain

In the initial NIH 6-month randomized controlled study, we found a significant reduction in pain scores, using the Brief Pain Inventory, in patients on ERT compared with those on placebo [11]. When the patients on placebo crossed over to receive agalsidase alfa, they exhibited a similar benefit (Figure 6) [12]. When followed over a longer

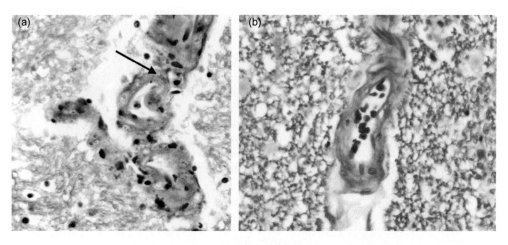

Figure 5. *Effect of 28 months of enzyme replacement therapy (ERT) using agalsidase beta on cerebral vasculature. Sections from the brain of a patient who died of an acute myocardial infarction after long-term ERT are stained with Luxol Fast Blue. (a) Blood vessel shows no storage material in the endothelial cells but there are numerous glycolipid deposits in the rest of the vessel wall (arrow). (b) A normal control shows no deposits (×40 magnification).*

period of time, however, there was no further reduction in pain scores (Figure 6). For these studies, patients were selected for severe neuropathic pain, and medication for neuro-pathic pain was stopped 1 week prior to pain scoring [12]. Our clinical impression

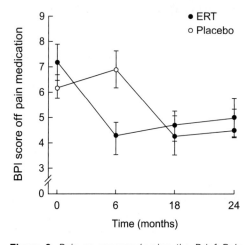

Figure 6. *Pain as assessed using the Brief Pain Inventory (BPI) in patients given enzyme replacement therapy (ERT) with agalsidase alfa for 24 months and those given placebo for the first 6 months followed by ERT for the next 18 months. Values are means ± SEM. Adapted with permission from [12].*

since then supports these initial findings. Neuropathic pain is reduced in patients, including children (authors' unpublished data); however, it is not usually completely eliminated and patients often need to continue with their pain medication, albeit at a lower dose.

Peripheral nerve sensory function

Using a well-established biophysical method based on computerized automated sensory testing equipment (CASE IV, WR Medical, Rochester, MN, USA) to measure detection thresholds for warmth and cold in the foot, thigh and hand, patients with Fabry disease were found to have significantly elevated detection thresholds for warm and cold stimuli in the foot, and for cold stimuli in the hand, compared with controls. Warm sensation was found to be normal in the hand [12]. ERT with agalsidase alfa had no significant effect on these sensory para-meters over the 6-month period of the ran-domized controlled trial. Over the 3 years of open-label treatment, however, there was a significant but modest reduction in the cold (Figure 7) and warm detection thresholds in the foot in patients receiving ERT and for

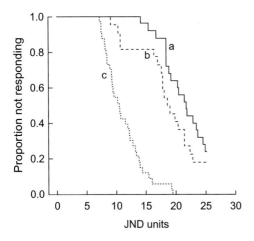

Figure 7. *Thermal sensation in patients with Fabry disease on enzyme replacement therapy (ERT). Kaplan–Meier curves show the proportion of patients not responding to cold stimulus in the foot as a function of the stimulus threshold. The solid line (a) represents patients at initiation of ERT, the broken line (b) represents patients after 3 years of ERT, and the dotted line (c) represents normal controls. JND (just noticeable difference) are units representing perception threshold values. Reproduced with permission from [12].*

warm perception in the thigh. There was also a trend for reduction of cold detection thresholds in the hand [12]. This effect took about 18 months to occur and sensory function seemed to stabilize thereafter. Similar results, looking particularly at heat pain thresholds, were obtained by a group treating patients with agalsidase beta [13]. These authors also described an improvement in vibration detection thresholds. In two separate studies, we found that patients with Fabry disease had a normal vibration detection threshold. However, over time there was no change in vibration threshold in the hand, but a significant increase in the foot threshold, possibly reflecting uraemic neuropathy in some patients. The vibration detection function, however, remained within the normal range for the patient group as a whole [12]. The functional improvement in cold perception of about 10% was not associated with an increase in epidermal innervation density [14].

Overall, although these findings are encouraging, they do not suggest complete normalization of peripheral nerve function. It may be that early treatment before irreversible axonal damage, or higher and more frequent dosing, may be more effective. Alternatively, as mentioned above for the Fabry vascular diathesis, perhaps the infused enzyme has insufficient access to affected sensory nerves and ganglia.

Sweat gland function

Sweat gland function in Fabry disease is of particular interest, as it is possible to measure sweat gland function directly. Moreover, as the capillaries around the sweat glands are fenestrated, it might be expected that ERT would improve sweat gland function relatively early in the course of therapy [15]. We studied sweat gland function using the quantitative sudomotor sweat test (QSART) [16]. As we did not have this technique at our disposal at the start of our initial randomized controlled study, the study of sweat gland function was started at the 3-year time point for this patient cohort. Sweat gland function was found to improve 24–48 hours after enzyme infusion compared with pre-infusion values (Figure 8), while the QSART response normalized in four anhidrotic patients [12]. We also observed a significant improvement in sweat response over time in another study (Figure 9). To date, however, some patients have remained anhidrotic despite years of ERT.

Hearing

There is little information about the effect of ERT with agalsidase alfa on auditory function [17] (see Chapter 25). In this study, the first 6 months consisted of a randomized controlled period, followed by an additional 24 months in which all subjects received ERT. At 6 months, there was an average decline in high-frequency pure-tone thresholds of 4.3 dB for both ERT and placebo groups. Extended monitoring over the next 24 months for ten of the subjects revealed a small, but statistically significant, improvement in high-

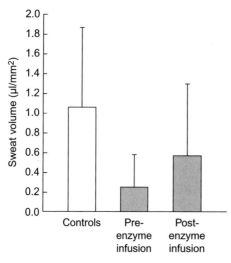

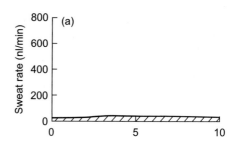

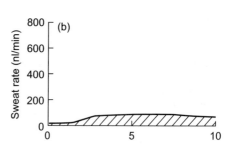

Figure 8. *Quantitative sudomotor axon reflex test (QSART) in patients with Fabry disease and controls. The QSART response is shown in controls (n = 38) and in patients 3 years after the start of enzyme replacement therapy both immediately before an infusion and 24–48 hours after an infusion. Values are means ± SD.*

frequency hearing from baseline in 80%. The mean improvement of 4.9 dB is less than that considered clinically significant and is within the accepted range of test–retest variability and learning effects [18–20]. Subjects in the NIH cohort were monitored over 30 months of ERT. Although we did not systematically examine hearing in our patients beyond this, hearing loss appeared to progress in our patient population, with instances of sudden hearing loss and the need for hearing aids in a number of patients on ERT (M Ries *et al.*, unpublished data).

Conclusions

ERT has shown promise in ameliorating some of the neurological manifestations of Fabry disease. However, this form of therapy needs to be optimized in the future (e.g. by testing more frequent administration of the enzyme). Structural modification of the infused protein to allow better delivery of enzyme within organs and tissues should be attempted. Controlled trials should be

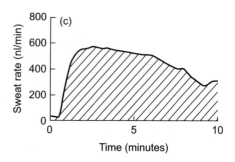

Figure 9. *Quantitative sudomotor axon reflex test in a patient (a) prior to initiation of enzyme replacement therapy (ERT) with agalsidase alfa, (b) after 6 months of ERT and (c) after 3 years of ERT. This patient became extremely sensitive to acetylcholine stimulation and started sweating as soon as the acetylcholine was deposited on the skin. The shaded area under the curve at each time point indicates the total amount of sweat excreted over 10 minutes.*

performed to assess whether initiating ERT in early childhood will further improve the neurological outcome of patients with Fabry disease.

References

1. Ries M, Gupta S, Moore DF, Sachdev V, Quirk JM, Murray GJ et al. Pediatric Fabry disease. *Pediatrics* 2005;115:e344–55

2. Bradberry JC, Fagan SC, Gray DR, Moon YS. New perspectives on the pharmacotherapy of ischemic stroke. *J Am Pharm Assoc (Wash DC)* 2004;44: S46–56; quiz S56–7

3. Chong JY, Mohr JP. Anticoagulation and platelet antiaggregation therapy in stroke prevention. *Curr Opin Neurol* 2005;18:53–7

4. Moore DF, Scott LT, Gladwin MT, Altarescu G, Kaneski C, Suzuki K et al. Regional cerebral hyperperfusion and nitric oxide pathway dysregulation in Fabry disease: reversal by enzyme replacement therapy. *Circulation* 2001;104:1506–12

5. Moore DF, Altarescu G, Herscovitch P, Schiffmann R. Enzyme replacement reverses abnormal cerebrovascular responses in Fabry disease. *BMC Neurol* 2002;2:4

6. Moore DF, Ye F, Brennan ML, Gupta S, Barshop BA, Steiner RD et al. Ascorbate decreases Fabry cerebral hyperperfusion suggesting a reactive oxygen species abnormality: an arterial spin tagging study. *J Magn Reson Imaging* 2004;20:674–83

7. Moore DF, Altarescu G, Ling GS, Jeffries N, Frei KP, Weibel T et al. Elevated cerebral blood flow velocities in Fabry disease with reversal after enzyme replacement. *Stroke* 2002;33:525–31

8. Settakis G, Molnar C, Kerenyi L, Kollar J, Legemate D, Csiba L et al. Acetazolamide as a vasodilatory stimulus in cerebrovascular diseases and in conditions affecting the cerebral vasculature. *Eur J Neurol* 2003;10:609–20

9. Wang Y, Russo TA, Kwon O, Chanock S, Rumsey SC, Levine M. Ascorbate recycling in human neutrophils: induction by bacteria. *Proc Natl Acad Sci USA* 1997; 94:13816–19

10. Wilcox WR, Banikazemi M, Guffon N, Waldek S, Lee P, Linthorst GE et al. Long-term safety and efficacy of enzyme replacement therapy for Fabry disease. *Am J Hum Genet* 2004;75:65–74

11. Schiffmann R, Kopp JB, Austin HA 3rd, Sabnis S, Moore DF, Weibel T et al. Enzyme replacement therapy in Fabry disease: a randomized controlled trial. *JAMA* 2001;285:2743–9

12. Schiffmann R, Floeter MK, Dambrosia JM, Gupta S, Moore DF, Sharabi Y et al. Enzyme replacement therapy improves peripheral nerve and sweat function in Fabry disease. *Muscle Nerve* 2003;28:703–10

13. Hilz MJ, Brys M, Marthol H, Stemper B, Dutsch M. Enzyme replacement therapy improves function of C-, Aδ-, and Aβ-nerve fibers in Fabry neuropathy. *Neurology* 2004;62:1066–72

14. Schiffmann R, Hauer P, Freeman B, Ries M, Scott LJC, Polydefkis M et al. Enzyme replacement therapy and intra-epidermal innervation density in Fabry disease. *Muscle Nerve* 2006; Mar 31 [Epub ahead of print]

15. Quick DC, Kennedy WR, Yoon KS. Ultrastructure of the secretory epithelium, nerve fibers, and capillaries in the mouse sweat gland. *Anat Rec* 1984;208:491–9

16. Low PA, Opfer-Gehrking TL. The autonomic laboratory. *Am J Electroneurodiagnostic Technol* 1999; 39:65–76

17. Hajioff D, Enever Y, Quiney R, Zuckerman J, Mackermot K, Mehta A. Hearing loss in Fabry disease: the effect of agalsidase alfa replacement therapy. *J Inherit Metab Dis* 2003;26:787–94

18. Laitakari K, Uimonen S. The Finnish speech in noise test for assessing sensorineural hearing loss. *Scand Audiol Suppl* 2001:52:165–6

19. Lemkens N, Vermeire K, Brokx JP, Fransen E, Van Camp G, Van De Heyning PH. Interpretation of pure-tone thresholds in sensorineural hearing loss (SNHL): a review of measurement variability and age-specific references. *Acta Otorhinolaryngol Belg* 2002;56:341–52

20. Schmuziger N, Probst R, Smurzynski J. Test–retest reliability of pure-tone thresholds from 0.5 to 16 kHz using Sennheiser HDA 200 and Etymotic Research ER-2 earphones. *Ear Hear* 2004;25:127–32

40 Effects of enzyme replacement therapy on pain and overall quality of life

Björn Hoffmann

Department of General Pediatrics, Heinrich-Heine-University, Moorenstrasse 5, D-40225 Düsseldorf, Germany

Pain is one of the first symptoms of Fabry disease, often beginning in childhood. Up to 90% of children and approximately 70% of all patients with Fabry disease report pain. Only a very small number of patients enrolled in FOS – the Fabry Outcome Survey – reported no 'pain on average' or no 'worst pain' before treatment. Acroparaesthesia in Fabry disease involves a burning, stabbing or tingling pain, predominantly located in the palms of the hands and soles of the feet. Pain may be aggravated by an elevated body or ambient temperature, as well as concurrent illness or certain dietary components. After 1 year of enzyme replacement therapy (ERT) with agalsidase alfa, pain was significantly reduced in both men and women with Fabry disease in FOS. These reductions were maintained after 2 and 3 consecutive years of treatment. Together with other symptoms, pain has a marked impact on health-related quality of life (HRQoL). Prior to ERT, the European Quality of Life Questionnaire (EQ-5D) score in men was 0.64 ± 0.33, while women rated their HRQoL only slightly better (0.66 ± 0.36). For women, this was 0.20 lower than a normal sample of the population, while for men it was 0.27 lower (p < 0.05 for both sexes). Compared with a range of other diseases, only patients with non-small-cell lung cancer reported lower EQ-5D scores than patients with Fabry disease. In patients receiving ERT with agalsidase alfa, the deviation in EQ-5D score from normal improved from –0.33 in men and –0.31 in women, to –0.13 in men and –0.22 in women (p < 0.05). These improvements were maintained during continued treatment. It is suggested that, in the absence of objective markers of disease severity, patient-reported HRQoL can be used to evaluate the benefits of ERT.

Introduction

The pain experienced by patients as a result of chronic disease, for example Fabry disease, has a significant impact on their quality of life (QoL). Any reduction in pain is therefore likely to have a positive effect on the overall QoL of affected individuals. This chapter examines the impact of pain on patients' lives and how enzyme replacement therapy (ERT) with agalsidase alfa not only reduces the symptoms of Fabry disease neuropathy but also improves overall health-related QoL (HRQoL).

Pain in Fabry disease

Pain is one of the first symptoms of Fabry disease and may already be a burden for the patient in childhood [1–4]. During the first decade of life, more than 20% of hemizygous males and more than 60% of heterozygous females develop pain [3]. Up to 90% of all children and approximately 70% of all patients with Fabry disease report pain [1, 3]. Despite the early presentation of this symptom of Fabry disease, data from the total population in FOS – the Fabry Outcome Survey – show that the mean time from first symptoms to diagnosis is still more than 13 years [3].

Typically, pain is located in the hands and feet and is therefore incorporated within the diagnostic term acroparaesthesia. However, nearly 25% of adult patients also complain of headache [5]. During childhood, 72% of children complain of diffuse recurrent abdominal pain [4], which is also reported to be a problem in adults [1, 6, 7]. Acroparaesthesia in Fabry disease is described as a burning, stabbing or tingling sensation. Predominantly located in the palms of the hands and soles of the feet, these sensations may radiate from distal to proximal sites. One-third of patients suffer from permanent pain, while the majority of patients report both constant background pain and excruciating pain attacks lasting several days [1].

An elevated body or ambient temperature, as well as concurrent illness, may trigger pain attacks. Other factors inducing pain include physical exercise (> 50% of patients), emotional stress and certain foods, including eggs, meat, coffee or alcohol [1, 5, 8]. Besides acute or long-lasting pain, hyperalgesia to heat or cold has been described in Fabry disease [9, 10]. Pain may become less severe with age [1], and one patient with Fabry disease reported that pain was reduced after a successful pregnancy [11].

The impact of the specific symptoms of Fabry disease and their influence on QoL were investigated before the introduction of ERT [1, 12, 13]. It was shown that pain not only reduces QoL but may substantially interfere with normal daily activities [12]. Pain medication, including morphine and anticonvulsants, was needed by the majority of patients suffering from Fabry neuropathy. Children with Fabry disease may avoid participation in physical education in school or in their leisure time, as physical exertion can initiate painful attacks [8]. Additionally, school attendance may be negatively affected [14]. Due

to their symptoms, children with Fabry disease and accompanying neuropathy may be wrongly labelled as neurotic [15].

Pain data from FOS

In FOS, patients are asked to answer questionnaires about pain and their QoL on a regular basis. The pain questionnaire used in FOS is the Brief Pain Inventory (BPI), a validated instrument for evaluation of pain and its impact on QoL. Although originally designed for assessing pain in patients with cancer, the BPI has also been used in other painful conditions [16–18]. Patients score their pain on a scale from 0 (no pain at all) to 10 (worst imaginable pain).

Pain attacks were reported in both males and females with Fabry disease. The mean age at onset of pain was 18.7 years in females ($n = 337$) and 13.1 years in males ($n = 318$).

BPI data on the severity of pain at baseline are currently available for 40 women (mean age, 44.4 ± 13.7 [SD] years) and 67 men (mean age, 35.7 ± 10.6 years). At baseline, only 12 (4 females, 8 males) of the patients in FOS reported no pain at all for the item 'pain on average', while eight patients (2 females, 6 males) reported no pain at all for the item 'worst pain' in the BPI questionnaire. Patients under the age of 18 years were excluded from this analysis, as the BPI is not validated for use in children. Interestingly, women with Fabry disease reported higher BPI scores than men ('worst pain' score, 5.45 in women versus 4.75 in men; not significant). Moreover, women complained of more severe 'pain on average' (mean score, 4.51 versus 3.71; not significant).

Information about the impact of pain on daily activities was available from 48 females (mean age, 46.6 ± 13.7 years) and 70 males (mean age, 35.5 ± 9.3 years). There were no differences observed between women and men regarding the impact of pain on daily activities. Pain had a greater impact on general activity, mood, normal work and enjoyment of life than it did on the ability to walk, social relations and sleep (Figure 1).

BPI scores for pain at its worst after 1 year of ERT in 40 patients (15 females, 25 males) fell from 5.5 ± 0.3 to 4.6 ± 0.4 (mean ± SEM). The improvement was markedly better in men than in women (–1.04 versus –0.6, respectively). Improvements in 'pain on average' scores were the same (–0.9) in males and females over 1 year of treatment.

Thirty-one patients (10 females, 21 males) had documented information about pain after 2 years of ERT. These results confirmed the 1-year observations, with a reduction in pain at its worst and in average pain. The BPI score for pain on average was reduced by a mean of 1.1 (–1.4 in males and –0.6 in females) and for pain at its worst by a mean of 1.2 (–1.3 in males and –0.9 in females).

Only limited data are available for 3-year pain evaluations. Seventeen patients (2 females, 15 males) continued to report less pain on average (–1.2 in both genders) as well as a

reduction in worst pain (–0.5 in both genders) compared with baseline (Figure 2).

The reduction of pain during ERT was reflected in improvements in the impact of pain on daily activities (Figure 3). In 34 patients given ERT for 1 year, reductions in the impact of pain were greatest for normal work, general activity and social relations.

QoL in Fabry disease

The European Quality of Life Questionnaire (EQ-5D) is used to evaluate HRQoL in FOS. The questionnaire covers the five dimensions of mobility, pain/discomfort, self-care, anxiety/depression and activities of daily living. The questionnaire is validated for use in different languages and generates a cardinal index of health. An EQ-5D score of 1 means the best imaginable HRQoL. A health state of 0 is equivalent to being dead. By calculation, it is possible to achieve an EQ-5D score below 0 [19, 20].

In addition to the physical impairment associated with Fabry disease, there are reports of psychiatric problems [21, 22], with a high incidence of suicide and depression.

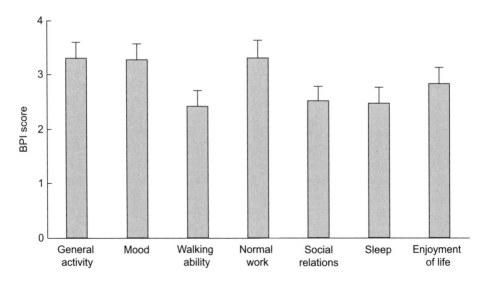

Figure 1. *Interference of pain in activities of daily life in 118 patients (48 females, 70 males) with Fabry disease prior to enzyme replacement therapy. Values are means ± SEM. High Brief Pain Inventory (BPI) scores indicate a high impact of pain on daily activities.*

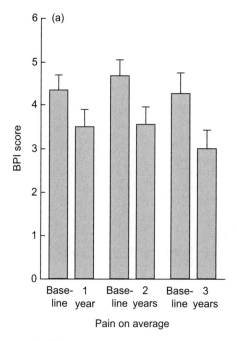

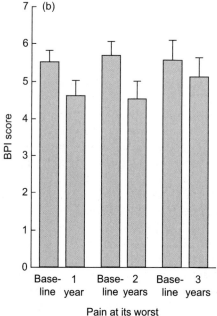

Figure 2. *Changes in Brief Pain Inventory (BPI) scores for (a) pain on average and (b) pain at its worst in patients with Fabry disease at baseline and after 1, 2 and 3 years of enzyme replacement therapy. Values are means ± SEM. Results are given for males and females combined.*

Improvements in a patient's perception of the impact of disease may result in improvements in mood and HRQoL. There may be a close link between mental and physical health in Fabry disease, and improvements in either one of these health aspects may be associated with improvements in the other.

Before the initiation of ERT, HRQoL is markedly reduced in patients with Fabry disease [12, 13]. Using the Short Form 36 (SF-36) health status questionnaire and the EQ-5D, Miners and colleagues found that before starting ERT, HRQoL in 38 male patients with Fabry disease was significantly lower than in the general population [13]. The item 'general health' from the SF-36 showed the greatest deviation from normal, while the 'mental component summary scores' showed the smallest deviation from general population data. Comparing scores from the visual analogue scale of the EQ-5D in the same patients with general UK population data revealed a significantly lower HRQoL in patients with Fabry disease (24.3 for Fabry disease versus 85.14 for the normal UK population). Similar results were described by Gold and co-workers, who reported HRQoL in 53 male patients with Fabry disease before the onset of ERT [12]. The greatest deviation from the general US population was observed for 'role physical', whereas the smallest deviation was found for mental health. Compared with the HRQoL reported in patients with renal disease, a history of stroke or AIDS, Gold *et al.* found that patients with Fabry disease tended to have lower SF-36 scores, particularly for 'general health', 'role physical' and 'vitality' [12]. However, neither of these reports described the evolution of HRQoL during ERT, nor did they report HRQoL in female patients with Fabry disease.

HRQoL data from FOS

Baseline data on HRQoL in FOS are available for 62 women and 81 men. As for the evaluation of pain, patients under the age of 18

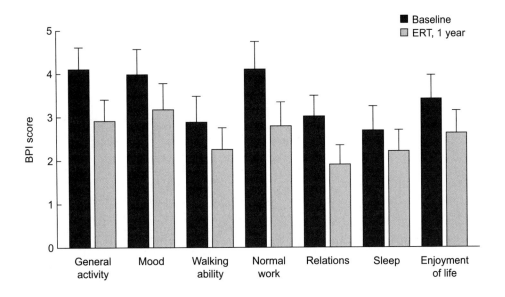

Figure 3. *Interference of pain in activities of daily life in 34 patients with Fabry disease at baseline and after 1 year of enzyme replacement therapy (ERT). Values are means ± SEM. As there were no gender differences, results are given for males and females combined. High Brief Pain Inventory (BPI) scores indicate a high impact of pain on daily activities.*

years were excluded from this analysis, as the EQ-5D is not validated for use in children.

Prior to the initiation of ERT, EQ-5D scores were similar in men and women. Men with Fabry disease rated their HRQoL as 0.64 ± 0.04 (mean ± SEM), while women showed only slightly better EQ-5D scores (0.66 ± 0.05). Compared with normal UK population data [23], this is a deviation of −0.20 in women and −0.27 in men (Figure 4).

These results become more meaningful when compared with EQ-5D scores reported by patients with other diseases (Figure 5). Interestingly, only patients with non-small-cell lung cancer report lower (worse) EQ-5D scores than patients with Fabry disease [24]. Patients with a kidney or liver transplant, breast cancer or diabetes mellitus have higher EQ-5D scores [25–28].

Follow-up data for HRQoL were evaluated in 51 patients (18 females, 33 males) after 1 year of ERT. The mean baseline EQ-5D score for these patients was −0.32 (females, −0.31; males, −0.33) when compared with the normal population value, and improved to −0.16 (females, −0.22; males, −0.13) after 12 months of ERT (Figure 6; $p < 0.05$). These significant improvements were maintained in 40 patients (11 females, 29 males) after 2 consecutive years of therapy (Figure 6). There are only limited follow-up data on HRQoL after 3 years of ERT. However, 14 men showed an improvement of 0.21 in EQ-5D scores (from a deviation of −0.39 compared with normal population data, to a deviation of −0.18).

Considerations relating to pain reduction and improved HRQoL

Several mechanisms may account for the reduction of pain during ERT. Pain in Fabry

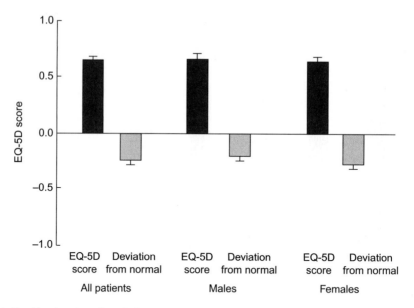

Figure 4. *Health-related quality of life, as assessed using the European Quality of Life Questionnaire (EQ-5D), in 143 patients with Fabry disease (62 females, 81 males) at baseline, and the deviation from normal UK population data. Values are means ± SEM.*

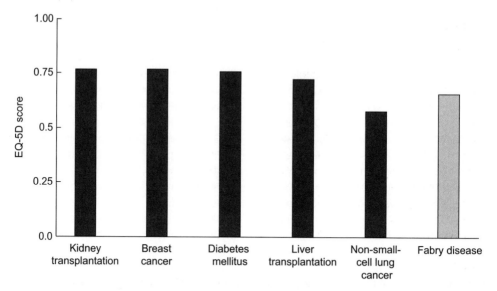

Figure 5. *Comparison of health-related quality of life, as assessed using the European Quality of Life Questionnaire (EQ-5D), in different diseases, including Fabry disease.*

disease is neuropathic; that is, it is due to damaged nerve fibres. Several reports have demonstrated both a reduction in pain perception and an improvement in general nerve function following ERT [29, 30].

Therefore, it is unlikely that pain reduction is due only to psychological or placebo effects. Complete abolition of pain would require regeneration of the damaged nerve fibres, which may require long-term treat-

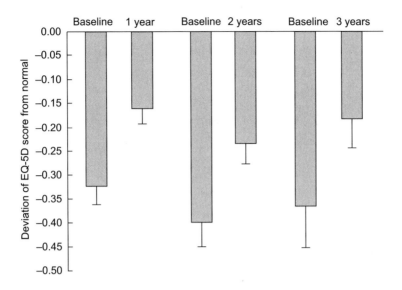

Figure 6. *Deviation of health-related quality of life scores, obtained using the European Quality of Life Questionnaire (EQ-5D), from normal population values in patients with Fabry disease after 1, 2 and 3 years of enzyme replacement therapy. Values are mean ± SEM.*

ment. During nerve fibre regeneration there may be periods of hypersensitivity, explaining the residual pain despite prolonged treatment.

In accordance with these findings, there may also be significant improvements in the perception of non-noxious thermal sensations. This may be explained by epidermal nerve regeneration, functional improvement in sensory nerves and ganglia, or recovery in other components of the peripheral nervous system [29, 30]. In untreated patients with Fabry disease, different authors have reported small-fibre derangement and vascular dysfunction [10, 31, 32]. Small myelinated axons transmitting cold perception are also severely altered in Fabry disease [31]. Unmyelinated C-fibres transmitting warmth perception are less severely affected, and large myelinated fibres seem to be relatively spared [31].

Globotriaosylceramide (Gb_3) deposits have been described in nerve fibres, dorsal root ganglia and sympathetic ganglia in several studies [15, 33, 34]. Hence, there is no reason why Gb_3 storage may not occur in nerve tissue. Clearance of Gb_3 has been described following ERT (e.g. in patients with Fabry disease with severe renal involvement [35, 36]). Additionally, reduction of the Gb_3 load in cardiac endothelial cells was observed by Eng *et al.* without any functional effects [36]. Furthermore, Schiffmann and co-workers observed a decrease in QRS duration, suggesting a reduction in left ventricular hypertrophy [35].

Structural changes in nerve fibres have not yet been described in Fabry disease. However, clinical improvements provide evidence that destruction of nerve fibres is halted and suggest that regeneration may take place [29]

Pain reduction and improvements in QoL should not be considered in isolation, but in the context of the patient's life in general. For children, one can speculate that a reduction in pain will result in an improvement in school attendance; however, psychological effects and cognitive improvements have yet to be proven. Adults may be able to attend work more regularly, with fewer days off due to fewer pain crises and reduced pain.

Possible use of patient-reported outcomes as surrogate markers

The words from the Hippocratic oath are still pertinent today. "Into whatever houses I enter, I will go into them for the benefit of the sick…". However, it is not always possible to define or evaluate this benefit clearly. In a few diseases, there are specific and sensitive markers that correlate well with disease severity. Some such markers also change during therapeutic interventions and may therefore be used as indicators of the benefit to the sick. One example is the use of the biomarker chito-triosidase in Gaucher disease. This marker not only reflects the total body load of storage material, but also changes during ERT, there-fore allowing an objective assessment of treatment effects.

Attempts have been made to identify bio-chemical [37] or clinical [38] markers of the progression of Fabry disease and the effects of ERT; however, results to date have not been convincing. In the absence of an objective marker, it is pertinent to ask the patients whether they feel any benefit from ERT. Certainly, such improvements are individual, as each patient has a different environment, cultural background and value system. Finally, the individual's goals and expectations, as well as his or her particular concerns, must be taken into account before deciding whether that individual has benefited from treatment. The World Health Organization takes all these factors into consideration when defining QoL [39]. However, this definition is too com-plex to show improvements by therapeutic interventions alone, as there are too many contributory factors that may not be influ-enced by an individual's health state. Hence, the definition of HRQoL is used to evaluate those aspects of QoL that may be influenced by health or disease.

In summary, when there is no marker that objectively reflects the disease burden or changes in disease severity following an intervention in patients with Fabry disease, it is suggested that patient-reported outcome measures can be useful, such as evaluation of HRQoL using the EQ-5D.

Conclusions

Fabry disease is a painful multisystemic disease that is already well established during childhood and adolescence, and is associated with a significant reduction in QoL. Evaluation of FOS data clearly reveals that ERT with agalsidase alfa significantly reduces pain, significantly improves QoL and is of overall benefit for both female and male patients with Fabry disease.

References

1. MacDermot KD, Holmes A, Miners AH. Anderson–Fabry disease: clinical manifestations and impact of disease in a cohort of 98 hemizygous males. J Med Genet 2001;38:750–60

2. MacDermot KD, Holmes A, Miners AH. Anderson–Fabry disease: clinical manifestations and impact of disease in a cohort of 60 obligate carrier females. J Med Genet 2001;38:769–75

3. Mehta A, Ricci R, Widmer U, Dehout F, Garcia de Lorenzo A, Kampmann C et al. Fabry disease defined: baseline clinical manifestations of 366 patients in the Fabry Outcome Survey. Eur J Clin Invest 2004; 34:236–42

4. Ries M, Gupta S, Moore DF, Sachdev V, Quirk JM, Murray GJ et al. Pediatric Fabry disease. Pediatrics 2005;115:e344–55

5. Hoffmann B, Basalla D, Walther A. The patient's perspective of pain in Fabry disease. Acta Paediatr Suppl 2005;447:118

6. Dehout F, Roland D, Treille de Granseigne S, Guillaume B, Van Maldergem L. Relief of gastro-intestinal symptoms under enzyme replacement therapy in patients with Fabry disease. J Inherit Metab Dis 2004;27:499–505

7. Banikazemi M, Ullman T, Desnick RJ. Gastrointestinal manifestations of Fabry disease: clinical response to enzyme replacement therapy. Mol Genet Metab 2005;85:255–9

8. Ries M, Ramaswami U, Parini R, Lindblad B, Whybra C, Willers I et al. The early clinical phenotype of Fabry disease: a study on 35 European children and adolescents. Eur J Pediatr 2003;162:767–72

9. Leder AA, Bosworth WC. Angiokeratoma corporis diffusum universale (Fabry's disease) with mitral stenosis. Am J Med 1965;38:814–19

10. Hilz MJ, Stemper B, Kolodny EH. Lower limb cold exposure induces pain and prolonged small fiber dysfunction in Fabry patients. *Pain* 2000;84:361–5

11. Lacomis D, Roeske-Anderson L, Mathie L. Neuropathy and Fabry's disease. *Muscle Nerve* 2005;31:102–7

12. Gold KF, Pastores GM, Botteman MF, Yeh JM, Sweeney S, Aliski W et al. Quality of life of patients with Fabry disease. *Qual Life Res* 2002;11:317–27

13. Miners AH, Holmes A, Sherr L, Jenkinson C, MacDermot KD. Assessment of health-related quality-of-life in males with Anderson–Fabry disease before therapeutic intervention. *Qual Life Res* 2002; 11:127–33

14. Mehta A. New developments in the management of Anderson–Fabry disease. *QJM* 2002;95:647–53

15. Kahn P. Anderson–Fabry disease: a histopathological study of three cases with observations on the mechanism of production of pain. *J Neurol Neurosurg Psychiatry* 1973;36:1053–62

16. Cleeland CS, Ryan KM. Pain assessment: global use of the Brief Pain Inventory. *Ann Acad Med Singapore* 1994;23:129–38

17. Davison SN. Pain in hemodialysis patients: prevalence, cause, severity, and management. *Am J Kidney Dis* 2003;42:1239–47

18. Tan G, Jensen MP, Thornby JI, Shanti BF. Validation of the Brief Pain Inventory for chronic nonmalignant pain. *J Pain* 2004;5:133–7

19. The EuroQol Group. EuroQol – a new facility for the measurement of health-related quality of life. *Health Policy* 1990;16:199–208

20. Macran S, Kind P. "Death" and the valuation of health-related quality of life. *Med Care* 2001;39:217–27

21. Grewal RP. Psychiatric disorders in patients with Fabry's disease. *Int J Psychiatry Med* 1993; 23:307–12

22. Wendrich K, Whybra C, Ries M, Kampmann C, Baehner F, Miebach E et al. Neurological manifestation of Fabry disease in male patients. *J Inherit Metab Dis* 2001;24 (Suppl 2):139

23. Kind P, Hardman G, Macran S. UK population norms for EQ-5D. York Centre for Health Economics Discussion Paper 1999;172

24. Trippoli S, Vaiani M, Lucioni C, Messori A. Quality of life and utility in patients with non-small cell lung cancer. Quality-of-life Study Group of the Master 2 Project in Pharmacoeconomics. *Pharmacoeconomics* 2001;19:855–63

25. Bryan S, Ratcliffe J, Neuberger JM, Burroughs AK, Gunson BK, Buxton MJ. Health-related quality of life following liver transplantation. *Qual Life Res* 1998; 7:115–20

26. Cleemput I, Kesteloot K, De Geest S, Dobbels F, Vanrenterghem Y. Health professionals' perceptions of health status after renal transplantation: a comparison with transplantation candidates' expectations. *Transplantation* 2003;76:176–82

27. Conner-Spady B, Cumming C, Nabholtz JM, Jacobs P, Stewart D. Responsiveness of the EuroQol in breast cancer patients undergoing high dose chemotherapy. *Qual Life Res* 2001;10:479–86

28. Koopmanschap M. Coping with type II diabetes: the patient's perspective. *Diabetologia* 2002;45:S18–22

29. Schiffmann R, Floeter MK, Dambrosia JM, Gupta S, Moore DF, Sharabi Y et al. Enzyme replacement therapy improves peripheral nerve and sweat function in Fabry disease. *Muscle Nerve* 2003; 28:703–10

30. Hilz MJ, Brys M, Marthol H, Stemper B, Dutsch M. Enzyme replacement therapy improves function of C-, Aδ-, and Aβ-nerve fibers in Fabry neuropathy. *Neurology* 2004;62:1066–72

31. Luciano CA, Russell JW, Banerjee TK, Quirk JM, Scott LJ, Dambrosia JM et al. Physiological characterization of neuropathy in Fabry's disease. *Muscle Nerve* 2002;26:622–9

32. Dutsch M, Marthol H, Stemper B, Brys M, Haendl T, Hilz MJ. Small fiber dysfunction predominates in Fabry neuropathy. *J Clin Neurophysiol* 2002; 19:575–86

33. Gadoth N, Sandbank U. Involvement of dorsal root ganglia in Fabry's disease. *J Med Genet* 1983; 20:309–12

34. Hozumi I, Nishizawa M, Ariga T, Inoue Y, Ohnishi Y, Yokoyama A et al. Accumulation of glycosphingolipids in spinal and sympathetic ganglia of a symptomatic heterozygote of Fabry's disease. *J Neurol Sci* 1989;90:273–80

35. Schiffmann R, Kopp JB, Austin HA 3rd, Sabnis S, Moore DF, Weibel T et al. Enzyme replacement therapy in Fabry disease: a randomized controlled trial. *JAMA* 2001;285:2743–9

36. Eng CM, Guffon N, Wilcox WR, Germain DP, Lee P, Waldek S et al. Safety and efficacy of recombinant human α-galactosidase A replacement therapy in Fabry's disease. *N Engl J Med* 2001;345:9–16

37. Whitfield PD, Calvin J, Hogg S, O'Driscoll E, Halsall D, Burling K et al. Monitoring enzyme replacement therapy in Fabry disease – role of urine globotriaosylceramide. *J Inherit Metab Dis* 2005;28:21–33

38. Whybra C, Kampmann C, Krummenauer F, Ries M, Mengel E, Miebach E et al. The Mainz Severity Score Index: a new instrument for quantifying the Anderson–Fabry disease phenotype, and the response of patients to enzyme replacement therapy. *Clin Genet* 2004;65:299–307

39. The World Health Organization Quality of Life assessment (WHOQOL): position paper from the World Health Organization. *Soc Sci Med* 1995; 41:1403–9

41 Safety of enzyme replacement therapy

Frédéric Barbey[1] and Françoise Livio[2]

[1]Nephrology Department and [2]Clinical Pharmacology Department, University Hospital, Lausanne, Switzerland

One of the main aims of FOS – the Fabry Outcome Survey – is to monitor the long-term safety of enzyme replacement therapy with agalsidase alfa in patients with Fabry disease. Detailed reporting within FOS has revealed few serious adverse events. Only two of these were classified as possibly related to treatment, out of a total of 401 treated patients, corresponding to 940 patient-years. Most adverse events were mild infusion reactions, occurring in approximately 13% of patients (associated with about 1% of the estimated total number of infusions). Infusion-related reactions occurred much less frequently in female than in male patients. In most of the affected patients the infusion reactions occurred soon after the initiation of treatment and normally disappeared after the first few infusions. No IgE antibodies have been detected. The data in FOS confirm that agalsidase alfa has a good safety profile and is well tolerated in adults and children when used in a wide range of patients and in daily clinical practice, including home therapy.

Introduction

The recombinant enzyme agalsidase alfa is produced in a continuous human cell line through gene activation [1]. Use of human cells ensures that correct glycosylation of the protein occurs, identical to that of the natural enzyme. The cell-culture system has been tested extensively and found to be free of viral or microbial contamination [2–4].

In preclinical studies, a single intravenous administration of agalsidase alfa to rats and mice appeared to be well tolerated up to the highest doses given, which were 10 mg/kg in rats and 2.3 mg/kg in mice (i.e. 50 and 11 times the bi-weekly clinical dose, respectively). Intravenous dosing with agalsidase alfa caused no toxic effects during a 2-week exposure study in rabbits (using doses up to 1 mg/kg/day), 13- and 26-week studies in rats, and a 13-week study in cynomolgus

monkeys (using doses up to 1 mg/kg/week). Formal carcinogenicity and mutagenicity studies have not been conducted with agalsidase alfa, although the drug is intended for long-term treatment. However, carcinogenic potential is not anticipated, based on the nature of the compound.

As Fabry disease is a rare disorder, agalsidase alfa was granted orphan designation by the European Agency for Evaluation of Medicinal Products in 2000, followed by marketing authorization under exceptional circumstances in 2001 [5].

In a phase I trial, ten patients with Fabry disease received a single intravenous infusion of one of five escalating dose levels of the enzyme (0.007–0.1 mg/kg). No untoward effects associated with agalsidase alfa occurred in any of the patients, and none of the patients developed agalsidase A antibodies by day 28 post-infusion [6].

A single-centre, double-blind, placebo-controlled phase II/III trial of agalsidase alfa involved 26 male patients with neuropathic pain who received 0.2 mg/kg every 2 weeks for 22 weeks (12 doses) [7]. In the treated group, the vast majority of adverse events (e.g. constipation, abdominal pain crises and hearing loss) were signs or symptoms that are typically observed during progression of Fabry disease [8, 9]. The most common side effects (in 8 of 14 treated patients) attributed to treatment were mild infusion-related reactions, consisting primarily of chills. These side effects decreased in frequency and severity over time, either spontaneously or following the introduction of appropriate premedication (antihistamines and/or low-dose corticosteroids). An IgG antibody response was observed in three patients. There was evidence of immunological tolerance, based on progressive reduction in antibody titres. Subset analyses demonstrated that the low-titre antibodies appeared to have no clinically significant effects on the safety or efficacy of agalsidase alfa. Finally, no patient developed IgE, IgA or IgM antibodies to agalsidase alfa.

In a phase III study involving heterozygous females, 15 patients received between eight and 20 infusions of agalsidase alfa [10]. Most of the adverse events reported were signs or symptoms that would be expected to occur in patients with Fabry disease. There were no apparent treatment-related adverse events detected by clinical laboratory tests, physical examination, electrocardiography or monitoring of vital signs. None of the patients experienced an infusion reaction or developed agalsidase alfa antibodies at any time during the study. The results indicated that the safety profile of agalsidase alfa was similar in both male and female patients with Fabry disease, except that no IgG antibodies have been detected and no infusion-

related reactions have been reported in female patients receiving agalsidase alfa.

Data from animal studies do not indicate any direct or indirect harmful effects with respect to fertility and embryonic/fetal development as a result of exposure to agalsidase alfa before pregnancy and during organogenesis [5]. Furthermore, three successful pregnancies, resulting in healthy offspring, have been reported in women treated with agalsidase alfa [11, 12]. It is not known whether agalsidase alfa crosses the placenta or is excreted in human milk; however, such passage of the drug can be expected to be limited. Safety data in children are still limited [13].

While the preclinical and early clinical observations depict a satisfactory safety and tolerability profile for agalsidase alfa, the prospective follow-up of adverse events in the patient population targeted for long-term therapy represents an invaluable source of safety information. Such follow-up is essential to assess the frequency of the more common side effects and to estimate the incidence of rare but serious adverse reactions. The Fabry Outcome Survey (FOS) was designed to provide such information, and the results of adverse events monitoring during the first 5 years of the survey are presented below.

Definitions in FOS

An adverse event was defined as any noxious, pathological or unintended change in anatomical, physiological or metabolic function, indicated by physical signs, symptoms and/or laboratory changes, which occurred after the introduction of agalsidase alfa, whether or not the event was related to the administration of the drug. This definition therefore includes exacerbation of any pre-existing conditions.

Adverse events were categorized as being unrelated to dosing with agalsidase alfa or possibly or probably related as follows.
● Not related: a clinical event or laboratory abnormality was considered to be unre-

lated to agalsidase alfa treatment if there was a highly plausible alternative cause or the absence of any chronological link.

- Possibly related: a clinical event or laboratory abnormality was deemed to be possibly related to agalsidase alfa treatment if there was a reasonable time sequence between its occurrence and administration of the drug, but the event could also be explained by concurrent disease or use of other drugs/chemicals.
- Probably related: a clinical event or laboratory abnormality was considered to be probably related to agalsidase alfa treatment if it occurred a reasonable amount of time after administration of the drug, was unlikely to be attributable to concurrent disease or other drugs/chemicals, and there was a clinically reasonable response on de-challenge.

An adverse event was defined as serious if it resulted in one or more of the following:
- death
- life-threatening reaction (i.e. immediate risk of death)
- in-patient hospitalization or prolongation of current hospitalization
- congenital anomaly or birth defect.

Adverse events were also considered to be serious if, based on medical judgement, they could have jeopardized the patient or have required medical or surgical intervention to prevent one of the serious outcomes listed above.

Patients were monitored for the following serious adverse events that fulfil the above criteria and are known to occur in Fabry disease.
- Cerebrovascular events: stroke, transient ischaemic attacks, and prolonged reversible ischaemic neurological disease.
- Cardiac events: left ventricular hypertrophy, myocardial infarction, heart failure, angina, valve disease, conduction abnormalities, arrhythmias and congenital heart disease.

- Renal events: microalbuminuria, proteinuria, haematuria, renal failure, haemodialysis, peritoneal dialysis and transplantation.

All adverse events – whether serious or not – were classified into one of three groups according to severity. Mild events were defined as those placing no limitations on usual activities. Moderate events were those that limited usual activities. Severe events indicated that the individual was unable to carry out usual activities.

Special reporting procedures in FOS

If a serious adverse event occurs that is considered to be possibly or probably drug related, the pharmacovigilance manager has to be contacted immediately by telephone.

Investigators have to report adverse events occurring in patients receiving treatment by entering the data into the FOS database. In the event of a suspected serious adverse drug reaction, investigators have to complete a detailed questionnaire, which can be printed from the FOS application and faxed to the pharmacovigilance manager. For patients participating in FOS who are not receiving agalsidase alfa treatment, any changes in health that meet the adverse event definition are reported to the FOS database in the examination section. However, if the patient has previously received agalsidase alfa therapy within 1 month of the adverse event, the event must be reported as an adverse event.

Results

As of 7 March 2005, the data available in the FOS database related to 401 patients (241 males and 160 females) who had received treatment with agalsidase alfa. These included 55 children or adolescents below 18 years of age (31 males, 24 females). The total exposure equated to approximately 940 patient-years and an estimated 24 537 infusions (8001 in females, 16 536 in males). The drug was administered by intravenous infusion at the

Table 1. *Serious adverse events observed in FOS – the Fabry Outcome Survey.*

Serious adverse event	Frequency	Serious adverse event	Frequency
Cardiac events	11	Infections	6
Atrial flutter/fibrillation	5	Pain at various locations	6
Sinus node dysfunction	2	Vascular events	6
Tachyarrhythmia	1	Respiratory events	5
Atrioventricular block	1	Trauma	5
Aortic valve stenosis	1	Neoplasm	3
Coronary artery stenosis	1	Gastrointestinal events	2
Cerebrovascular accidents	10	Psychiatric events	2
Transient ischaemic attacks	2	Others	3
Renal events, including chronic failure and proteinuria	9*		

*Five patients began dialysis after receiving ERT

standard dose of 0.2 mg/kg every other week, usually over a period of 40 minutes.

Serious adverse events

In total, 72 serious adverse events were reported in 54 patients (13.5% of the patient cohort). Two of these were considered to be potentially drug-related and were subsequently reported to the relevant health authorities. The first event was atrial fibrillation with anginal pain, which occurred 9 hours after agalsidase alfa infusion in a 54-year-old female patient (causality reported as possible). The other event was an infusion reaction with rigors, pyrexia and vomiting in a 42-year-old male patient after 2.5 years of treatment (causality deemed probable). At the time of the infusion, this patient suffered from a cold and sinusitis, and he subsequently developed a pericardial effusion that resolved without sequelae.

The other 70 serious adverse events observed to date in the FOS cohort are shown in Table 1. As expected, the most frequent events were consistent with cardiac, cerebrovascular and renal complications of Fabry disease.

Deaths

Five deaths have been reported in patients receiving agalsidase alfa therapy; all were attributed to complications of Fabry disease or concurrent diseases. The cause of death was cerebrovascular accident in two cases (subarachnoid haemorrhage due to cerebral aneurysm and multiple ischaemic lesions with cachexia), end-stage renal failure in one case, sepsis with endocarditis in one case and bronchopneumonia in a severely debilitated patient. Enzyme replacement therapy had been stopped 4 and 12 months before death in two of these cases.

Non-serious adverse events

In total, 192 non-serious adverse events were reported in 85 patients (21.2% of the patient cohort). Of these, 50 were considered to be unrelated to treatment. The most frequent unrelated adverse events were cold symptoms (9 cases), pain (7), hearing impairment (5), gastrointestinal events (7), renal manifestations (5) and cerebrovascular events (4, comprising 2 cerebrovascular accidents and 2 transient ischaemic attacks).

Of the 142 treatment-related adverse events, most (128) were deemed to be infusion-related reactions, because they occurred shortly after an infusion (on the same or the following day). The remaining events comprised impaired renal function (10), gastro-

Table 2. *Number and percentage of infusion-related adverse events in FOS – the Fabry Outcome Survey – according to sex.*

	Patients		Infusions	
	Total number	Number with adverse events (%)	Total number	Number of adverse events (%)
Females	160	9 (5.6%)	8001	38 (0.5%)
Males	241	42 (17.4%)	16 536	202 (1.2%)

enteritis (2), exacerbation of gastrointestinal symptoms (1) and polycythaemia (1).

Infusion-related reactions
Overall, 51 patients (12.7% of the patient cohort) reported infusion-related reactions (including the serious case already described). Because the same reaction recurred following several infusions in some patients, a total of 240 infusions were involved (i.e. about 1% of the estimated number of infusions administered to the patient cohort). The reactions were much more frequent in male than in female patients (Table 2).

The distribution of the age at first reaction roughly matched the age distribution of the whole patient population at the start of therapy. Therefore, the risk of developing an infusion-related reaction does not appear to be correlated with age.

In 31 of the 51 patients (60.8%), the first reaction occurred within 3 months of initiation of therapy (Figure 1). In seven cases (13.7%), however, the first reaction occurred after more than 12 months of therapy.

Forty-one patients (80.4%) experienced a limited number (1–5) of infusion-related reactions; such reactions did not then recur following subsequent infusions (Figure 2).

Figure 3 shows the relationship between treatment duration and use of premedication. A total of 44 patients received

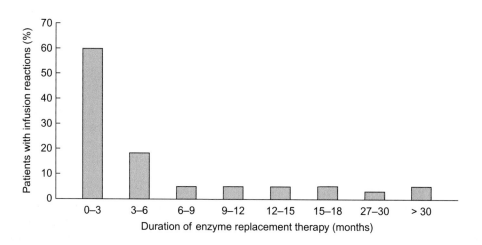

Figure 1. *Relationship between treatment duration and occurrence of infusion reactions in FOS – the Fabry Outcome Survey.*

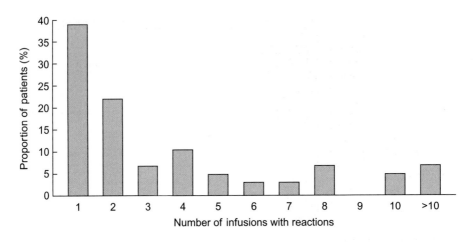

Figure 2. *Percentage of patients in FOS – the Fabry Outcome Survey – with one or more instances of infusion reactions.*

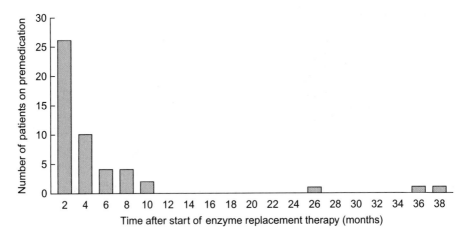

Figure 3. *Relationship between treatment duration and use of premedication in FOS – the Fabry Outcome Survey.*

premedication (38 males, 6 females). The most common premedications used were paracetamol and/or antihistamines and/or corticosteroids.

The type and frequency of infusion-related reactions experienced by the 51 patients are shown in Figure 4. The maximum number of symptoms experienced by a patient on one or more occasions was nine, with a median of two symptoms per patient. As shown in

clinical trials, the most frequent symptoms were rigors, flushing, headache, pyrexia, digestive manifestations (nausea, vomiting, abdominal pain) and dyspnoea.

The majority of infusion-related reactions were of mild intensity (31 patients; 61%), while only five severe reactions were reported in three patients (6%). One of these patients developed urticaria with itching after four consecutive infusions. The first reaction was moderate,

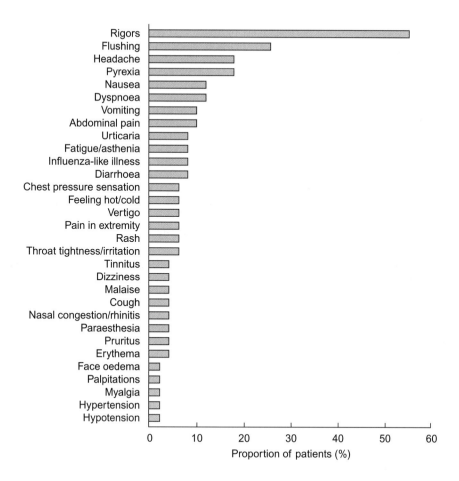

Figure 4. *Type of infusion-related reactions experienced by 51 patients in FOS – the Fabry Outcome Survey.*

but the second and third reactions were severe, necessitating intravenous corticosteroid injections. A mild reaction was reported on the fourth occasion, after the introduction of premedication. The second patient with a severe reaction was a boy who experienced rigors, fever, trismus and hypertension after three consecutive infusions. The first reaction was moderate, but the second and third were severe, requiring intravenous corticosteroid infusions (despite premedication with intravenous antihistamine before the third reaction). This patient was subsequently withdrawn from agalsidase alfa therapy. The third patient developed severe

dyspnoea with bronchospasm after the fourth infusion of agalsidase alfa. Subsequently, with premedication and a slower infusion rate, a similar reaction recurred only once and was of moderate severity.

Home therapy

Of the 401 patients in FOS at the time of analysis, 86 (21.4%) were being treated at home. The majority of these (56 patients; 65.1%) were resident in the UK, where home therapy with agalsidase alfa has become standard practice. The others resided in Switzerland (13), Italy (6), France (4), Norway (3), Germany (2), Spain (1) and Sweden (1).

Paediatric patients

Of the 55 paediatric patients, 20 were children aged less than 12 years (13 males, 7 females), and 35 were adolescents aged 12–18 years (18 males, 17 females). They received an estimated total of 2366 infusions.

Eight of these paediatric patients (14.5%) reported 21 adverse events unrelated to treatment with agalsidase alfa. Most of these events (14) were infectious episodes (ear/nose/throat infections or gastroenteritis); one case of recurrent tonsillitis was considered serious. Six were exacerbations of abdominal pain or pain in the extremities related to Fabry disease; one was considered serious. One adverse event was anaemia due to iron deficiency.

Ten patients (18.2%; 9 males, 1 female) reported a total of 30 infusion-related reactions (1–8 per patient), giving an overall incidence of 1.3%. The most frequent of the infusion-related symptoms were rigors, flushing, pyrexia, dyspnoea, headache and nausea. These reactions occurred initially within the first 1–4 months of the start of treatment. As previously mentioned, although one patient discontinued therapy due to severe infusion reactions, the large majority of reactions were rated as mild (26 of 30; 86.7%). Seven (70%) of the ten paediatric patients with infusion reactions received premedication before their subsequent infusions.

Finally, two patients experienced a worsening of the primary disease, which was considered to be a possible adverse drug reaction. The deterioration in one of these patients was a progressive decrease in glomerular filtration rate (moderate), while in the other patient an exacerbation of gastrointestinal symptoms (severe) was observed.

Antibodies

As yet, no information about the development of antibodies has been recorded in FOS. However, combined analysis of long-term clinical trials has shown that approximately 24% of adult male patients developed anti-agalsidase IgG antibodies after 3–12 months of treatment. After 12–54 months of therapy, 17% of treated patients were still antibody positive, whereas 7% showed evidence of the development of immunological tolerance, based on the disappearance of IgG antibodies over time. The remaining 76% were antibody negative throughout. No IgE antibodies have been detected in any patient receiving agalsidase alfa [5].

Discussion

Although FOS is an open-label observational outcomes database, which is potentially liable to ascertainment bias and incomplete data collection, it is able to provide safety data on greater numbers of patients than have been studied in clinical trials. Based on these data, it can be concluded that agalsidase alfa has a good safety profile. Home therapy can be authorized rapidly, after six to ten infusions in the hospital setting. The safety profile of agalsidase alfa appears to be as good in children as in adults.

As expected, the majority of serious adverse events were attributed to the primary disease, such as cardiac, cerebrovascular and renal manifestations. Only two were considered to be possibly/probably related to treatment. Five patients died while on therapy, all from complications of Fabry disease or concurrent pathology.

In fewer than 15% of patients, the drug has been associated with mild acute infusion effects, during or within 1 hour of infusion. The most common symptoms are chills and facial flushing; these reactions are usually transient. In the majority of cases, infusion-related reactions are managed conservatively. Mild and transient effects may not require medical treatment or discontinuation of the infusion. In cases of more severe and persistent reactions, the infusion can be interrupted temporarily (5–10 minutes) until symptoms subside, and then restarted.

Premedication, generally with paracetamol, oral antihistamines and/or corticosteroids given 1–24 hours before the infusion, has prevented subsequent reactions in patients in whom symptomatic treatment was required. If severe allergic or anaphylactic-type reactions occur, immediate discontinuation of the infusion should be considered and the current medical standards for emergency treatment must be observed. As of 7 March 2005, only three patients in FOS have had a severe treatment-related infusion reaction. Symptoms reported included pyrexia, rigors, urticaria and dyspnoea with bronchospasm. Such reactions generally occur within the first 2–4 months of initiation of treatment with agalsidase alfa. Only one patient has stopped agalsidase alfa therapy due to recurrent reactions.

Infusion-related reactions may occur in patients developing IgG antibodies against the infused recombinant enzyme or may be idiosyncratic non-specific reactions. The therapeutic use of proteins, derived either from human or from non-human sources, has always been associated with the problem of immunogenicity [14]. Absence of residual enzymatic activity is considered to be the cause of the lack of tolerance in patients with Fabry disease, as infusion-related reactions are more frequent in patients with little or no residual galactosidase A activity. Males are therefore more likely than females to experience such reactions. In contrast to type 1 Gaucher disease, in which only 15% of patients develop non-neutralizing IgG antibodies against the normal enzyme [15], up to 90% of male patients with the classic form of Fabry disease who are treated with agalsidase beta and approximately 24% of those receiving agalsidase alfa develop IgG antibodies [5, 16].

IgG antibodies appear to develop after approximately 3 months of therapy. After 12–18 months of therapy, 83% of patients treated with agalsidase alfa are antibody free, and about 30% of patients who were antibody positive showed evidence of the development of immunological tolerance, based on the reduction of antibody titres over time [5]. The observed decline in antibody titres over time suggests that the appearance of IgG antibodies may not prove to have therapeutic implications. In a recent paper, however, Linthorst and colleagues reported the emergence of antibodies with neutralizing capacities *in vivo* in 18 patients (16 men, 2 women) treated with agalsidase alfa (0.2 mg/kg biweekly; $n = 7$) or agalsidase beta (0.2 mg/kg biweekly, $n = 6$ or 1.0 mg/kg biweekly, $n = 5$) [17]. After 6 months of treatment, all male IgG-negative patients showed a significant reduction in urinary globotriaosylceramide concentrations compared with IgG-positive patients, suggesting a negative effect of circulating antibodies on renal tubular cells. Moreover, IgG antibodies cross-reacted *in vitro* similarly with both recombinant enzymes, which suggests that it is unlikely that switching from one to the other recombinant protein would prevent the immune response and related effects. However, this requires further follow-up [18].

Conclusions

The data collected from this extensive European post-marketing follow-up survey confirms that agalsidase alfa is safe and well tolerated in adults and children when used in a wide range of patients and in daily clinical practice, including home therapy. The safety profile appears consistent with data previously obtained from clinical trials. Precise clinical guidelines for treatment are currently under development.

References

1. Lemansky P, Bishop DF, Desnick RJ, Hasilik A, von Figura K. Synthesis and processing of α-galactosidase A in human fibroblasts. Evidence for different mutations in Fabry disease. *J Biol Chem* 1987;262:2062–5

2. Products. CFPM. Note for guidance on minimising the risk of transmitting animal spongiform en-

cephalopathy agents via medicinal products. Committee for Proprietary Medicinal Products (CPMP). European Agency for the Evaluation of Medicinal Products (EMEA), September 2000. http://www.emea.eu.int/

3. Draft of points to consider in the characterization of cell lines used to produce biologicals. Bethesda: Food and Drug Administration, 1993. http:www.fda.gov/cber/gdlns/ptccell.pdf

4. International Conference on Harmonisation Expert Working Group. Viral safety evaluation of biotechnology products derived from cell lines of human or animal origin. ICH Expert Working Groups, Step 4, 5 March 1997. ICH Q5A. Food and Drug Administration, 1998. http://www.ich.org/LOB/media/MEDIA392.pdf

5. European Agency for the Evaluation of Medicinal Products (EMEA). Product overview. Replagal. www.emea.eu.int/humandocs/Humans/EPAR/replagal/replagal.htm

6. Schiffmann R, Murray GJ, Treco D, Daniel P, Sellos-Moura M, Myers M *et al*. Infusion of α-galactosidase A reduces tissue globotriaosylceramide storage in patients with Fabry disease. *Proc Natl Acad Sci USA* 2000;97:365–70

7. Schiffmann R, Kopp JB, Austin HA 3rd, Sabnis S, Moore DF, Weibel T *et al*. Enzyme replacement therapy in Fabry disease: a randomized controlled trial. *JAMA* 2001;285:2743–9

8. MacDermot KD, Holmes A, Miners AH. Anderson–Fabry disease: clinical manifestations and impact of disease in a cohort of 60 obligate carrier females. *J Med Genet* 2001;38:769–75

9. MacDermot KD, Holmes A, Miners AH. Anderson–Fabry disease: clinical manifestations and impact of disease in a cohort of 98 hemizygous males. *J Med Genet* 2001;38:750–60

10. Bähner F, Kampmann C, Whybra C, Miebach E, Wiethoff CM, Beck M. Enzyme replacement therapy in heterozygous females with Fabry disease: results of a phase IIIB study. *J Inherit Metab Dis* 2003;26:617–27

11. Wendt S, Whybra C, Kampmann C, Teichmann E, Beck M. Successful pregnancy outcome in a patient with Fabry disease receiving enzyme replacement therapy with agalsidase alfa. *J Inherit Metab Dis* 2005;28:787–8

12. Dehout F, Roland D, Henry F, Langlois A, van Maldergem L. Successful pregnancy in a patient with Fabry disease receiving enzyme replacement therapy. *Acta Paediatr* Suppl 2006;451:137–8

13. Ramaswami U, Wendt S, Parini R, Pintos G Léon JA, Santus F *et al*. Safety of enzyme replacement therapy with agalsidase alfa in children with Fabry disease. *J Inherit Metab Dis* 2005; 28 (Suppl 1):330-P

14. Jacquemin MG, Saint-Remy JM. Factor VIII immunogenicity. *Haemophilia* 1998;4:552–7

15. Grabowski GA, Barton NW, Pastores G, Dambrosia JM, Banerjee TK, McKee MA *et al*. Enzyme therapy in type 1 Gaucher disease: comparative efficacy of mannose-terminated glucocerebrosidase from natural and recombinant sources. *Ann Intern Med* 1995;122:33–9

16. Eng CM, Guffon N, Wilcox WR, Germain DP, Lee P, Waldek S *et al*. Safety and efficacy of recombinant human α-galactosidase A – replacement therapy in Fabry's disease. *N Engl J Med* 2001;345:9–16

17. Linthorst GE, Hollack CEM, Donker-Koopman WE, Strijland A, Aerts JMFG. Enzyme therapy for Fabry disease: neutralizing antibodies toward agalsidase alfa and beta. *Kidney Int* 2004;66:1589–95

18. Schellekens H. Bioequivalence and the immunogenicity of biopharmaceuticals. *Nat Rev Drug Discov* 2002;1:457–62

42 Monitoring and follow-up of patients

Atul Mehta[1], Michael Beck[2], Aleš Linhart[3] and Gere Sunder-Plassmann[4]

[1]Lysosomal Storage Disorders Unit, Department of Academic Haematology, Royal Free and University College Medical School, Rowland Hill Street, London NW3 2PF, UK; [2]Universitäts-Kinderklinik, Langenbeckstrasse 1, D-55101 Mainz, Germany; [3]2nd Department of Internal Medicine, 1st School of Medicine, Charles University, U Nemocnice 2, CZ-128 08 Prague 2, Czech Republic; [4]Division of Nephrology and Dialysis, Department of Medicine III, Medical University Vienna, Währinger Gürtel 18–20, A-1090 Vienna, Austria

The availability of enzyme replacement therapy for Fabry disease has had a major impact on the organization of patient care. Many countries have produced expert guidelines outlining the recommended requirements for investigation, treatment and follow-up of patients and their families. This chapter summarizes the standards of care that operate in some of the major centres that contribute patient data to the FOS – Fabry Outcome Survey – database.

Introduction

The successful use of enzyme replacement therapy (ERT) in Gaucher disease, where it is now the standard of care [1], has led to the recognition of its potential role in treating other lysosomal disorders, such as Fabry disease [2]. Drug development was also given further impetus by legislation in the USA and the European Union, which provided commercial incentives to companies producing 'orphan' drugs. ERT for Fabry disease was licensed in August 2001 (see Chapter 36), and is now widely available within Europe. However, the cost of treatment means that prescriptions are subject to rigorous scrutiny. This has made it necessary to develop explicit guidelines for the diagnosis, assessment, treatment and follow-up of patients and their families. There is no internationally centralized process for preparing such guidelines, and the USA, Australia, Canada and countries in Europe have produced their own [3–6].

There is considerable diversity within Europe with regard to how such treatments are funded.

In some countries the main source of funding is private medical insurance. In most countries, however, there is a greater or lesser involvement of the state in funding these expensive treatments. Some countries are very specific in terms of the arrangements for the care of patients. For example, in the UK only nationally designated centres are able to prescribe therapy. The UK guidelines are multidisciplinary to reflect the need to involve the 'commissioners' – the agencies that fund therapy. In countries where there is substantial involvement of the state in funding treatment, the funds come from local government agencies representing the area of residence of the patient or from a central government source.

Assessment of patients

Once a diagnosis is confirmed, the aim of further investigations is to provide a precise assessment of the severity of the clinical manifestations of the disease. This will determine the requirement for specific and adjunctive therapies, and will provide the baseline against which the effectiveness of such therapies can be assessed. The results of clinical assessment and investigations may be used to calculate a disease-specific severity score, such as the Mainz Severity Score Index [7], to allow sequential monitoring of overall disease severity. Recommended investigations are listed in Table 1.

There is often a requirement for patients to attend specialist centres (e.g. UK, Australia and Canada) to receive treatment according to approved protocols. It is expected that patient details will be entered into outcomes databases and reports made available to funding agencies.

Criteria for starting ERT

A previous attempt at producing expert guidelines [4] has been well received by clinicians, patients and carers worldwide. The main criteria for initiating ERT are listed in Table 2. There are four critical areas to consider when assessing whether ERT should be started in patients with Fabry disease: pain, renal disease, cardiac disease and cerebrovascular disease.

We believe that ERT should be available for all symptomatic adult males, even if they do not have evidence of organ disease. Women and children require special consideration, and the criteria for initiating ERT therefore include

Table 1. *Recommended investigations for patients presenting with Fabry disease.*

- **General investigations**
  - Medical history and family pedigree
  - Clinical examination
  - Vital signs
  - Pain score (Brief Pain Inventory)*
  - Quality-of-life score (SF-36 or EQ-5D)*
  - Assessment of disease severity score index, e.g. Mainz Severity Score Index [7]

- **Cardiac investigations**
  - Electrocardiography (ECG)
  - 24-hour ECG
  - Echocardiogram
  - Exercise testing, if appropriate

- **Renal investigations**
  - Glomerular filtration rate (e.g. ^{51}Cr-EDTA)
  - 24-hour urinary creatinine clearance
  - 24-hour urinary albumin and/or protein excretion
  - 24-hour urinary globotriaosylceramide (Gb_3) excretion
  - Spot urine – albumin:creatinine ratio
  - Urinary sediment
  - Renal ultrasound
  - Renal biopsy – at the discretion of the renal physician

- **Neurology**
  - Magnetic resonance imaging of the brain
  - Quantitative sudomotor axon reflex test, where available
  - Electromyogram where neuropathy is clinically apparent

- **Ophthalmology**
  - Slit-lamp examination (cornea verticillata)
  - Retroillumination (Fabry cataract)
  - Retinal examination (vascular abnormalities)

- **Audiology**
  - Pure-tone audiogram

- **Laboratory investigations**
  - Full blood count
  - Creatinine and electrolytes
  - Liver function tests
  - Fasting lipid profile
  - Plasma Gb_3

*For children, it is recommended to use age-appropriate scores; for example, Varney–Thompson for pain and KINDL for quality of life.

Table 2. *Criteria for initiating enzyme replacement therapy.*

General symptoms of Fabry disease
- Uncontrolled pain leading to impaired quality of life

Evidence of renal disease
- Clinically significant reduction in glomerular filtration rate (< 90 ml/min/1.73 m^2)
- Proteinuria > 300 mg/24 hours in the absence of other causes (renal biopsy may be required)

Evidence of cardiac disease
- Electrocardiography (ECG) signs of left ventricular hypertrophy or conduction abnormalities
- Echocardiographic abnormalities
  - Increased left ventricular mass (in patients with concentric remodelling or hypertrophy)
  - Increased left ventricular wall thickness (≥ 13 mm in any segment)
  - Left atrial enlargement
  - Valvular thickening/insufficiency
  - Systolic impairment (regional wall motion abnormality or reduction in left ventricular ejection fraction [< 50%])
  - Diastolic dysfunction (using age-corrected Doppler assessment)

- Arrhythmia
  - 24-hour ECG (or other documented electrocardiographic evidence) showing bradyarrhythmia, atrial arrhythmia or ventricular tachycardia
- Ischaemic heart disease: positive exercise test, positron emission tomography in the absence of angiographically significant coronary artery disease

Evidence of neurovascular disease
- Previous stroke or transient ischaemic attack in the absence of other risk factors
- Abnormal cerebral magnetic resonance imaging scans

Gastrointestinal symptoms
- Including pain, vomiting or altered bowel habits, which have a significant negative impact on quality of life and are not attributable to other pathologies

Other symptoms
- Vertigo or hearing loss sufficient to interfere with quality of life (in adults, these symptoms by themselves would not be sufficient to warrant enzyme replacement therapy, but they may be sufficient in children)

evaluation of organ systems where disturbances will not cause life-threatening complications or where it is perceived that symptoms cause limited impairment of quality of life (e.g. dermatological changes, sensory organ disturbance and gastrointestinal disease). A challenge for the future is to question these assumptions and perceptions and to refine the criteria for initiating ERT accordingly.

Some countries give very specific guidelines on the degree of organ impairment, and some have developed major and minor criteria in an attempt to reflect the various effects of different disease manifestations on quality of life. Major criteria are typically significant renal, cardiac and cerebro-

vascular disease and pain; minor criteria are transient ischaemic attacks or abnormal brain magnetic resonance imaging with no other cause identified, gastrointestinal symptoms and sensory organ abnormalities.

Follow-up of patients

Follow-up should be at 6-monthly intervals in patients receiving ERT. For those patients not receiving ERT, follow-up should be every 12 months. The recommended evaluations are listed in Table 3.

An important aim of follow-up is to assess treatment efficacy, which involves evaluating the current status of signs and symptoms against the baseline assessment, with partic-

Table 3. Recommended evaluations at follow-up.

At each infusion (unless patients self-administer enzyme at home)
- Vital signs
- Adverse events
- Concomitant medications

Every 6 months
- Medical history and concomitant medications
- Clinical examination
- Vital signs
- Pain score (Brief Pain Inventory)
- Quality-of-life score (SF-36 or EQ-5D)
- Assessment of overall disease severity, such as the Mainz Severity Score Index [7]
- Blood tests (full blood count, creatinine and electrolytes, liver function, fasting lipid profile)
- Urine tests (albumin:creatinine ratio, urinary protein)
- Electrocardiography (ECG)

Every 12 months – as for 6 months with addition of the following
- Glomerular filtration rate (GFR)
- 24-hour urinary protein

- Echocardiogram
- 24-hour ECG
- Magnetic resonance imaging (MRI) scan if abnormal at baseline (every 2 years if normal at baseline)
- Audiology
- Assay for α-galactosidase A antibodies
- Plasma and urinary globotriaosylceramide
- In children: GFR, 24-hour ECG, 24-hour urinary protein, and MRI brain scan (if practical)

Efficacy endpoints: improvement in or a prevention of deterioration in the following
- Renal function (defined by GFR or 24-hour urine creatinine clearance or proteinuria)
- Pain scores
- Age-appropriate quality-of-life measurement
- Cardiac structure and function
- Neurological status
- Growth and development in children

ular reference to the disease manifestations that led to the initiation of therapy.

A further major aim of follow-up is to assess the safety of treatment. ERT appears to be well tolerated by patients with Fabry disease. Antibody formation has been reported with both the available enzyme preparations, but there is no clear evidence that these antibodies impact on the clinical efficacy of treatment [8]. Antibody measurements should be made at regular intervals (e.g. every 12 months) and an extra sample should be taken if there are any clinical indicators of allergy (e.g. skin rash). Regular follow-up also allows the prescriber to confirm compliance with treatment. In addition, follow-up provides an opportunity to confirm that the patient is taking optimal adjunctive therapy in terms of renoprotective, cardioprotective and vasculoprotective medication.

Funding agencies in most countries require written information on the outcome of treatment as a prerequisite for continued funding of ERT.

Home therapy
The first ERT infusion should always be given in hospital. Subsequent infusions can be given in the home setting provided the patient tolerates treatment well and the carers consider it appropriate. Home therapy is frequently practised in the UK and Switzerland. A recent report from The Netherlands [9] gives practice guidelines for home therapy. Thirty of 36 patients eligible for home therapy in this study were able to receive it. Women tolerated treatment better than men (presumably because of a lower incidence of antibodies) and in men agalsidase alfa at its licensed dose of 0.2 mg/kg was easier to administer at home

than agalsidase beta at its licensed dose of 1 mg/kg. Experience from the UK in delivering home treatment for patients with lysosomal storage diseases is generally very positive and has recently been reported [10].

Criteria for stopping treatment

Guidelines should also stipulate the criteria for stopping treatment. These would include intolerable adverse effects, development of complications as a result of ERT, or disease progression to such an extent that further ERT would be very unlikely to have a significant long-term impact on the disease (e.g. a severe cerebrovascular event). Treatment should be reviewed during pregnancy; although there are case reports of successful treatment during pregnancy, pregnancy and lactation are generally considered exclusion criteria.

Criteria for ERT in children under 18 years of age

The criteria for commencing ERT in adults and children differ, as it is very rare for children to develop cardiomyopathy, significant proteinuria or arrhythmias. Pain (including abdominal pain), impaired quality of life and abnormalities of growth and development are more important and relevant indications for initiating treatment in children. It is important to use age-appropriate pain scores in children; for example, those derived from the paediatric-specific Brief Pain Inventory and the Varney–Thompson Paediatric Pain Questionnaire. Age-appropriate quality-of-life scores, such as those derived from the KINDL, Short-Form-36 (SF-36) and European Quality of Life (EQ-5D) questionnaires, are also available.

Conclusions

The practice of evidence-based medicine requires written guidelines that are easily accessible, frequently updated and have ownership by all interested parties. As healthcare costs continue to rise, it is particularly important that available resources are optimally utilized. The two principal health economic arguments

against funding orphan drugs are that the criteria for determining cost-effectiveness of therapies should be rigidly applied regardless of whether a condition is common or rare; and funding for expensive drugs for one indication inevitably incurs an 'opportunity cost' which will mean denying treatment provision for other indications [11, 12]. In this threatening environment, it becomes crucially important to have an evidence base for all interventions. The provision of guidelines and protocols, together with audit of practice against these documents, is likely to become an increasingly important aspect of medicine.

References

1. Grabowski GA, Leslie N, Wenstrup R. Enzyme therapy for Gaucher disease: the first 5 years. *Blood Rev* 1998;12:115–33

2. Pastores GM, Thadhani R. Advances in the management of Anderson–Fabry disease: enzyme-replacement therapy. *Expert Opin Biol Ther* 2002; 2:325–33

3. Hughes DA, Ramaswami U, Elliott P, Deegan P, Lee P, Waldek S *et al*. Guidelines for the diagnosis and management of Anderson–Fabry disease. www.dh.gov.uk/PublicationsAndStatistics/Publications/PublicationsPolicyAndGuidance/PublicationsPolicyAndGuidanceArticle/fs/en?CONTENT_ID=4118404&chk=oSyxOB

4. Desnick RJ, Brady R, Barranger J, Collins AJ, Germain DP, Goldman M *et al*. Fabry disease, an under-recognized multisystemic disorder: expert recommendations for diagnosis, management, and enzyme replacement therapy. *Ann Intern Med* 2003;138:338–46

5. Guidelines for eligibility to receive treatment with agalsidase through life saving drugs program. 31 July 2004. www.health.gov.au/internet/wcms/publishinng.nsf/content/health-pbs-general-supply-othersupply-copy2/$file/fabryguide.pdf

6. Clarke LA, Clarke JTR, Sirrs S *et al*. Fabry disease: Recommendations for diagnosis, management and enzyme replacement therapy in Canada. Revised November 2005. www.garrod.ca/pdf-files/canadian%20Fabry%guidelines%20%20november%202005.doc

7. Whybra C, Kampmann C, Krummenauer F, Ries M, Mengel E, Miebach E *et al*. The Mainz Severity Score Index: a new instrument for quantifying the Anderson–Fabry disease phenotype, and the response of patients to enzyme replacement therapy. *Clin Genet* 2004;65:299–307

8. Linthorst GE, Hollak CE, Donker-Koopman WE, Strijland A, Aerts JM. Enzyme therapy for Fabry disease: neutralizing antibodies toward agalsidase alpha and beta. *Kidney Int* 2004;66:1589–95

9. Linthorst GE, Vedder AC, Ormel EE, Aerts JM, Hollak CE. Home treatment for Fabry disease: practice guidelines based on three years experience in The Netherlands. *Nephrol Dial Transplant* 2006;21:355–60

10. Milligan A, Hughes D, Goodwin S, Richfield L, Mehta A. Intravenous enzyme replacement therapy: better in home or hospital? *Br J Nurs* 2006;15:330–3

11. McCabe C, Claxton K, Tsuchiya A. Orphan drugs and the NHS: should we value rarity? *BMJ* 2005; 331:1016–19

12. Burls A, Austin D, Moore D. Commissioning for rare diseases: view from the frontline. *BMJ* 2005; 331:1019–21

43 Possible future therapies for Fabry disease

Roscoe O Brady and Raphael Schiffmann

Developmental and Metabolic Neurology Branch, National Institute of Neurological Disorders and Stroke, Building 10, Room 3D04, National Institutes of Health, Bethesda, Maryland 20892-1260, USA

It is anticipated that enzyme replacement therapy (ERT) will be the major approach to the treatment of patients with Fabry disease for the foreseeable future. Various strategies to improve the efficacy of ERT may be required, however, for optimal patient benefit. Furthermore, other approaches to the treatment of patients with lysosomal storage disorders have been conceived and merit consideration. These strategies may be used alone or in conjunction with ERT. Among the potential options are molecular chaperones that increase α-galactosidase A activity in patients with demonstrable residual catalytic activity, substrate reduction therapy, gene editing, gene therapy, structural modification of α-galactosidase A and therapies targeting the downstream mechanism of the disease. Each of these avenues is presently under laboratory investigation, and a molecular chaperone is close to being tested in a clinical trial.

Introduction

Following the original descriptions of patients with 'angiokeratoma corporis diffusum' by the dermatologists Johannes Fabry and William Anderson in 1898, many years passed before therapeutic trials began for patients with what is now known as Fabry disease. The first impediment was the unknown nature of the storage material that accumulated in the blood vessels and elsewhere throughout the body. An investigation by Sweeley and Klionsky in 1963 identified ceramidetrihexoside, now called globotriaosylceramide (Gb_3), as the major accumulating glycosphingolipid in patients with this disorder [1]. Several years later, the defect was established as insufficient activity of the enzyme ceramidetrihexosidase (α-galactosidase A) that catalyses the hydrolytic cleavage of the terminal molecule of galactose from Gb_3 [2]. α-Galactosidase A was initially purified from the small intestine [3] and later from human placental tissue [4]. Intravenous injections of the latter enzyme

preparation into two patients with Fabry disease caused brief, but significant, reductions of Gb_3 in the blood [5]. Further investigations into enzyme replacement therapy (ERT) for Fabry disease were delayed for many years until improved procedures were developed for the production and purification of α-galactosidase A. Eventually, two preparations of α-galactosidase A became available, and the effects of their administration in patients with Fabry disease have been examined. Meanwhile, other potential forms of therapy for Fabry disease have begun to emerge, which will be discussed here.

Molecular chaperone therapy

It has been reported that galactose, one of the products of the enzymatic hydrolysis of Gb_3, can stabilize the protein products of some missense mutations of the α-galactosidase A gene [6]. In the absence of such a stabilizing agent (chaperone), many proteins produced by altered genes are misfolded and become subject to quality control surveillance mechanism(s) in the endoplasmic reticulum (ER). The abnormal proteins are extruded from the ER and, after ubiquitination, are biodegraded in the proteasome [7]. It has been reported that administration of galactose brought about clinical improvement in a patient with Fabry disease with the cardiac phenotype who had significant residual α-galactosidase A activity [8]. Another strategy employed to stabilize mutated α-galactosidase A involves the use of 1-deoxygalactonojirimycin (DGJ; 1,5-dideoxy-1,5-imino-D-galactitol), a competitive inhibitor of the enzyme [9]. Chaperones of this type are used at: "concentrations lower than that usually required for intracellular inhibition of the enzyme" [10]. We have confirmed the augmentation of residual α-galactosidase A activity in patients in whom glutamine has been substituted for arginine at position 301 (R301Q) and patients in whom valine is found at amino acid residue 97 instead of alanine (A97V). Following appropriate safety and dose–response studies, we shall examine the clinical effects of DGJ in patients with these mutations as well as others in whom residual catalytic activity of α-galactosidase A is augmented with DGJ. Active-site chemical chaperones have a theoretical advantage over ERT because they are small molecules that are widely distributed to all types of cells, primarily by diffusion, and may cross the blood–brain barrier.

Substrate reduction therapy

Substrate reduction therapy is a potential alternative or supplement to ERT. Instead of augmenting the catabolic activity of cells in which Gb_3 accumulates, the agents used in substrate reduction therapy block the formation of accumulating glycosphingolipids. The most extensively investigated example of this approach has been the use of the glucose analogue N-butyldeoxynojirimycin to reduce the biosynthesis of glucocerebroside in patients with type 1

(non-neuronopathic) Gaucher disease [11]. We have shown that the ceramide analogues 4'-hydroxy-1-phenyl-2-palmitoylamino-3-pyrrolidino-1-propanol and ethylenedioxy-1-phenyl-2-palmitoylamino-3-pyrrolidino-1-propanol (EtDO-P4), which are very potent inhibitors of glucosylceramide synthase, reduced the formation of Gb_3 in lymphoblasts derived from patients with Fabry disease [12]. Administration of EtDO-P4 to the α-galactosidase A knockout mouse model of Fabry disease [13] caused a significant reduction of accumulated Gb_3 in the kidney, liver and heart [14]. Several considerations arise from these demonstrations. The first is that there is a possibility that inhibitors of Gb_3 formation may be given by mouth to patients with Fabry disease, similar to the administration of N-butyldeoxynojirimycin to patients with Gaucher disease. The second is that EtDO-P4, or similarly acting compounds, may cause a uniform reduction of accumulated Gb_3 in organs such as the kidney, where only specific types of cells appear to respond favourably to intravenously administered α-galactosidase A [15]. This accomplishment may enhance the effect of ERT on kidney function in patients with Fabry disease in whom, to date, the most consistent benefit has been stabilization of renal function (Schiffmann et al., unpublished data). Therefore, an effective oral agent to reduce Gb_3 formation may overcome the limitations of enzyme delivery to renal cells. This approach may also augment therapeutic responses in other organs. As most patients with Fabry disease have no residual α-galactosidase activity, it is unlikely that substrate reduction therapy alone will be sufficient in these patients to achieve a therapeutic effect. Perhaps substrate reduction therapy in combination with ERT may be required to produce a significant benefit.

Gene editing

Two strategies appear to be on the horizon to correct nucleotide alterations. The first is the use of aminoglycosides to override stop codons. This approach has been examined in a murine model [16] and in patients with Duchenne muscular dystrophy [17], as well as in patients with cystic fibrosis [18–20]. Such an approach seems attractive in the large cohort of patients with Fabry disease who have premature stop codons in the α-galactosidase A gene and are negative for cross-reactive immunological material. However, two clinical trials of aminoglycosides in patients with muscular dystrophy did not result in improvement [21, 22]. A recent study has indicated that the response varies with the patient's stop codon mutation. Some are refractory to treatment with amino-glycosides, and the response, which when present is actually very modest, depends on the individual agent employed [23]. We infer from these reports that induced readthrough of stop codons as presently achieved may provide limited or no benefit to patients with Fabry disease.

A second gene-editing strategy utilizes various nucleotide constructs. Some are single-stranded DNA; others are chimeric single-stranded RNA–DNA oligonucleotides that are self-complementary and fold into a double hairpin conformation [24, 25]. Lu et al. reported that they were able to increase α-glucosidase activity in cultured fibroblasts derived from a patient with Pompe disease using a single-stranded oligonucleotide flanked by phosphorothiolated sequences [26]. In addition, the authors developed a transgenic mouse model of Pompe disease by inserting a nonsense mutation into the murine α-glucosidase gene in mouse liver and kidney. Accumulation of glycogen was observed only in the liver. It is surprising that no mention was made of correcting the defect in the transgenic mouse in vivo. A follow-on literature search was unrevealing. Perhaps one is forced to conclude that the investigators were unsuccessful in this regard. If that is true, it currently leaves a gap with regard to the application of gene

editing for the correction of lysosomal storage disorders.

Gene therapy

Spectacular results have been obtained in gene therapy experiments with the murine model of Fabry disease. Early investigations employed retroviral vectors to introduce the normal α-galactosidase A gene into bone marrow haematopoietic stem and progenitor cells and stromal cells derived from patients with Fabry disease [27]. α-Galactosidase A was delivered into the circulation from the transduced bone marrow cells [28], and was able to reduce levels of accumulated Gb_3 in this murine model [29]. More striking results were obtained by pre-selecting cells that contained the transgene [30]. Recent investigations using adeno-associated viral vectors revealed long-term enzymatic and functional correction in multiple organs of the Fabry mouse [31, 32]. It was noted that no immune response was elicited in the knock-out mice [31] that produce no α-galactosidase A, similar to a major proportion of patients with Fabry disease. An even longer beneficial response in Fabry mice was reported by another study, where the α-galactosidase A gene was also administered by adeno-associated viral vector transfer [33]. Moreover, induction of immune tolerance to α-galactosidase A was observed in this study. These findings seem to augur well for gene therapy for Fabry disease. However, it has been reported that mice that lack α-glucuronidase activity, similar to patients with mucopolysaccharidosis type VII, which were injected with adeno-associated viral vectors containing the human glucuronidase gene, were found to have hepatocellular carcinomas and angiosarcomas [34]. Transgenic mice that over-expressed α-glucuronidase were produced in a subsequent investigation [35]. In one line of mice, several types of neoplasms were found. The cause of the tumours is presently unclear. Recombinant adeno-associated viral vectors with the same promoter employed in both of these studies have been used in a number of investigations with other genes without evidence of tumour formation [36]. Tumour production appears to depend on the over-expression of glucuronidase, as well as the strain of mouse employed. Nevertheless, hot spots for the integration of adeno-associated viral vectors have been identified, including chromosomal DNA breaks [37] and a preference for integration near gene regulatory sequences [38]. Possible cancer-related genes were hit at a frequency of 3.5%. Considerably more information is obviously required concerning the safety of such vectors. Hopefully, methods will be forthcoming to target such vectors to non-deleterious sites.

Infusions of structurally modified α-galactosidase A

ERT has been very effective in Gaucher disease, because the infused enzyme has direct access to macrophages, the cell type that is solely responsible for the non-neurological manifestations of the disease. In Fabry disease, on the other hand, many types of cells are involved, and therefore the infused enzyme must be much more widely distributed in cells of various organ systems. The infused α-galactosidase A in patients with Fabry disease is taken up mostly by vascular endothelial cells, thus limiting its effectiveness. Development of methods to expand the delivery of α-galactosidase A to all of the various types of cells in the kidney may require the production of several specifically targeted glycoforms of the enzyme. Another approach would be to modify α-galactosidase A by adding the TAT protein transduction domain that allows for receptor-independent uptake by a variety of cell types [39, 40]. Other peptide carrier delivery systems, such as VP22 [41, 42] and Pep-1, have been proposed [43].

Therapies based on the down-stream mechanism of disease

In recent years, a growing emphasis has been placed on understanding the mecha-

nisms by which increased levels of glycolipids can cause cellular dysfunction. For example, increased glucocerebroside in the brains of patients with type 2 Gaucher disease has been shown to enhance calcium release markedly through the ryanodine receptor [44]. In theory, the use of inhibitors of this receptor may diminish the harmful effect of glucocerebroside. Our current hypothesis regarding a possible mechanism underlying the vasculopathy of Fabry disease is that increased release of reactive oxygen species (ROS), such as superoxide, possibly via uncoupled endothelial nitric oxide synthase (eNOS), plays a central role [45]. If so, molecules that serve as scavengers for ROS or that favour coupling of eNOS may significantly interfere with the putative toxic effects of Gb_3 [46].

In addition, other pathogenic mechanisms that allow relatively simple and cost-effective interventions may be discovered and become useful therapeutic modalities for patients with Fabry disease.

Conclusions

The incomplete response to ERT in Fabry disease is thought to be related mostly to the inability of the enzyme to be distributed to all cells in any given organ or system [47]. There is therefore a need to consider improving enzyme delivery by modifying the α-galactosidase A molecule or by developing other approaches that are based on small-molecule therapy. Small molecules should be more widely distributed throughout the body than large proteins. The small-molecule approach may be based on a number of different mechanisms, which include enzyme enhancement, substrate reduction or interference with the deleterious mechanism of the offending glycolipid(s) in Fabry disease. It remains to be seen which therapeutic strategy will be the most successful. In general, however, prevention is likely to be more effective than attempting to reverse already damaged organs in patients with Fabry disease.

Acknowledgements

The authors are particularly grateful for the excellent help of Mary E Ryan, Biomedical Librarian/Informationist.

References

1. Sweeley CC, Klionsky B. Fabry's disease: classification as a sphingolipidosis and partial characterization of a novel glycolipid. *J Biol Chem* 1963;238:3148–50

2. Brady RO, Gal AE, Bradley RM, Martensson E, Warshaw AL, Laster L. Enzymatic defect in Fabry's disease. Ceramidetrihexosidase deficiency. *N Engl J Med* 1967;276:1163–7

3. Brady RO, Gal AE, Bradley RM, Martensson E. The metabolism of ceramide trihexosides. I. Purification and properties of an enzyme that cleaves the terminal galactose molecule of galactosylgalactosylglucosylceramide. *J Biol Chem* 1967;242:1021–6

4. Johnson W, Brady RO. Ceramidetrihexosidase from human placenta. *Methods Enzymol* 1972;XXVIII: 849–56

5. Brady RO, Tallman JF, Johnson WG, Gal AE, Leahy WR, Quirk JM et al. Replacement therapy for inherited enzyme deficiency. Use of purified ceramidetrihexosidase in Fabry's disease. *N Engl J Med* 1973; 289:9–14

6. Okumiya T, Ishii S, Takenaka T, Kase R, Kamei S, Sakuraba H et al. Galactose stabilizes various missense mutants of α-galactosidase in Fabry disease. *Biochem Biophys Res Commun* 1995; 214:1219–24

7. Kuznetsov G, Nigam SK. Folding of secretory and membrane proteins. *N Engl J Med* 1998;339:1688–95

8. Frustaci A, Chimenti C, Ricci R, Natale L, Russo MA, Pieroni M et al. Improvement in cardiac function in the cardiac variant of Fabry's disease with galactose-infusion therapy. *N Engl J Med* 2001;345:25–32

9. Legler G, Pohl S. Synthesis of 5-amino-5-deoxy-D-galactopyranose and 1,5-dideoxy-1,5-imino-D-galactitol, and their inhibition of α- and β-D-galactosidases. *Carbohydr Res* 1986;155:119–29

10. Fan JQ, Ishii S, Asano N, Suzuki Y. Accelerated transport and maturation of lysosomal α-galactosidase A in Fabry lymphoblasts by an enzyme inhibitor. *Nat Med* 1999;5:112–15

11. Cox T, Lachmann R, Hollak C, Aerts J, van Weely S, Hrebicek M et al. Novel oral treatment of Gaucher's disease with N-butyldeoxynojirimycin (OGT 918) to decrease substrate biosynthesis. *Lancet* 2000;355: 1481–5

12. Abe A, Arend LJ, Lee L, Lingwood C, Brady RO, Shayman JA. Glycosphingolipid depletion in Fabry disease lymphoblasts with potent inhibitors of glucosylceramide synthase. *Kidney Int* 2000;57:446–54

13. Ohshima T, Murray GJ, Swaim WD, Longenecker G, Quirk JM, Cardarelli CO et al. α-Galactosidase A deficient mice: a model of Fabry disease. *Proc Natl Acad Sci USA* 1997;94:2540–4

14. Abe A, Gregory S, Lee L, Killen PD, Brady RO, Kulkarni A et al. Reduction of globotriaosylceramide in Fabry disease mice by substrate deprivation. *J Clin Invest* 2000;105:1563–71

15. Eng CM, Banikazemi M, Gordon RE, Goldman M, Phelps R, Kim L et al. A phase 1/2 clinical trial of enzyme replacement in Fabry disease: pharmacokinetic, substrate clearance, and safety studies. *Am J Hum Genet* 2001;68:711–22

16. Barton-Davis ER, Cordier L, Shoturma DI, Leland SE, Sweeney HL. Aminoglycoside antibiotics restore dystrophin function to skeletal muscles of mdx mice. *J Clin Invest* 1999;104:375–81

17. Politano L, Nigro G, Nigro V, Piluso G, Papparella S, Paciello O et al. Gentamicin administration in Duchenne patients with premature stop codon. Preliminary results. *Acta Myol* 2003;22:15–21

18. Wilschanski M, Famini C, Blau H, Rivlin J, Augarten A, Avital A et al. A pilot study of the effect of gentamicin on nasal potential difference measurements in cystic fibrosis patients carrying stop mutations. *Am J Respir Crit Care Med* 2000;161:860–5

19. Wilschanski M, Yahav Y, Yaacov Y, Blau H, Bentur L, Rivlin J et al. Gentamicin-induced correction of CFTR function in patients with cystic fibrosis and CFTR stop mutations. *N Engl J Med* 2003;349:1433–41

20. Clancy JP, Bebok Z, Ruiz F, King C, Jones J, Walker L et al. Evidence that systemic gentamicin suppresses premature stop mutations in patients with cystic fibrosis. *Am J Respir Crit Care Med* 2001;163:1683–92

21. Wagner KR, Hamed S, Hadley DW, Gropman AL, Burstein AH, Escolar DM et al. Gentamicin treatment of Duchenne and Becker muscular dystrophy due to nonsense mutations. *Ann Neurol* 2001;49:706–11

22. Serrano C, Moore S, King W et al. Gentamicin treatment for muscular dystrophy patients with stop codons. *Neurology* 2001;56 (Suppl 3):A79

23. Howard MT, Anderson CB, Fass U, Khatri S, Gesteland RF, Atkins JF et al. Readthrough of dystrophin stop codon mutations induced by aminoglycosides. *Ann Neurol* 2004;55:422–6

24. Rice MC, Czymmek K, Kmiec EB. The potential of nucleic acid repair in functional genomics. *Nat Biotechnol* 2001;19:321–6

25. Liu L, Parekh-Olmedo H, Kmiec EB. The development and regulation of gene repair. *Nat Rev Genet* 2003;4:679–89

26. Lu IL, Lin CY, Lin SB, Chen ST, Yeh LY, Yang FY et al. Correction/mutation of acid α-D-glucosidase gene by modified single-stranded oligonucleotides: *in vitro* and *in vivo* studies. *Gene Ther* 2003;10:1910–16

27. Takenaka T, Hendrickson CS, Tworek DM, Tudor M, Schiffmann R, Brady RO et al. Enzymatic and functional correction along with long-term enzyme secretion from transduced bone marrow hematopoietic stem/progenitor and stromal cells derived from patients with Fabry disease. *Exp Hematol* 1999;27: 1149–59

28. Takenaka T, Qin G, Brady RO, Medin JA. Circulating α-galactosidase A derived from transduced bone

marrow cells: relevance for corrective gene transfer for Fabry disease. *Hum Gene Ther* 1999;10:1931–9

29. Takenaka T, Murray GJ, Qin G, Quirk JM, Ohshima T, Qasba P *et al.* Long-term enzyme correction and lipid reduction in multiple organs of primary and secondary transplanted Fabry mice receiving transduced bone marrow cells. *Proc Natl Acad Sci USA* 2000; 97:7515–20

30. Qin G, Takenaka T, Telsch K, Kelley L, Howard T, Levade T *et al.* Preselective gene therapy for Fabry disease. *Proc Natl Acad Sci USA* 2001;98:3428–33

31. Jung SC, Han IP, Limaye A, Xu R, Gelderman MP, Zerfas P *et al.* Adeno-associated viral vector-mediated gene transfer results in long-term enzymatic and functional correction in multiple organs of Fabry mice. *Proc Natl Acad Sci USA* 2001;98:2676–81

32. Park J, Murray GJ, Limaye A, Quirk JM, Gelderman MP, Brady RO *et al.* Long-term correction of globotriaosylceramide storage in Fabry mice by recombinant adeno-associated virus-mediated gene transfer. *Proc Natl Acad Sci USA* 2003;100:3450–4

33. Ziegler RJ, Lonning SM, Armentano D, Li C, Souza DW, Cherry M *et al.* AAV2 vector harboring a liver-restricted promoter facilitates sustained expression of therapeutic levels of α-galactosidase A and the induction of immune tolerance in Fabry mice. *Mol Ther* 2004;9:231–40

34. Donsante A, Vogler C, Muzyczka N, Crawford JM, Barker J, Flotte T *et al.* Observed incidence of tumorigenesis in long-term rodent studies of rAAV vectors. *Gene Ther* 2001;8:1343–6

35. Vogler C, Galvin N, Levy B, Grubb J, Jiang J, Zhou XY *et al.* Transgene produces massive overexpression of human β-glucuronidase in mice, lysosomal storage of enzyme, and strain-dependent tumors. *Proc Natl Acad Sci USA* 2003;100:2669–73

36. Kay MA, Nakai H. Looking into the safety of AAV vectors. *Nature* 2003;424:251

37. Miller DG, Petek LM, Russell DW. Adeno-associated virus vectors integrate at chromosome breakage sites. *Nat Genet* 2004;36:767–73

38. Nakai H, Wu X, Fuess S, Storm TA, Munroe D, Montini E *et al.* Large-scale molecular characterization of adeno-associated virus vector integration in mouse liver. *J Virol* 2005;79:3606–14

39. Schwarze SR, Ho A, Vocero-Akbani A, Dowdy SF. *In vivo* protein transduction: delivery of a biologically active protein into the mouse. *Science* 1999;285: 1569–72

40. Wadia JS, Stan RV, Dowdy SF. Transducible TAT-HA fusogenic peptide enhances escape of TAT-fusion proteins after lipid raft macropinocytosis. *Nat Med* 2004;10:310–15

41. Elliott G, O'Hare P. Intercellular trafficking and protein delivery by a herpesvirus structural protein. *Cell* 1997; 88:223–33

42. Lai Z, Han I, Zirzow G, Brady RO, Reiser J. Intercellular delivery of a herpes simplex virus VP22 fusion protein from cells infected with lentiviral vectors. *Proc Natl Acad Sci USA* 2000;97:11297–302

43. Morris MC, Depollier J, Mery J, Heitz F, Divita G. A peptide carrier for the delivery of biologically active proteins into mammalian cells. *Nat Biotechnol* 2001;19:1173–6

44. Pelled D, Trajkovic-Bodennec S, Lloyd-Evans E, Sidransky E, Schiffmann R, Futerman AH. Enhanced calcium release in the acute neuronopathic form of Gaucher disease. *Neurobiol Dis* 2005;18:83–8

45. Moore DF, Scott LT, Gladwin MT, Altarescu G, Kaneski C, Suzuki K *et al.* Regional cerebral hyperperfusion and nitric oxide pathway dysregulation in Fabry disease: reversal by enzyme replacement therapy. *Circulation* 2001;104:1506–12

46. Moore DF, Ye F, Brennan ML, Gupta S, Barshop BA, Steiner RD *et al.* Ascorbate decreases Fabry cerebral hyperperfusion suggesting a reactive oxygen species abnormality: an arterial spin tagging study. *J Magn Reson Imaging* 2004;20:674–83

47. Schiffmann R, Rapkiewicz A, Abu-Asab M, Ries M, Askari H, Tsokos M *et al.* Pathological findings in a patient with Fabry disease who died after 2.5 years of enzyme replacement. *Virchows Arch* 2006; 448:337–43

44 Concluding remarks

Atul Mehta[1], Michael Beck[2], Aleš Linhart[3] and Gere Sunder-Plassmann[4]

[1]Lysosomal Storage Disorders Unit, Department of Academic Haematology, Royal Free and University College Medical School, Rowland Hill Street, London NW3 2PF, UK; [2]Universitäts-Kinderklinik, Langenbeck-strasse 1, D-55101 Mainz, Germany; [3]2nd Department of Internal Medicine, 1st School of Medicine, Charles University, U Nemocnice 2, CZ-128 08 Prague 2, Czech Republic; [4]Division of Nephrology and Dialysis, Department of Medicine III, Medical University Vienna, Währinger Gürtel 18–20, A-1090 Vienna, Austria

Remarkably, it is less than 50 years since Christian de Duve first described the lysosome and proposed the concept of enzyme replacement therapy (ERT) for lysosomal storage diseases (LSDs). Following his groundbreaking discovery, tremendous advances have been made in our understanding of lysosomal physiology. In particular, we have gained insight into the function and trafficking of the many lysosomal enzymes and associated proteins that are involved in the cellular recycling of complex macromolecules. Despite these advances, and the increased appreciation of the role of lysosomes and lysosomal enzymes in health and disease, it is only recently that ERT has become available. Even now, ERT has been developed for only a small number of the approximately 50 recognized LSDs.

Initial approval of the use of ERT in Fabry disease 5 years ago was based on the short-term response to treatment in a small number of patients. Post-approval surveillance of the outcome of ERT in larger numbers of patients in normal clinical practice was therefore mandatory and led, in 2001, to the initiation of FOS – the Fabry Outcome Survey. At that time, it would have been difficult to predict the success and clinical value of the FOS database. Building on its primary objective of documenting the outcome of ERT with agalsidase alfa in terms of safety and efficacy,

FOS is also actively promoting research into the natural history of Fabry disease, the effects of treatment in specific patient subgroups, and how best to detect, manage and monitor individuals with Fabry disease. Thus, analyses of the FOS database have:

- defined the multisystemic progressive nature of Fabry disease
- described the presence and extent of clinical signs and symptoms in female heterozygotes
- demonstrated the early onset of signs and symptoms of the disease in both boys and girls
- confirmed the beneficial effects of ERT with agalsidase alfa on
  - renal function
  - cardiac structure and function
  - pain and quality of life.

These have been considerable achievements; however, there remain numerous unanswered questions concerning the long-term treatment of patients with Fabry disease.

- To what extent is treatment able to reverse the progressive organ damage seen in patients with Fabry disease?
- When should ERT be commenced if we are to prevent major organ damage?
- What is the optimum dose and time schedule for ERT?
- What signs and symptoms should trigger consideration of ERT in females who are

heterozygous for Fabry disease?

- How far is it possible to predict the clinical phenotype from the genotype, and what are the epigenetic and environmental factors that affect the progression of Fabry disease?

There is little doubt that the increasingly large FOS database will be instrumental in providing many of the answers to these questions. Looking to the immediate future, the merging of FOS with FIRE – the Fabry International Research Exchange – will expand the current database to some 1200 patients from 18 countries and add greatly to the power of FOS in addressing these complex issues. In the longer term, it is possible that small-molecule therapies, such as the use of molecular chaperones, or gene therapy, may also prove to have a role in the management of patients with Fabry disease, although ERT is likely to remain the treatment of choice for some considerable time.

To conclude, we have gained a great deal of knowledge of Fabry disease and its treatment from analysis of data from the first 5 years of FOS. This outcomes survey has provided much more clinically relevant information on large numbers of patients than could possibly have been obtained from formal clinical trials. The growth of FOS in the next 5 years and beyond should see continued advances in our understanding of Fabry disease to the further benefit of patients and their families.

Subject index